Practical Issues in Geriatrics

Series Editor
Stefania Maggi, Aging Branch, CNR-Neuroscience Institute, Padua, Italy

This practically oriented series presents state of the art knowledge on the principal diseases encountered in older persons and addresses all aspects of management, including current multidisciplinary diagnostic and therapeutic approaches. It is intended as an educational tool that will enhance the everyday clinical practice of both young geriatricians and residents and also assist other specialists who deal with aged patients. Each volume is designed to provide comprehensive information on the topic that it covers, and whenever appropriate the text is complemented by additional material of high educational and practical value, including informative video-clips, standardized diagnostic flow charts and descriptive clinical cases. Practical Issues in Geriatrics will be of value to the scientific and professional community worldwide, improving understanding of the many clinical and social issues in Geriatrics and assisting in the delivery of optimal clinical care.

Indexed in Scopus

Virginia Boccardi • Luigi Marano
Editors

The Frail Surgical Patient

A Geriatric Approach Beyond Age

Springer

Editors
Virginia Boccardi
Division of Gerontology and Geriatrics
University of Perugia
Perugia, Italy

Luigi Marano
Department of Medicine
Academy of Applied Medical and Social Sciences - AMiSNS
Elbląg, Poland

ISSN 2509-6060 ISSN 2509-6079 (electronic)
Practical Issues in Geriatrics
ISBN 978-3-031-77709-7 ISBN 978-3-031-77707-3 (eBook)
https://doi.org/10.1007/978-3-031-77707-3

This Springer imprint is published by the registered company Springer Nature Switzerland AG
The registered company address is: Gewerbestrasse 11, 6330 Cham, Switzerland

Foreword

The Essence of Geriatrics for Frailty

Geriatrics has long recognized the significance of frailty as a critical clinical phenomenon in older adults, particularly after the age of 75. Frailty extends beyond the mere accumulation of diseases; it represents an intrinsic vulnerability associated with aging. Identifying frailty is not only essential for diagnosis but also plays a crucial role in prevention and therapeutic management, profoundly influencing resource allocation and care planning.

Frailty in geriatrics should be viewed not merely as a condition but as an opportunity for a more personalized therapeutic approach. This makes it particularly relevant in the surgical context, where geriatricians and surgeons must collaborate to explore intervention possibilities for frail older patients. This process includes debunking outdated myths and developing treatment plans that are both clinically appropriate and sensitive to individual needs within an integrated network of health and social services.

The geriatric surgeon operating in this field utilizes a comprehensive array of tools, including updated guidelines, risk stratification techniques, and minimally invasive procedures. These tools extend care beyond the hospital, integrating local resources to ensure safe and effective interventions.

Yet, it is essential to recognize that these techniques and strategies do not include the full meaning of "frailty." Frailty remains a central dimension of the human experience, reflecting the complexity of aging and vulnerability. This enriched understanding requires an approach that integrates psychological, physical, functional, and socio-environmental aspects, creating a truly person-centered care framework. Thus, frailty invites a broader reflection on human vulnerability, encouraging physicians, patients, and families to consider health and well-being in a more interconnected manner, even in advanced age.

This book aims to guide the reader from theoretical understanding to clinical practice, demonstrating how frailty can be addressed not only as a challenge but as an opportunity for deeper, more respectful care of each older individual's uniqueness. This text is not just a technical manual for specialists; it serves as a fundamental reference for all who interact daily with the complex reality of geriatric frailty.

A combined vision that integrates psycho-physical assessments with functional and socio-environmental data is crucial for understanding frailty in geriatrics. This holistic approach not only enhances medical treatment but also encourages caregivers to consider every aspect of the patient's existence, recognizing the complexity of interactions between mind, body, and environment.

In this foreword, I wish to convey that the term "frailty" should not be interpreted solely in a biomedical sense, focusing on the reduction of functional reserves, nor purely in a bio-psycho-social mode, expanding the concept to the loss of functional domains. The term "frailty" indeed resonates with the original meaning of an intrinsic condition of every human being. Thus, frailty is not merely a negative prognostic indicator but also represents the precious nature of every living being.

Frailty, therefore, transcends its characterization as a medical condition described through biomedical or bio-psycho-social paradigms. It embodies a quality intrinsic to being human, present from birth to death. This concept, while seemingly foreign or even inappropriate in the context of geriatric surgery, is vital. When a physician refers to a patient as "frail," it touches on the very essence of the patient's humanity.

The words "frail" and "vulnerable" evoke a universal dimension, suggesting a reflection that extends beyond their clinical use. In this sense, the geriatric surgeon is called to incorporate these notions into daily practice, adopting an attitude that fully considers the person as a whole.

Recognizing frailty as a fundamental aspect of human existence transforms our approach to geriatric surgery. Frailty should not be seen merely as a risk factor or a limitation to be circumvented to prevent therapeutic failures. Instead, frailty and vulnerability should be understood as essential elements that define our shared humanity. This perspective transforms frailty from a mere problem to be managed into a profound point of reflection on the human condition.

Viewing frailty and vulnerability not as defects but as intrinsic aspects of our humanity reveals their "preciousness." As moral philosopher Luigi Alici taught, it is not about saying "precious but frail" or "precious although frail" but "frail therefore precious."

This intrinsic understanding of frailty and vulnerability allows us to see beyond the "negative prognostic indicator" and recognize the inherent value of every human being. It invites us to respond ethically, practicing care that honors the dignity and preciousness of each person, thereby promoting a truly healing and humanizing approach to health.

From this understanding, it becomes clear that even the most "technical" chapter of this volume is infused with an ethical stance that enriches the experience of older adults by acknowledging their frailty. This perspective transforms every surgical intervention, risk assessment, and therapeutic decision into an act of deep humanity, where frailty is not seen as a limitation but as an element that, when correctly understood and managed, enhances patient care and guides us toward more thoughtful and personalized care.

The multidisciplinary approach that characterizes this volume is not just an advanced clinical methodology but also a testament to professional humility. This attitude reflects the awareness that adequately caring for the person, and appreciating the value they represent, requires collaborative and integrated work among various specialists.

The health of older person, complex in its facets, can be effectively safeguarded only through the joint contribution of diverse expertise—from medicine to psychology, from physiotherapy to social support.

Finally, the discussion on intermediate care, physiotherapeutic treatments, community assistance, and palliative care is significant. These topics represent not just practical aspects of managing frailty; they embody a care ethic that never abandons the patient but accompanies them at every stage of their health journey. Addressing these forms of assistance acknowledges that every stage of life, even those closest to the end, has intrinsic value and deserves attention and respect.

Approaching the frail means being willing to listen to and understand their stories, woven with ideas, expectations, desires, and feelings at any age. This perspective, derived from narrative medicine, underscores that every frail person possesses a unique and irreplaceable narrative identity deserving of respect and value. Actively listening to our patients' stories allows us not only to better understand their medical conditions but also to address their fears, expectations, and hopes, integrating these dimensions into treatment planning and daily care.

In this context, the role of family members and caregivers becomes crucial as they significantly contribute to the care narrative, providing indispensable support to the patient's frailty. They offer not only emotional and practical assistance but also enrich the medical team's understanding of the patient's life context, allowing for more personalized and attentive care. Even in situations of cognitive impairment, where the patient may struggle to express themselves fully, family members can help weave that net of mutual understanding vital for a true therapeutic alliance.

It is my hope that this vision will enrich your reading of this book, encouraging all those dedicated to the care of frail individuals and providing support to those who love and assist them in their often complex journey through the world of geriatric surgery.

Study Center of the Italian Society
of Narrative Medicine
Milan, Italy

Massimiliano Marinelli

Contents

Part III Post-operative Management

Part I

Background

The Epidemiology of Aging in Surgical Settings

1

Alfredo Matano, Angela Annecchiarico, Carlo Manzi, Gina Varricchio, Mario Virgilio Papa, Joanna Polom, and Raffaele Pagliuca

1.1 Introduction

Epidemiology, the fundamental cornerstone of public health, represents an indispensable aspect of the field. Its critical function is to identify the determinants or causes of health-related conditions or events [1]. The term "cause" refers to a specific event, condition, or characteristic that precedes the occurrence of a health outcome and is essential for it to happen. The identification of causal associations is a complex process that involves the use of valid statistical associations, the time sequence of events, biological plausibility, and consistency among studies. Moreover, epidemiology goes beyond the study of diseases and also examines events, behaviors, and conditions associated with health, as encapsulated by the term "health-related states or events." The insights gained through epidemiological investigations have the potential to inform the implementation of effective health programs and to guide individuals toward making informed decisions about their

A. Matano · A. Annecchiarico
Department of Public Health, A.O.R.N. Caserta, Caserta, Italy
e-mail: alfredo.matano@aorncaserta.it

C. Manzi
Department of Public Health, A.S.L. Caserta, Caserta, Italy

G. Varricchio · R. Pagliuca (✉)
Department of Geriatric Medicine, A.O.R.N. Caserta, Caserta, Italy
e-mail: gina.varricchio@aorncaserta.it; raffaele.pagliuca@aorncaserta.it

M. V. Papa
Department of Medical and Surgical Sciences, University of Padua, Padua, Italy

J. Polom
Department of Medical Laboratory Diagnostics – Fahrenheit Biobank BBMRI.pl, Medical University of Gdansk, Gdansk, Poland

Department of Medicine, Academy of Applied Medical and Social Sciences - AMiSNS: Akademia Medycznych I Spolecznych Nauk Stosowanych, Elbląg, Poland

V. Boccardi, L. Marano (eds.), *The Frail Surgical Patient*, Practical Issues in Geriatrics, https://doi.org/10.1007/978-3-031-77707-3_1

health behaviors [2]. Epidemiological research typically focuses on key demographic characteristics, including age, gender, race/ethnicity, marital status, occupation, and education. Among these factors, age is particularly important as it exerts a strong influence on health outcomes and disease incidence. Life expectancy is a fundamental measure of health, providing valuable insights into the causal mechanisms of disease. As people age, they become more susceptible to a range of debilitating conditions, including diabetes, Alzheimer's disease, Parkinson's disease, cardiovascular disease, chronic obstructive pulmonary disease, osteoporosis, and osteoarthritis. These conditions can lead to significant disability, reduced quality of life, and increased public health costs, as depicted in Fig. 1.1 [3, 4].

Therefore, we must develop policies to ensure that older adults receive appropriate and sustainable healthcare, including necessary surgical interventions. Indeed, as the population ages, the demand for surgical procedures among older patients is rising at an alarming rate. While older patients may face greater risks during surgery, healthcare providers and policymakers must explore new approaches to prioritize the needs of older adults and ensure they receive suitable pre- and post-operative care. The challenges posed by an aging population demand a professional and proactive response from the medical community [5, 6]. Medical technology has come a long way, and now more older individuals are undergoing surgery around the world. However, the risks involved can vary depending on the location. As the number of older people increases, there is a corresponding rise in health problems that may require surgery. A significant portion of the surgery recipients comprises old people. Scientists have extensively studied how surgery affects the older population, including its impact on heart risk, brain function, and overall health status [7]. However, we also need to consider whether the location and specific surgical procedures make a difference. While some of the risks are attributed to aging, others may

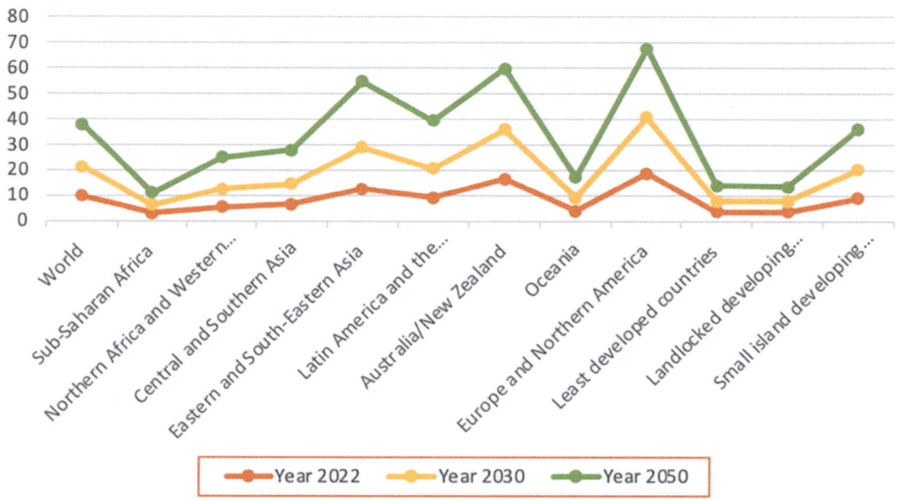

Fig. 1.1 Projected increase in older population in various regions of the world by the year 2050

be linked to a weaker immune system. Post-surgery complications can result in the need for intensive care unit (ICU) treatment or even lead to death. Due to the higher prevalence of health problems among older individuals, they are more likely to encounter challenges during the recovery process [8–10]. European countries are home to some of the oldest populations in the world, with Italy being particularly notable. According to the World Bank, Italy's population over 65 years old was 23.3% in 2015, surpassing the world average of 8.9%. This highlights the significance of comprehending the risks associated with surgery in older people in Italy and other European countries. A study analyzed data from more than 1.5 million patients undergoing surgery in 58 health districts of the countries, and the results are presented in Table 1.1 The study found that the risk of death in the month after surgery increases with age, especially in patients over 80 years old [11]. The study also revealed significant differences in surgical risk between countries, with high-income countries having a lower surgical risk compared to low-income countries. However, older patients in European countries may still encounter challenges such as longer hospital stays, a higher incidence of postoperative complications, and an increased risk of readmission [12] (Fig. 1.2).

A comprehensive preoperative evaluation is essential to minimize surgical risk in such vulnerable population. The ideal model of preoperative care for this complex population should include the assessment, optimization, and management of issues related to surgical stress while considering the contextual evaluation and management of underlying chronic pathologies and geriatric syndromes. This comprehensive assessment can provide valuable information to identify potential risks and determine the most appropriate surgical plan. It involves reviewing the assessment,

Table 1.1 Data gathered from England between 1995 and 2015, showing % of the total surgical population, and estimated cost in each group, i.e., age 60–74 and age ≥75 (the cost in the bracket represents the %)

	Age 60–74		Age ≥ 75	
Year	Surgical patients (%)	Cost	Surgical patients (%)	Cost
1999	10.5	1398.6 (24)	14.9	1104.3 (18.9)
2000	10.7	1430 (24.5)	15.5	1139.3 (19.5)
2001	10.7	1444.3 (24.7)	15.5	1161.9 (19.8)
2002	11.2	1526.7 (24.9)	16.1	1227 (20)
2003	11.5	1587.9 (25.4)	16.6	1275.6 (20.4)
2004	11.6	1647.3 (25.8)	16.8	1312.9 (20.5)
2005	12.1	1731.7 (25.9)	17.2	1375.2 (20.6)
2006	12.7	1858.5 (26.6)	17.7	1442.2 (20.6)
2007	13.5	2069.1 (27.5)	19	1561.5 (20.8)
2008	14.1	2227.1 (28.1)	20.5	1670.9 (21.1)
2009	14.3	2279 (28)	21.2	1723.7 (21.2)
2010	14.5	2344.1 (28.2)	21.5	1775.6 (21.4)
2011	14.5	2382.5 (28.4)	21.7	1812.2 (21.6)
2012	14.4	2389.3 (28.6)	21.5	1819.1 (21.8)
2013	14.9	2493.4 (28.8)	22.4	1915.3 (22.1)
2014	15.1	2552.1 (28.9)	23	1980.8 (22.5)
2015	15	2575.8 (29.1)	22.9	990.5 (22.5)

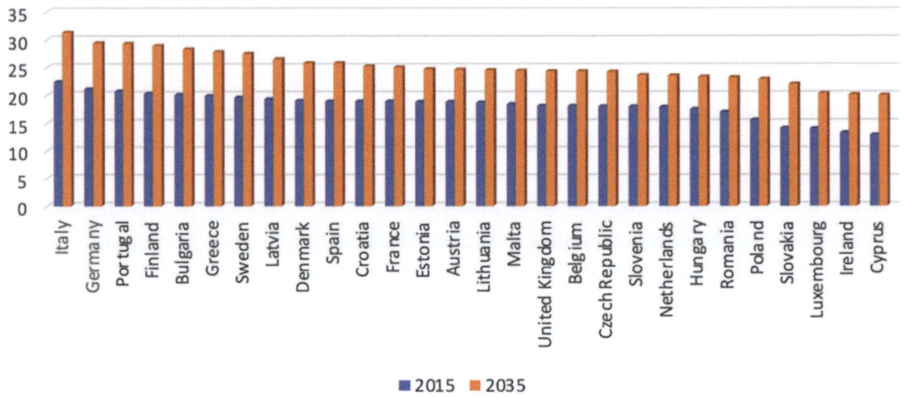

Fig. 1.2 Percentage of population aged 85 years and over, EU countries, 2015 and 2035 (projected)

assessing organ-specific risk, overall risk of morbidity and mortality, risk of postoperative functional loss/cognitive impairment, optimizing known comorbidities, and engaging in proactive communication with patients, relatives, surgeons, anesthesiologists, service teams, and primary care providers [13–16].

1.2 Aging and Surgical Volume Across Countries

As the number of older people continues to increase worldwide, concerns have been raised in several countries regarding the potential impact of aging on the frequency of surgeries. Studies have shown that not only is the proportion of older people in the general population increasing but also the likelihood of older individuals undergoing surgery is rising. These trends significantly affect health systems, especially in countries with a high proportion of older individuals [17]. Studies conducted in Europe and Italy have shed light on the relationship between aging and surgical volume. In 2020, Europe had the highest proportion of people aged 65 and over, accounting for 19.8% of the population. This percentage is projected to reach nearly 30% by 2050. In Italy, the population aged 65 and over now represents over 23% of the total population, making it the second oldest country in Europe after Greece [18]. As the population ages, the rate of surgical procedures in the older population is rising. For example in England, 2.5 million people over the age of 75 years underwent surgery between years 2014 and 2015, as opposed to just under 1.5 million between 2006 and 2007. Nearly 30% of these 2.5 million were over 85 years old [9]. In the US population, studies have estimated that approximately 53% of all surgical procedures are performed on patients over the age of 65. Projections estimate that approximately half of the population over the age of 65 will require surgery once in their lives [19].

1.2.1 Correlation Between Aging and Surgical Procedures

When considering the association between aging and receiving surgical procedures, researchers reveal that as people get older, they are more likely to require surgery. This is attributed to several causes, including the incidence of acute infections and natural body deterioration. According to Vaduganathan et al., the incidence of hip and knee replacements (common procedures among older people) increased by 25% in Europe between 2005 and 2015, with older adults accounting for a higher proportion of such medical procedures [20]. Data indicates that the share of the older population undergoing surgery in Italy has been steadily increasing. More than 15% of individuals treated surgically in Italy were 75 years old or older, according to an examination, and this percentage is expected to rise in the future. Following the survey, between 2005 and 2015, Italy's surgical volume reached 35%, with older individuals comprising a significant portion of the surgeries (Fig. 1.3). This aligns with international trends where aging is associated with a higher prevalence of chronic medical conditions requiring surgery [22–24].

1.2.2 Technological Advancement and Surgical Care

Technological innovation in medical services has extended the average lifespan globally, leading to an aging population in many countries. Surgeries are more frequently performed on individuals over the age of 65 than on younger patients, a trend observed in both developed and developing nations. The report also highlights national disparities in surgery volume, with advanced countries conducting more

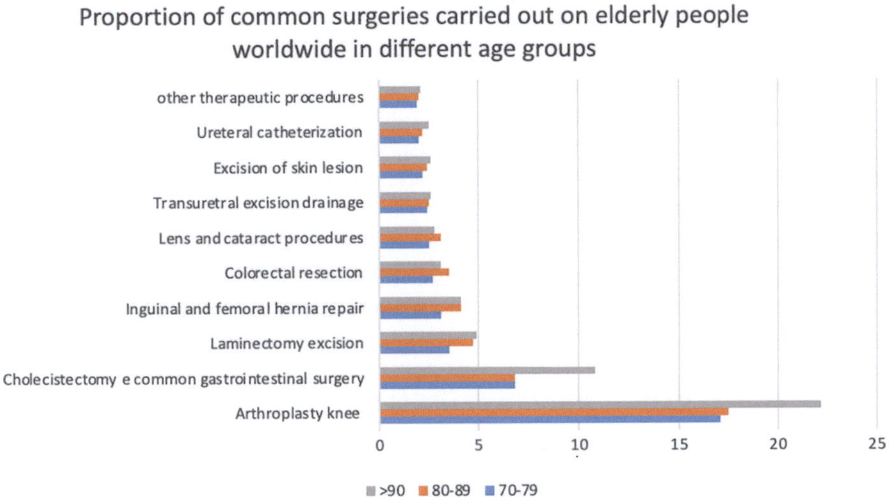

Fig. 1.3 Proportion of common surgeries carried out on older people worldwide in different age groups [21]

procedures compared to less developed nations. Specifically, Europe possesses a larger surgical volume, with Italy ranking as the country with the highest number of surgeries [25]. These developments raise concerns about medical services' capacity to meet the growing need for therapeutic services in nations with significant old populations. Issues such as excessive surgery prices, a scarcity of clinical infrastructure, and deficient healthcare systems are challenges faced by older individuals worldwide. In Italy, for instance, concerns have been raised about the accessibility of specially designed geriatric surgery facilities to meet the demands of older and frail patients. This is particularly crucial because older people are at a higher risk of facing complex healthcare demands and difficulties after surgery. Addressing these issues will require innovative healthcare delivery methods and investments in specialized services to cater to the needs of older patients [26].

1.3 Aging and Surgical Procedures Across Countries

The growing older population and the global prevalence of chronic illnesses are closely related. Age-specific disorders are becoming more prevalent, particularly in older age groups. The mortality rate from coronary artery disease has been declining across all age groups. However, the burden of cardiovascular disease has shifted to older age groups due to the rising median age of initial occurrence and mortality [27]. With improved healthcare and living conditions, an increasing number of older individuals are now encouraged to pursue procedures that were previously deemed too risky (Fig. 1.4). In the USA, for instance, cataract surgery surpassed joint replacement surgery and heart treatments as the most popular surgeries performed on older patients, accounting for approximately 2.1 million surgical procedures in 2019. In Europe, joint replacement surgery was the most frequently performed procedure on old patients (over 1.5 million surgeries in 2018), followed by heart surgeries (over 1 million) and cataract surgery (1.2 million). Meanwhile, in Asia, cataract surgery ranked as the most common surgical procedure, with over 6 million operations performed in 2019, surpassing gastrointestinal operations (over 1 million) and heart surgeries (over 900,000). In Africa, due to limited resources and accessibility to healthcare, older patients rarely undergo surgeries. However, cataract surgery (more than 300,000 treatments per year) and joint replacement surgery (more than 60,000 procedures per year) are becoming increasingly popular. In summary, these data support that the most frequent surgical procedures performed on older individuals around the world vary based on geographic location [28].

1.3.1 Impact of Post-operative Outcomes

The need for procedures that may cause serious injury to individuals is expected to increase as the global population of older persons grows. Negative postoperative outcomes may be more likely if geriatric syndromes, such as cognitive decline, are more common in older individuals. Postoperative complications, such as

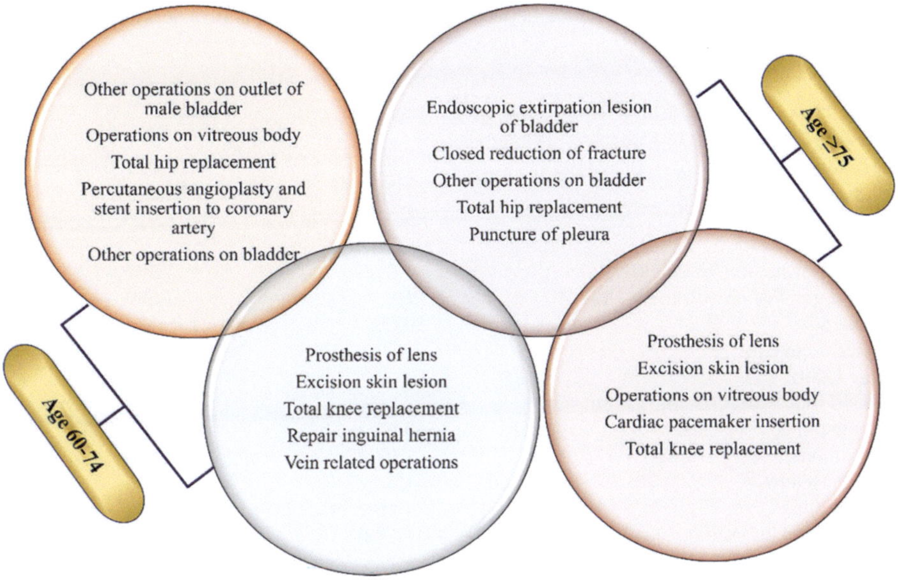

Fig. 1.4 Common surgical procedures performed in the older population grouped according to age distribution

pneumonia, wound infection, and venous thromboembolism, were most frequently documented as a composite [29]. Across all surgical specialties, the combined prevalence of complications following the operation was 25.16%, with cardiac surgery accounting for 9.46%, abdominal surgery at 24.73%, and thoracic surgery at 33.97%. Poor performance status, as measured by the Eastern Cooperative Oncology Group (ECOG) score [30], was the predictive variable most closely linked to the emergence of postoperative complications [31, 32]. Risk factors that predispose frail patients to diseases make them more susceptible to postoperative issues. Delirium appears to be the leading postoperative problem in frail surgical patients, with an incidence ranging from 15% to 50% in this population (Table 1.2). Preexisting cognitive decline and dementia are the two main risk factors for delirium. Other risk factors that should be taken into account before surgery include drug dependency, anxiety, poor general functional status, impaired hearing or vision, polypharmacy, and visual impairment. Studies suggest that up to 40% of surgical delirium in hospitalized older persons can be prevented. Therefore, it is crucial to establish evidence-based treatments and understand the patient's delirium-associated factors [33, 34].

1.3.2 Significance of Patient-Centered-Care

Compared to younger patients, older adult patients require a higher level of medical attention during the pre-, peri-, and post-operative phases. One of the key goals of

Table 1.2 Analysis of the association between risk factors and postoperative delirium in different age groups

	95% CI	
Risk factors	Lower	Upper
60–69 years old		
Arteriosclerosis	1.483	18.021
Coronary heart disease	1.719	18.683
Dementia	66.37	1428.9
70–79 years old		
Blood transfusion volume (0u)	1.518	5.307
Blood transfusion volume (1–4u)	1.4	7.689
Dementia	50.05	155.78
Arteriosclerosis	1.71	5.808
Age (>80)		
Blood transfusion volume (5–8u)	2.389	10.487
Dementia	59.65	116.07
Pneumonia	2.078	4.656
Arteriosclerosis	1.5	2.906
Arrhythmia	1.16	2.555
Myocardial infarction	1.288	5.986
Cerebral infarction	1.486	2.828

The upper and lower values are presented with a 95% Confidence Interval (CI)

the post-operative phase is early mobilization, which necessitates early weight-bearing. This can impact the therapy options available to older population. It is crucial to carefully monitor a patient's physical status, particularly blood pressure, pulse rate, and the presence of dyspnea. Pre-operative identification of dementia is essential for risk assessment and has implications for post-operative delirium assessment [35]. Nevertheless, certain age-biased laws and medical practices must be maintained and developed to provide older people with essential benefits. The Association of Anesthetists of Great Britain and Ireland, the British Geriatric Society, and the American Society of Anesthesiologists/American Geriatrics Society have all produced protocols for the perioperative care of older people. It is widely acknowledged that older surgical patients require perioperative care teams to oversee them during and after surgery [36, 37]. Compared to "usual care," regular geriatric consultation and focused guidance have shown to reduce delirium following hip fracture restoration by up to 50%. The care models have evolved, transitioning from geriatric assessment of patients assigned for treatment to integrated joint care provided by orthopedic and geriatric specialists [38]. For these patients facing surgery, proactive perioperative care teams offer a multidimensional strategy for creating an individual patient route of integrated treatment, which reduces the proportion of canceled surgeries and improves outcomes. Perioperative assessments include recognizing health abnormalities that can be treated or anticipated and planning for postoperative discharge requirements, along with relevant input from social services. Patient education (and involvement of the patient's family), as seen in conventional accelerated recovery programs, is of utmost importance [39]. Several studies have shown that in postoperative elective orthopedic patients, this post-operative care method has led to a significant reduction in the incidences of pneumonia, wound infection, and pressure sores. There is no universally accepted care model, and various versions have been reported worldwide. While major surgery patients benefit the most from these services, older surgical patients participating in minor or ambulatory surgery can also benefit from them [40].

1.4 Aging and Healthcare Utilization Across Countries

The aging of the world's population is leading to an increased need for healthcare services among older individuals, encompassing both surgical and nonsurgical treatments. Recent statistics indicate that between 2015 and 2030, worldwide healthcare use by older individuals is expected to rise by more than 50%. The most common procedures performed on older patients include coronary artery bypass surgery, cataract surgery, and joint replacement surgery. Globally, older adults frequently utilize nonsurgical treatments such as prescription drugs and physical therapy. The number of older individuals requiring various medications to manage chronic illnesses is on the rise, and this trend is expected to continue in the coming years. Another crucial non-surgical strategy used by older persons to maintain mobility and independence is physical therapy and rehabilitation services [41, 42].

1.5 Medical Interventions Across Different Countries

Around the world, older people are receiving more medical interventions, leading to a larger portion of healthcare spending being allocated to their care. In the USA, the older population accounts for one-third of healthcare spending. Among older individuals in the USA, joint replacement procedures, with approximately 1 million surgeries conducted each year, constitute the most frequently performed surgical interventions. In Canada, seniors make up 45% of the population receiving healthcare. Nonsurgical therapies are commonly used by older individuals in Canada, with estimates indicating that more than 90% of senior citizens consistently use at least one medicine. Similarly, in the UK, nonsurgical treatments are the most popular among older persons [43]. In Japan, older individuals frequently undergo surgical procedures, with estimates indicating that more than 1 million cataract operations are performed yearly. In China, traditional Chinese medicine is commonly used by older individuals, with studies indicating that more than 80% of older adults consistently use at least one prescription [44].

1.6 Access to Healthcare Facilities

The impact of healthcare use on outcomes in older individuals is significantly influenced by the standard of healthcare provided, access to treatment, and coordination of care. Aging-related outcomes have been linked, in several nations, to healthcare fragmentation, which refers to the absence of collaboration and consistency of treatment. For instance, research conducted in the USA indicated that older persons who received treatment from various providers or in different venues were more likely to experience negative outcomes, including hospitalization [45]. Conversely, results for older persons have been better in nations with integrated and patient-centered care strategies. For example, the introduction of comprehensive geriatric evaluations and care coordination programs in the UK has been associated with better outcomes for older individuals, such as reduced hospitalizations and an improvement in quality of life. The adoption of comprehensive healthcare models has also been linked to improved results for older individuals in Japan and Canada, including fewer hospitalizations and an increased functional status [46].

1.7 Approaches for Patient-Centered Care

In many areas, patient-centered care is essential for older persons to maximize healthcare utilization and improve outcomes. This approach involves tailoring medical treatments to meet each person's unique requirements and preferences and involving both the individuals receiving treatment and their families in the decision-making process. By reducing unnecessary procedures and avoiding adverse outcomes, this strategy can enhance results and reduce healthcare expenses. Many nations, including the USA, Canada, and the UK, have implemented policies to support patient-centered care for older adults, such as comprehensive geriatric assessments and coordinated healthcare programs. Japan has also established coordinated care approaches, with a focus on preventative medicine and early intervention. Studies indicate that coordinated approaches to care can lead to improved outcomes and lower healthcare costs for older people. However, the percentage of older adults receiving coordinated care varies across nations [14].

1.8 International, European, and Italian Perspectives

Numerous physiological changes brought on by aging are known to increase the risk of postoperative complications and fatalities. To improve patient satisfaction and lower costs, various specialized services have recently been established to care for elderly patients before surgery. Healthcare professionals must consider these factors while providing treatment to older persons because the unique characteristics of aging and surgical treatment vary across different geographical regions. The ability of older persons to access medical treatment may be severely hampered in low- and middle-income nations where medical facilities are scarce. For instance, in sub-Saharan Africa, a lack of surgeons, limited access to surgical materials and equipment, and an inefficient healthcare system can significantly impact how well older patients are treated during surgery. This can lead to high rates of death and morbidity due to restricted access to surgical treatment [44].

Table 1.3 Proportion of patients not undergoing surgery or experiencing delayed surgery, from both patients' and physicians' perspectives

	Proportion of patients		
Reasons	USA	Europe	Japan
Patients' perspective			
Unwillingness to have surgery	35	28	60
Feeling of not having surgery	56	50	41
Fear of surgery	39	36	49
Cost of surgery	1	13	2
Unsure about surgical success	1	2	1
Fear of surgical risks and complications	1	0	4
Physician's perspective			
Patient reluctance	74	69	79
Patient health	66	63	42
Patient age	56	60	53
Cost to patient	30	7	38
Cost to healthcare system	10	16	12
Others	13	6	4

In high-income nations with ample healthcare resources, older and frail persons may encounter distinct difficulties. For example, a study conducted in Japan, USA, and Europe on patients suffering from osteoarthritis reported various reasons for not undergoing surgery (see Table 1.3). Due to the frequency of comorbidities and age-associated physiological changes, patients are also susceptible to negative consequences. For instance, the incidence of comorbidities, such as diabetes and cardiovascular disease, increases with aging, which may complicate operations and raise the possibility of unfavorable outcomes. Healthcare professionals must also take into account the special psychosocial needs of older persons, which include a requirement for social support and the potential effects of cognitive decline on decision-making and consent. Research indicates that older Americans are more likely than younger Americans to experience negative consequences from surgery, such as higher mortality rates and prolonged hospital admissions. In older patients suffering from circulatory disease, the death rate in various countries is represented in Fig. 1.5 [48].

Recommendations for the care of older persons undergoing surgical operations have been developed in Italy by the Italian Society of Geriatric Surgery, taking into account the specific physiological, psychological, and social needs of this group. Additionally, programs like the "Silver Code," which provides guidelines for the management of elderly people in emergency rooms, have been implemented to improve healthcare accessibility and treatment outcomes for this population [49].

1.9 Conclusion

The need to continue identifying common surgical treatments in older persons, along with related challenges, postoperative outcomes, and complications, is one of the most pressing issues. By highlighting potential improvement areas, this research

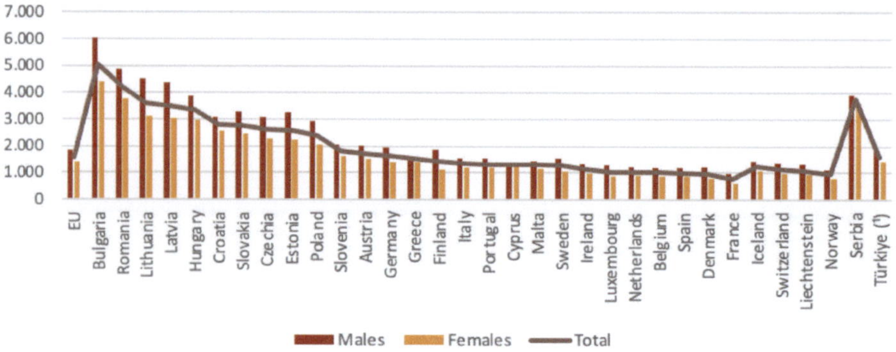

Fig. 1.5 Standardized death rate/100,000 inhabitants, resulting from circulatory disease in people aged ≥65

can help raise the standard of surgical treatment provided to older patients. Furthermore, as technology advances, it is crucial to understand how these developments can be utilized to enhance the outcomes of surgeries performed on older patients. Future studies should focus on expanding older persons' access to surgical treatment, especially in areas with limited accessibility. To ensure that older persons receive the excellent medical care they require to preserve their physical and mental well-being, it is essential to identify access barriers and devise ways to overcome them through the work described below. To further advance our knowledge of geriatric surgical treatment, continued collaboration between global, European, and Italian researchers is essential. Most interesting is the EUropean PErioperative MEdical networking (EUPMEN) project [47]. The EUPEMEN project aims to incorporate the expertise and clinical experience of national clinical specialists into the development of perioperative rehabilitation protocols. Providing special recommendations for all aspects of patient perioperative care and the participation of diverse specialists, the EUPEMEN protocol aims to provide faster postoperative recovery and reduce the length of hospital stay, postoperative morbidity, and mortality rate. The Eupemen project has been carried out by Fundación Instituto de Investigación Sanitaria Aragón-IISA as coordinator and Azienda Unità Sanitaria Locale Ferrara—AUSLFE, Univerzita Karlova—CUNI, Universidad Miguel Hernández de Elche—UMH and "G. Papanikolaou—GPAP" General Hospital of Thessaloniki as partners. The development of this field can be accelerated, and surgical outcomes for senior citizens around the world can be improved by exchanging data and knowledge between different geographic regions. Future healthcare advancements are expected to expand options for the treatment of senior citizens in European medical systems with constrained resources and address current issues by ensuring an acceptable standard of healthcare services for all senior citizens. Embracing a medical policy of personalized care for patients, geriatricians have the opportunity to take the initiative and contribute to improvements on every front. Therefore, maintaining a strong geriatric medicine specialty will be a crucial strategy. Future research should focus on evaluating the clinical and economic effectiveness of preoperative geriatric optimization clinics and perioperative surgical cooperation in surgical specialties.

References

1. Merrill RM. Foundations of epidemiology. In: Introduction to epidemiology. Burlington, MA: Jones & Bartlett Learning; 2017. p. 1–15.
2. Friis RH, Sellers TA. History and scope of epidemiology. In: Epidemiology for public health practice. Burlington, MA: Jones & Bartlett Learning; 2021. p. 1–45.
3. Dhama K, Patel SK, Kumar R, Rana J, Yatoo MI, Kumar A, Tiwari R, Dhama J, Natesan S, Singh R, Harapan H. Geriatric population during the COVID-19 pandemic: problems, considerations, exigencies, and beyond [mini review]. Front Public Health. 2020;8:8. https://doi.org/10.3389/fpubh.2020.574198.
4. Guo J, Huang X, Dou L, Yan M, Shen T, Tang W, Li J. Aging and aging-related diseases: from molecular mechanisms to interventions and treatments. Signal Transduct Target Ther. 2022;7(1):391.
5. Amarya S, Singh K, Sabharwal M. Ageing process and physiological changes. In: Gerontology. IntechOpen; 2018.
6. Gjorgjievski M, Ristevski B. Postoperative management considerations of the elderly patient undergoing orthopaedic surgery. Injury. 2020;51:S23–7.
7. Artiles-Armas M, Roque-Castellano C, Conde-Martel A, Marchena-Gómez J. The comprehensive complication index is related to frailty in elderly surgical patients. J Surg Res. 2019;244:218–24.
8. Fröhlich M, Caspers M, Lefering R, Driessen A, Bouillon B, Maegele M, Wafaisade A, TraumaRegister DGU. Do elderly trauma patients receive the required treatment? Epidemiology and outcome of geriatric trauma patients treated at different levels of trauma care. Eur J Trauma Emerg Surg. 2020;46:1463–9.
9. Lin H-S, Watts J, Peel N, Hubbard R. Frailty and post-operative outcomes in older surgical patients: a systematic review. BMC Geriatr. 2016;16(1):1–12.
10. Masutani R, Pawar A, Lee H, Weissman JS, Kim DH. Outcomes of common major surgical procedures in older adults with and without dementia. JAMA Netw Open. 2020;3(7):e2010395.
11. de Jesus Neves Silva D, Casimiro LGG, de Oliveira MIS, da Cunha Ferreira LB, Abelha FJPA. The very elderly surgical population in a critically ill scenario: clinical characteristics and outcomes. Rev Bras Anestesiol. 2020;70:3–8.
12. Tjeertes EK, van Fessem JM, Mattace-Raso FU, Hoofwijk AG, Stolker RJ, Hoeks SE. Influence of frailty on outcome in older patients undergoing non-cardiac surgery-a systematic review and meta-analysis. Aging Dis. 2020;11(5):1276.
13. Janssen T, Alberts A, Hooft L, Mattace-Raso F, Mosk C, van der Laan L. Prevention of postoperative delirium in elderly patients planned for elective surgery: systematic review and meta-analysis. Clin Interv Aging. 2019;14:1095–117.
14. Jarzebski MP, Elmqvist T, Gasparatos A, Fukushi K, Eckersten S, Haase D, Goodness J, Khoshkar S, Saito O, Takeuchi K, Theorell T, Dong N, Kasuga F, Watanabe R, Sioen GB, Yokohari M, Pu J. Ageing and population shrinking: implications for sustainability in the urban century. NPJ Urban Sustain. 2021;1(1):17. https://doi.org/10.1038/s42949-021-00023-z.
15. Jaul E, Barron J. Age-related diseases and clinical and public health implications for the 85 years old and over population. Front Public Health. 2017;5:335.
16. Ko FC. Preoperative frailty evaluation: a promising risk-stratification tool in older adults undergoing general surgery. Clin Ther. 2019;41(3):387–99.
17. Rose J, Weiser TG, Hider P, Wilson L, Gruen R, Bickler SW. Estimated need for surgery worldwide based on prevalence of diseases: implications for public health planning of surgical services. Lancet Glob Health. 2015;3(Suppl 2):S13.

18. Demir E, Southern D, Rashid S, Lebcir R. A discrete event simulation model to evaluate the treatment pathways of patients with cataract in the United Kingdom. BMC Health Serv Res. 2018;18(1):1–15.
19. Yang R, Wolfson M, Lewis MC. Unique aspects of the elderly surgical population: an Anesthesiologist's perspective. Geriatr Orthop Surg Rehabil. 2011;2(2):56–64. https://doi.org/10.1177/2151458510394606. PMID: 23569671; PMCID: PMC3597305.
20. Vaduganathan M, Mensah GA, Turco JV, Fuster V, Roth GA. The global burden of cardiovascular diseases and risk: A compass for future health, vol. 80. Washington, DC: American College of Cardiology Foundation; 2022. p. 2361–71.
21. Deiner S, Westlake B, Dutton RP. Patterns of surgical care and complications in elderly adults. J Am Geriatr Soc. 2014;62(5):829–35. https://doi.org/10.1111/jgs.12794. Epub 2014 Apr 14. PMID: 24731176; PMCID: PMC4024102.
22. Barbabella F, Cela E, Socci M, Lucantoni D, Zannella M, Principi A. Active ageing in Italy: A systematic review of national and regional policies. Int J Environ Res Public Health. 2022;19(1):600.
23. Fowler A, Abbott T, Prowle J, Pearse R. Age of patients undergoing surgery. J Br Surg. 2019;106(8):1012–8.
24. Monika K, Del Mar NAM, Maria N, Martina NC, Christiaan VL. Demographic outlook for the European Union 2022. Think Tank; 2022.
25. Prado CM, Ford KL, Gonzalez MC, Murnane LC, Gillis C, Wischmeyer PE, Morrison CA, Lobo DN. Nascent to novel methods to evaluate malnutrition and frailty in the surgical patient. J Parenter Enter Nutr. 2023;47:S54–68.
26. Bader AM. Geriatric surgery centers: the way forward. Int Anesthesiol Clin. 2023;61(2):55–61.
27. Carling Cheung M, Meissner MA, Garg T. Incorporating outcomes that matter to older adults into surgical research [editorial]. J Am Geriatr Soc. 2021;69(3):3. https://doi.org/10.1111/jgs.17028.
28. Isaacs AM, Riva-Cambrin J, Yavin D, Hockley A, Pringsheim TM, Jette N, Lethebe BC, Lowerison M, Dronyk J, Hamilton MG. Age-specific global epidemiology of hydrocephalus: systematic review, metanalysis and global birth surveillance. PLoS One. 2018;13(10):e0204926.
29. Cooper L, Abbett SK, Feng A, Bernacki RE, Cooper Z, Urman RD, Frain LN, Edwards AF, Blitz JD, Javedan H. Launching a geriatric surgery center: recommendations from the Society for Perioperative Assessment and Quality Improvement. J Am Geriatr Soc. 2020;68(9):1941–6.
30. Zubrod C, et al. Appraisal of methods for the study of chemotherapy in man: comparative therapeutic trial of nitrogen mustard and thiophosphoramide. J Chronic Dis. 1960;11:7–33.
31. Chawan AP, Rathore YS, Chumber S, Kataria K. Surgical diseases and surgical outcomes in geriatric patients. Int Surg J. 2020;7(10):6. https://doi.org/10.18203/2349-2902.isj20204129.
32. Desserud K, Veen T, Søreide K. Emergency general surgery in the geriatric patient. J Br Surg. 2016;103(2):e52–61.
33. Nagaratnam K. Delirium in the oldest of old. In: Nagaratnam N, Nagaratnam K, Cheuk G, editors. Advanced age geriatric care: a comprehensive guide. Cham: Springer; 2019. p. 287–96.
34. Wang T, Guo J, Hou Z, Zhang Y. Risk factors of postoperative delirium in elderly patients with intertrochanteric fracture: an age-stratified retrospective analysis of 2307 patients. Geriatr Orthop Surg Rehabil. 2022;13:21514593221081779.
35. Fagard K, Deschodt M, Geyskens L, Willems S, Boland B, Wolthuis A, Flamaing J. Geriatric care for surgical patients: results and reflections from a cross-sectional survey in acute Belgian hospitals. Eur Geriatr Med. 2023;14:1–11.
36. Ellis G, Gardner M, Tsiachristas A, Langhorne P, Burke O, Harwood RH, Conroy SP, Kircher T, Somme D, Saltvedt I. Comprehensive geriatric assessment for older adults admitted to hospital. Cochrane Database Syst Rev. 2017;9:CD006211.
37. Partridge J, Sbai M, Dhesi J. Proactive care of older people undergoing surgery. Aging Clin Exp Res. 2018;30(3):253–7. https://doi.org/10.1007/s40520-017-0879-4.
38. Vitiello R, Bellieni A, Oliva MS, Di Capua B, Fusco D, Careri S, Colloca GF, Perisano C, Maccauro G, Lillo M. The importance of geriatric and surgical co-management of elderly in muscoloskeletal oncology: a literature review. Orthop Rev. 2020;12(Suppl 1):8662.

39. Wirtz D, Kohlhof H. The geriatric patient: special aspects of peri-operative management. EFORT Open Rev. 2019;4(6):240.
40. Cheuk G, Nagaratnam N. End-of-life care in geriatric population. In: Nagaratnam N, Nagaratnam K, Cheuk G, editors. Advanced age geriatric care: a comprehensive guide. Cham: Springer; 2019. p. 11–7.
41. Miller IT, Boyle S, Kopolovich H, Shah A, Wiener DE. Emergency medicine management of the elderly. In: Latifi R, editor. Surgical decision making in geriatrics: a comprehensive multidisciplinary approach. Cham: Springer; 2020. p. 23–44.
42. Watt J, Tricco AC, Talbot-Hamon C, Pham B, Rios P, Grudniewicz A, Wong C, Sinclair D, Straus SE. Identifying older adults at risk of harm following elective surgery: a systematic review and meta-analysis. BMC Med. 2018;16(1):2. https://doi.org/10.1186/s12916-017-0986-2.
43. Stuck AE, Masud T. Health care for older adults in Europe: how has it evolved and what are the challenges? Age Ageing. 2022;51(12):afac287.
44. Howdon D, Pasali S. The impact of ageing on accessibility, affordability and availability of healthcare services in Asia and the Pacific. ESCAP Working Paper. 2022;
45. Zayas CE, He Z, Yuan J, Maldonado-Molina M, Hogan W, Modave F, Guo Y, Bian J. Examining healthcare utilization patterns of elderly middle-aged adults in the United States. In: Proceedings of the … International Florida AI Research Society Conference. Florida AI Research Symposium; 2016.
46. Potter JF, Harper GM. Screening tools for geriatric assessment by specialists. In: Lee AG, Potter JF, Harper GM, editors. Geriatrics for specialists. 2nd ed. Cham: Springer Nature; 2021. https://doi.org/10.1007/978-3-030-76271-1_8.
47. Ioannidis O, Ramirez JM, Ubieto JM, Feo CV, Arroyo A, Kocián P, Sánchez-Guillén L, Bellosta AP, Whitley A, Enguita AB, et al. The EUPEMEN (EUropean PErioperative MEdical networking) protocol for bowel obstruction: recommendations for perioperative care. J Clin Med. 2023;12:4185. https://doi.org/10.3390/jcm12134185.
48. Reece G, Poojara L. The elderly in intensive care. In: Nagaratnam N, Nagaratnam K, Cheuk G, editors. Advanced age geriatric care: a comprehensive guide. Springer; 2019. p. 101–9. https://doi.org/10.1007/978-3-319-96998-5_14.
49. Melchiorre MG, Socci M, Quattrini S, Lamura G, D'Amen B. Frail older people ageing in place in Italy: use of health services and relationship with general practitioner. Int J Environ Res Public Health. 2022;19(15):9063.

2 Implications of Population Aging for Societies and Governments

Erica Eugeni, Maria Roberta De Blasiis, Chiara De Marchi, Francesco Enrichens, Elisa Guglielmi, Enrico Coscioni, and Giovanni Baglio

2.1 Introduction: The Current Situation

Health demography presents a scenario for Western countries characterized by the prevalence of chronic and degenerative diseases, which lack possibilities of cure or resolution in the short term, due to the general aging of the population, the success of medicine in addressing numerous infectious diseases, the development of new healthcare technologies, but also due to exposure to health risk factors (such as smoking, high-calorie diet, alcohol abuse, physical inactivity, and sedentary lifestyle).

Specifically, Italy is among the European Union countries with the oldest population, presenting on January 1, 2023, an old-age index—calculated as the percentage ratio between the age group over 64 years and the one under 15 years—of 193.1% [18]. Within the country, marked territorial variability is evident: the index indeed shows values of 200.6% in the Northwest, 195.5% in the Northeast, 204.1% in the Center, 175.8% in the South, and 188.5% in the Islands. Among individuals over 64 years old, the so-called "oldest old" (those who have surpassed 80 years of age) show a higher growth rate. Life expectancy is higher for women than for men, to the extent that women constitute 56% of the elderly population overall and about 62% of those who have surpassed 80 years [18].

The older age groups are the most affected by chronic degenerative diseases: among those over 65, 59% of the population suffers from at least one chronic disease, while above 85 years, the percentage rises to 72% [17]. Among the most

E. Eugeni · M. R. De Blasiis · C. De Marchi · F. Enrichens · E. Guglielmi · E. Coscioni
G. Baglio (✉)
Italian National Agency for Regional Healthcare Services – Agenas, Rome, Italy
e-mail: direzionericerca@agenas.it; mariaroberta.deblasiis@uniroma1.it; chiara.demarchi@uniroma1.it; enrichens@agenas.it; guglielmi@agenas.it; coscioni@agenas.it; baglio@agenas.it

V. Boccardi, L. Marano (eds.), *The Frail Surgical Patient*, Practical Issues in Geriatrics, https://doi.org/10.1007/978-3-031-77707-3_2

common chronic diseases are heart diseases (28%), diabetes (21%), chronic respiratory diseases (17%), and cancer (14%).

Patients are thus increasingly affected by multimorbidity and increasingly complex needs, with impacts both in economic and bioethical terms (consider, for example, end-of-life issues), and require greater collaboration between the healthcare and social sectors in terms of care delivery [22]. Healthcare needs, closely related to the need to reduce costs associated with care demand and increase its sustainability, therefore require new management methods for patients and people in discomfort, an emphasis on care continuity and socio-health integration, and a rethinking of patient care approaches, as medical hyper-specialization has often restricted a whole-person approach, diverting attention from patient's life and suffering experience [29].

2.2 Risk Stratification as a Tool for Planning

Effective healthcare planning in light of the current demographic and epidemiological asset necessitates the adoption of tools and strategies for managing available resources economically and professionally while ensuring equitable care. Among these tools, risk stratification facilitates the implementation of targeted and personalized interventions, optimizing resource allocation and enhancing overall health outcomes. This strategy involves categorizing the population into homogeneous groups based on the characteristics such as disease risk, care needs, and socio-economic conditions. It aligns with the *Chronic Care Model (CCM)* [3, 30] and *Population Health Management (PHM)*, which aims to enhance the health of defined populations and reduce disparities in service access and health outcomes [16].

In PHM programs, a crucial aspect is assigning individual beneficiaries a predetermined risk level, enabling both treating physicians and caregivers, and healthcare and social services to guide and tailor care accordingly. This includes setting up healthcare facilities and developing public health strategies commensurate with risk, considering sustainability, equity, appropriateness, and intervention effectiveness. The stratification process ensures timely activation of appropriate services for patients, following the "initiative healthcare" model based on their risk factors, before conditions worsen, and irrespective of patient-initiated requests [1].

Various international stratification models exist, as outlined in the National Chronicity Plan 2016 [21]. For instance, the *Kaiser* US pyramid categorizes populations with chronic conditions into subgroups based on condition development stages, with defined prevalence percentages for subclasses. An intriguing adaptation is the *King's Fund* model in the UK, which stratifies populations based on health and social needs. The US *Adjusted Clinical Groups (ACG)* system, on the other hand, categorizes the population by the level of healthcare complexity based on combinations of diagnoses present simultaneously in the same patient.

In Italy, stratification models have been developed in various regions. One of the most recent experiments, based on the integration of numerous socio-health information systems, is the "modular methodology" developed by the Lazio Region. This methodology involves dividing the population into the following categories based on different levels of care intensity: categorizing populations based on care intensity levels: healthy, single chronic condition, multiple chronic conditions, and high clinical complexity/multiple chronic conditions with socio-economic vulnerability factors [20]. However, to date, the completeness and quality of data in the current healthcare information flows in various regions, particularly those related to territorial assistance, are lacking. This shortfall sometimes prevents stratification of the reference population according to models similar to that proposed by Lazio or other regions that have developed similar systems [9]. Additionally, Ministry of Health Decree No. 77 of May 23, 2022 [8], has adopted a stratification model based on the identification of six levels of care complexity to be implemented nationwide. However, for such mapping activity to be initiated and extended to the entire reference population, it will be necessary to enhance the reliability and completeness of information available in current information flows, also promoting the interconnection processes of socio-health data collection systems.

Overall, population stratification can enhance the more efficient use of available resources, identifying subgroups needing greater assistance or at risk of poorer health outcomes. This can lead to both reducing overall healthcare costs and improving access to care for those most in need, contributing to ensuring equity in access and health outcomes through the identification of socio-economic disparities and the implementation of targeted interventions to overcome them.

2.3 Integrated Care Models

This new care landscape prioritizes organizational models focused on continuity of care and guiding citizens within the service system [13]. More generally, attention shifts from Clinical Pathways for Disease Management (Percorsi Diagnostici Terapeutici Assistenziali—PDTA), constructed and calibrated for individual pathologies, to multidisciplinary and multiprofessional care pathways characterized by a high level of competence and integration. There is an emphasis on abandoning a monodisciplinary approach, focused on a single disease or organ, in favor of embracing the person in their entirety and complexity. A *multifaceted* intervention mode is promoted, based on teamwork and integration of viewpoints, through collaboration among different professions, particularly from social and healthcare fields, working jointly in the assessment and treatment of so-called "complex" cases.

In recent years, there has also been a re-emergence of focus on the individual within their living environment and more broadly, in the social context, along with a strong promotion of primary care. The significant budget contractions faced by healthcare, social healthcare, and social services; the desire to reduce institutionalization of individuals with chronic and degenerative diseases, which encourages discharge from specialized facilities and reintegration into the social network, and the reduction of hospital stays in favor of the development of community services; and the aim to keep the older persons in their homes for as long as possible: all of these factors are leading to an increasing amount of care and assistance provided in the home environment or in spaces close to where the individual lives, and to the coexistence of multiple actors from the public, nonprofit private, and purely private sectors. National and regional healthcare planning has shifted toward a reorganization of services providing care and assistance, with a significant downsizing of the hospital's role in resolving the population's health problems and a greater emphasis on territorial healthcare and social healthcare activities and services. The latter include facilities and personnel resources related to basic social healthcare assistance, home care, and care provided by residential and semi-residential facilities. Home care, in particular, involves the intervention of general practitioners or family pediatricians, and various professionals (nurses, physiotherapists, specialist doctors, social workers, and social assistants) who provide first- and second-level services, nursing and rehabilitative assistance, and domestic help.

In the Italian context, the Project PON GOV Chronicity [23], for which Agenas held the technical-scientific coordination, has made it possible to define at the national level tools, technologies, and professionalism based on best practices and aimed at supporting a person-centered care model, which prioritizes patient's maintenance in their own life context.

The community of practice, born from the collaboration among all operators, stakeholders, and regional representatives, is still a valuable operational tool for participants to achieve the same goals and objectives, through discussion and sharing of best local experiences on Telemedicine and care for people with chronic conditions [1, 10, 11].

2.4 The Role of *Caregiver*

This shift of focus from the hospital to the community, from treatment to care pathways, from pathology to discomfort, involves new professional figures, such as home care workers and community nurses, linked to health management and socio-assistance, often working in "alternative" spaces of care and support, such as the intimate space of households. Such ways of care delivery do not exclusively involve the public sector and patients accessing care, but they foster the creation of a complex and articulated field [14], within which a significant role is played by families, although there is no formal recognition of the caregiving work done in the domestic space [5, 6] by neighborhood communities, and by those intermediary organizations called upon in various capacities to respond to the needs of a growing segment of the population.

Within the field of extra-institutional or "informal" resources, first and foremost, are caregivers or family collaborators, namely individuals (typically women) who spend the entire day and sometimes even the night with the older persons and may not necessarily receive a salary in exchange for their presence in the home but may instead exchange the assistance they provide for the hospitality the older persons are able to offer. Secondly, there are all those relationships within and outside the family network that can be helpful for older persons in the perspective of an overall improvement in the quality of their life, as well as for handling small tasks they may not be able to cope with individually [7, 12]. The ensemble of personal relationships that the older persons are able to mobilize to pursue a specific goal or improve their condition, and the resources derived from these relationships, constitute a form of "social capital" [4], useful for complementing the care provided by services and family members.

The Italian welfare system, in particular, assigns families an important role in caregiving and assistance, yet without providing adequate support through family policies capable of recognizing and supporting caregiving work. For this reason, in the Italian case and more generally in the "Southern European familistic system," there is talk of passive subsidiarity [19]. Policies aimed at supporting older persons in their living environment pose challenges for families related to the domestic management of illness and discomfort, requiring particular attention to the experience of caregivers who day by day care for older persons, sick, nonself-sufficient, or disabled individuals, whose role is often inadequately considered, both practically and socially [5, 15]. The management of chronic illness and its consequences, as well as aging, combines and mobilizes "high-level technical and professional acts and interventions, with a more common function of care and assistance in daily life, which largely falls on those who are close [to the sick or older persons]" [5]. Therefore, the therapeutic and caregiving space in this case not only involves specialists but also transforms the household into a "consumer" of practices provided by third parties and by institutions and services responsible for managing discomfort, as well as all those who provide care or receive care in daily life [27]. They are involved not only as caregivers to their loved ones but also often as individuals actively engaged at different levels in the care provided by services—sometimes trained in administering therapies or managing emergencies. They serve as valuable resources through which it is possible to ensure that older persons remain in the environment they have always lived in and avoid institutional care.

The field of care and assistance, especially in a territorial context, is predominantly female-oriented. Women are at the core of the domestic sphere and the caregiving provided within it: they are generally tasked with taking care of and providing assistance to those in need within the family setting. However, the support and assistance provided by these women are not institutionally recognized, as caregiving within the family realm is associated with social invisibility and unpaid work [15, 26–28]. As emphasized by Muehlebach [25], even if a woman is employed outside the domestic space, her life cycle is always structured around caregiving, often unrecognized and frequently unpaid. Women provide care without receiving compensation to their children, and subsequently to their parents and often to their spouses: thus, their life cycle is characterized by a continuum of various types of unpaid caregiving. The role of women as caregivers is extremely flexible and capable of adapting to the limitations and specificities of professional interventions, which they are often called upon to compensate for [5]. In this sense, from the perspective of care and health services, it is a role conceived as a "deficiency," as Bungener [5] underscores since it presupposes an adaptation afterward to the resources that the public sector can make available to address each individual's situation of discomfort or illness.

The immigrant population is also personally involved, partly tasked with supporting the epidemiological shift, due to the increased demand for workers employed in caregiving activities [24]. In many cases, these individuals perform a significant portion of the activities aimed at support, assistance, and accompaniment, which ensure the older persons can remain within the home environment. If home care indeed provides older individuals in discomfort the opportunity to remain in their familiar living environment, it can only be activated by relying on resources other than institutional ones, particularly those upon which an older person can depend. It is therefore required that all those involved with an older individual in discomfort contribute to their well-being, utilizing a one-on-one intervention model. In this sense, home care renders caregiving difficult to sustain, especially for caregivers, as it individualizes the management of discomfort, making it an individual burden. While this mode of delivering care contributes to the need to reduce the economic burden on the service system, serving as a valid tool to address the challenges stemming from the evolving scenario of illness and discomfort, it also increases the costs endured by families in physical and emotional terms. In this regard, caring for the individual in their living environment risks perpetuating the inequalities that the overall reorganization of the system aims to mitigate, to the extent that only those with economic means can afford to be relieved of the burden of care, for example, by hiring private support, and only those with useful social relationships to support or replace the presence of family members, integrating service provision, can guarantee the possibility of remaining in the home environment.

Moreover, if insufficient consideration is given to the context within which the individual is situated and the fact that the condition of discomfort can also impact those who perform caregiving duties on a daily basis, the intervention of services itself ends up, albeit indirectly, facilitating the emergence of further vulnerability [12].

2.5 Development Perspectives: Proximity and Telemedicine

In Italy, the National Health Service (NHS) represents the historically determined attempt to build a healthcare system that is more attentive to people's needs and more oriented toward the pursuit of the common good, the fight against inequalities, and the recognition of health as a universal right, without exclusion. The direction must be toward increasing attention to people in conditions of vulnerability, which requires the NHS to make greater efforts in protection, including older persons.

Increasingly central to healthcare planning is the dimension of "proximity." In recent years, significant experiences have been developed to protect vulnerable groups of the population, especially migrants and the homeless, and to support accessibility to social and healthcare services. These experiences have helped outline the features of a "practical philosophy of proximity," which now serves as a reference paradigm for the entire population [2] and can be understood in at least three ways: positional, postural, and participatory.

Proximity as a position relates to the "where" of delivering care or placing services. In this sense, proximity healthcare involves physical closeness to people, achieved through decentralization of part of the care delivery or by "shoe-leather" activities, such as directly visiting people's living, working, or gathering places in favor of those being assisted. An example of this is represented by active offer programs or home care activities. Proximity as a posture, on the other hand, refers to the "how" care is delivered. It implies understanding the healthcare needs of people living in the territories, especially those who may not have the strength or ability to translate into demand and therefore may not reach services, along with the system's ability to rethink itself in terms of greater accessibility and equity. The third aspect is participation, which concerns "with whom." It involves creating synergies with care resources and assistance different from those provided by services, with society, and with the social capital of the territories, starting from third-sector organizations and patient associations [2].

Proximity and integration must go hand in hand with digital transformation, which is central to the projects of the National Recovery and Resilience Plan (PNRR), promoting the widespread adoption of telemedicine solutions, as well as the design and implementation of an information technology platform for the delivery of digital services aimed at supporting, innovatively and through the use of artificial intelligence techniques and algorithms, doctors and their patients in the context of primary care and territorial assistance delivery [23]. From the perspective of proximity, especially benefiting the most deprived areas, marginalized segments of the population, and those in conditions of greater fragility such as older persons, the use of digital health represents an extraordinary opportunity to support and accompany the care relationship.

References

1. Agenas. Le Centrali Operative: standard di servizio, modelli organizzativi, tipologia di attività ed esperienze regionali. 2022. https://www.agenas.gov.it/comunicazione/primo-piano/2029-le-centrali-operative-standard-di-servizio,-modelli-organizzativi,-tipologie-di-attivit%C3%A0-ed-esperienze-regionali. Accessed 21 Feb 2024.
2. Baglio G, Eugeni E. Ripensare la sanità pubblica in chiave di prossimità: un obiettivo condiviso. Quaderni dell'ASviS. 2022;6:49–51. https://www-2020.asvis.it/public/asvis2/files/Pubblicazioni/QuadernoASVISGoal3.pdf. Accessed 21 Feb 2024.
3. Bodenheimer T, Wagner EH, Grumbach K. Improving primary care for patients with chronic illness: the chronic care model, part 2. JAMA. 2002;288(15):1909–14. https://doi.org/10.1001/jama.288.15.1909.
4. Bourdieu P. Le capital social: notes provisoires. Actes de la Recherche en Science Sociales. 1980;31:2–3.
5. Bungener M. Une gestion des corps malades et vieillissants. Le transfert domestique des activités de soins. In: Fassin D, Memmi D, editors. Le gouvernement des corps. Paris: Éditions de l'École des hautes études en sciences sociales; 2004. p. 109–33.

6. Comelles JM. La importancia cresciente de los no professionales en los procesos asistenciales. Canelobre: Revista del Instituto Alicantino de Cultura "Juan Gil-Albert"; 1987. p. 11–8.
7. Corin E, Tremblay J, Sherif T, Bergeron L. Entre le services professionales e les réseaux sociaux: les stratégies d'existence des personnes âgées. Sociologie et société. 1984;2:89–104.
8. Decreto Ministero della Salute 23 maggio 2022. n. 77. GU n.144 del 22-06-2022. https://www.gazzettaufficiale.it/eli/gu/2022/06/22/144/sg/pdf. Accessed 21 Feb 2024.
9. Di Martino M, Furfaro S, Mulas MF, Mataloni F, Santurri M, Paris A, Maritati A. La stratificazione della popolazione come strumento per rimodulare la rete assistenziale sul territorio: il ruolo determinante dei sistemi informativi socio-sanitari. Recenti Prog Med. 2022;113(2):97–104. https://doi.org/10.1701/3748.37313.
10. Enrichens F. I pilastri di una nuova rete territoriale. Recenti Prog Med. 2021;Suppl Forward 22:S12–3.
11. Enrichens F, Borghini A, Furfaro S, Cosentino M. La casa come primo luogo di cura per il cittadino - centrali operative territoriali e assistenza domiciliare. Monitor. Elementi di analisi e osservazione del sistema salute. 2021;45:27–35.
12. Eugeni E. Dalla riproduzione alla manipolazione dello "Stato": gli usi del capitale sociale nel welfare che cambia. Il caso dell'assistenza domiciliare sociale. AM Rivista della società italiana di antropologia medica. 2013;35-36:225–45.
13. Eugeni E. Culture in sanità. Politiche e pratiche dell'accesso e della presa in carico in un Distretto sanitario romano. AM Rivista della società italiana di antropologia medica. 2015;37-38:537–54.
14. Fassin D. L'espace politique de la santé. Essai de généalogie, vol. 5. Paris: Presses Universitaires de France; 1996. p. 85.
15. Gagnon E, Saillant F. De la dépendance et de l'accompagnement. Soins à domicile et liens sociaux. Paris e Québec: L'Harmattan e Les Presses de l'Université Laval; 2000.
16. Girwar SM, Jabroer R, Fiocco M, Sutch SP, Numans ME, Bruijnzeels MA. A systematic review of risk stratification tools internationally used in primary care settings. Health Sci Rep. 2021;4(3):e329. https://doi.org/10.1002/hsr2.329.
17. ISS - Istituto Superiore di Sanità. Sorveglianza Passi d'Argento. Patologie croniche, dati 2021–2011. https://www.epicentro.iss.it/passi-argento/dati/croniche. Accessed 21 Feb 2024.
18. ISTAT. Demo - Statistiche demografiche. https://demo.istat.it/. Accessed 21 Feb 2024.
19. Kazepov Y. La dimensione territoriale delle politiche sociali in Italia. Roma: Carocci editore; 2009.
20. MaCroScopio (Osservatorio sulla Cronicità). StratificaPDTA. Roma: Il Pensiero Scientifico Editore; 2021.
21. Ministero della Salute. Piano Nazionale della Cronicità. 2016. https://www.salute.gov.it/imgs/C_17_pubblicazioni_2584_allegato.pdf. Accessed 21 Feb 2024.
22. Ministero della Salute/Consiglio Superiore di Sanità - Sezione I. Invecchiamento della popolazione e sostenibilità del SSN. 2020. https://www.salute.gov.it/portale/documentazione/p6_2_2_1.jsp?id=3094. Accessed 21 Feb 2024.
23. Ministero della Salute/Agenas. PON GOV Cronicità - Sostenere la sfida alla cronicità con il supporto dell'ICT - Logiche e strumenti gestionali e digitali per la presa in carico della cronicità - Manuale operativo e buone pratiche per ispirare e supportare l'implementazione del PNRR. 2023. https://www.agenas.gov.it/comunicazione/primo-piano/2313-pubblicata-la-versione-aggiornata-del-manuale-operativo-pon-gov-cronicità. Accessed 21 Feb 2024.
24. Muehlebach A. The enemy in the house: economies of intimacy in an era of privatization. Cahiers Parisiens/Parisian Notebooks. 2007;3:590–603.
25. Muehlebach A. The moral neoliberal. Welfare and citizenship in Italy. Chicago and London: The University of Chicago Press; 2012.
26. Saillant F. Femmes, soins domestiques et espace thérapeutique. Anthropologie et société. 1999;23(2):15–39.
27. Saillant F, Gagnon E. Présentation. Vers une anthropologie des soins. Anthropologie et société. 1999;23(2):5–11.

28. Saillant F, Gagnon E. Responsabilité pour autrui et dépendance dansa modernité avancée. Le cas de l'aide aux proches. Lien social 7et Politiques. 2001;46:55–69. https://doi.org/10.7202/000323ar.
29. Tognetti Bordogna M. I grandi anziani tra definizione sociale e salute. Milano: Franco Angeli Editore; 2007.
30. Wagner EH. The role of patient care teams in chronic disease management. BMJ. 2000;320(7234):569–72. https://doi.org/10.1136/bmj.320.7234.569.

The Impact of Aging Population on General Surgical Workforce Needs

3

Giovanni Aprea, Marianna Capuano, and Giuseppe Palomba

Over the years, the older population over the age of 65 has been rapidly growing and is increasingly diversified. Currently, 13% of the population is aged 65 years or older, and 1.9% is between 80 and 99 years old. According to data reported by the WHO, by the end of the Decade of Healthy Ageing (2021–2030), the number of people aged 60 years and older will be 34% higher. By 2050, the global population of older people will have more than doubled. The proportion of older people will increase, from one in eight people aged 60 years or over in 2017 to one in six by 2030 and one in five by 2050 (Table 3.1).

According to the Italian National Statistical Institute (ISTAT) data, the number of individuals aged 65 and older increased from 4.6 million in 1960 (9.3%) to 7.4 million in 1980 (13.1%), to 10.3 million in 2000 (18.1%). In 2009 they were close to 12 million and constituted 20.3%, while in 2019 they increased to 13.8 million or 22.8% of the total population.

The older population will increasingly be composed of individuals of diverse races and ethnicities, better socioeconomic conditions, higher levels of education, and lower levels of poverty. These factors can affect health status and use of health services. Older adults require more health care than younger adults and often more complex care. The healthcare system often fails to provide adequate care to these patients and it is necessary to develop strategies to meet these demands and ensure quality care.

With an increase in life expectancy and an aging population, an increasing number of older adults will develop surgical diseases, as well as chronic conditions. Older patients have increasing access to surgery. The peak incidence rate of surgery in the whole population is among 80–84 years old [1]. Nearly 40% of colorectal cancers are diagnosed after age 75, and most of them are operated [2]. Moreover,

G. Aprea (✉) · M. Capuano · G. Palomba
Department of Clinical Medicine and Surgery, University of Naples "Federico II", Naples, Italy
e-mail: aprea@unina.it

V. Boccardi, L. Marano (eds.), *The Frail Surgical Patient*, Practical Issues in Geriatrics, https://doi.org/10.1007/978-3-031-77707-3_3

Table 3.1 Percentage of population over the age of 60 to the total population over time

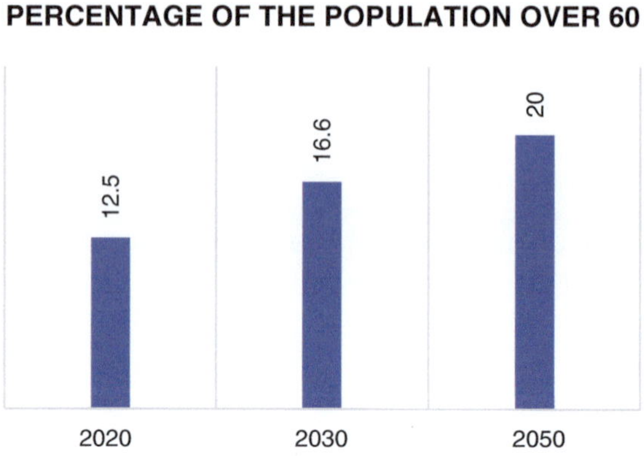

about 85% of the American population over 65 years of age have at least one chronic morbidity and 60% have at least two chronic conditions, such as cardiovascular diseases, cancers, chronic respiratory diseases, diabetes, degenerative joint disease, and visual impairment [3]. Reducing smoking could lead to a lower demand for healthcare while conversely increasing obesity rates could require more assistance.

Older adults have significantly higher rates of inpatient, outpatient surgical, and non-surgical procedures than other age groups. It is estimated that geriatric patients account for 47% of all hospital outpatient visits, one—third of all inpatient procedures, and greater than 40% of hospital stays. They need more ambulatory care, hospital services, nursing home services, and home healthcare services than younger people [1].

Soon, the aging population will lead to a significant increase (14–47%) in the demand for surgical services. It is necessary to strike the proper balance between surgeon productivity and the quality of care provided to respond to this increased workload. A multidisciplinary team with adequate preparation for the management of older patients is essential to simplify and improve the work of the surgeon and the entire team [4]. In addition, to increase the productivity of surgical activity, nonphysician clinicians, such as specialized nurses, could play an increasing role in supporting part of the workload.

The increase in surgical services needed to address the ever-increasing demand is not equally distributed among the various surgical specialties. Specialties that treat older and frail patients have greater increases in workloads. The projected growth in procedure-based work closely parallels the growth in the number of procedures performed by each specialty. Greater growth is expected in specialties that provide care for patients over age 65, such as ophthalmology or cardiothoracic surgery, than in other specialties that care for younger patients. Orthopedic, urological, and neurosurgical surgeries are also increasing. Otolaryngology is the only specialty that does not see an increase because only a small proportion of the surgeries (around 8%) involve older patients. Like other branches, even in general surgery, there is an increase in procedures performed on older and frail patients [4].

A 2004 study published in JAMA showed that general surgery rates in patients over the age of 65 were 3 times higher than those performed in patients between 15 and 44 years and 1.6 times higher than those performed in individuals between 45 and 64 years. This trend was observed in all types of surgery. Gastrointestinal tract surgery was 5 and 3.2 times greater in older patients than in the other two age groups. Hepatobiliary surgery was 3 and 1.3 times more frequent in older adults than in the two younger groups. Breast, soft tissue, and hernia surgery were also 4 and 1.5 times greater than in the other two populations, respectively [5]. Frail persons are the main patients of general surgery, and the number of older people is increasing much faster than the overall population. So, the general surgery workload will increase faster than population growth (Table 3.2).

An increasing number of cancer patients will need surgical care. The number of general surgeons needed in the next decade will be smaller than these needs. This situation will lead to an increase in the workload for each surgeon. A 2017 analysis estimated a 56% increase in cancers treated by general surgeons from 2010 to 2035. In the United States in 2010 the number of cancer patients treated by general surgeons was 23 patients per surgeon, assuming an equal distribution of cases among surgeons. It is estimated that this ratio will increase by 34% in 2035 with 31 potential patients per general surgeon. The United States would need nearly 35,000 general surgeons available to provide the necessary care to maintain the same distribution, an increase of nearly 10,000 over what is expected from current training numbers and population growth. In addition, the incidence of disease in different areas of the country and the uneven distribution of the number of surgeons practicing in different parts of the country must be considered [6]. However, the increase in the number of surgeons only partially solves the increase in operative work per surgeon. Moreover, as the population ages, the proportion of surgical procedures performed on an emergency/urgent basis is sure to increase, and it is important that the general surgical workforce is sufficient to meet the demands for elective services and still provide coverage for urgent conditions (Table 3.3).

Older adults present unique challenges in surgical management and decision-making. Advanced age, especially as biological aging is associated with increased surgical risk [7]. Several studies on large databases show that operative mortality of gastrointestinal surgery is higher in elderly patients despite adjustment for comorbidity conditions. The association of multiple comorbidities and the physiological vulnerability status that occurs with age puts older adults at high risk in terms of morbidity, mortality, and poor functional recovery after surgery. In addition, surgery in older patients can result in increased complications, prolonged hospital stays, increased access to the emergency room, readmission rates, post-discharge care requirements, and healthcare costs [8, 9]. Particularly, reduced life expectancy and physical function in frail and older patients are associated with a two-fold increased

Table 3.2 Increased rates of general surgery in people over 65 compared with other age groups

	Increased rates of surgery in age over 65 compared to	
Operative category	Age 15–44	Age 45–64
General surgery (total)	3x	1.6x
Gastrointestinal	5x	3.2x
Hepatobiliary	3x	1.3x
Brest/soft tissue	4x	1.2x
Hernia	4x	1.5x

Table 3.3 Increase in General Surgery Work for cancer patients

	2010	2035
Cancer patients surgical treated	511,450	798,070 (+56%)
Cancer patients treated per surgeon	23	31 (+34%)
General surgeons required	25,500	34,698 (+9198)

risk of postoperative complications. Postoperative delirium with cognitive impairment hampers functional recovery after surgery resulting in a three-fold increase in hospital stay or admissions to rehabilitation facilities [10].

The demand for healthcare services risks overloading the system if models are not implemented to increase and improve supply. Surgeons and all healthcare professionals must approach this population with specific skills and knowledge to provide optimal care. A competent healthcare workforce and effective models of care are needed. In 2008, in response to the crisis in providing health services to older patients, the American Institute of Medicine published a report in which the Committee on the Future Health Care Workforce for Older Americans established healthcare needs and workforce for patients over the age of 65. The goals of this commission were to improve the competence of the entire health workforce in working with geriatric patients, increase geriatric specialists, and improve methods of delivering health care. The Board of Surgery with the support of the American Geriatrics Society, focused on the skills needed in all surgical specialties. Geriatric patient care has been incorporated into the training of future surgeons and other healthcare professionals. All healthcare professionals must be adequately trained to provide appropriate care and improve the entire workforce. Healthcare provided to older patients needs to be timely, efficient, safe, effective, and patient-centered. The era of "geriatric surgery" is increasingly relevant. Therefore, in addition to specific training toward the elderly patient, there should be the figure of "geriatric surgeon." This purpose requires a specific organization of training, using part of general surgeons for geriatric surgery. However, given the increasing number of older patients and the shortage of surgeons, it is essential that all surgeons have the knowledge to deal with the specific challenges of these patients [11].

In addition, much of the daily care is performed by informal caregivers, relatives, and others, who often have very little training. Even these important figures would need adequate education on the part of health workers (Box 3.1).

Box 3.1 Aims of Healthcare Workforce to Address Healthcare Needs of Geriatric Patients

- Improve the competence of the entire healthcare workforce.
- Increase geriatrics specialists.
- Improve healthcare delivery methods.
- Incorporate geriatric content into the training examinations of future specialists and all other healthcare professionals.
- Recognize the figure of the geriatric surgeon.
- Education of informal caregivers.

A comprehensive understanding of the unique vulnerabilities of older adults' geriatric syndromes and risk factors is required to accurately estimate surgical risk, inform surgical decision-making, and guide perioperative management [12]. Physiologic changes, multicomorbidities, polypharmacy, and psychosocial problems unique to the older and frail patients require skills beyond those of the surgeon so a multidisciplinary approach is needed. Perioperative management of the those patient begins with the choice of surgical treatment and continues until postoperative recovery. This approach should be managed not only by the surgeon and anesthesiologist but also by doctors of other specialties working with the patient and family members.

The management of the frail patient begins with the preoperative work-up that must adapt to their specific needs. Surgical indications in the frail patient are not always clear (Fig. 3.1). The surgical decision should be adapted to the clinical condition, the patient's specific operational risk, achievable outcomes, and life expectancy. Decision-making must be properly aligned between surgeon and patient, so the patient and his or her family must be clearly informed about operative risks, effects of potential complications on quality of life, and expected outcomes of the surgery. Conversely, the patient's personal goals of care must be incorporated into any assessment and treatment decisions. Often elderly patients are more concerned

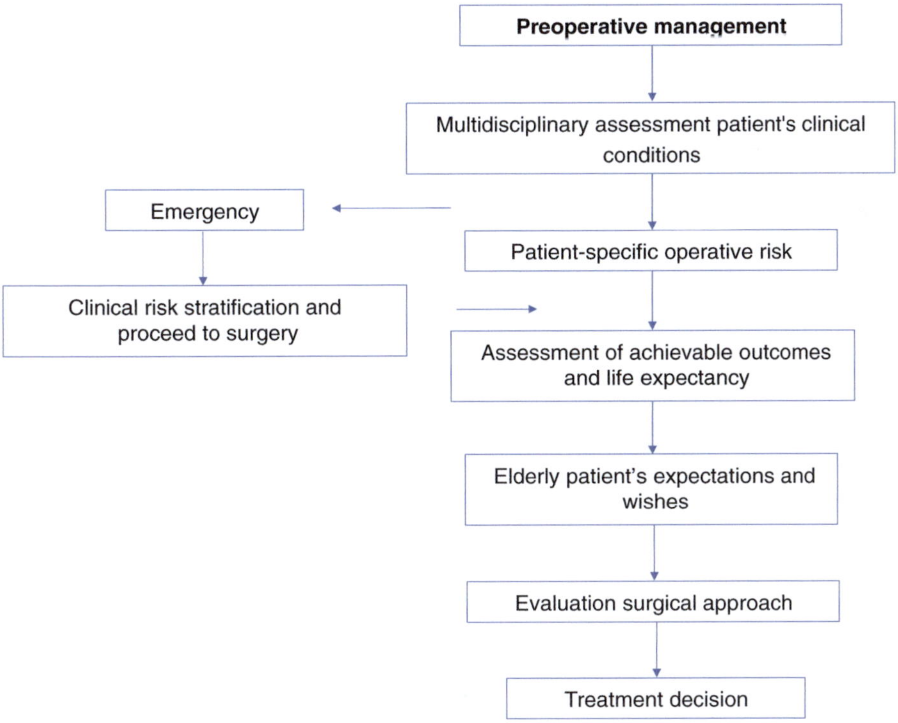

Fig. 3.1 Preoperative management flowchart

about the risk of functional impairment that can drastically affect quality of life and would require ongoing care in rehabilitation centers or nursing homes, than about the risk of mortality. Sometimes it may also be necessary to modify the surgical approach to ensure better functional outcomes, and the geriatric surgeon must be able to meet these challenges.

Surgery in older adults requires careful consideration and a co-management program is necessary to deliver comprehensive geriatric care with individualized care plan including co-morbidity management, reduction of delirium, nutritional assessment, physiotherapy support, and postoperative follow-up. Surgeons need to know when more surgery is needed in older patients, especially in emergency conditions or cancer patients with a reduced life expectancy. Surgical treatment in these patients should improve life expectancy by achieving safe treatment without compromising functional status or quality of life. Frail patients often have common problems in response to surgical stress and perioperative management needs to be standardized to deal with them better (Fig. 3.2).

The enhanced recovery after surgery (ERAS) protocol is effective in reducing surgical patient morbidity and hospital stay but should be complemented by a geriatric care protocol [12]. The main component of the comprehensive geriatric care model is the comprehensive geriatric assessment (CGA) [13]. The CGA is an established system that evaluates the physiological, social, psychological, and functional status of frail patients. It consists in a multidisciplinary team that includes surgeons, anesthesiologists, geriatricians, as well as cardiologists, geriatric nurses, dietitians, and physical therapists. It is still unclear whether there are significant improvements in decreasing adverse outcomes, length of stay, prevalence of delirium, rate of 30-day admission, and mortality, possibly geriatric care models result in better outcomes than standard care to elderly patients [14].

A holistic approach to perioperative care should be ensured that assesses both specific surgical care, cognitive and emotional well-being, good communication,

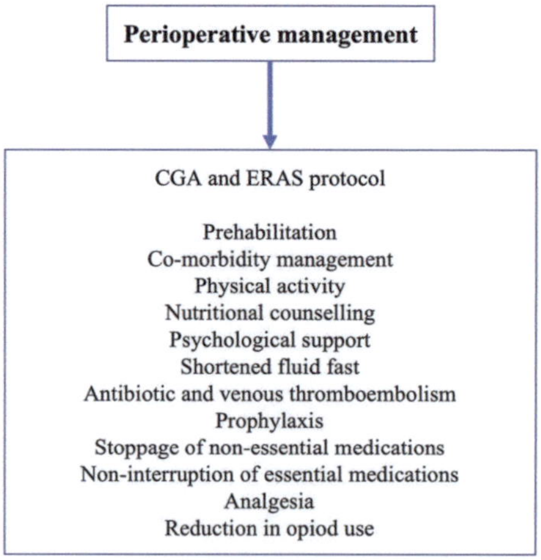

Fig. 3.2 Perioperative management flowchart

and shared decision-making, ensuring fewer outpatient checks and a smoother transition between primary care and hospital services. Specific organizations were created for this purpose. The Centre for Perioperative Care (CPOC) is an inter-organizational entity established in the United Kingdom to bring together the entire workforce involved in perioperative management. It has developed guidelines, programs, and training for the multispecialty approach of elderly patients [15]. The CPOC and the British Geriatrics Society (BGS) published in 2021 the first guideline on perioperative care for frail individuals undergoing elective and emergency surgery [16]. Although frailty is not an age-based concept, frequently the older adults are considered frail, characterized by a higher vulnerability to external factors and increased risk of functional decline, institutionalization, and death. CPOC/BGS guidelines support the dissemination of perioperative services based on CGA.

Moreover, in parallel with the development of holistic perioperative services based on CGA, prehabilitation in perioperative care has also been studied. Prehabilitation is a patient-tailored intervention designed to improve an individual's resilience prior to elective surgery. The process of optimal management of the older surgical patient must begin with prehabilitation, for improvement of functional capacity prior to planned surgery, aimed at improving the patient's tolerance to physiological stress. Despite evidence that nutritional support and physical exercise reduce frailty and functional dependence, there is not yet evidence that prehabilitation programs improve postoperative outcomes for frail persons [17]. However, prehabilitation has demonstrated results in cardiovascular surgery by improving cardiovascular status, respiratory function and postoperative outcomes, and most recent findings underscore its usefulness also in abdominal surgery, combining moderate physical activity, nutritional counseling with protein supplementation, and psychological support to increase patient compliance [18].

The American College of Surgeons National Surgical Quality Improvement Program (ACS NSQIP/AGS) in a 2014 geriatric surgery pilot project evaluated several outcomes. These results have made it possible to develop a Geriatric Risk calculator. This calculator is a great tool for predicting surgical risk in terms of complications such as pneumonia, surgical site infections, and cognitive and functional decline. Given the importance of surgery for older adults and the need for standardization, the ACS with The John A. Hartford Foundation created the Coalition for Quality in Geriatric Surgery. The aim of this group was to improve outcomes for surgical care through multidisciplinary and patient-centered care and with practical guidelines for perioperative management. They emphasize the importance of shortened fluid fast, antibiotic and venous thromboembolism prophylaxis, stoppage of nonessential medications and conversely non-interruption of essential ones, analgesia, to reduce opioid use and to prevent functional and cognitive decline. These patients are very susceptible to the adverse effects of many drugs used during hospitalization (for example, analgesics, antiemetics, and anxiolytics). Opioids should be avoided because they are associated with cognitive impairment, delirium, and constipation. The ACS Geriatric Surgery Verification Program in addition to opioid-sparing techniques, has indicated other rules for the management of postoperative pain such as avoiding Beer's list of drugs and titrating medication.

Postoperative management of frail patients also requires multispecialty care and assessment of risks of delirium, functional deterioration, and medical and surgical complications (Fig. 3.3). This organization determines the most appropriate place for postoperative care and the possible need for a period of intensive or sub-intensive care. Those who do not need or refuse this treatment should be placed in appropriate care units. Functional recovery should be promoted by reducing postoperative pain, and its management should consider the relationship between frailty, pain, analgesics, dementia, and delirium [19]. Healthcare professionals should anticipate, prevent, identify, and manage medical complications early, which are more common in frail patients. In addition, the patient's hydration and nutrition devices, anti-decubitus beds, and supports for getting out of bed and walking should also be included in the care. Nursing care plays a very important role in the care of frail patient through mobilization, fall prevention, nutrition, continence, and surgical wound dressing.

Postoperative care hospital readmission rate is higher in older patients than in young patients regardless of the type of surgery. Unfortunately, in 25–30% of cases, rehospitalization takes place in a different hospital resulting in negative outcomes.

Discharge communications should take place in a clear, bidirectional, and precise manner with the patient, family members, caregivers, and with the postoperative care or rehabilitation facility. This information could solve many common problems.

Palliative care requires expertise from the surgeon and health care personnel. The surgeon both as a leader and as a member of an interdisciplinary team must be able to scale the objectives from curative to palliative by communicating effectively and compassionately with patients and their families. From the beginning of the perioperative period, it is necessary to discuss the expectations in terms of length stay, nursing, postoperative rehabilitation, and functional results. In addition, family involvement, physical therapy assessment, and home adequacy should be

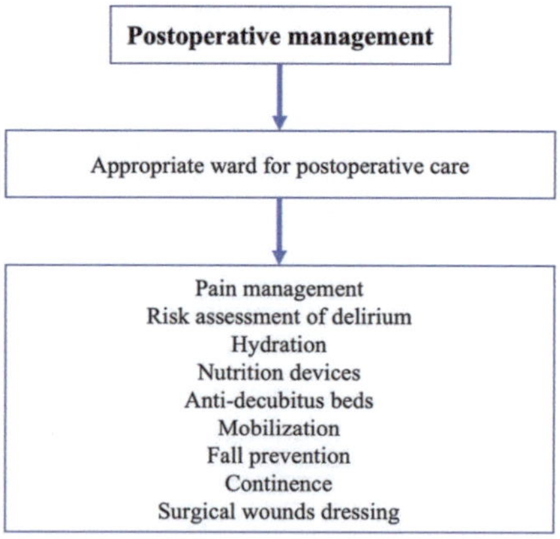

Fig. 3.3 Postoperative management flowchart

considered in discharge planning. There are several studies that have shown how advanced discharge planning and tighter nursing follow-up can improve outcomes, treat complications early, and reduce the readmission rate. Many older and frail people at the end of life express a desire to die at home, although invasive procedures or ICU admissions are common at this phase. Palliative care aims to relieve pain and suffering maintaining the highest quality of life [20].

In conclusion, geriatric surgery is becoming an essential part of the surgical activity. It is necessary that general surgery becomes increasingly interesting and attractive for new medical doctors, in order to increase the workforce over the years. Geriatric patient management should be integrated into the training of all healthcare professionals and should include a multidisciplinary team. Specific guidelines should be applied for these patients that aid the best perioperative decisions.

References

1. Omling E, Jarnheimer A, Rose J, Björk J, Meara JG, Hagander L. Population-based incidence rate of inpatient and outpatient surgical procedures in a high-income country. Br J Surg. 2018;105(1):86–95. https://doi.org/10.1002/bjs.10643. Epub 2017 Nov 13. PMID: 29131303; PMCID: PMC5765448.
2. Cheema FN, Abraham NS, Berger DH, Albo D, Taffet GE, Naik AD. Novel approaches to perioperative assessment and intervention may improve long-term outcomes after colorectal cancer resection in older adults. Ann Surg. 2011;253(5):867–74. https://doi.org/10.1097/SLA.0b013e318208faf0. PMID: 21183846.
3. Fong JH. Disability incidence and functional decline among older adults with major chronic diseases. BMC Geriatr. 2019;19(1):323. https://doi.org/10.1186/s12877-019-1348-z. PMID: 31752701; PMCID: PMC6873710.
4. Etzioni DA, Liu JH, Maggard MA, Ko CY. The aging population and its impact on the surgery workforce. Ann Surg. 2003;238(2):170–7. https://doi.org/10.1097/01.SLA.0000081085.98792.3d. PMID: 12894008; PMCID: PMC1422682.
5. Liu JH, Etzioni DA, O'Connell JB, Maggard MA, Ko CY. The increasing workload of general surgery. Arch Surg. 2004;139(4):423–8. https://doi.org/10.1001/archsurg.139.4.423.
6. Ellison CE, et al. The impact of the aging population and incidence of cancer on future projections of general surgical workforce needs. Surgery. 2017;163:553–8.
7. McVeigh TP, Al-Azawi D, O'Donoghue GT, Kerin MJ. Assessing the impact of an ageing population on complication rates and in-patient length of stay. Int J Surg. 2013;11(9):872–5. https://doi.org/10.1016/j.ijsu.2013.07.016. Epub 2013 Aug 2. PMID: 23917211.
8. Merani S, Payne J, Padwal RS, Hudson D, Widder SL, Khadaroo RG. Predictors of in-hospital mortality and complications in very elderly patients undergoing emergency surgery. World J Emerg Surg. 2014;9:43. https://doi.org/10.1186/1749-7922-9-43. PMID: 25050133; PMCID: PMC4105124.
9. Mistry PK, Gaunay GS, Hoenig DM. Prediction of surgical complications in the elderly: Can we improve outcomes? Asian J Urol. 2017;4(1):44–9. https://doi.org/10.1016/j.ajur.2016.07.001. Epub 2016 Aug 18. PMID: 29264206; PMCID: PMC5730906.
10. Rinaldi P, Mecocci P, Benedetti C, Ercolani S, Bregnocchi M, Menculini G, Catani M, Senin U, Cherubini A. Validation of the five-item geriatric depression scale in elderly subjects in three different settings. J Am Geriatr Soc. 2003;51(5):694–8. https://doi.org/10.1034/j.1600-0579.2003.00216.x. PMID: 12752847.
11. Chia CL, Tan KY. The era of geriatric surgery. Ann Acad Med Singap. 2019;48(11):345–6. PMID: 31960013.

12. Greco M, Capretti G, Beretta L, Gemma M, Pecorelli N, Braga M. Enhanced recovery program in colorectal surgery: a meta-analysis of randomized controlled trials. World J Surg. 2014;38(6):1531–41. https://doi.org/10.1007/s00268-013-2416-8. PMID: 24368573.
13. Partridge JS, Harari D, Martin FC, Peacock JL, Bell R, Mohammed A, Dhesi JK. Randomized clinical trial of comprehensive geriatric assessment and optimization in vascular surgery. Br J Surg. 2017;104(6):679–87. https://doi.org/10.1002/bjs.10459. Epub 2017 Feb 15. PMID: 28198997.
14. Saripella A, Wasef S, Nagappa M, Riazi S, Englesakis M, Wong J, Chung F. Effects of comprehensive geriatric care models on postoperative outcomes in geriatric surgical patients: a systematic review and meta-analysis. BMC Anesthesiol. 2021;21(1):127. https://doi.org/10.1186/s12871-021-01337-2. PMID: 33888071; PMCID: PMC8061210.
15. Centre for Perioperative Care [Internet]. CPOC. [cited 21 June 2022]. Available from: https://cpoc.org.uk.
16. Partridge JSL, Ryan J, Dhesi JK. CPOC-BGS perioperative frailty guideline group. New guidelines for the perioperative care of people living with frailty undergoing elective and emergency surgery-a commentary. Age Ageing. 2022;51(11):afac237. https://doi.org/10.1093/ageing/afac237. PMID: 36436009.
17. Han CY, Miller M, Yaxley A, Baldwin C, Woodman R, Sharma Y. Effectiveness of combined exercise and nutrition interventions in prefrail or frail older hospitalised patients: a systematic review and meta-analysis. BMJ Open. 2020;10(12):e040146. https://doi.org/10.1136/bmjopen-2020-040146. PMID: 33318114; PMCID: PMC7737105.
18. Kow AW. Prehabilitation and its role in geriatric surgery. Ann Acad Med Singap. 2019;48(11):386–92. PMID: 31960020.
19. Justins DM. The Faculty of Pain Medicine of the Royal College of Anaesthetists. Br J Anaesth. 2008;101(1):4–7. https://doi.org/10.1093/bja/aen104. PMID: 18556696.
20. Ballou JH, Brasel KJ. Palliative care and geriatric surgery. Clin Geriatr Med. 2019;35(1):35–44. https://doi.org/10.1016/j.cger.2018.08.004. Epub 2018 Sep 28. PMID: 30390982.

Aging Trajectories and Phenotypes

4

Liliana Mazza

4.1 Introduction

Aging is a physiological process that starts when growth has been completed and ends with death. It is defined by relatively predictable changes, appearing progressively over time, whose impact on biological processes and systems causes relevant modifications. These may appear in different moments of life and in a heterogeneous way, finally causing the deterioration of organic systems.

The process of aging has always been of interest to the humankind. Ancient Greeks considered aging as an incurable disease, defined by specific symptoms: dry skin, whitening of hair, joint pain and weakness in the legs, vision problems, depression, and a death wish. In Ancient Rome a similar definition of aging can be found by Terenzio ("Ipsa senectus morbus," aging is itself a disease), whereas other authors proposed a different approach to older life: for instance, Seneca considered old age as positive and essential for those around the older adults. Similarly, Cicero in his "De Senectute" described the measures necessary to maintain one's health (such as exercising, eating, and drinking adequately), strengthening that old age is worthy of honor [16].

Nowadays, the massive presence of older people in society requires a reflection on aging. Medical technologies, timeliness of treatments, and global improvement in healthcare services have contributed to longevity. From another perspective, older patients are becoming increasingly complex and vulnerable [15]. The challenge for clinicians is to understand and value the characteristics of older patients, adapting treatments and care to each individual in a patient-tailored sense. In this sense, geriatricians play a key role in the evaluation and management of both "fit" and "frail" older patients.

L. Mazza (✉)
Unit of Geriatrics, Maggiore Hospital, Department of Integration, Azienda USL di Bologna, Bologna, Italy

V. Boccardi, L. Marano (eds.), *The Frail Surgical Patient*, Practical Issues in Geriatrics, https://doi.org/10.1007/978-3-031-77707-3_4

The aim of this chapter is to provide a narrative literature review concerning various aspects of aging. In particular, aging will be discussed from different points of view. Firstly, a brief description of the most relevant biological theories of aging will be furnished. Then, the concept of aging trajectories will be proposed, according to the literature. Finally, different phenotypes of older age will be described.

4.2 Biological Theories of Aging

Many biological theories of aging have been proposed in the literature through the past decades, and can be formally divided into two groups [13]:

1. Programmed theories
2. Damage or error theories

4.2.1 Programmed Aging Theories

In this field, aging is considered a scheduled process. Three different categories can be distinguished:

(a) *Programmed longevity*: Aging is related to genetic instability, as senescence appears when certain specific age-related genes are regulated (switched on or switched off, based on their activity). A more stable genome is implicated in longevity [8].
(b) *Endocrine theory*: Hormones play a relevant role in controlling the aging pace. Studies have been conducted especially on Insulin/Insulin-line growth factor (IGF) signaling (IIS), whose downregulation appears to be associated with human longevity [25].
(c) *Immunological theory*: The immune system seems to be implicated in aging in two different ways. On one hand, its programmed decline over time is responsible for increased vulnerability to infections, which can lead to disability and death [7]. On the other hand, the dysregulation of immune response is related to some diseases typically seen in older age, such as cancer, cardiovascular disease, and Alzheimer's disease [22].

4.2.2 Damage or Error Theories

In this context, aging is perceived as the sum of multiple and subsequent genetic and biological errors. Multiple theories can be enumerated in this category:

(a) *Wear and tear theory*: Vital components of cells and tissues wear out over time, causing aging.

(b) *Rate of living theory*: The life span of an organism is inversely proportional to its oxygen basal metabolism [19].
(c) *Cross-linking theory*: Aging is due to the slowdown of body processes consequent to the accumulation of cross-linked proteins, which damages cells and tissues [2].
(d) *Free radicals theory*: Cells and organs stop functioning because of free radicals damage, which affects macromolecules such as proteins, sugars, lipids, and nucleic acids. Intrinsic antioxidant enzymes are able to limit free radicals' impact, otherwise life expectancy would be naturally shorter [12]. An extension to this theory is based on the antioxidative action caused by calorie restriction, which apparently contributes to the reduction of oxidative stress, especially implicated in vascular diseases related to aging [1].
(e) *Somatic DNA damage theory*: DNA damages, which occur constantly during cell replication, are generally repaired by specific proteins. Aging is associated with the accumulation of genetic errors and mutations, which happen so quickly that they cannot be corrected, causing cell deterioration and malfunction [11].

4.2.3 The Role of Telomeres

Telomeres are nucleoprotein structures located at the end of chromosomes. Their role is to protect chromosomes from inadequate DNA repair activities secondary to cell replication. This task is performed by their progressive erosion with every cell replication. As long as they reach a critical or dysfunctional length, cell replication is blocked, leading to senescence. For this peculiar behavior, telomeres are also considered as "biological clocks," as they actually limit the number of cell replications [9].

A recent study identified that telomeres shortening is not only due to the so-called and aforementioned "end replication problem," but can also be reconducted to multiple factors, including telomeric replication stress and incomplete telomere replication [3]. Telomeres shortening and cell senescence appear strictly related to age and lifestyle factors that increase inflammation and oxidative stress.

4.3 Aging as a Complex Process

Multiple changes in biological processes are observed with advanced age. Every organ and apparatus is implicated in aging with its own peculiarity, in a way that is not necessarily uniform or homogeneous. Altogether, in the context of aging a loss of complexity is observed, resulting in the reduced variability of vital parameters (heart rate, blood pressure, etc.) and in the poor adaptive response to stress [14]. What is more, aging can affect different individuals in different ways, being influenced not only by genetic factors but also by lifestyle choices and environmental exposures. Considering that aging appears a multifaceted process and not all aging is the same. Starting from these reflections, different trajectories of aging have been described in the literature in the last decades.

4.3.1 Aging Trajectories

Up to the early 1980s, aging had been considered a progressive process in which changes could be attributed either to age itself or to specific diseases. In the first case, aging was considered "normal" and the progressive deterioration of physiological functions was only ascribed to the passing years. In the second case, aging was defined as "pathological": the impact of one or more illnesses on organs or systems was responsible for aging.

According to this perspective, the older population could be distinguished into two categories: "diseased" and "normal." However, this concept had serious and non-negligible limitations. First, the emphasis on normality could mislead to the consideration that those "normal" older people were in a riskless condition. Moreover, it could lead to the easy assumption that "normal" is equal to natural, not necessary nor worthy to be changed, supporting the ageism stereotype that older adults are undeserving of treatment or care [4].

Starting from these considerations, a different vision of aging was proposed. Rowe and Kahn [20] distinguished the abovementioned concept of "normal" aging into two different trajectories: (1) "usual" aging and (2) "successful" aging. On one hand, in "usual" aging extrinsic factors heighten the effects of aging alone. On the other hand, "successful" aging is characterized by a neutral or positive impact of extrinsic factors on aging.

This brand-new point of view added a special focus not only on the heterogeneity of aging within age groups but above all encouraged a positive and propositive approach to aging, enlightening the role of explanatory variables for different trajectories. In fact, a transition from usual to successful aging can be optimized by managing extrinsic factors. In this sense, the role of living habits, social behaviors, and external factors' exposure has been validated as relevant elements for the definition of aging pathways.

Ten years later, Rowe and Kahn [21] expanded the concept of success in aging by considering three elements for its fulfillment: low probability of disease, good physical and mental functioning, and active engagement with life. This further clarification is particularly relevant as it highlights the role of aging on the global health of an individual, considering functional, cognitive, and social aspects of life. Figure 4.1 summarizes the three different trajectories of aging described above.

4.3.2 Homeostenosis

Aging is a multifaceted process and multiple factors can be involved in its variability and heterogeneity among individuals. Nevertheless, all aging trajectories share a relevant physiological component. Whatever the trajectory of aging, physiologic

Pathological aging	A progressive process determined by the impact of one or more diseases on specific physiological functions
Usual aging	The physiological process of aging heightened by extrinsic factors
Successful aging	The physiological process of aging with a neutral or positive impact of extrinsic factors

Fig. 4.1 Three different "trajectories" of aging

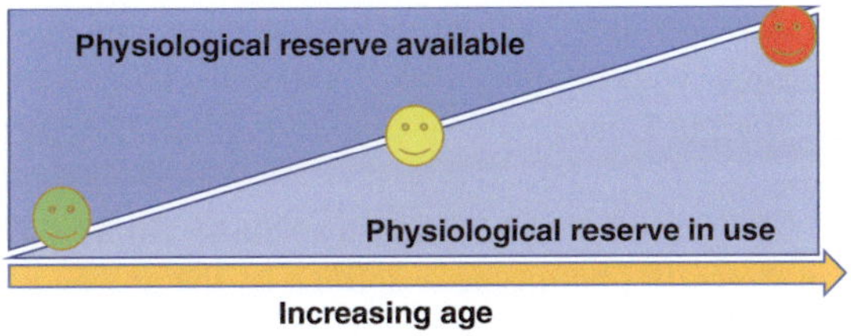

Fig. 4.2 Homeostenosis

reserves tend to reduce over time, so that the ability to face challenges (e.g., infections, trauma) fades. This concept is known as "homeostenosis": in other words, the ability of an older person to react to happenings in life and, consequentially, to maintain homeostasis narrows [24].

In Fig. 4.2 homeostenosis is represented graphically. According to the increasing age, the physiological reserve available to react to stressors becomes thinner. At the same time, physiological reserve in use is higher even for minimal insults. At the endpoint, the capability to deal with insults is totally ineffective, and adverse outcomes are frequently consequent even to minor stress, and can be interpreted as frailty. That is, physiological reserve reduces over time, and the vulnerability to stress increases.

4.4 A Modern Approach to Aging

The different combinations of aging patterns lead to different profiles of older individuals, according to physiological and pathological status. In this context, different phenotypes of aging have been described in the literature in the last decades. One big distinction can be made between "fit," those healthy-aged patients, and "frail," whose definition needs to be explored in detail.

4.4.1 Frailty: One Syndrome, Multiple Phenotypes

Frailty is an aging-related syndrome, highly prevalent in the geriatric population (a.k.a. *geriatric syndrome*), characterized by marked vulnerability to stressors such as acute illnesses, surgical interventions, or trauma. This vulnerability is due to the decrease in physiological reserves (see above) and it is responsible for adverse outcomes such as procedural complications, falls, institutionalization, disability, and death [6].

Frailty has been variously described in the literature. Two relevant and shared definitions are those by Fried et al. [10] and Rockwood et al. [17, 18].

Fried et al. identified five core symptoms of frailty, described as follows:

1. **F**atigue, as indicated by self-report of exhaustion.
2. Low **R**esistance or weakness, as defined by low grip strength.
3. Low physical **A**ctivity, considered as low kcal spent per week.
4. Slow walk**i**ng pace (>6–7 s to walk 15 ft).
5. Weight **L**oss (≥5% of body weight in last year).

The presence of ≥3 criteria accounts for a *Frail* phenotype, while an *Intermediate* (or *Prefrail)* phenotype is defined by the presence of 1 or 2 of the enlisted symptoms.

In their work, Fried et al. [10] demonstrated that frailty is an independent predictor of risk of adverse outcomes such as falls, hospitalizations, disability, and death. Interestingly, even the prefrail phenotype is at intermediate risk for these outcomes, as well as at risk of subsequent frailty.

From a different perspective, Rockwood et al. [17] considered multiple aspects for the definition of frailty in their "Frailty Index." They defined a list of 70 illnesses, deficits, or pathological conditions, whose combination is supposed to be related to frailty (Fig. 4.3). They demonstrated the strong predictive validity of summing the number of deficits or impairments to individuate frailty in older patients.

Because of the large number of conditions taken into account, this approach appeared time-consuming and not easily applicable in clinical practice. As a consequence, Rockwood et al. [18] continued their work defining the "Clinical Frailty Scale" (CFS), an instrument for the identification of frailty based on clinical judgement. It distinguishes nine categories of patients, mixing items such as comorbidity, cognitive impairment, and disability (Fig. 4.4).

The first three phenotypes are three different steps of healthy aged (Very Fit, Well, and Managing Well), characterized by an active life and few symptoms. In the middle, mild and moderate aspects of frailty are introduced (Vulnerable, Mildly Frail, and Moderately Frail). The last three points of the scale are dedicated to older patients with high-care necessities and risk of dying (Severely Frail, Very Severely Frail, and Terminally Ill) (Fig. 4.5).

Since its introduction, CFS has been widely adopted in different contexts and in a variety of settings all around the world. It represents a useful tool for clinicians to provide more informed and rational shared decision-making [5].

4.5 The Role of the Geriatrician

Considering its many facets, aging appears to be a process full of unknowns and variables that can be only partially predictable and identifiable. Whereas genetic factors and biological pathways are undoubtedly implicated in aging, the role of

70-item CSHA Frailty Index		
Changes in everyday activities	Mood problems	Seizures, partial complex
Head and neck problems	Feeling sad, blue, depressed	Seizures, generalized
Poor muscle tone in neck	History of depressed mood	Syncope or blackouts
Bradykinesia, facial	Tiredness all the time	Headache
Problems getting dressed	Depression (clinical impression)	Cerebrovascular problems
Problems with bathing	Sleep changes	History of stroke
Problems carrying out personal grooming	Restlessness	History of diabetes mellitus
Urinary incontinence	Memory changes	Arterial hypertension
Toileting problems	Short-term memory impairment	Peripheral pulses
Bulk difficulties	Long-term memory impairment	Cardiac problems
Rectal problems	Changes in general mental functioning	Myocardial infarction
Gastrointestinal problems	Onset of cognitive symptoms	Arrhythmia
Problems cooking	Clouding or delirium	Congestive heart failure
Sucking problems	Paranoid features	Lung problems
Problems going out alone	History relevant to cognitive impairment or loss	Respiratory problems
Impaired mobility	Family history relevant to cognitive impairment or loss	History of thyroid disease
Muscoloskeletal problems	Impaired vibration	Skin problems
Bradykinesia of the limbs	Tremor at rest	Malignant disease
Poor muscle tone in limbs	Postural tremor	Breast problems
Poor limb coordination	Intention tremor	Abdominal problems
Poor coordination, trunk	History of Parkinson's disease	Presence of snout reflex
Poor standing posture	Family history of degenerative disease	Presence of palmomental reflex
Irregular gait pattern	Falls	Other medical history

Fig. 4.3 Seventy-item CSHA Frailty Index proposed by Rockwood et al. [17]

lifestyle choices, environmental exposures, and other extrinsic factors is not negligible and must be considered.

In a preventive logic, focusing on risk factors (such as smoking, alcoholic habit, and sedentary life) during youth and middle life is a valuable strategy in order to favor healthy and successful aging. Nonetheless, patients whose aging trajectory is deficient need even more attention and dedicated support. These patients are often complex, vulnerable, and frail, needing a multidimensional approach with the aim of identifying all the needs to be answered. For these patients, the geriatricians play a key role and the Comprehensive Geriatric Assessment represents the most appropriate tool for the definition of objectives and targets [23]. The cooperation of geriatricians with other medical specialists is fundamental for the classification of the patient and the evaluation of the most appropriate treatment path.

1. Very Fit - People who are robust, active, energetic and motivated. These people commonly exercise regularly. They are among the fittest for their age.	**4. Vulnerable** - While not dependent on others for daily help, often symptoms limit activities. A common complaint is being "slowed up", and/or being tired during the day.	**7. Severely Frail** - Completely dependent for personal care, from whatever cause (physical or cognitive). Even so, they seem stable and not at high risk of dying (within 6 months).
2. Well - People who have no active disease symptoms but are less fit than cat.1. Often, they exercise or are very active occasionally, e.g. seasonally.	**5. Mildly Frail** - These people often have more evident slowing, and need help in high order IADLs (finances, transportation, heavy housework, medications). Typically, mild frailty progressively impairs shopping and walking outside alone, meal preparation and housework.	**8. Very Severely Frail** - Completely dependent, approaching the end of life. Typycally, they could not recover even from a minor illness.
3. Managing Well - People whose medical problems are well controlled, but are not regularly active beyond routine walking.	**6. Moderately Frail** - People need help with all outside activities and with keeping house. Inside, they often have problems with stairs and need help with bathing and might need minimal assitance (cuing, standy) with dressing.	**9. Terminally Ill** - Approaching the end of life. This category applies to people with a life expectancy <6 months, who are not otherwise evidently frail.

Fig. 4.4 Clinical Frailty Scale (CFS) according to Rockwood et al. [18]

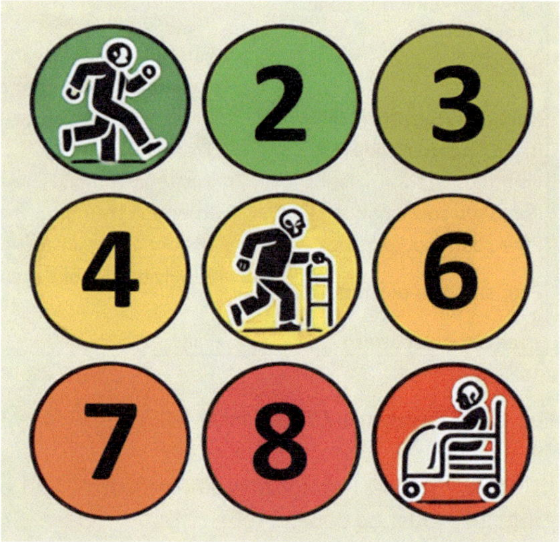

Fig. 4.5 A graphical representation of CFS phenotypes

4.6 Conclusions

In this chapter aging was defined starting from its biological processes and theories, through its different trajectories, and finally describing different phenotypes of older people. The role of clinicians should be on the one hand to support in identifying and preventing risk factors in order to favor healthy aging. On the other hand, understanding and interpreting health conditions in those vulnerable and frail older patients is fundamental in order to favor patient-tailored treatments, with respect to the universality of treatments.

References

1. Afanas'ev I. Signaling and damaging functions of free radicals in aging-free radical theory, hormesis, and TOR. Aging Dis. 2010;1(2):75–88. Epub 2010 Jul 12. PMID: 22396858; PMCID: PMC3295029.
2. Bjorksten J. The crosslinkage theory of aging. J Am Geriatr Soc. 1968;16(4):408–27. https://doi.org/10.1111/j.1532-5415.1968.tb02821.x.
3. Boccardi V, Cari L, Nocentini G, Riccardi C, et al. Telomeres increasingly develop aberrant structures in aging humans. J Gerontol A. 2020;75(2):230–5.
4. Bülow MH, Söderqvist T. Successful ageing: A historical overview and critical analysis of a successful concept. J Aging Stud. 2014;31:139–49.
5. Church S, Rogers E, Rockwood K, Theou O. A scoping review of the clinical frailty scale. BMC Geriatr. 2020;20(1):1–18.
6. Clegg A, Young J, Iliffe S, Rikkert MO, Rockwood K. Frailty in elderly people. Lancet. 2013;381(9868):752–62.
7. Cornelius E. Increased incidence of lymphomas in thymectomized mice—evidence for an immunological theory of aging. Experientia. 1972;28(4):459. https://doi.org/10.1007/BF02008340.
8. Davidovic M, Sevo G, Svorcan P, Milosevic DP, Despotovic N, Erceg P. Old age as a privilege of the "selfish ones". Aging Dis. 2010;1(2):139–46. Epub 2010 Jul 30. PMID: 22396861; PMCID: PMC3295027.
9. Fagagna F, Reaper PM, Clay-Farrace L, et al. A DNA damage checkpoint response in telomere-initiated senescence. Nature. 2003;426(6963):194–8.
10. Fried LP, Tangen CM, Walston J, et al. Frailty in older adults: evidence for a phenotype. J Gerontol A Biol Sci Med Sci. 2001;56(3):M146–57.
11. Gensler HL, Bernstein H. DNA damage as the primary cause of aging. Quarter Rev Biol. 1981;56(3):279–303.
12. Harman D. Aging: a theory based on free radical and radiation chemistry. J Gerontol. 1956;11(3):298–300. https://doi.org/10.1093/geronj/11.3.298.
13. Jin K. Modern biological theories of aging. Aging Dis. 2010;1(2):72–4. PMID: 21132086; PMCID: PMC2995895.
14. Lipsitz LA, Goldberger AL. Loss of 'complexity'and aging: potential applications of fractals and chaos theory to senescence. JAMA. 1992;267(13):1806–9.
15. Mazza L, Ievoli R. Sustainability and Well-being in Geriatrics: proposing a performance-based approach for the implementation of geriatric care activities. Geriatric Care. 2021;7(2) https://doi.org/10.4081/gc.2021.9764.
16. Memini F. Ipsa senectus morbus? La vecchiaia nella letteratura greco-latina; 2019. https://www.agingproject.uniupo.it/ipsa-senectus-morbus-la-vecchiaia-nella-letteratura-greco-latina/.
17. Rockwood K, Mitnitski AB, MacKnight C. Some mathematical models of frailty and their clinical implications. Rev Clin Gerontol. 2002;12(2):109–17.
18. Rockwood K, Song X, MacKnight C, Bergman H, et al. A global clinical measure of fitness and frailty in elderly people. CMAJ. 2005;173(5):489–95.
19. Rollo CD. Aging and the Mammalian regulatory triumvirate. Aging Dis. 2010;1(2):105–38. Epub 2010 Sep 10. PMID: 22396860; PMCID: PMC3295031.
20. Rowe JW, Kahn RL. Human aging: usual and successful. Science. 1987;237(4811):143–9.
21. Rowe JW, Kahn RL. Successful aging. Gerontologist. 1997;37(4):433–40.
22. Rozemuller AJ, van Gool WA, Eikelenboom P. The neuroinflammatory response in plaques and amyloid angiopathy in Alzheimer's disease: therapeutic implications. Curr Drug Targets CNS Neurol Disord. 2005;4(3):223–33. https://doi.org/10.2174/1568007054038229. PMID: 15975026.
23. Stuck AE, Siu AL, Wieland GD, et al. Comprehensive geriatric assessment: a meta-analysis of controlled trials. The Lancet. 1993;342(8878):1032–6.

24. Taffett GE. Physiology of aging. In: Geriatric medicine: an evidence-based approach. New York: Springer; 2003. p. 27–35.
25. van Heemst D. Insulin, IGF-1 and longevity. Aging Dis. 2010;1(2):147–57. Epub 2010 Aug 26. PMID: 22396862; PMCID: PMC3295030.

Understanding Aging, Frailty, and Resilience

5

Carmelinda Ruggiero

5.1 Unveiling the Role of Frailty in Surgical Care for Older Adults

With the extension of life expectancy and remarkable medical advancements gained over the last decades, the demand for surgical interventions has risen, particularly in the aging population. Surgical procedures are now commonplace among older and oldest-old patients, both in elective and urgent settings. Despite advances in refining technical approaches and interdisciplinary attempts to reduce peri-operative complications, unique challenges persist in managing older and oldest-old adults undergoing surgery, especially in urgent scenarios.

The coexistence of acute and chronic multi-systemic changes often triggers pathological issues making older patients more vulnerable to medical and surgical complications. Surgical and anesthesiologist procedures continue to strive healthcare professionals in the geriatric field, often generating complex medical and surgical care pathways more than those required based on the patient's characteristics. The complexity of the care processes in older adults usually unveils a poor understanding of real patients' medical and surgical needs. As a consequence, additional unneeded medical processes and activities are initiated, potentially raising the responsibility of not being able to accomplish the priorities in a timely fashion, exposing older patients to elevated risks of both medical and surgical complications, and clinicians to legal issues. To date, the general consensus is that healthcare for older adults requires the spreading of geriatric culture, and the integration of

C. Ruggiero (✉)
Associate Professor of Geriatrics, Department of Medicine and Surgery,
University of Perugia, Perugia, Italy

Head Orthogeriatric Unit, Geriatric Unit, Teaching Hospital S. Maria Misericordia Perugia,
Perugia, Italy
e-mail: carmelinda.ruggiero@unipg.it

V. Boccardi, L. Marano (eds.), *The Frail Surgical Patient*, Practical Issues in Geriatrics, https://doi.org/10.1007/978-3-031-77707-3_5

surgical and medical competencies, built and validated in this growing subgroup of patients.

Indeed, frailty, rather than age itself, is the main independent risk factor for complications in older adults [16]. Frailty is a condition characterized by increasing compromised body homeostasis, which in the established phase usually reveals itself with the atypical clinical presentation of the acute health changes. These are the geriatric syndromes, i.e., delirium, falls and fragility fractures, functional decline, adverse drug reactions, etc. When frail patients undergo surgery, it could become difficult to maintain their body's homeostasis and, as a consequence, these patients fully manifest their "unsteady state" or "increased vulnerability" activating a cascade of adverse events up to the failure-to-thrive [23]. Even a simple diagnostic or surgical procedure added to an acute health change in an unrecognized frailty condition may represent the final straw, inducing a critical turning point and significant or fatal consequences. Noteworthy, frailty acts as an effect modifier of well-established procedures and interventions, usually developed and validated among robust adults or older adults, but daily adopted in managing frail patients.

The tendency to generate less favorable outcomes in frail and pre-frail older individuals is particularly relevant in surgical urgent scenarios as compared to elective procedures, where decision-making time is not constrained, and comprehensive patient information is available. Critical to this setting is the preoperative assessment of surgical and medical conditions and risks, including reasons and options of surgical and anesthetic procedures, than the adoption of perioperative patients' co-management of medical and surgical aspects, including coexisting multimorbidity, disability, and personal goals.

To comply with the urgent need to focus on and manage the frailty of older adults approaching surgical procedures, several scoring systems exist for the stratification of risks [36]. The main limitation of these tools lies in the impact of chronological age, often generating poor stratification power with floor or ceiling effects. Categorizing older and oldest-old patients as high risk mainly based on age is an oversimplification, as the risk is not primarily determined by chronological age, while pre-existing comorbidities (metabolic, cardiovascular, and neurological) or prior functional performance often better summarize their prognosis.

Achieving an optimal balance between surgical proficiency and medical expertise is of paramount importance in managing frail older adults. The window of opportunity opens from sharing the awareness of the high standards of proficiency reached in the surgical and anesthetist fields, and the many cultural and methodological obstacles we are facing in the medical management of frail older adults. The gold standard for the management of older adults is the early adoption of the comprehensive geriatric assessment (CGA). The CGA is pivotal for identifying the individual's frailty, unveiling the real needs and potential pitfalls in the assessment process due to coexistent multisystemic alterations, and enhancing the decision-making process about diagnostic approaches and therapeutic solutions at the individual level, ultimately minimizing appropriate care delays.

Frailty also poses organizational dilemmas in the pathway and transition of care for older adults. Detecting frailty at the population level and stratifying individuals based on their frailty status are essential for planning future health and social care demands, with a focus on the promotion of successful aging, quality of life, and dignity treatments, as well as the sustainability of healthcare systems. In achieving these results, interdisciplinary joint care models are warranted for effectively managing older frail people. Orthogeriatrics have been extensively developed and validated for the acute care management of older people facing major fragility fractures and hospitalized for surgical repair of fragility fractures. Orthogeriatrics improves patient and system outcomes and mitigates adverse events in their entire care pathway. Then, oncogeriatrics has made huge progress in the evaluation and treatment of older adults with solid and hematological forms of cancer, reducing the risk of geriatric syndromes and impaired quality of life.

5.2 Frailty: A Linkage Between Aging, Disease, and Quality of Life

5.2.1 Frailty as a Stand-Alone Condition with Underlying Multi-Organ Dysregulation

The study of frailty is increasingly dominating the scientific and clinical scene. Frailty is a multisystemic geriatric syndrome posing older adults in a health condition of increasing vulnerability to develop adverse events triggered by physiological or pathological stressors. Frailty could be envisioned as a crucial link in the continuum chain of aging. It consists of an intermediate health status positioning the body between optimal and poor levels of functioning, with an impaired efficiency in basal conditions therefore at risk of failure when facing an additional stressor. From a physiological perspective in the clinical setting, frailty could be envisioned as a continuum from robustness to failure-to-thrive (Fig. 5.1). When in their clinically advanced phase, frail individuals exhibit a high demand for basal energetic availability even to accomplish daily functioning, and beyond what is expected based on the body's overall characteristics [34, 40].

Conceptualized as a homeostatic status requiring additional energy compared to robust individuals in basic functioning, frailty progression to failure-to-thrive implies a poor resilience of the body to counteract or adapt to the intensity of the stressors, where the energetic requirements for the recovery of the homeostasis are progressively higher compared to the intensity of faced stressors. Indeed, moving from robustness to pre-frail, and terminal illness subjects, the physio-pathological compensatory mechanisms become slower and less effective over time, and the capacities to adapt or counteract acute external insults or stressors impoverish exponentially (Fig. 5.2). Consequently, the combination of stressors and physiological decline across multiple systems generates atypical and unexpected complications, adverse events that may trigger fatal consequences. The above reasons mainly help in explaining some of the unexpected adverse outcomes occurring during acute illnesses or surgical interventions in frail patients, including delirium, infections, impaired functional recovery, prolonged healing processes, heightened risk for falls,

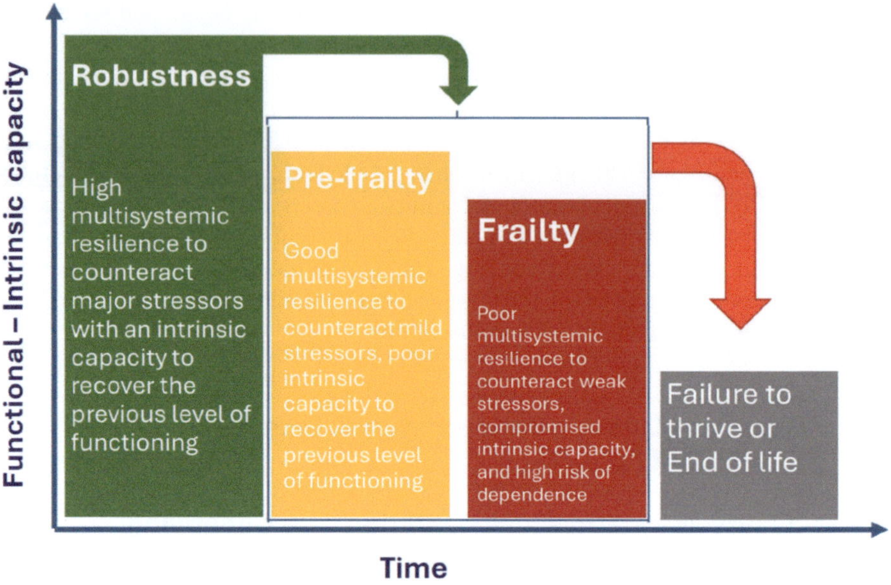

Fig. 5.1 Transitioning from robustness to frailty and disability

admission to nursing homes, and increased mortality. Geriatric syndromes are only partially related to reasons and types of surgery while strongly recognizing frailty and its management as the main underlying causal factors in the presence of surgical stressors [38].

From the clinical and healthcare service viewpoint, it has been a long time clear the urge to abandon the disease-oriented approach and embrace a much-integrated approach to the health of older adults outlined as a determinant of well-being, functioning, and quality of life [6]. From a scientific perspective, the adoption of a multiorgan approach and overall body's functioning may leverage the development of technologies for quantifying organ structure and functioning, and ultimately may present an opportunity to achieve comprehensive health outcomes [37].

5.2.2 Frailty Is Not Advanced Age, Simply Emerges When Intrinsic Capacities Fail

One important concept about frailty is that increasing age is correlated with increased frailty, but frailty is not restricted to, nor defined by advanced age. There are many patients younger than 65 who would meet the criteria and definition of frailty, and on the contrary, not all older individuals are frail [13]. These observations suggest the existence of common but not identical pathways between aging and frailty. They share many features but are distinct entities, and frailty may, to some extent, be amenable to interventions [7]. Aging entails a decline in physiological reserves, still maintaining adequate functioning in basal and stressful conditions

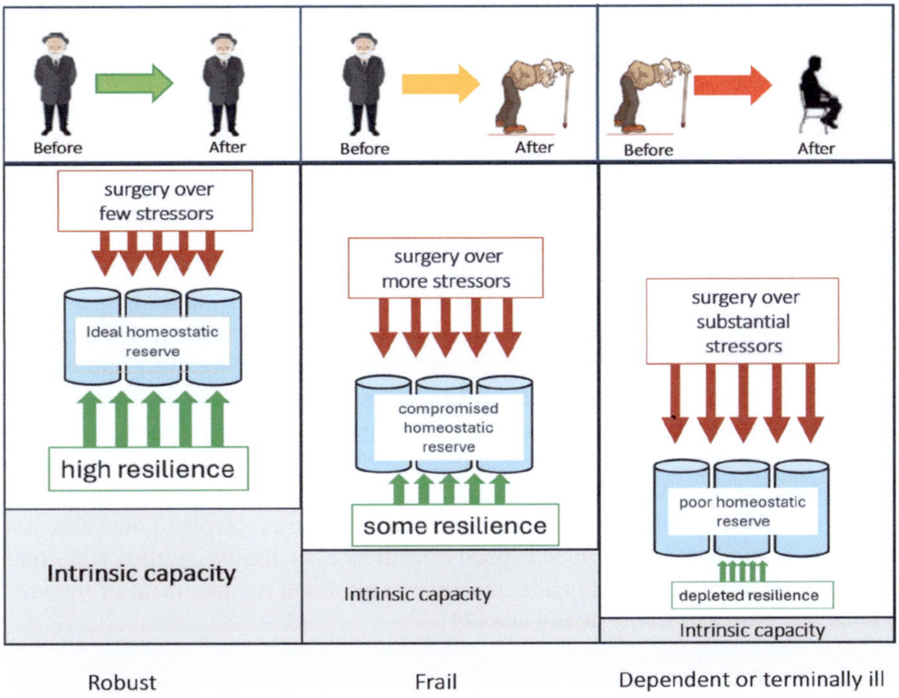

Fig. 5.2 Surgical outcomes according to pre-surgical clinical phenotype and underlying balance between the type of stressors and resilience

and leading to adaptative physio-pathological compensatory changes detectable as minor alterations at clinical levels. Aging is associated with organ- and system physiological changes, mainly considered adaptive, which include the structural, anatomic, biochemical, metabolic, and vascular modification of organs. When these changes overcome a certain threshold, they also lead to preclinical endothelial dysfunction, neurodegeneration, energy imbalance, hormonal dysregulation, and altered body composition.

On top of the aging process, frailty adds a progressive and accelerated dysregulation of body's homeostasis and hemodynamics. Frailty-related changes make the organism progressively less resilient, unable to compensate or counteract damages, eventually leading to a state of "exhaustion" in facing even minor stressors, and causing in the clinical field to the onset of geriatric syndromes, the cascade of complications up to failure-to-thrive [12].

The extent of aging's impact hinges on the intrinsic reserve capacities of different physiological systems, which are currently termed "intrinsic capacity." From a clinical standpoint, intrinsic capacity is a central mainstay for aging, it marks a shift from the paradigm of vulnerability to that of positive attributes of healthy aging [5].

The main attributes of intrinsic capacity are those sustaining older adults' well-being and functional ability, while counteracting the onset of frailty, diseases, and mobility disability [3]. Indeed, the construct of intrinsic capacity intends to transcend the constraints of the disease-centered approach and frailty complexity. At the individual level, intrinsic capacity represents the composite physical and mental capacities that enable older adults to engage with environmental factors and pursue valuable activities. Cognition, locomotion, sensory functions, vitality, and psychological domains reflect an individual's intrinsic capacity [21, 41], which ultimately helps in capturing part of the heterogeneity among older individuals [15]. Intrinsic capacity and frailty are upper-layer complementary phenomena, detectable at the phenotypical level and predictors of multi-organ alterations, exhibiting interwoven physio-pathological pathways [24], and both associated with the biological hallmarks of aging. The hallmarks of aging, either primary (epigenetic alterations, disabled autophagy, telomere attrition, genomic instability, and loss of proteostasis), integrative (stem cell exhaustion, altered intercellular communication, chronic inflammation, and dysbiosis), or antagonistic (mitochondrial dysfunction, cellular senescence, and deregulated nutrient sensing), represent biomolecular mechanisms deeply interconnected and influencing each other substantially, they are also affected by the internal milieu and the environmental factors. The exact role of the hallmarks of aging in modulating intrinsic capacity, resilience, or frailty requires additional research, however, to date it is undeniable they represent the basement of the individual's vitality and frailty at any age [22].

5.2.3 Frailty's Intricate Connection Between Aging and Diseases

Frailty phenotype often presents without co-existing diseases but can also co-occur with multimorbidity and disability. Frailty and diseases are bidirectionally connected. Comorbidities like congestive heart failure, myocardial infarction, rheumatoid arthritis, peripheral vascular diseases, diabetes, and hypertension heighten the risk of developing frailty [18]. Frailty has been also identified as a predictive factor for dementia, encompassing Alzheimer's disease, vascular dementia, and all types of dementia in community-dwelling older populations [19]. Then, in advanced stages of many conditions, such as severe congestive heart failure or advanced renal failure, the development of the features of frailty is virtually an inevitable outcome of the disease [28].

Moreover, multimorbidity, commonly defined as two or more chronic conditions coexisting within the same individual, coexists with frailty. Frailty and multimorbidity are closely correlated because of a certain degree of biological overlap [4, 39]. In these persons, sorting out disease from frailty may be possible only at an early stage if at all. However, not all older individuals with multimorbidity become frail, and conversely, not all who meet the criteria for frailty exhibit discernible underlying medical conditions. Therefore, the terms "primary" and "secondary" frailty have been proposed to distinguish frailty occurring in the absence or presence of chronic illnesses, respectively [10].

Frailty may precede the onset of the diseases in a subclinical fashion, acting as a crucial link to the onset and progression of sarcopenia, osteoporosis, malnutrition, and other diseases increasing susceptibility to falls, fragility fractures, infections, and ultimately to functional decline. In addition, frailty may become clinically apparent concurrently with the emergence of acute or chronic diseases when resilience is eventually overwhelmed. From this perspective, frailty can be recognized as a susceptibility factor that highly predisposes individuals to developing chronic diseases. However, the clinical impact of such a distinction remains uncertain, as the number of individuals with primary frailty is small.

Perhaps more important is the development of acute diseases with the ability to precipitate frailty. In this scenario, the onset of an acute condition or stressor requires the organism to mobilize available resources with the potential consequence of exhausting the intrinsic functional reserves of systems, leading firstly to the failure of noble body's functions, i.e., physical and cognitive performance, since they are not essential for survival, and later to the impairment of basic vital functions. This implies that the relationship between frailty and comorbidities could evolve into a causal connection and extend to the clinical manifestation observed in geriatric syndromes when additional factors come into play, such as acute stressors or the accumulation of multiple deficits [11, 25].

5.3 Detection of Frailty for Preventing Its Consequences

Although a long-standing debate, in clinical settings a pragmatic determinant of patients' robustness or frailty remains the way in which the organism responds and recovers after facing an acute health change or challenge. The poor healing and unexpected sequels of interventions allow us to understand "a posteriori" that we should have better assessed and adopted a different approach to managing such a subject compared to the majority of adults. However, at this stage, the opportunities for recovery remain scanty, and revisions will potentially add more issues. In older populations, our goal is to identify frailty or pre-frailty in their pre-clinical stage and manage them appropriately to save patients' life and, most of all, their quality of life.

The main theories underlying the development of tools for detecting frailty are the "phenotypic frailty" and the "deficit accumulation model" frailty index. According to the former, frailty marks a distinct clinical syndrome with underlying multifactorial pathophysiology [12], while in the latter, frailty identifies the accumulation of multiple clinically identified deficits, diseases, consequences, and risk factors and summarizes it into a composite index for risk prediction [25]. Although they are distinct conceptualizations, in terms of etiologies, measures, and possibly processes, both predict a high risk of adverse events, mainly geriatric syndromes, institutionalization, and mortality, but they also identify different targets of interventions. Further definitions of frailty have also integrated additional constructs, particularly cognitive frailty, the ability to perform activities of daily living independently, and clinical appearance from robustness to terminal illness [17, 30].

Studies have not shown a high correlation between the different tools, possibly because they evaluate different manifestations or types of frailty in different health status conditions and settings of presentation, i.e., admission to the Emergency Department in case of acute healthcare changes or to the General Practitioner during healthcare monitoring. In community-dwelling older adults, evidence suggests that frailty exhibits a robust association with mortality risk, with a likelihood more than two-fold higher in frail than that in nonfrail counterparts, and several adverse events, including physical restrictions, falls and fractures, hospitalization, institutionalization, and the development of disabilities in basic activities of daily living [38].

While approaching older adults in diagnosing frailty and estimating risk for adverse events, we should acknowledge that this is a crucial step in the process of care and it is specific to the time and context clinicians encounter older adults. From a pragmatic standpoint, looking for frailty requires specific tools as well as managing frailty depends on intervention strategies adequate to the context of care.

Indeed, having multiple definitions and scales for frailty should not appear perplexing when we agree with the principle of that "one-size-fits-all" and we cannot use the same tool in every situation, just because the recipients are simply older adults. The one-size-fits-all approach is untenable among frail older adults, particularly when considering that acute health conditions require distinct assessments and management strategies, markedly different from those applied in chronic healthcare scenarios. Although this is a fundamental principle of general medicine, it deserves more attention and emphasis in the context of older adults. Indeed, frail older adults have numerous multi-systemic impairments and varying levels of resilience at body levels during acute or chronic conditions, these factors coupled with the influential role of social-environmental factors require explicit acknowledgment and tailored management to be successful at individual's and system's levels.

5.3.1 Different Tools for Detecting Clinical Frailty

Frailty becomes readily apparent when it reaches a severe stage, aligning with profound negative consequences for an individual's well-being and healthcare systems' burdens. The recognition of established frailty is relatively straightforward among older adults experiencing geriatric syndromes, like delirium or falls, during the onset of acute physiological or pathological stressors. Geriatric syndromes are "clinical signs" of an established frailty, indicating the imperative for urgent CGA driving management. Conversely, identifying frailty among community-dwelling older individuals with comorbidities, mild mobility disabilities, and without previous geriatric syndromes poses a challenge.

To identify frailty at an early stage, different approaches have been proposed to meet the most appropriate criteria for individuals living in the community. This effort is sustained by the general consensus about the opportunity that recognizing frailty at its early stage is amenable to modifications in its trajectory.

Fried et al.'s phenotype or physical frailty is the most popular approach in defining physical frailty, and it was derived from the Cardiovascular Health Study. The frail phenotype describes age-related decline in physical capacities based on the following criteria: unintentional weight loss; self-reported exhaustion; weakness based on low grip strength; low physical activity; and slow walking speed.

According to this model, the presence of one or two of the above criteria indicates pre-frail status, the presence of three or more indicates frailty status, and the absence of any indicates robust status. People defined as pre-frail or frail must be supported to manage their health and well-being as they age, as they are eligible for interventions preventing frailty progression as well as reversal when they live in stable healthcare conditions.

Early detection of frailty in community-dwelling older people holds particular significance as these individuals may face a higher risk of falls, mobility disability, functional decline, hospitalization, and adverse events culminating in long-term admission and mortality within the subsequent 2–3 years. Then, they could be ideal target sub-groups for prevention interventions in the community. At the time of acute care issues, they could be eligible for dedicated diagnostic and therapeutic pathways based on multidisciplinary and integrated care. Those identified as living with severe frailty, given the burden of severe disability, could be properly supported according to their needs [26]. Lastly, the description of the frailty phenotype in the past two decades allowed the identification of several layers of biological determinants, conveying aging as a complex phenomenon, whose pace and phenotype occur heterogeneously [31].

The Frailty Index was proposed as a proxy measure of aging and mortality by Mitnitski and Rockwood, building on the data gathered from the Canadian Study of Health and Aging [25]. The frailty index is strongly associated with the risk of death, long-term care placement, and worsening health and functional status. The Frailty Index describes the proportion of accumulated deficits in individuals at the time of their health appraisal, focusing first on the number of their health deficits and then on the nature of those deficits. Deficits are identified in a list of variables (related to symptoms, signs, activities of daily living, disease, cognitive impairment, etc.) on the assumption that they support an individual's health and independence. According to a standard procedure for creating and operationalize a frailty index, at least 30 health variables should be included, to reflect properties "at the level of the whole organism rather than any given functional deficiency." The categorical, ordinal, and interval variables can be coded so that 0 = absence of a deficit and 1 = full expression of the deficit [35]. The frailty index shows a consistent, sub-maximal limit at about two-thirds of the considered deficits. For example, if a frailty index comprises 60 items, the most that anyone will have wrong with them is not 60, but 40 [33]. The Frailty Index has been validated in several countries and different settings, including acute, chronic, and community care.

The Clinical Frailty Scale (CFS) is another validated and widely used measure and it focuses on evaluating patient function, including mobility, physical activity, and daily tasks. The CFS assesses the patient's ability to perform activities like bathing, dressing, housework, and managing medications, with increasing frailty severity at higher levels. The CFS aids in identifying patients with functional limitations and susceptibility to adverse outcomes, enabling healthcare providers to implement timely preventive strategies. However, its application requires clinical judgment, leading to potential inter-observer variation. The CFS proves valuable in triage, predicting adverse outcomes in emergency department patients. It finds application across various care settings, including nursing homes, intensive care units, emergency rooms, hospital admissions, and preoperative evaluations.

Some criticisms highlight a potential "ableism" bias correlated with the FI and CFS, emphasizing deficit accumulations or patient functioning, and overlooking variations in baseline health status, which could impact resource allocation decisions, particularly in critical care settings [1, 9].

5.3.2 The Frail Older Adults in the Surgical Setting

People living with frailty have a greater risk for adverse events in case of acute changes of their health conditions and those who need to undergo surgery can have less successful outcomes if their frailty has not been identified prior to the surgical procedure. Frailty is intricately linked to various health issues in older individuals as illustrated in Fig. 5.3. These health issues often contribute to and result from the progression of frailty until the emergence of terminal illnesses, creating a bidirectional relationship that may accelerate the downward spiral.

Applied to the perioperative period, frailty generates a state of exquisite vulnerability and predisposes frail subjects to several adverse consequences, including delay of surgery, increased postoperative morbidity and mortality, prolonged length of stay, functional dependence, disability, and increased need for long-term care admissions. In a frail individual, the exposure to stressors results in a disproportionate decline in multisystemic functional capacity and failure to return to the baseline level of daily functioning. Stressors can be categorized as iatrogenic (for example, surgery) or pathological; the latter is caused by acute illness or chronic disease.

In older surgical patients, mainly aged 75 and more, undergoing cardiac, oncological, general, vascular, and orthopedic surgeries, frailty is consistently associated

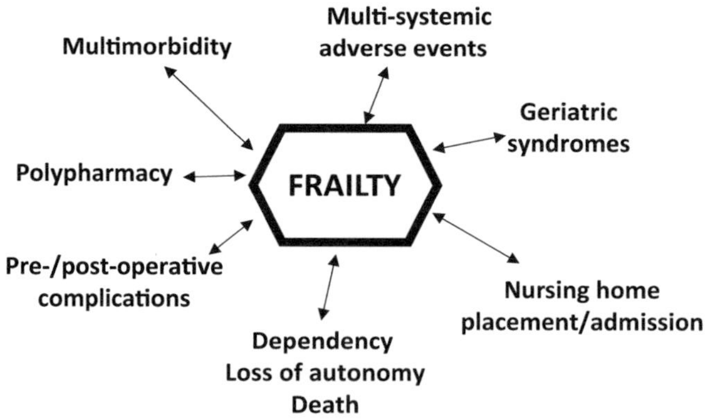

Fig. 5.3 Adverse health outcomes of frailty

with increased mortality, post-operative complications, prolonged hospital stays, and discharge to residential care facilities. The most significant evidence of this association is observed in the context of 30-day mortality, and the correlation holds across different frailty assessment tools and is independent of the type of surgery. The connection between frailty and outcomes such as the return to pre-morbid function, discharge destination, and postoperative quality of life warrants further investigation [20].

5.4 The Comprehensive Geriatric Assessment for Managing Frailty in the Surgical Setting

Older chronological age and more extensive comorbidity profiles are still widely used to assess eligibility for surgical procedures and predict outcomes following medical or surgical treatment. Surgical and oncologic care remains no exception, with patient series demonstrating poorer outcomes among the old-old and oldest-old patient cohorts. However, the paradigm has evolved to recognize that not all older patients are the same and that stratification by their personal risk profile adds value in the evaluation of medical-surgical treatment strategies. Consequently, a more precise means of predicting the risk of poor outcomes has been sought, leading in recent times to the incorporation of frailty into therapeutic decision-making.

The gold standard for identifying and managing frailty in the surgical setting is the CGA. Originating from geriatric medicine, CGA denotes a specialized multidisciplinary assessment tailored to the individual medical, cognitive, and psychological needs of older patients [British Geriatrics Society]. This clinical management strategy provides a framework for the identification of interventions that address relevant issues for each patient. Following CGA, a comprehensive list of needs and issues is generated, leading to the formulation of an individualized care and support plan that aligns with the patient's needs, wants, and priorities (Fig. 5.4). CGA encompasses various domains, as outlined in Table 5.1, and involves a thorough, time-consuming, and holistic assessment conducted by a team of multidisciplinary specialists, including doctors, occupational therapists, physiotherapists, and speech and language therapists. Subsequently, tools measuring the individual's level of frailty can be employed.

Research indicates that the proactive application of CGA to elective surgical patients reduces post-operative complications and shortens hospital stays. In hospital settings, CGA has been shown to enhance independence, increase the likelihood of returning home after discharge, and reduce mortality compared to standard medical care. Notheworthy, the adoption of a CGA to mange older adults has an estimated number needed to treat of 33, meaning that a physician can expect to benefit and avoid negative outcomes in one out of 33 patients managed by using CGA, therefore proving its effectivenes in a practical way [8].

Furthermore, routine frailty assessment during the preoperative evaluation of cancer patients is recommended to accurately stratify risks, transparently counsel patients, and support individualized oncologic care. This approach to understanding and identifying frailty in oncologic settings has prompted the investigation of

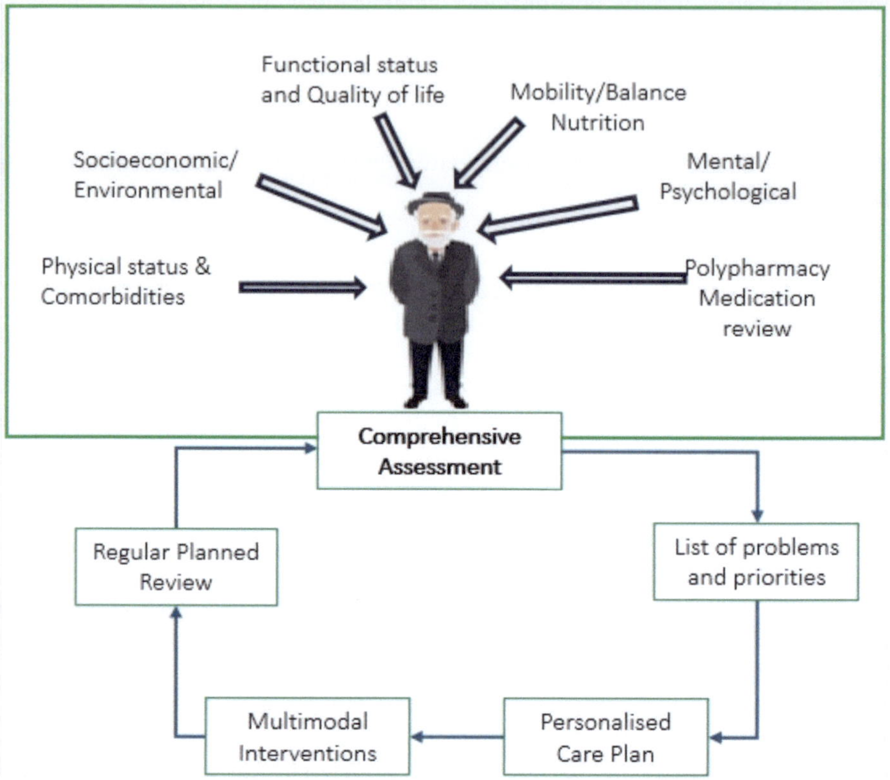

Fig. 5.4 The Comprehensive Geriatric Assessment informing and driving the patients' management

personalized risk reduction strategies to minimize treatment-associated toxicities and maximize survival among this at-risk population. Extensive evidence supports the adoption of CGA in community settings, suggesting that implementing CGA focused on older individuals identified with frailty in the community could effectively reduce hospital admissions.

5.5 Elevating Surgical Quality Through Integrated Model of Care

Incorporating measures of frailty and CGA into clinical and surgical practice is essential for developing effective interventions and personalized care plans that consider frailty, multimorbidity, and disability, as well as the unique goals and preferences of older individuals. The CGA provided by an interprofessional coordinated approach enables the management of patients' complex needs supporting preventive, patient-centered, time-dependent, and transmural strategies. Several

Table 5.1 Domains of the comprehensive geriatric assessment

Physical domain	Illnesses and diseases, including pain, falls, functional decline, drug adverse events, and polypharmacy
Mental health domain	Memory, mood and complaints of poor organization, underlying illnesses, and diseases, including dizziness, delirium, and polypharmacy
Functioning in daily activity	Level of function for personal care (washing, dressing, grooming continence, and mobility) and life functions (communication, cooking, shopping using the phone, etc.), including social role
Social support	Networks currently available, both informal (family, friends, and neighbors) and formal (social services carers, meals, day care), including the social dynamic between the individual and his/her family and carers (while trying to avoid too much judgement)
Living environment	State of housing, facilities, and comfort; ability and tendency to use technology; and availability and ability to use local transport
Level of participation	Individual concerns, i.e., the degree to which the person has active roles and things they have determined are of significance to them (people, activities, functions, and memories). Individual anxieties, for example, fear of "cancer" or "dementia." knowledge of these will help frame the developing care and support plan
Resilience	The compensatory mechanisms and intrinsic and extrinsic resources that the individual uses to counteract frailty. Knowing these resources will allow to enhance care and support health programs that incorporate strategies to enhance resilience efforts

compelling reasons support the implementation and activation of integrated care models of care based on interprofessional healthcare teams and transmural services (Table 5.2). These models of care have demonstrated effectiveness in enhancing the quality of life and health-related outcomes for diverse categories of geriatric patients within surgical settings. Among integrated models of care for frail older adults, orthogeriatrics and oncogeriatrics stand out as the most well established, both relying on CGA as a foundation.

Orthogeriatrics aligns with the principles of patient-centered and interdisciplinary care and contributes to the overall well-being of older adults hospitalized because of fragility fractures, especially hip and humeral fractures. Older patients with fragility fractures are suffering from biomechanical issues, i.e., bone fragility which has allowed the fracture after minimal trauma, and from physiological issues, i.e., frailty associated with chronic and acute comorbidities that extremely weaken their capacity to respond to the stressors. Therefore, they need the application of both skill sets if they are to emerge from the experience with good health and function. The basic argument of orthogeriatric co-management is the CGA informing the management of patients in a personalized, goal-oriented and time-dependent fashion from hospital admission to discharge. In the pathway of care, orthopedic surgeons are trained to deal with fragility, and geriatricians are trained to address frailty, but it is also expanded to include other disciplines in a multidisciplinary team, particularly anesthetists, nurses, and physiotherapists. Orthogeriatrics covers the entire post-fracture care pathway, including medical optimization, surgery, rehabilitation, and secondary prevention, and has led to the development of local pathways and protocols to standardize and improve care and to ensure communication

Table 5.2 Main characteristics and advantages of the integrated models of care

Holistic approach for the promotion of independence	Adopting a holistic approach overcomes cancer as a physical health problem, and includes mental, social, and functional aspects potentially related to frailty, which may interfere with health-related outcomes. This comprehensive perspective facilitates a thorough understanding of individual needs. Through personalized care plans and targeted interventions, the aim is to maximize functional abilities, supporting individuals in living independently for as long as possible
Early interventions to prevent adverse outcomes	Emphasizing early identification and interventions to prevent frailty trajectories. Identifying and addressing signs of frailty across multisystemic functional decline allows timely adaptation of cancer treatment protocols and implementation of interventions to prevent multisystemic deterioration, enhancing the quality of life. Preventive measures, including regular screenings, health assessments, and personalized care plans, mitigate the risks of adverse events related to frailty, medical, and surgical treatments, promoting overall Well-being while managing frailty-related complications
Patient-centered care	Prioritizing patient-centered care by tailoring interventions to the preferences, goals, and values of frail older adults. This approach fosters a stronger doctor–patient relationship, encouraging shared decision-making and empowering individuals to actively participate in their care
Coordination of services, information exchange, and efficient resource utilization	Facilitating better coordination among different providers, ensuring that medical, social, and support services align with the unique individuals' needs. Additionally, it reduces fragmented care and redundancies, leveraging health information exchange systems to ensure relevant health information is shared among different care providers. This information sharing enhances care coordination, reduces duplication of tests, and supports evidence-based decision-making. While optimizing healthcare resource use, this model can result in cost savings and improved resource allocation
Community engagement and caregiver support	Engaging with community-based resources enhances the social connection of frail older adults, recognizes the importance of caregiver support, and incorporates mechanisms to assess and address caregiver needs, including education, respite services, and emotional support. Addressing the social determinants of health contributes to improved outcomes

between all specialists involved. Orthogeriatric co-management as a dedicated ward adds a significant value to both patients and healthcare services by improving patient outcomes, tailoring care plans, reducing complications, and fostering collaboration among healthcare professionals [14, 27].

Oncogeriatrics is a specialized field, also known as geriatric oncology, integrating the principles from both geriatrics and oncology and emphasizing the consideration of functional age over chronological age when selecting patients for standard or modified treatments for cancer [2]. Older oncology patients constitute an exceedingly diverse demographic, wherein chronological age, while serving as a recognized risk factor for the tumor itself, remains insufficient in determining patient prognosis. In the interdisciplinary collaborative model of care, oncology physicians focus is the assessment of cancer variables, such as tumor biology and stage, and develop cancer-specific treatment plans, while geriatricians assess physiologic age and functional status, and focus on optimizing an individual's independence. The CGA emerges as indispensable for a thorough evaluation of the holistic health challenges facing elderly cancer patients. CGA is strongly recommended in cancer patients aged over 70 who are potential candidates for aggressive therapeutic interventions facilitating the formulation of personalized treatment plans. It guides the clinical decision-making process by bringing to light unknown problems in domains that may clearly interfere with cancer treatment decision-making, reduce the potential toxicities, and improve patient tolerance to available treatments, i.e., surgical interventions, systemic treatments, and radiation therapy, preserve the functionality and quality of life of older adults, heighten patients' satisfaction, and positively affect treatment completion, while helping professionals to ascertain a patient's functional status and then tailor cancer treatment to avoid over-treatment in patients at high risk of functional decline. Moreover, waiting for an improved representation of older adults in research, CGA furnishes critical prognostic insights that inform treatment decisions and enables the planning of tailored interventions geared toward enhancing overall quality of life, mitigating age-related biases in treatment decisions [29, 32].

5.6 Conclusions

Effective management of frail older adults in the surgical setting demands a nuanced understanding of frailty's impact on surgical outcomes. Prioritizing comprehensive geriatric assessment, employing interdisciplinary care models, and stratifying based on frailty status are imperative for optimizing patient care, fostering successful aging, and ensuring the sustainability of healthcare systems. Addressing frailty in the surgical context is not only a clinical imperative but also a pivotal step toward enhancing the quality of life and dignity of older adults.

References

1. Aucoin SD, Hao M, Sohi R, Shaw J, Bentov I, Walker D, McIsaac DI. Accuracy and feasibility of clinically applied frailty instruments before surgery: a systematic review and meta-analysis. Anesthesiology. 2020;133(1):78–95. https://doi.org/10.1097/ALN.0000000000003257.
2. Barrault-Couchouron M, Micheli N, Soubeyran P. Exploring determinants of interdisciplinary collaboration within a geriatric oncology setting: a mixed-method study. Cancers [Basel]. 2022;14(6):1386. https://doi.org/10.3390/cancers14061386.
3. Belloni G, Cesari M. Frailty and intrinsic capacity: two distinct but related constructs. Front Med. 2019;6:462264.
4. Cesari M, Pérez-Zepeda MU, Marzetti E. Frailty and multimorbidity: different ways of thinking about geriatrics. J Am Med Dir Assoc. 2017;18(4):361–4. https://doi.org/10.1016/j.jamda.2016.12.086. Epub 2017 Mar 6. PMID: 28279606.
5. Cesari M, De Carvalho IA, Thiyagarajan JA, Cooper C, Martin FC, Reginster J-Y, et al. Evidence for the domains supporting the construct of intrinsic capacity. J Gerontol A Biol Sci Med Sci. 2018;73:1653–60.

6. Daly RM, Iuliano S, Fyfe JJ, Scott D, Kirk B, Thompson MQ, Dent E, Fetterplace K, Wright ORL, Lynch GS, Zanker J, Yu S, Kurrle S, Visvanathan R, Maier AB. Screening, diagnosis and management of sarcopenia and frailty in hospitalized older adults: recommendations from the Australian and New Zealand Society for Sarcopenia and Frailty Research [ANZSSFR] Expert Working Group. J Nutr Health Aging. 2022;26(6):637–51. https://doi.org/10.1007/s12603-022-1801-0.
7. De Lepeleire J, Iliffe S, Mann E, Degryse JM. Frailty: an emerging concept for general practice. Br J Gen Pract. 2009;59(562):e177–82. https://doi.org/10.3399/bjgp09X420653.
8. Eamer G, Taheri A, Chen SS, Daviduck Q, Chambers T, Shi X, Khadaroo RG. Comprehensive geriatric assessment for older people admitted to a surgical service. Cochrane Database Syst Rev. 2018;1(1):CD012485. https://doi.org/10.1002/14651858.CD012485.pub2.
9. Falk Erhag H, Guðnadóttir G, Alfredsson J, Cederholm T, Ekerstad N, Religa D, Nellgård B, Wilhelmson K. The association between the clinical frailty scale and adverse health outcomes in older adults in acute clinical settings - a systematic review of the literature. Clin Interv Aging. 2023;18:249–61. https://doi.org/10.2147/CIA.S388160.
10. Fried LP, Walston J. Frailty and failure to thrive. In: Hazzard WR, Blass JP, Halter JB, et al., editors. Principles of geriatric medicine and gerontology, vol. 5. New York: McGraw Hill; 2003. p. 1487–502.
11. Fried LP, Xue QL, Cappola AR, Ferrucci L, Chaves P, Varadhan R, Guralnik JM, Leng SX, Semba RD, Walston JD, Blaum CS, Bandeen-Roche K. Nonlinear multisystem physiological dysregulation associated with frailty in older women: implications for etiology and treatment. J Gerontol A Biol Sci Med Sci. 2009;64(10):1049–57. https://doi.org/10.1093/gerona;glp076.
12. Fried LP, Cohen AA, Xue QL, Walston J, Bandeen-Roche K, Varadhan R. The physical frailty syndrome as a transition from homeostatic symphony to cacophony. Nat Aging. 2021;1(1):36–46. https://doi.org/10.1038/s43587-020-00017-z.
13. Gordon SJ, Baker N, Kidd M, Maeder A, Grimmer KA. Pre-frailty factors in community-dwelling 40-75 year olds: opportunities for successful ageing. BMC Geriatr. 2020;20(1):96. https://doi.org/10.1186/s12877-020-1490-7.
14. Grigoryan KV, Javedan H, Rudolph JL. Orthogeriatric care models and outcomes in hip fracture patients: a systematic review and meta-analysis. J Orthop Trauma. 2014;28(3):e49–55. https://doi.org/10.1097/BOT.
15. Gutiérrez-Robledo LM, García-Chanes RE, Pérez-Zepeda MU. Screening intrinsic capacity and its epidemiological characterization: a secondary analysis of the Mexican Health and Aging Study. Rev Panam Salud Publica. 2021;45:e121. https://doi.org/10.26633/RPSP.2021.121. PMID: 34531905; PMCID: PMC8437155.
16. Joseph B, Pandit V, Zangbar B, Kulvatunyou N, Hashmi A, Green DJ, O'Keeffe T, Tang A, Vercruysse G, Fain MJ, Friese RS, Rhee P. Superiority of frailty over age in predicting outcomes among geriatric trauma patients: a prospective analysis. JAMA Surg. 2014;149(8):766–72. https://doi.org/10.1001/jamasurg.2014.296.
17. Kelaiditi E, Cesari M, Canevelli M, van Kan GA, Ousset PJ, Gillette-Guyonnet S, Ritz P, Duveau F, Soto ME, Provencher V, Nourhashemi F, Salvà A, Robert P, Andrieu S, Rolland Y, Touchon J, Fitten JL, Vellas B, IANA/IAGG. Cognitive frailty: rational and definition from an [I.A.N.A.;I.A.G.G.] international consensus group. J Nutr Health Aging. 2013;17(9):726–34. https://doi.org/10.1007/s12603-013-0367-2.
18. Klein BE, Klein R, Knudtson MD, Lee KE. Frailty, morbidity and survival. Arch Gerontol Geriatr. 2005;41(2):141–9. https://doi.org/10.1016/j.archger.2005.01.002.
19. Kojima G, Taniguchi Y, Iliffe S, Walters K. Frailty as a predictor of alzheimer disease, vascular dementia, and all dementia among community-dwelling older people: a systematic review and meta-analysis. J Am Med Dir Assoc. 2016;17(10):881–8. https://doi.org/10.1016/j.jamda.2016.05.013.
20. Lin HS, Watts JN, Peel NM, Hubbard RE. Frailty and post-operative outcomes in older surgical patients: a systematic review. BMC Geriatr. 2016;16(1):157. https://doi.org/10.1186/s12877-016-0329-8.

21. Liu M, Hou T, Nkimbeng M, Li Y, Taylor JL, Sun X, Tang S, Szanton SL. Associations between symptoms of pain, insomnia and depression, and frailty in older adults: A cross-sectional analysis of a cohort study. Int J Nurs Stud. 2021;117:103873. https://doi.org/10.1016/j.ijnurstu.2021.103873. Epub 2021 Jan 12. PMID: 33621722; PMCID: PMC9940903.
22. López-Otín C, Blasco MA, Partridge L, Serrano M, Kroemer G. Hallmarks of aging: an expanding universe. Cell. 2023;186(2):243–78. https://doi.org/10.1016/j.cell.2022.11.001.
23. Merten H, Johannesma PC, Lubberding S, Zegers M, Langelaan M, Jukema GN, Heetveld MJ, Wagner C. High risk of adverse events in hospitalised hip fracture patients of 65 years and older: results of a retrospective record review study. BMJ Open. 2015;5(9):e006663.
24. Meng LC, Hsiao FY, Huang ST, Lu WH, Peng LN, Chen LK. Intrinsic Capacity Impairment Patterns and their Associations with Unfavorable Medication Utilization: A Nationwide Population-Based Study of 37,993 Community-Dwelling Older Adults. J Nutr Health Aging. 2022;26(10):918–25. https://doi.org/10.1007/s12603-022-1847-z. PMID: 36259580.
25. Mitnitski AB, Mogilner AJ, Rockwood K. Accumulation of deficits as a proxy measure of aging. Sci World J. 2001;1:323–36. https://doi.org/10.1100/tsw.2001.58. PMID: 12806071; PMCID: PMC6084020.
26. Morley JE, Vellas B, van Kan GA, Anker SD, Bauer JM, Bernabei R, Cesari M, Chumlea WC, Doehner W, Evans J, Fried LP, Guralnik JM, Katz PR, Malmstrom TK, McCarter RJ, Gutierrez Robledo LM, Rockwood K, von Haehling S, Vandewoude MF, Walston J. Frailty consensus: a call to action. J Am Med Dir Assoc. 2013;14(6):392–7. https://doi.org/10.1016/j.jamda.2013.03.022.
27. Moyet J, Deschasse G, Marquant B, Mertl P, Bloch F. Which is the optimal orthogeriatric care model to prevent mortality of elderly subjects post hip fractures? A systematic review and meta-analysis based on current clinical practice. Int Orthop. 2019;43(6):1449–54. https://doi.org/10.1007/s00264-018-3928-5.
28. Newman AB, Gottdiener JS, Mcburnie MA, Hirsch CH, Kop WJ, Tracy R, Walston JD, Fried LP, Cardiovascular Health Study Research Group. Associations of subclinical cardiovascular disease with frailty. J Gerontol A Biol Sci Med Sci. 2001;56(3):M158–66. https://doi.org/10.1093/gerona;56.3.m158.
29. Ninomiya K, Inoue D, Sugimoto K, Tanaka C, Murofushi K, Okuyama T, Watanuki S, Imamura CK, Sakai D, Sakurai N, Watanabe K, Tamura K, Saeki T, Ishiguro H. Significance of the comprehensive geriatric assessment in the administration of chemotherapy to older adults with cancer: recommendations by the Japanese geriatric oncology guideline committee. J Geriatr Oncol. 2023;14(5):101485. https://doi.org/10.1016/j.jgo.2023.101485.
30. Oviedo-Briones M, Laso ÁR, Carnicero JA, Cesari M, Grodzicki T, Gryglewska B, Sinclair A, Landi F, Vellas B, Checa-López M, Rodriguez-Mañas L. A comparison of frailty assessment instruments in different clinical and social care settings: the frailtools project. J Am Med Dir Assoc. 2021;22(3):607.e7–607.e12. https://doi.org/10.1016/j.jamda.2020.09.024.
31. Polidori MC, Ferrucci L. Frailty from conceptualization to action: the biopsychosocial model of frailty and resilience. Aging Clin Exp Res. 2023;35(4):725–7. https://doi.org/10.1007/s40520-022-02337-z.
32. Reid-Agboola C, Klukowska A, Malcolm FL, Harrison C, Parks RM, Cheung KL. Comprehensive geriatric assessment for older women with early-stage (non-metastatic) breast cancer-an updated systematic review of the literature. Curr Oncol. 2023;30(9):8294–309. https://doi.org/10.3390/curroncol30090602.
33. Rockwood K, Mitnitski A, Song X, Steen B, Skoog I. Long-term risks of death and institutionalization of elderly people in relation to deficit accumulation at age 70. J Am Geriatr Soc. 2006;54(6):975–9. https://doi.org/10.1111/j.1532-5415.2006.00738.x.
34. Schrack JA, Knuth ND, Simonsick EM, Ferrucci L. "IDEAL" aging is associated with lower resting metabolic rate: the Baltimore longitudinal study of aging. J Am Geriatr Soc. 2014;62(4):667–72. https://doi.org/10.1111/jgs.12740.
35. Searle SD, Mitnitski A, Gahbauer EA, Gill TM, Rockwood K. A standard procedure for creating a frailty index. BMC Geriatr. 2008;8:24. https://doi.org/10.1186/1471-2318-8-24.

36. Suskind AM, Finlayson E. A call for frailty screening in the preoperative setting. JAMA Surg. 2017;152(3):240–1. https://doi.org/10.1001/jamasurg.2016.4256.
37. Taylor JA, Greenhaff PL, Bartlett DB, Jackson TA, Duggal NA, Lord JM. Multisystem physiological perspective of human frailty and its modulation by physical activity. Physiol Rev. 2023;103(2):1137–91. https://doi.org/10.1152/physrev.00037.2021.
38. Vermeiren S, Vella-Azzopardi R, Beckwée D, Habbig AK, Scafoglieri A, Jansen B, Bautmans I, Gerontopole Brussels Study Group. Frailty and the prediction of negative health outcomes: a meta-analysis. J Am Med Dir Assoc. 2016;17(12):1163.e1–1163.e17. https://doi.org/10.1016/j.jamda.2016.09.010.
39. Vetrano DL, Palmer K, Marengoni A, Marzetti E, Lattanzio F, Roller-Wirnsberger R, Lopez Samaniego L, Rodríguez-Mañas L, Bernabei R, Onder G, Joint Action ADVANTAGE WP4 Group. Frailty and multimorbidity: a systematic review and meta-analysis. J Gerontol A Biol Sci Med Sci. 2019;74(5):659–66. https://doi.org/10.1093/gerona/gly110.
40. Zampino M, AlGhatrif M, Kuo PL, Simonsick EM, Ferrucci L. Longitudinal changes in resting metabolic rates with aging are accelerated by diseases. Nutrients. 2020;12(10):3061. https://doi.org/10.3390/nu12103061.
41. Zhao J, Chhetri JK, Chang Y, Zheng Z, Ma L, Chan P. Intrinsic Capacity vs. Multimorbidity: A Function-Centered Construct Predicts Disability Better Than a Disease-Based Approach in a Community-Dwelling Older Population Cohort. Front Med (Lausanne). 2021;8:753295. https://doi.org/10.3389/fmed.2021.753295. PMID: 34651003; PMCID: PMC8505775.

6 Surgical Risk Assessment: From Chronological Age to Frailty Status

Gianmario Edoardo Poto, Francesco Antonio Ciarleglio, Silvia Malerba, Alice Bombino, Daniele Fusario, Benito Sepe, Antonio Brillantino, Jarosław Skokowski, Leszek Kalinowski, and Ludovico Carbone

G. E. Poto · D. Fusario
Unit of Surgery, USL Toscana SudEst, Valtiberina Hospital, Sansepolcro, Italy

F. A. Ciarleglio
Department of General Surgery, APSS Trento, Trento, Italy
e-mail: francesco.ciarleglio@apss.tn.it

S. Malerba
Academic General Surgery Unit, Department of Biomedical Sciences and Human Oncology, Policlinico di Bari, Bari, Italy

A. Bombino
Department of Neurologic Surgery, Institute of Neurological Sciences of Bologna, Bologna, Italy

B. Sepe · L. Carbone (✉)
Unit of Surgery, USL Toscana SudEst, Campostaggia Hospital, Poggibonsi, Italy

A. Brillantino
3rd Division of General Surgery, A. Cardarelli Hospital, Naples, Italy

J. Skokowski
Department of Medicine, Academy of Applied Medical and Social Sciences-AMiSNS: Akademia Medycznych I Spolecznych Nauk Stosowanych, Elbląg, Poland

Department of General Surgery and Surgical Oncology, "Saint Wojciech" Hospital, "Nicolaus Copernicus" Health Center, Gdańsk, Poland

L. Kalinowski
Department of Medical Laboratory Diagnostics - Fahrenheit Biobank BBMRI.pl, Medical University of Gdansk, Gdańsk, Poland

BioTechMed Centre/Department of Mechanics of Materials and Structures, Gdansk University of Technology, Gdańsk, Poland

V. Boccardi, L. Marano (eds.), *The Frail Surgical Patient*, Practical Issues in Geriatrics, https://doi.org/10.1007/978-3-031-77707-3_6

6.1 Aging Population and Frailty

Advancements in surgical procedures, new insights into preoperative therapy, centralization of rare conditions, and recent developments in health technology have significantly improved patient outcomes, allowing for the successful treatment of a variety of medical conditions. Two key issues arise from this evidence. First, the world's population is aging more rapidly than at any time in history. The number of individuals aged 65 years and older has tripled over the last 50 years, and it is projected to more than triple again over the next 50 years. By then, the older people will represent nearly 20% of the total population [1] (see Fig. 6.1). In 2020, the World Health Organization reported that life expectancy in Italy was 80.9 years for males and 84.9 for females, resulting in an overall life expectancy of 83.0 years [2] (see Fig. 6.2). The increased longevity suggests that aging is a biological process rather than merely a chronological one.

Therefore, the second theme concerns the increasing number of complex surgeries being performed on older persons. The shifting demographics have compelled surgeons to revise and customize their care strategies while identifying new prognostic indicators to assess "Surgical Risk." Relying solely on age as a predictor of surgical outcomes oversimplifies the complexity of a patient's health [3]. Chronological age does not provide insight into an individual's physiological condition, functional status, or comorbidities, which biological age does [4]. Recent studies have investigated how advanced age per se is a risk factor for patients undergoing major surgery, although with conflicting results [5, 6]. While age can offer a rough estimate of functional reserves, the mechanisms by which age-associated clinical

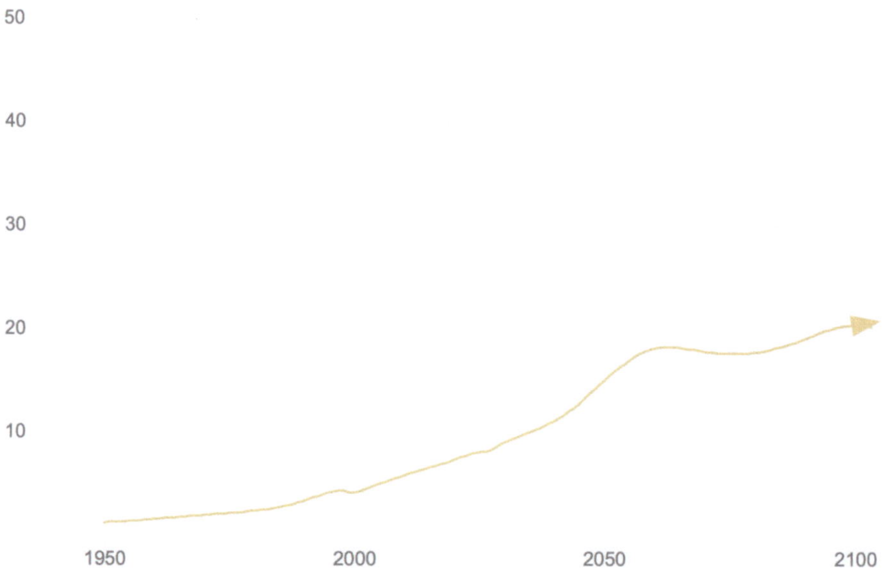

Fig. 6.1 Percentage of Italian population aged over 80 years old. World Health Organization 2023

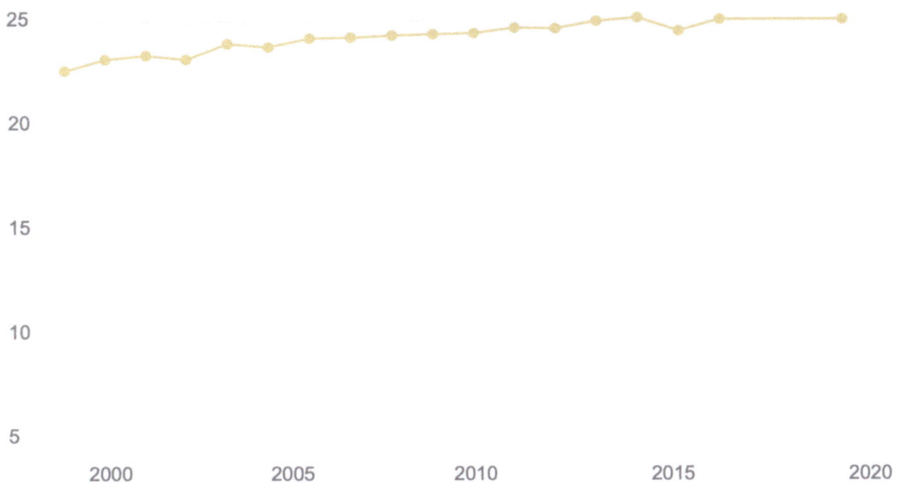

Fig. 6.2 Life expectancy (in years) at age 60 in the Italian population. World Health Organization 2023

and epigenetic changes contribute to an increased risk of premature or pathological aging are not fully understood [7, 8]. As a result, over the years, extensive research endeavors have been dedicated to the identification of potential biological markers of aging. However, it is imperative to underscore that, as of the present, the establishment of a definitive biomarker for the aging process remains elusive. Consequently, there has been a paradigm shift within the scientific community, emphasizing the transition from a mere consideration of chronological age to a more intricate examination of biological age. This paradigmatic shift encompasses the amalgamation of a spectrum of biological and functional markers, facilitating the identification of aging trajectories, each corresponding to a rate of response and adaptation to lifelong stressors, leading to healthy, normal, or unsuccessful aging [9]. Rowe and Kahn (1997) described healthy or successful aging as "low risk and high function," while usual aging is "nonpathological but at high risk" of disease/disability [10]. Frailty degrees could quantify the risk that the aging trajectory may vary and predict susceptibility to adverse outcomes independently of chronological age. The utility of this model has been demonstrated across a range of clinical contexts. In the cardiovascular setting, frailty has been validated to predict disease-specific risks, replacing standardized age-based risk calculators [11]. Growing evidence suggests that frailty is a biological syndrome of decreased reserves in multiple systems that results from dysregulation, which generally occurs with aging. Biomarkers of biological aging, such as telomeres or DNA methylation, are improving in accuracy, with the potential to identify unsuccessful or aberrant aging trajectories before the onset of clinically manifest frailty [12].

Frailty encompasses a comprehensive assessment of physical, cognitive, and psychosocial factors, considering the ability to withstand stressors, also referred to as resilience [13], including surgical procedures. Exploring the etymology of "frail," it connects with "frangible," meaning something inherently prone to break, including an increased risk of morbidity, mortality, and loss of independence in the perioperative period. In other words, frailty strongly aids in identifying individuals at risk for adverse surgical outcomes, regardless of their chronological age. As the Italian writer Alessandro D'Avenia debated, "Being frail forces one to rely on someone… This requires courage and patience." Also "the art to be learned is not to be invincible and perfect, but to knowing how to be as one is, invincibly frail and imperfect."

6.2 Surgical Risk Assessment

Frailty syndrome results from the dysregulation of multiple homeostatic systems, leading to a state of decreased physiological reserve and increased vulnerability to stressors [14–16]. Various validated tools, such as the Fried Frailty Phenotype and the Clinical Frailty Scale (CFS), assist in assessing frailty. These tools evaluate factors like unintentional weight loss, exhaustion, low physical activity, slowness, and weakness, providing a comprehensive picture of an individual's susceptibility to surgical stressors. Approximately 10% of surgical patients, particularly geriatric ones, exhibit frailty characteristics, while the prevalence estimate ranges from 30% to 45% for pre-frailty, a subset of individuals are at a high risk of progressing to frailty based on Fried's clinical phenotype.

In emergency settings, the prevalence of frailty is significantly higher, with 1 in 4 patients already frail upon admission. Furthermore, the risk of adverse clinical outcomes appears to be higher after operations performed within the realm of general surgery [17]. A growing body of research has shown that frailty is associated with higher rates of postoperative complications, longer hospital stays, increased mortality, and reduced functional recovery [18]. By incorporating frailty status into surgical risk assessment and routine clinical practice, healthcare professionals can better customize perioperative care and interventions to optimize patient outcomes beyond merely considering chronological age. The role of the geriatrician is pivotal in addressing these needs, as they can identify, through the Comprehensive Geriatric Assessment (CGA), the multifaceted demands of the older population. These demands are phenotypically distinct from those of adults, often eluding conventional medical assessments. The geriatrician serves as a crucial clinical link between specialists such as surgeons, anesthesiologists, and other relevant healthcare professionals. They help optimize patient selection, develop the most effective diagnostic and therapeutic care pathways, and provide support for the patient's needs during the postoperative period. This is why the concept of "Gerosurgery" has emerged, albeit cautiously. The role of the geriatrician can be likened to that of a choreographer, ensuring that each planned step occurs correctly and at the right time, resulting in a well-coordinated dance, with the general surgeon as the main character. A clear example of this collaboration is the Italian intersociety consensus endorsed by the Italian Society of Geriatrics and Gerontology (SIGG) concerning orthogeriatric co-management for the care of older individuals with hip fractures [19].

As a result, numerous indices and scores have been proposed and rigorously validated in patient cohorts undergoing general surgery. One of the most renowned prognostic scores in this context is the P-Possum. Extensive research studies have sought to validate its effectiveness in both elective and emergency general surgery. Notably, it has been acclaimed as the most accurate model for predicting post-operative mortality following colorectal cancer surgery [20]. In the realm of gero-surgery, P-Possum has emerged as a crucial predictor of 90-day mortality after emergency laparotomy in geriatric patients [21].

In more recent times, the Multidimensional Prognostic Index (MPI), designed by Pilotto et al. (2008) as a prognostic tool for predicting short- and long-term mortality in older patients, has shown a close association with major post-operative complications in older colorectal patients [22, 23].

The application of several geriatric scores to the surgical population has ensured an increasingly rapid transition from the concept of aging to the clinical syndrome of frailty. Fried (2003) hypothesized frailty as being at the center of a cycle of physiological decline. "Clinically, such a cycle appears self-perpetuating once initiated, ultimately leading to a spiral of decline and death." [24]. Undernutrition, sarcopenia and weight loss, weakness, lower exercise tolerance, slowed motor performance, and low activity levels all contributed to aberrant aging and a clinically apparent state. The presence of only one or two of the major components of the clinical phenotype of frailty predicts the development of the full syndrome soon, suggesting the existence of a previous pre-frail status.

The Toledo Study of Healthy Aging which included 1611 participants of 65 years or more, indicated that the prevalence of frailty among persons with sarcopenia ranged from 8.2% to 15.7%. Furthermore, among frail persons, the prevalence of sarcopenia ranged from 40.27% to 72.2%. Consequently, sarcopenia showed low sensitivity but high specificity for the diagnosis of frailty, suggesting that they are interrelated conditions [25]. For this reason, in the absence of a standardized and validated method for assessment or screening in the peri-operative context, the assessment of sarcopenia through a simple, inexpensive, and easy-to-repeat instrument such as the handgrip strength could be a valid measure of frailty degree in the surgical patient [26–28].

The key is to assess the state of pre-frailty. In other words, early detection and surveillance of the pre-frail patient will increase the likelihood of physical recovery and regaining their functional capacity, ultimately improving their outcomes.

When considering calculators that integrate information related to planned surgical procedures, two prominent tools stand out: the American College of Surgeons National Surgical Quality Improvement Program (ACS NSQIP) Surgical Risk Calculator and the Surgical Outcome Risk Tool v2 (SORT). The ACS NSQIP collects data that offers a comprehensive and insightful analysis, aiding surgeons and hospitals in gaining a better understanding of their quality of care in comparison to similar facilities with similar patient profiles. The primary objective of the ACS NSQIP risk calculator is to furnish accurate, patient-specific risk information to guide both surgical decision-making and the informed consent process [29]. This valuable tool was developed based on data from over 4.3 million operations stored in the ACS NSQIP database. More recently, a joint effort between the ACS NSQIP and the ACS Geriatric Task Force (GTF) resulted in the Geriatric Surgery ACS NSQIP Collaborative, a data registry capturing additional variables pertinent to patients 75 years of age or older [30].

On the other hand, SORT serves as a preoperative risk prediction tool designed to estimate the risk of death within 30 days of inpatient surgery. The original SORT model and associated website were developed through collaboration between the National Confidential Enquiry into Patient Outcome and Death (NCEPOD), the Surgical Outcomes Research Centre (SOuRCe), and clinicians affiliated with the University College London Surgical Outcomes Research Centre. The second version of SORT incorporates data collected from patients in the UK, Australia, and New Zealand, showcasing enhanced accuracy, particularly in the fields of neurological/spinal and cardiothoracic surgery [31].

6.3 Perioperative Optimization

The frail phenotype carries several implications:

1. Increased Surgical Risks: Frail individuals are more susceptible to surgical complications, spanning from surgical site infections to postoperative delirium and vascular thrombosis.
2. Prolonged Hospitalization: Frailty often results in longer hospital stays, leading to higher healthcare costs and exposing patients to healthcare-associated infections.
3. Functional Decline: Surgery can exacerbate frailty, resulting in a decline in functional abilities, reduced quality of life, and increased dependence on caregivers.
4. Mortality Risk: Elevated postoperative mortality risk has been documented in primarily retrospective studies.

Prehabilitation and rehabilitation are two critical phases in the management of surgical patients. The first one involves interventions such as exercise, physical therapy, nutritional assessment, and interventions to correct any deficiencies, as well as the management of comorbidities. These interventions help patients improve their physical health before surgery, enhancing their ability to withstand the surgical stress and expediting their postoperative recovery. Prehabilitated patients often experience shorter hospitalizations and a quicker return to their normal daily activities. This step is still the subject of debate due to its limited clinical applicability, especially in emergency settings or among cancer patients who require prompt surgery scheduling, and the results remain mixed [32].

After surgery, rehabilitation aims to restore the patient's functional abilities. This may include physical rehabilitation to regain muscle strength and mobility. Rapid rehabilitation can help prevent immobilization-related complications, such as pressure ulcers and deep vein thrombosis. It also aids in managing postoperative pain through pharmacological and nonpharmacological therapies, thus improving the overall quality of life for patients. Both rehabilitation and pre-rehabilitation can incorporate ongoing psychological support to address issues such as anxiety, depression, or isolation [33]. Similarly, Enhanced Recovery After Surgery (ERAS) protocols can be adapted for frail patients, with a focus on minimizing surgical stress and optimizing postoperative recovery.

6.4 International Record Database and Organization

Several working groups have embarked on extensive explorations into the impact of frailty within surgical settings, both in Italy and on an international scale (see Fig. 6.3):

- The premier European prospective cohort study addressing the prevalence of frailty in surgical patients is presently the FRAGILE study (FRAilty inciDence in surGIcal European patients). It has received endorsements from the Spanish Multimodal Rehabilitation Group (GERM), REDGERM, and the Spanish Society of Anesthesiology (SEDAR). The data collection phase has already concluded, and further information is available at https://grupogerm.es/fragile/.
- The International Database Inquiry on Frailty (FrData) represents the first phase of a CIHR-funded team program titled "Understanding frailty and frail older persons' needs, to design innovative models of care" (Frailty-Research.ca). This

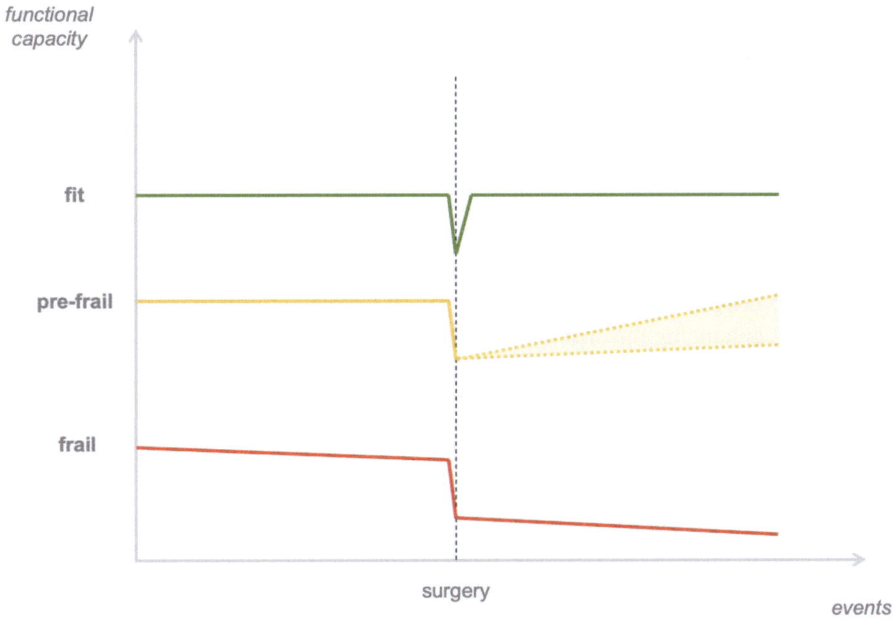

Fig. 6.3 Impact of surgical stress on functional status trajectories in fit, pre-frail and frail patients

program investigates the predictive validity of several frailty domains selected by the Canadian Initiative on Frailty and Aging.
- The Italian multicentric Marjory group has designed a prospective study with the aim of determining the prevalence of frailty in an abdominal surgery setting, irrespective of age, and identifying straightforward markers for frailty. These markers can assist surgeons in making decisions regarding appropriate health-care plans. Recent data analysis from this group has shown that muscle strength, as measured by handgrip dynamometry, can provide important prognostic information for surgical outcomes, including the length of hospital stay, even after adjustment for age and gender [28].

In the context of emergency situations:

- The Emergency Laparotomy and Frailty study (ELF) is a UK multicenter prospective cohort study led by the Northwest Research Collaborative and supported by the Older Persons Surgical Outcomes Collaboration (OPSOC), the Northwest Surgical Trials Centre, and the Bowel Disease Research Foundation [34].
- In Italy, there is a prospective, multicenter study aimed at evaluating perioperative outcomes in frail individuals known as the Frailty and Emergency Surgery in the Elderly (FRAILESEL Study) [35, 36]. This study was proposed by the ERASO (Elderly Risk Assessment And Surgical Outcome) Collaborative Study Group, representing Italian surgical societies such as the Italian Society for Emergency and Trauma Surgery (SICUT), Italian Hospital Surgeons Association (ACOI), Italian Society for Geriatric Surgery (SICG), Italian Society for Endoscopic Surgery (SICE), and the Italian Chapter of the World Society of Emergency Surgery (WSES).

Apart from these initiatives, there are notable organizations:

- The American College of Surgeons (ACS) and the National Institute on Aging (NIA) are prominent professional organizations in the United States, conducting research and offering guidelines for the treatment of frail patients. The Canadian Frailty Network (CFN) is a national initiative aimed at improving care for older patients, enhancing the efficiency of the healthcare system, promoting evidence-informed policy and practice, and advancing research in the field of frailty. Europe has also shown a growing interest in frailty in general surgery, with various research efforts focused on understanding the incidence and impact of frailty in surgical patients. Finally, the Centre for Perioperative Care (CPOC), led by the Royal College of Anaesthetists, and the British Geriatrics Society (BGS) have collaborated to develop comprehensive guidelines for perioperative care in frail individuals undergoing both elective and emergency surgery. These guidelines offer recommendations for healthcare professionals across the entire care pathway, as well as for patients, their caregivers, managers, and commissioners (Fig. 6.4).

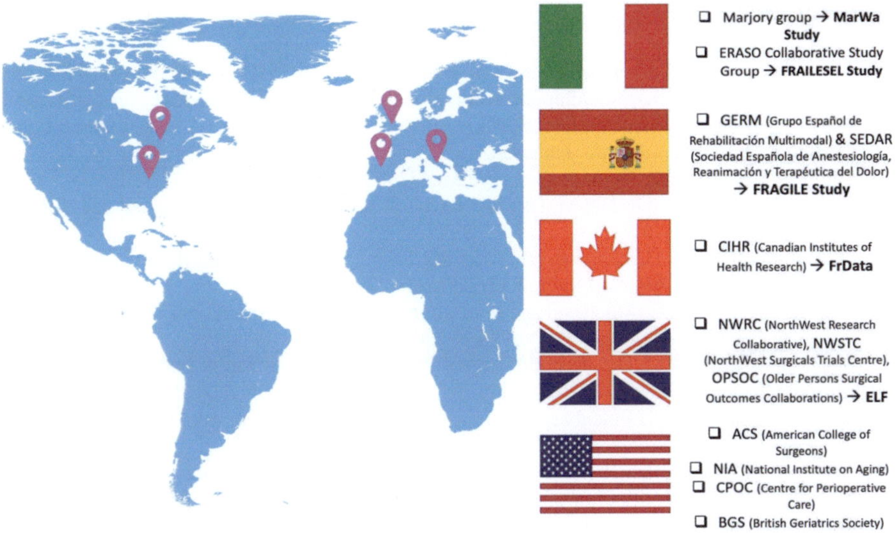

Fig. 6.4 Main worldwide ongoing data registries on the prevalence of frailty in surgical patients

6.5 Challenges and Future Directions

Frailty in general surgery presents a complex challenge that demands a holistic approach to patient care. In 2016, the Royal Marsden introduced the Marsden Surgical Frailty Programme, proposing a five-stage quality improvement project. Its primary goal is to implement frailty screening for all surgical patients and identify those at high risk who can benefit from targeted interventions. While recognizing frailty as a key determinant of surgical risk marks significant progress, there are lingering challenges. Frailty assessment tools require further validation and standardization to ensure consistent and reliable results. Additionally, integrating frailty assessment into clinical workflows and gaining acceptance among healthcare providers are essential. Research should prioritize the development of interventions and perioperative strategies specifically tailored to frail individuals to enhance patient-centered care. Prehabilitation and rehabilitation remain integral components of surgical care for frail patients. Furthermore, incorporating frailty assessments into shared decision-making empowers patients and their families to make informed choices based on a comprehensive evaluation of surgical risks and benefits. Resilience is of exceptional importance for surgical patients. Frail patients who exhibit resilience are more likely to adhere to post-operative instructions, which can expedite their healing, reduce complications, and ultimately enhance their overall quality of life. "To be resilient, it is essential to experience frailty," Virginia Boccardi.

References

1. Suzman R, Beard J. Global health and aging: preface. In: National Institute on Aging website; 2011. www.nia.nih.gov/research/publication/global-health-and-aging/preface.
2. World Health Organization. WHO Life Expectancy; 2020. www.who.int/gho/mortality_burden_disease/life_tables/en.
3. Lubin MF. Is age a risk factor for surgery? Med Clin North Am. 1993;77:327–33.
4. Preston SD, Southall AR, Nel M, Das SK. Geriatric surgery is about disease, not age. J R Soc Med. 2008;101:409–15.
5. Turrentine FE, Wang H, Simpson VB, Jones RS. Surgical risk factors, morbidity, and mortality in elderly patients. J Am Coll Surg. 2006;203:865–77.
6. Blair SL, Schwarz RE. Advanced age does not contribute to increased risks or poor outcome after major abdominal operations. Am Surg. 2001;67:1123–7.
7. Boccardi V, Marano L. The geriatric surgery: the importance of frailty identification beyond chronological age. Geriatrics. 2020;5:12.
8. Gerstorf D, Bertram L, Lindenberger U, Pawelec G, Demuth I, Steinhagen-Thiessen E, Wagner GG. Editorial. Gerontology. 2016;62:311–5.
9. Franceschi C, Garagnani P, Morsiani C, Conte M, Santoro A, Grignolio A, Monti D, Capri M, Salvioli S. The continuum of aging and age-related diseases: common mechanisms but different rates. Front Med (Lausanne). 2018;5:61. https://doi.org/10.3389/fmed.2018.00061.
10. Rowe JW, Kahn RL. Successful Aging. Gerontologist. 1997;37:433–40.
11. Farooqi MAM, Gerstein H, Yusuf S, Leong DP. Accumulation of deficits as a key risk factor for cardiovascular morbidity and mortality: a pooled analysis of 154 000 individuals. J Am Heart Assoc. 2020;9:e014686. https://doi.org/10.1161/JAHA.119.014686.
12. Diebel LWM, Rockwood K. Determination of biological age: geriatric assessment vs biological biomarkers. Curr Oncol Rep. 2021;23:104.
13. Han B, Li Q, Chen X. Effects of the frailty phenotype on post-operative complications in older surgical patients: a systematic review and meta-analysis. BMC Geriatr. 2019;19:141.
14. Pilotto A, Custodero C, Maggi S, Polidori MC, Veronese N, Ferrucci L. A multidimensional approach to frailty in older people. Ageing Res Rev. 2020;60:101047.
15. Morley JE, Vellas B, Abellan van Kan G, et al. Frailty consensus: a call to action. J Am Med Dir Assoc. 2013;14:392–7.
16. Xue Q-L. The frailty syndrome: definition and natural history. Clin Geriatr Med. 2011;27:1–15.
17. Sioutas G, Tsoulfas G. Frailty assessment and postoperative outcomes among patients undergoing general surgery. Surgeon. 2020;18:e55–66.
18. Lin H-S, Watts JN, Peel NM, Hubbard RE. Frailty and post-operative outcomes in older surgical patients: a systematic review. BMC Geriatr. 2016;16:157.
19. De Vincentis A, Behr AU, Bellelli G, et al. Orthogeriatric co-management for the care of older subjects with hip fracture: recommendations from an Italian intersociety consensus. Aging Clin Exp Res. 2021;33:2405–43.
20. Richards CH, Leitch FE, Horgan PG, McMillan DC. A systematic review of POSSUM and its related models as predictors of post-operative mortality and morbidity in patients undergoing surgery for colorectal cancer. J Gastrointest Surg. 2010;14:1511–20.
21. Cao Y, Bass GA, Ahl R, Pourlotfi A, Geijer H, Montgomery S, Mohseni S. The statistical importance of P-POSSUM scores for predicting mortality after emergency laparotomy in geriatric patients. BMC Med Inform Decis Mak. 2020;20:86.
22. Pilotto A, Ferrucci L, Franceschi M, et al. Development and validation of a multidimensional prognostic index for one-year mortality from comprehensive geriatric assessment in hospitalized older patients. Rejuvenation Res. 2008;11:151–61.
23. Pata G, Bianchetti L, Rota M, et al. Multidimensional Prognostic Index (MPI) score has the major impact on outcome prediction in elderly surgical patients with colorectal cancer: the FRAGIS study. J Surg Oncol. 2021;123:667–75.

24. Fried LP, Darer J, Walston J. Frailty. In: Geriatric medicine. New York: Springer; 2003. p. 1067–76.
25. Davies B, García F, Ara I, Artalejo FR, Rodriguez-Mañas L, Walter S. Relationship between sarcopenia and frailty in the Toledo study of healthy aging: a population based cross-sectional study. J Am Med Dir Assoc. 2018;19:282–6.
26. Guo C-B, Zhang W, Ma D-Q, Zhang K-H, Huang J-Q. Hand grip strength: an indicator of nutritional state and the mix of postoperative complications in patients with oral and maxillofacial cancers. Br J Oral Maxillofac Surg. 1996;34:325–7.
27. Chen C-H, Ho-Chang HY-Z, Hung T-T. Hand-grip strength is a simple and effective outcome predictor in esophageal cancer following esophagectomy with reconstruction: a prospective study. J Cardiothorac Surg. 2011;6:98.
28. Marano L, Carbone L, Poto GE, et al. Handgrip strength predicts length of hospital stay in an abdominal surgical setting: the role of frailty beyond age. Aging Clin Exp Res. 2022;34:811. https://doi.org/10.1007/s40520-022-02121-z.
29. Bilimoria KY, Liu Y, Paruch JL, Zhou L, Kmiecik TE, Ko CY, Cohen ME. Development and evaluation of the universal ACS NSQIP surgical risk calculator: a decision aid and informed consent tool for patients and surgeons. J Am Coll Surg. 2013;217:833–842e3.
30. Ma M, Zhang L, Rosenthal R, Finlayson E, Russell MM. The American College of Surgeons geriatric surgery verification program and the practicing colorectal surgeon. Semin Colon Rectal Surg. 2020;31:100779.
31. Wong DJN, Harris S, Sahni A, et al. Developing and validating subjective and objective risk-assessment measures for predicting mortality after major surgery: an international prospective cohort study. PLoS Med. 2020;17:e1003253.
32. Carli F, Bousquet-Dion G, Awasthi R, et al. Effect of multimodal prehabilitation vs postoperative rehabilitation on 30-day postoperative complications for frail patients undergoing resection of colorectal cancer. JAMA Surg. 2020;155:233.
33. Xiangting Y, Meichun Z, Huiying Q. Supportive care needs and related factors among colorectal cancer patients with stoma in the postoperative rehabilitation period from a bio-psycho-social perspective: a cross-sectional study. Support Care Cancer. 2023;31:599.
34. Parmar KL, Law J, Carter B, Hewitt J, Boyle JM, Casey P, Maitra I, Farrell IS, Pearce L, Moug SJ. Frailty in older patients undergoing emergency laparotomy. Ann Surg. 2021;273:709–18.
35. Poillucci G, Podda M, Pisanu A, et al. Risk factors for postoperative morbidity following appendectomy in the elderly: a nationwide prospective cohort study. Eur J Trauma Emerg Surg. 2021;47:1729–37.
36. Costa G, Massa G. Frailty and emergency surgery in the elderly: protocol of a prospective, multicenter study in Italy for evaluating perioperative outcome (The FRAILESEL Study). Updat Surg. 2018;70:97–104.

7 Integrating Geriatrics Principles into Surgical Care Setting: A "Surgery for Frails" Novel Model

Virginia Boccardi, Sergii Girnyi, Tomasz Cwalinski, Karol Polom, Patrizia Mecocci, and Luigi Marano

7.1 Introduction

In the past five decades, significant advancements in social and health conditions have led to unprecedented increases in human lifespan. Italy has experienced a remarkable rise in the older population, attributed to scientific progress and a decrease in natality rates. Some key factors have contributed to the increase in lifespan and including improved healthcare, disease prevention, nutrition, vaccination programs, advance in medicine, and education. As medical advancements continue, the older population is benefiting from better healthcare and improved quality of life, leading to an overall increase in average lifespan. As of 2018, the World Health

V. Boccardi · P. Mecocci
Section of Gerontology and Geriatrics, Department of Medicine and Surgery, University of Perugia, Perugia, Italy
e-mail: virginia.boccardi@unipg.it; patrizia.mecocci@unipg.it

S. Girnyi · T. Cwalinski
Department of General Surgery and Surgical Oncology, "Saint Wojciech" Hospital, "Nicolaus Copernicus" Health Center, Gdańsk, Poland

K. Polom
Department of Medicine, Academy of Applied Medical and Social Sciences - AMiSNS: Akademia Medycznych I Spolecznych Nauk Stosowanych, Elbląg, Poland

Department of Gastrointestinal Surgical Oncology, Greater Poland Cancer Centre, Poznan, Poland
e-mail: k.polom@amisns.edu.pl

L. Marano (✉)
Department of General Surgery and Surgical Oncology, "Saint Wojciech" Hospital, "Nicolaus Copernicus" Health Center, Gdańsk, Poland

Department of Medicine, Academy of Applied Medical and Social Sciences - AMiSNS: Akademia Medycznych I Spolecznych Nauk Stosowanych, Elbląg, Poland
e-mail: l.marano@amisns.edu.pl

V. Boccardi, L. Marano (eds.), *The Frail Surgical Patient*, Practical Issues in Geriatrics, https://doi.org/10.1007/978-3-031-77707-3_7

Organization (WHO) reported life expectancy in Italy as 80.5 years for males and 84.9 years for females, with an overall life expectancy of 82.9 years [1]. However, along with longer lifespans, aging has brought about an increase in chronic age-related conditions, polypharmacy, and disability [2]. A central concern in geriatric medicine revolves around addressing the needs of patients grappling with multiple concurrent chronic diseases, alongside physical and cognitive limitations. Frail individuals commonly contend with an extensive array of diagnoses, medications, impairments, social challenges, and financial constraints, thereby frequently presenting complex medical problems that are not easy to resolve [3]. This demographic shift has also led to a notable increase in surgical demands, with a growing number of complex operations performed on individuals over 85 years of age. While surgery remains an essential medical intervention, it poses unique challenges in older persons due to age-related changes in organs, tissues, and systems [4]. Surgery and anesthesia can exert greater stress on their bodies, leading to longer recovery times and higher complication rates. The evolving landscape of health, the complex interplay of biological and nonbiological factors, the aging demographic, and the variability in individual health priorities collectively underscore the inadequacy of focusing solely on diagnosing and treating specific diseases. Such an approach risks becoming obsolete at best and detrimental at worst. Focusing too much on the illness might accidentally cause not enough or too much treatment, or even the wrong treatment. While various strategies have emerged to address the limitations of the disease-focused model, they often cater only to certain groups thereby exacerbating fragmentation of care. Decision-making in clinical practice should prioritize achieving individual goals and addressing all modifiable biological and nonbiological factors, rather than solely concentrating on disease diagnosis, treatment, or prevention. Additionally, the perception of the disease model as an absolute truth rather than a previously useful framework poses a significant barrier [5]. Nevertheless, to effectively meet the healthcare needs of patients in the twenty-first century, medical care must adapt and evolve.

Determining whether a patient is too old for surgery remains a complex decision, as advancing age itself can be a significant risk factor for operative and postoperative morbidity and mortality [6]. However, age alone should not be the sole basis for surgical eligibility. Dr. Lubin's insightful article in 1993 succinctly highlighted that the impact of age on surgery is not absolute but depends on various factors such as physiologic changes, comorbidities, types of surgery, and surgical timing [7].

7.2 Aging Trajectories and Frailty Status for Surgical Patients

We commonly perceive human aging as a series of changes that happen as time passes, marking individuals as either "older" or "younger." Following the principles of biology, these changes occur across different levels: molecular, cellular, physiological, and functional. The body has mechanisms to maintain stability at the molecular level, delaying the effects on how aging shows up physically and functionally.

But when these disturbances become significant, they start affecting the body's structure and functions, leading to limitations in physical and cognitive abilities. The primary goals of geriatric medicine prioritize enhancing an individual's ability to function effectively within their surroundings as well as preserving independence and maximizing overall quality of life [8]. As we grow older, the likelihood of experiencing various age-related health issues rises, accompanied by a decline in both physical and cognitive functions. Nonetheless, aging is not solely determined by the number of years one has lived. There is a notable divergence between what we typically consider as "chronological age" and the concept of "biological age." The trajectories of aging differ greatly among individuals, prompting considerable research into the biological mechanisms influencing the rate of aging.

Recent studies have underscored that age itself is not the primary prognostic risk factor for complications after elective surgery in older patients; rather, cognitive or functional frailty plays a crucial role [9]. In the field of aging and its associated surgical challenges, it is evident that there exists considerable variability. Among those who age successfully, individuals may exhibit remarkable physical abilities, such as maintaining the agility of a gymnast at 80 or the speed of a track star at 90, indicating a substantial reserve capacity. In such instances, should surgery become necessary, these individuals typically possess enough reserve to endure the accompanying stress. For individuals experiencing less favorable aging outcomes, characterized by frailty and the depletion of reserves necessary for daily functioning and homeostasis, the stress induced by surgery can present a significant risk. This stress has the potential to exacerbate organ decline and elevate the likelihood of mortality for these individuals. Frailty is a condition characterized by a decline in functioning across multiple physiological systems, accompanied by an elevated vulnerability to stressors. It typically emerges as individuals age and is associated with a heightened likelihood of experiencing several detrimental health consequences. These may include hospitalization, falls, the need for institutional care, and ultimately, mortality. Frailty is conceptualized as the loss of harmonic interaction between domains (also referred to as dimensions) including genetic, biological, functional, cognitive, psychological, and socio-economic domain [10]. The aging process is influenced by factors such as the neuro-immuno-endocrine system, nutritional status, and levels of physical activity. In frail older individuals, these regulatory mechanisms tend to become less efficient, possibly due to the occurrence of low-grade inflammation, known as inflammaging, and excessive oxidative stress that is not adequately counteracted. Over the long term, the accumulation of damage at both somatic and stem cells may lead to a loss of their metabolic and functional activities, which includes the age-associated decline in immune function, the so called immunosenescence. Indeed, inflammaging and immunosenescence have been suggested as contributors to frailty, and sarcopenia defined as the progressive loss of skeletal muscle mass and strength associated with reduced physical performance, conditions that are generally considered characteristic components of physical frailty. Hence, not surprisingly, poor nutritional status may sustain directly and/or indirectly the downward cascade typical of frailty [10].

Fried LP et al. [11] introduced a standardized phenotype delineating frailty among older adults sourced from the general population (excluding those institutionalized or in end-stage conditions) and illustrated its ability to forecast adverse outcomes commonly associated with frailty, such as falls, hospitalizations, disability, and mortality, as recognized by geriatric specialists. Even after accounting for various factors including socioeconomic status, health condition, the presence of subclinical and clinical ailments, depressive symptoms, and baseline disability status, frailty persisted as an independent prognostic factor for these adverse events. Moreover, individuals categorized within the intermediate group, displaying one or two frailty characteristics, exhibited heightened yet moderate risks for these outcomes, along with susceptibility to subsequent frailty development. Consequently, older patients, including those with cancer, are sometimes less likely to be referred for surgery, despite evidence that post-operative recovery outcomes are not solely age dependent. To address this, when considering the metabolic and inflammatory alterations induced by surgery on top of frailty, it becomes apparent that meticulous attention to detail is essential to ensure favorable surgical outcomes for frail older patients. Furthermore, it is recognized that older adults and frail individuals encounter complications differing from typical issues like myocardial infarction and surgical site infections. They are more prone to aspiration, polypharmacy, undernutrition, malnutrition, deconditioning, fall-related injuries, pressure ulcers, and catheter-related urinary tract infections [12–14]. However, perhaps the most significant complications for older adults, which have often been overlooked, include delirium, cognitive decline, functional deterioration, and loss of independence [15–19]. These complications, particularly delirium, impose immense stress on patients and their caregivers [16]. These findings stem from the American College of Surgeons National Surgery Quality Improvement Program (NSQIP) Geriatric Surgery Pilot study, revealing significant disparities between patients who experience delirium during their hospitalization for surgery and those who do not. The data illustrate notably higher rates of post-discharge transfers to acute care facilities, serious morbidity, and mortality among delirious patients. Notably, the occurrence of delirium also imposes substantial costs on the healthcare system, ranging from $15,000 to $64,000 per patient episode. When extrapolated to encompass all instances of delirium, the potential economic burden amounts to $38 to $152 billion [20]. Crucially, it has been determined that 30% of postoperative delirium cases are preventable [17]. Implementing preventive measures could not only benefit patients but also alleviate the financial strain on the healthcare system. Additionally, patients express significant apprehension regarding the prospect of losing independence and becoming reliant on their families. Analysis of hospital data reveals that such loss of independence manifests as decreased function, mobility, and increased post-operative care requirements. Remarkably, 60% of patients experience some degree of independence loss, with a consequent almost seven-fold increase in mortality within 30 days post-discharge among affected individuals [21]. While the precise impact of interventions targeting independence loss remains unclear, evidence suggests that improving mobility can lead to better outcomes. Consequently, interventions aimed at preserving patients' independence during hospitalization hold promise.

Moreover, it should be highlighted that the treatment preferences of older individuals facing serious illness are significantly influenced by the burden of treatment, its outcomes, and the likelihood of those outcomes. Fried TR et al. [22] investigated older patients' treatment preferences in scenarios where adverse outcomes could occur. The analysis distinguished between high-burden interventions like surgery and lower-burden interventions such as medications. It was observed that the acceptance of treatment remained relatively high, even with a 50% likelihood of adverse outcomes for high-burden interventions. However, for low-burden interventions associated with functional or cognitive decline, acceptance declined more rapidly. This suggests that, for certain patients, the prospect of experiencing functional or cognitive decline outweighs the risk of death. Given these findings, it is imperative to engage older adults in discussions regarding their values and preferences. Another study examined several conditions to determine what older adults consider worse than death, revealing conditions such as bowel and bladder incontinence, reliance on a breathing machine, and immobility [23]. Therefore, it is crucial to have open discussions with patients to understand their priorities and preferences. This ensures that treatment plans align with their values and goals.

7.3 Is My Patient Frail?

Unfortunately, within the medical community, including surgeons, anesthesiologists, and patients alike, the Lake Wobegon effect often prevails. This phenomenon entails individuals perceiving themselves or their peers as above average in various aspects. Indeed, many patients express a belief in their above-average health and resilience. However, the challenge lies in identifying the minority who may not align with this perception [24]. Addressing this challenge in clinical settings presents unique obstacles. Time constraints limit extensive risk assessments, often necessitating rapid evaluations using straightforward methods. This urgency arises from the critical importance of identifying patients at heightened risk, particularly those who are frail and undergoing major surgical procedures. Robinson T et al. [25] underscored the significance of this identification process. Their findings demonstrate that frail patients undergoing major surgery face a staggering one in two chances of experiencing major post-operative complications. To illustrate the implications, the financial aspect should be pointed out. For instance, in a group of 24 nonfrail patients undergoing colorectal operations, the cost of care at 6 months amounts to $800,000. Conversely, for frail patients, the cost triples, with a majority requiring nonhome destinations for recovery and a significant readmission rate [25]. These notable differences underscore the profound impact of frailty on outcomes and healthcare costs. Hence, there arises an imperative for surgeons to consistently pose a singular question before every operation: "Is my patient frail?" This simple yet crucial inquiry holds the potential to significantly enhance patient care and outcomes in the operating room. To address this issue, decision-making should involve a Comprehensive Geriatric Assessment (CGA), which provides a comprehensive view of the patient, encompassing cognitive, functional, nutritional, socioeconomic, and affective aspects [26]. Healthcare professionals, especially surgeons, should shift their focus from chronological age to a holistic evaluation of each patient's overall health and well-being. Recognition of the significance of comorbidities and physiological changes is vital in improving outcomes for older surgical patients. The implementation of a multidisciplinary team (MDT) approach, involving geriatricians, anesthetists, critical care specialists, nurses, therapists, and dieticians, can be transformative in delivering individualized care to older surgical patients. Frailty has been conceptualized and a clear roadmap has emerged based on a recent consensus paper, dividing it into two models [27]. The first category is physical frailty, which necessitates the measurement of grip strength and walking speed. The second category is the cumulative deficit model proposing that the accumulation of health and functional problems reflects an individual's aging-related health state. This concept is operationalized through a "frailty index" assessment, which involves assessing a broad range of potential signs, symptoms, laboratory abnormalities, medical conditions, social settings, and disabilities. Each deficit is not considered individually but collectively indicates a higher risk for mortality at high levels of accumulated co-morbidity, surpassing what is expected given one's chronological age. Interestingly, a recent study indicates that frailty, as assessed by both the Accumulation of Deficits and Fried models, is prevalent even among younger adults aged 18–65 years old [28]. For instance, among several tools that have been developed to measure frailty, there is no standardized and validated method for assessment or screening in the peri operative context. A more accessible indicator of frailty holds the potential for immediate clinical application within the surgical domain. Within this framework, handgrip strength (HGS), recognized as a valuable marker of frailty, serves both as a practical and objective measure of overall muscle strength [29], and a constituent element of comprehensive geriatric assessment [30–32]. Extensive evidence demonstrates that HGS independently predicts adverse health outcomes and mortality across diverse older populations and clinical contexts [33]. Previous studies have highlighted preoperative HGS as a strong predictor of postoperative complications, including pneumonia, length of hospital stay (LOS), institutionalization, and mortality following esophagectomy [34]. Additionally, low HGS has been identified as a significant risk factor for morbidity after gastric cancer surgery [35]. Systematic reviews further support the association between impaired preoperative HGS and adverse postoperative outcomes, including morbidity, LOS, and mortality [36]. A unique study was conducted to characterize frailty in a general surgery and elective setting without a chronological age limit (age range 19–93 years old), offering further evidence that frailty status could be independent of chronological age in such a context. Marano et al. [37] investigated the prevalence of frailty and the predictive validity of handgrip strength (HGS) for LOS among patients undergoing abdominal surgery. A total of 108 adult and older patients were included, with their demographic and clinical characteristics recorded. Frailty status was assessed using Fried's criteria, and handgrip strength was measured objectively. The findings revealed that among a population with a mean age of 67.8 years, 53.7% and 30.6% of patients undergoing abdominal surgery were pre-frail or frail, respectively. Handgrip strength exhibited a significant correlation with LOS, irrespective of chronological age and sex. Furthermore, HGS was inversely associated with LOS even after adjusting for various covariates, including body mass index (BMI), overall frailty status, surgical type, and nutritional status, highlighting the potential of HGS as a valuable single marker for predicting LOS in surgical patients. Consequently, it may be considered a useful, easily obtainable, and objective marker of frailty. The study suggests that this factor plays a significant role in the decision-making process, serving as a reliable tool that could potentially impact preoperative counseling.

Additionally, another interesting topic of debate is whether the impact of frailty extends beyond major surgeries to all operations. The study by Shinall MC et al. [38] analyzed data from a large sample of half a million veteran patients over 4 years. They identified 566 Current Procedural Terminology (CPT) codes representing various surgical procedures and classified them according to their physiological stress level, ranging from low to high. The findings revealed that mortality rates were significantly higher among frail or very frail patients, regardless of the level of operative stress. While low-stress procedures showed relatively low mortality rates among average-risk patients, frail individuals faced mortality rates at least ten times higher. This discrepancy suggests that the stress of certain procedures may accelerate the decline of frail patients by depleting their reserves. Furthermore, the study highlighted the need for improved case selection, particularly for high-risk procedures, to mitigate mortality risks in frail patients. Ultimately, the findings underscored that there is no such thing as low-risk surgery for frail patients, with mortality rates far exceeding the thresholds commonly used to define high-risk procedures in the surgical literature [39, 40].

7.4 The "Surgery for Frails" Novel Model: Goals and Decision Making

It would be advisable to establish a standardized preoperative assessment focused on identifying frailty-related factors requiring attention and pinpointing patients at high risk for various outcomes, thus enabling patient involvement in decision-making processes [4, 37]. Additionally, we sought to implement interdisciplinary care protocols to address vulnerabilities, mitigate complications, and prevent decline [26]. Furthermore, improving care transitions through enhanced communication among healthcare providers, patients, and their caregivers is a priority. The clinical standards can be divided into the section on goals and decision-making, which has been emphasized as crucial. According to the standard, it is recommended to engage in discussions regarding treatment and overall healthcare objectives, aiming to understand the patient's priorities in their own words [18]. Furthermore, the discussion surrounding surgery should not solely focus on survival and symptoms, but also on postoperative function, living arrangements, and caregiver burden [17]. Other important aspects include addressing code status and advanced directives, designating a medical proxy, and discussing a life-sustaining therapy for individuals expected to require intensive care. Additionally, it is essential to ensure that every patient can review their decision-making process with a member of the surgical team, fostering confidence in their choices. What is equally crucial is that once all pertinent information is gathered and vulnerabilities for everyone are identified, a comprehensive care plan must be devised to address these vulnerabilities. Additionally, a multidisciplinary meeting should be convened to discuss the care of high-risk patients thoroughly and ensure everyone involved is aligned with the plan. This information must be shared not only with the patient and their family but also with the patient's designated primary care physician. Regarding postoperative management, standardization is imperative, particularly for frail patients with sensory impairments. To mitigate risks, it is essential to avoid medications known to pose problems for frail adults, such as those listed in the Beers Criteria [41], and instead utilize opioid-sparing pain management strategies [42]. Protocolized plans, like enhanced recovery protocols, ensure consistent and appropriate treatment for patients based on their vulnerabilities [43]. Additionally, the transition of care standards is crucial. Discharge documentation should reflect any preoperatively identified deficits and plans to address these deficits post-discharge should be outlined. Patients, families, and caregivers should also be educated about potential postoperative geriatric syndromes or complications. Furthermore, bidirectional communication between hospitals and post-acute care facilities is essential to ensure continuity of care and proper understanding of patient outcomes. These standards form the foundation of the "Surgery for Frails" novel model, ensuring comprehensive and improved patient care.

A systematic revision of the literature on frailty tools showed that they have excellent sensitivity, but very low specificity, limiting therefore their reliability in current clinical use for the identification and diagnosis of frailty [44]. Indeed, principal international guidelines from geriatric scientific societies discourage the use of "short" instruments as tools in community-based setting but rather recommend an approach centered on comprehensive geriatric assessment (CGA). Operatively, CGA is administered to the patient using specific scales that explore functional disability, cognition, depression, nutritional status, comorbidities, number of drugs used by the patient, falls and pressure sores risk, cohabitation status, and social and welfare context. We recommend CGA for all patients scheduled for surgery, implementing this along with handgrip strength (HGS) measurement as mandatory tasks for all surgeons. Prior to scheduling surgery, surgeons with a geriatrician co-management must understand and provide the patient's vulnerability-frailty status. Then a transdisciplinary team will be involved including an anesthesiologist, nutritionist, nurse, psychologist, and physiotherapist. Subsequently, weekly reviews should be conducted by the chief of the surgery office. Either the chief or a designated representative would review patients with high scores and engage with the medical team treating the patient, including anesthesiologists, surgeons, or residents. They would inquire, "What's your goal here? What are you hoping to accomplish? Is there anything I can do to assist you in ensuring an optimal outcome?". The aim is to ascertain treatment goals and aid optimize outcomes, a process we refer to as the surgical pause (Fig. 7.1). While 90% of patients could receive usual care, the remaining 10% identified as frail should undergo further risk assessment,

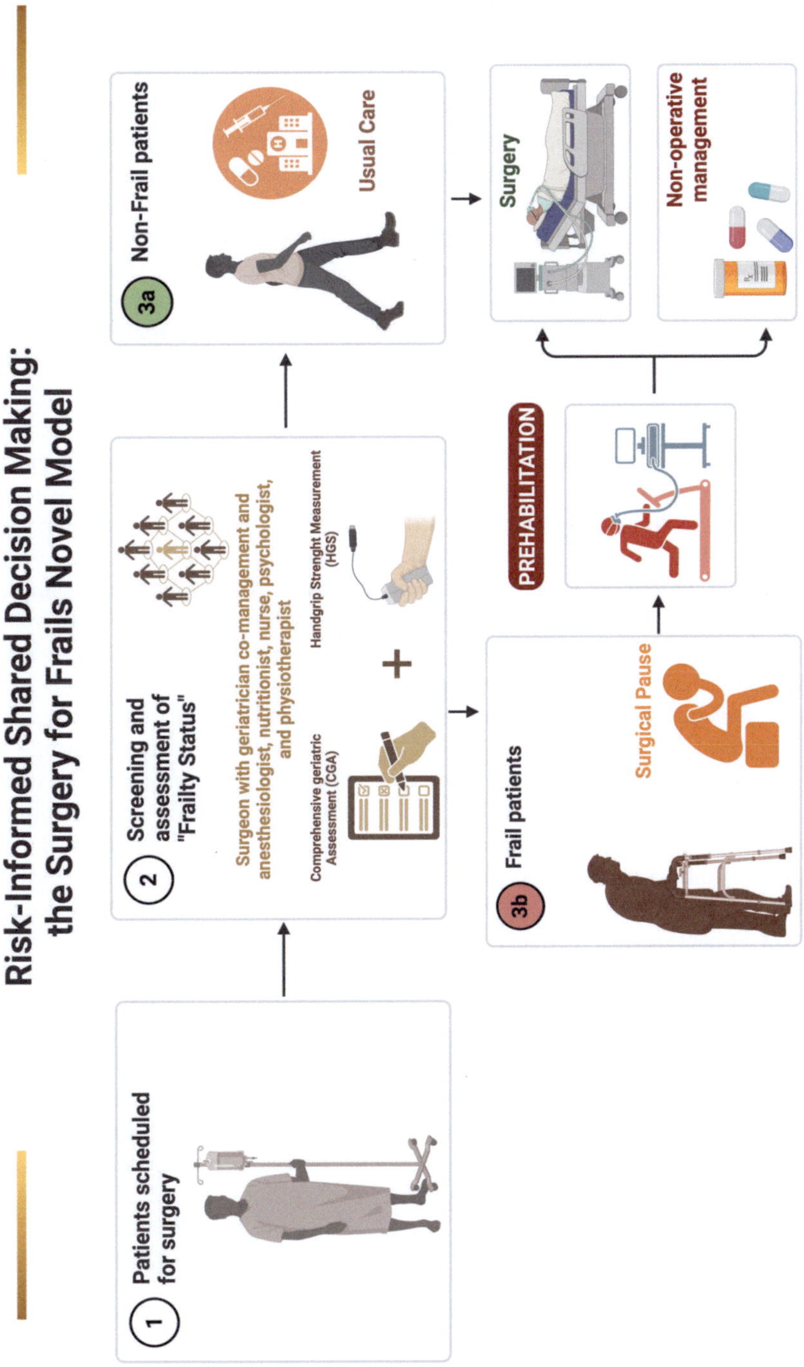

Fig. 7.1 Risk-informed shared decision making: the surgery for frails novel model

participate in risk-informed shared decision-making, prehabilitation, or could be advised against major surgery if deemed not in their best interest. The impact on the health system would be significant, with a notable decrease in mortality sustained over time. At this point, it is crucial to emphasize the significance of establishing a strong connection with the patient's surroundings to facilitate intermediate care, enabling a smoother transition for both patients and their families during the rehabilitation process, and ultimately ensuring a seamless return to their homes. Again, in some cases, palliative care integration should be restructured, with surgeons initiating palliative care consultations preoperatively to provide patients with a realistic understanding of their upcoming procedure, rather than reacting postoperatively to complications in the ICU. So, from a practical standpoint, we can break down the entire process into three distinct phases. The first phase involves screening for frailty using the proposed tools in co-management with a geriatrician, the expert of CGA and medicine for complexity. In the second phase, efforts are made to address frailty. Among the various standards discussed, three have been emphasized: interdisciplinary and transdisciplinary review for frail individuals, goal clarification sessions, and referral to care clinics where specialized training in palliative care communication techniques is available [45]. It has been observed that through these interventions, the care plan for one out of every five frail individuals who would have otherwise undergone surgery is altered, with one-fifth opting for nonsurgical alternatives [46]. For those who choose to proceed with surgery, there is an opportunity for prehabilitation. Several pilot studies have demonstrated that engaging in exercise and balance training in the three to 6 weeks leading up to surgery can improve endurance, gait speed, respiratory pressures, and overall functional performance [47–53]. In the third phase, a more comprehensive shared decision-making process is initiated, informed by the risks associated with frailty as identified by the GCA and HGS. Alternatively, patients may be referred to the interdisciplinary anesthesia-led preoperative medical home, such as the Center for Presurgical Care, or directed to their primary care provider for further risk assessment. Supporting this model is the study by Hall D et al. [54], which assessed the frailty screening initiative's impact on surgical outcomes. Frail patients were subject to administrative review, with perioperative plans adjusted based on multidisciplinary input. Among 9153 patients undergoing major, elective, noncardiac surgery, implementing frailty screening led to a significant reduction in 30-day mortality, from 1.6% to 0.7%. Mortality rates among frail patients notably decreased from 12.2% to 3.8%. Similar trends were observed at 180 and 365 days post-surgery. Multivariable analysis confirmed improved survival following FSI implementation, irrespective of age, frailty, and predicted mortality. These results underscore the potential benefits of preoperative frailty screening and system-level initiatives to enhance surgical outcomes, necessitating further research to establish causality definitively.

7.5 Conclusion

To contextualize, the Surgery for Frails model, while not universally adopted, has significantly impacted mortality rates. This underscores the challenge of not only improving our healthcare system but doing so at a pace that exceeds current advancements. It is clear that relying solely on subjective assessments, like visual evaluations by surgeons or oncologists using performance scales, is insufficient for identifying at-risk patients compared to standardized frailty assessment tools. These tools consistently yield better outcomes across various medical specialties. To highlight the need for structured assessments in risk stratification and future care decisions, a multidisciplinary disease board convened a meeting. Each site presented current efforts and future strategies to address mortality concerns, reflecting varied priorities. As our population ages, integrating geriatric principles into surgical care settings becomes imperative. This transformation demands a collective effort from the medical community, with a focus on a patient-centric approach to optimize surgical outcomes and reduce healthcare costs. The "Surgery for Frails" model, with its emphasis on multidisciplinary collaboration and comprehensive patient evaluation, represents a significant advancement in ensuring the well-being of older surgical patients in today's world.

References

1. Mortality and global health estimates. https://www.who.int/data/gho/data/themes/mortality-and-global-health-estimates. Accessed 18 Feb 2024.
2. McPhail SM. Multimorbidity in chronic disease: impact on health care resources and costs. Risk Manag Healthc Policy. 2016;9:143–56. https://doi.org/10.2147/RMHP.S97248.
3. Ferrucci L, Gonzalez-Freire M, Fabbri E, et al. Measuring biological aging in humans: a quest. Aging Cell. 2020;19:e13080. https://doi.org/10.1111/ACEL.13080.
4. Boccardi V, Marano L. The geriatric surgery: the importance of frailty identification beyond chronological age. Geriatrics (Basel). 2020;5:12. https://doi.org/10.3390/GERIATRICS5010012.
5. Tinetti ME, Fried T. The end of the disease era. Am J Med. 2004;116:179–85. https://doi.org/10.1016/j.amjmed.2003.09.031.
6. Turrentine FE, Wang H, Simpson VB, Jones RS. Surgical risk factors, morbidity, and mortality in elderly patients. J Am Coll Surg. 2006;203:865–77. https://doi.org/10.1016/J.JAMCOLLSURG.2006.08.026.
7. Lubin MF. Is age a risk factor for surgery? Med Clin North Am. 1993;77:327–33. https://doi.org/10.1016/S0025-7125(16)30254-1.
8. Ferrucci L, Levine ME, Kuo PL, Simonsick EM. Time and the metrics of aging. Circ Res. 2018;123:740. https://doi.org/10.1161/CIRCRESAHA.118.312816.
9. Han B, Li Q, Chen X. Effects of the frailty phenotype on post-operative complications in older surgical patients: a systematic review and meta-analysis. BMC Geriatr. 2019;19:141. https://doi.org/10.1186/S12877-019-1153-8.
10. Pilotto A, Custodero C, Maggi S, et al. A multidimensional approach to frailty in older people. Ageing Res Rev. 2020;60:101047. https://doi.org/10.1016/J.ARR.2020.101047.
11. Fried LP, Tangen CM, Walston J, et al. Frailty in older adults: evidence for a phenotype. J Gerontol A Biol Sci Med Sci. 2001;56:M146. https://doi.org/10.1093/GERONA/56.3.M146.

12. Vermeiren S, Vella-Azzopardi R, Beckwée D, et al. Frailty and the prediction of negative health outcomes: a meta-analysis. J Am Med Dir Assoc. 2016;17:1163.e1–1163.e17. https://doi.org/10.1016/j.jamda.2016.09.010.
13. Aprahamian I, Mamoni RL, Cervigne NK, et al. Design and protocol of the multimorbidity and mental health cohort study in frailty and aging (MiMiCS-FRAIL): unraveling the clinical and molecular associations between frailty, somatic disease burden and late life depression. BMC Psychiatry. 2020;20:573. https://doi.org/10.1186/S12888-020-02963-9.
14. Lv J, Li R, Yuan L, et al. Research on the frailty status and adverse outcomes of elderly patients with multimorbidity. BMC Geriatr. 2022;22:1–8. https://doi.org/10.1186/S12877-022-03194-1/TABLES/3.
15. Young J, Inouye SK. Delirium in older people. BMJ. 2007;334:842–6. https://doi.org/10.1136/BMJ.39169.706574.AD.
16. Berian JR, Zhou L, Russell MM, et al. Postoperative delirium as a target for surgical quality improvement. Ann Surg. 2018;268:93–9. https://doi.org/10.1097/SLA.0000000000002436.
17. Leslie DL, Inouye SK. The importance of delirium: economic and societal costs. J Am Geriatr Soc. 2011;59:S241–3. https://doi.org/10.1111/J.1532-5415.2011.03671.X.
18. American Geriatrics Society Expert Panel on Postoperative Delirium in Older Adults. Postoperative delirium in older adults: Best practice statement from the American geriatrics society. J Am Coll Surg. 2015;220:136–148.e1. https://doi.org/10.1016/J.JAMCOLLSURG.2014.10.019.
19. Hebert C. Evidence-based practice in perianesthesia nursing: application of the American Geriatrics Society clinical practice guideline for postoperative delirium in older adults. J Perianesth Nurs. 2018;33:253–64. https://doi.org/10.1016/J.JOPAN.2016.02.011.
20. Berian JR, Zhou L, Hornor MA, et al. Optimizing surgical quality datasets to care for older adults: lessons from the American College of Surgeons NSQIP geriatric surgery pilot. J Am Coll Surg. 2017;225:702–712.e1. https://doi.org/10.1016/J.JAMCOLLSURG.2017.08.012.
21. Berian JR, Mohanty S, Ko CY, et al. Association of loss of independence with readmission and death after discharge in older patients after surgical procedures. JAMA Surg. 2016;151:e161689. https://doi.org/10.1001/JAMASURG.2016.1689.
22. Fried TR, Bradley EH, Towle VR, Allore H. Understanding the treatment preferences of seriously ill patients. N Engl J Med. 2002;346:1061–6. https://doi.org/10.1056/NEJMSA012528.
23. Rubin EB, Buehler AE, Halpern SD. States worse than death among hospitalized patients with serious illnesses. JAMA Intern Med. 2016;176:1557–9. https://doi.org/10.1001/JAMAINTERNMED.2016.4362.
24. Teno JM, Ankuda C. The Lake Wobegon effect-where every medicare advantage plan is "above average". JAMA Health Forum. 2022;3:E224320. https://doi.org/10.1001/JAMAHEALTHFORUM.2022.4320.
25. Robinson TN, Wu DS, Stiegmann GV, Moss M. Frailty predicts increased hospital and six-month healthcare cost following colorectal surgery in older adults. Am J Surg. 2011;202:511–4. https://doi.org/10.1016/J.AMJSURG.2011.06.017.
26. Ellis G, Gardner M, Tsiachristas A, et al. Comprehensive geriatric assessment for older adults admitted to hospital. Cochrane Database Syst Rev. 2017;2017:CD006211. https://doi.org/10.1002/14651858.CD006211.PUB3/FULL.
27. Walston J, Bandeen-Roche K, Buta B, et al. Moving frailty toward clinical practice: NIA intramural frailty science symposium summary. J Am Geriatr Soc. 2019;67:1559–64. https://doi.org/10.1111/JGS.15928.
28. Kehler DS, Ferguson T, Stammers AN, et al. Prevalence of frailty in Canadians 18-79 years old in the Canadian Health Measures Survey. BMC Geriatr. 2017;17:28. https://doi.org/10.1186/S12877-017-0423-6.
29. Porto JM, Nakaishi APM, Cangussu-Oliveira LM, et al. Relationship between grip strength and global muscle strength in community-dwelling older people. Arch Gerontol Geriatr. 2019;82:273–8. https://doi.org/10.1016/J.ARCHGER.2019.03.005.
30. White JV, Guenter P, Jensen G, et al. Consensus statement: Academy of Nutrition and Dietetics and American Society for Parenteral and Enteral Nutrition: characteristics recommended for

the identification and documentation of adult malnutrition (undernutrition). JPEN J Parenter Enteral Nutr. 2012;36:275–83. https://doi.org/10.1177/0148607112440285.

31. Syddall H, Cooper C, Martin F, et al. Is grip strength a useful single marker of frailty? Age Ageing. 2003;32:650–6. https://doi.org/10.1093/AGEING/AFG111.
32. Norman K, Stobäus N, Gonzalez MC, et al. Hand grip strength: outcome predictor and marker of nutritional status. Clin Nutr. 2011;30:135–42. https://doi.org/10.1016/J.CLNU.2010.09.010.
33. Sasaki H, Kasagi F, Yamada M, Fujita S. Grip strength predicts cause-specific mortality in middle-aged and elderly persons. Am J Med. 2007;120:337–42. https://doi.org/10.1016/J.AMJMED.2006.04.018.
34. Colcord ME, Benbow JH, Trufan S, et al. Preoperative muscle strength is a predictor of outcomes after esophagectomy. J Gastrointest Surg. 2021;25:3040–8. https://doi.org/10.1007/S11605-021-05183-Y.
35. Sato T, Aoyama T, Hayashi T, et al. Impact of preoperative hand grip strength on morbidity following gastric cancer surgery. Gastric Cancer. 2016;19:1008–15. https://doi.org/10.1007/S10120-015-0554-4.
36. Sultan P, Hamilton MA, Ackland GL. Preoperative muscle weakness as defined by handgrip strength and postoperative outcomes: a systematic review. BMC Anesthesiol. 2012;12:1. https://doi.org/10.1186/1471-2253-12-1.
37. Marano L, Carbone L, Poto GE, et al. Handgrip strength predicts length of hospital stay in an abdominal surgical setting: the role of frailty beyond age. Aging Clin Exp Res. 2022;34:811–7. https://doi.org/10.1007/S40520-022-02121-Z.
38. Shinall MC, Arya S, Youk A, et al. Association of preoperative patient frailty and operative stress with postoperative mortality. JAMA Surg. 2020;155:e194620. https://doi.org/10.1001/JAMASURG.2019.4620.
39. Schwarze ML, Barnato AE, Rathouz PJ, et al. Development of a list of high-risk operations for patients 65 years and older. JAMA Surg. 2015;150:325–31. https://doi.org/10.1001/JAMASURG.2014.1819.
40. Shah R, Attwood K, Arya S, et al. Association of frailty with failure to rescue after low-risk and high-risk inpatient surgery. JAMA Surg. 2018;153:e180214. https://doi.org/10.1001/JAMASURG.2018.0214.
41. American Geriatrics Society. 2023 updated AGS Beers Criteria® for potentially inappropriate medication use in older adults. J Am Geriatr Soc. 2023;71:2052–81. https://doi.org/10.1111/JGS.18372.
42. Ghai B, Jafra A, Bhatia N, et al. Opioid sparing strategies for perioperative pain management other than regional anaesthesia: a narrative review. J Anaesthesiol Clin Pharmacol. 2022;38:3–10. https://doi.org/10.4103/JOACP.JOACP_362_19.
43. Ljungqvist O, Scott M, Fearon KC. Enhanced recovery after surgery: a review. JAMA Surg. 2017;152:292–8. https://doi.org/10.1001/JAMASURG.2016.4952.
44. Clegg A, Rogers L, Young J. Diagnostic test accuracy of simple instruments for identifying frailty in community-dwelling older people: a systematic review. Age Ageing. 2015;44:148–52. https://doi.org/10.1093/AGEING/AFU157.
45. Ernst KF, Hall DE, Schmid KK, et al. Surgical palliative care consultations over time in relationship to systemwide frailty screening. JAMA Surg. 2014;149:1121–6. https://doi.org/10.1001/JAMASURG.2014.1393.
46. Hall DE, Arya S, Schmid KK, et al. Development and initial validation of the risk analysis index for measuring frailty in surgical populations. JAMA Surg. 2017;152:175–82. https://doi.org/10.1001/JAMASURG.2016.4202.
47. She K, Huang L, Zhang H, et al. Effect of prehabilitation on postoperative outcomes in the frail older people: a systematic review and meta-analysis. Geriatr Nurs (Minneap). 2024;55:79–88. https://doi.org/10.1016/J.GERINURSE.2023.10.027.
48. Furyk C, Senthuran S, Nye D, et al. Prehabilitation for frail patients undergoing colorectal surgery: lessons learnt from a randomised feasibility study. Front Rehab Sci. 2021;2:650835. https://doi.org/10.3389/FRESC.2021.650835/BIBTEX.

49. Norris CM, Close JCT. Prehabilitation for the frailty syndrome: improving outcomes for our most vulnerable patients. Anesth Analg. 2020;130:1524–33. https://doi.org/10.1213/ANE.0000000000004785.
50. Schaller SJ, Kiselev J, Loidl V, et al. Prehabilitation of elderly frail or pre-frail patients prior to elective surgery (PRAEP-GO): study protocol for a randomized, controlled, outcome assessor-blinded trial. Trials. 2022;23:1–17. https://doi.org/10.1186/S13063-022-06401-X/TABLES/5.
51. Baimas-George M, Watson M, Elhage S, et al. Prehabilitation in frail surgical patients: a systematic review. World J Surg. 2020;44:3668–78. https://doi.org/10.1007/S00268-020-05658-0.
52. Macías-Valle A, Rodríguez-López C, González-Senac NM, et al. Exercise effects on functional capacity and quality of life in older patients with colorectal cancer: study protocol for the ECOOL randomized controlled trial. BMC Geriatr. 2023;23:1–14. https://doi.org/10.1186/S12877-023-04026-6/TABLES/2.
53. Brach JS, Perera S, Shuman V, et al. Effect of timing and coordination training on mobility and physical activity among community-dwelling older adults: a randomized clinical trial. JAMA Netw Open. 2022;5:e2212921. https://doi.org/10.1001/JAMANETWORKOPEN.2022.12921.
54. Hall DE, Arya S, Schmid KK, et al. Association of a frailty screening initiative with postoperative survival at 30, 180, and 365 days. JAMA Surg. 2017;152:233–40. https://doi.org/10.1001/JAMASURG.2016.4219.

8 The Role of a Multidisciplinary Team for Shared Strategies in Gerosurgery

Francesco Paolo Prete, Angela Gurrado, Silvia Malerba, and Mario Testini

8.1 Introduction

With improvements in health and social care in the preceding century, older persons, defined here as the over-65-year-old contingent, currently account for a quarter of the population in developed countries [1], and their number is projected to rise to nearly 2 billion or 16% of the global population in 2050 [2]. Over the recent decade, there has been a rise in geriatric surgery that can be attributed to increased life expectancy, improved socioeconomic conditions, and advances in surgical and anesthetic techniques. As aging is associated with an increase in the incidence of degenerative, neoplastic, and vascular conditions, it is increasingly common for surgical teams to provide treatment for older people: with approximately 45% of surgical interventions performed in the over-65 population in Italy in 2017 [3] it has been estimated that half of this age group will require some form of surgery at least once in their lives, so this change in the structure of society is likely to impact the delivery of healthcare [4]. Benefits of surgical intervention include control of symptoms and increased life expectancy; however, despite numerous advances in surgical and anesthetic techniques, older people continue to have higher rates of perioperative morbidity and mortality in comparison to younger patients after both elective and emergency surgeries and incur higher health and social care costs [5, 6]. Hence there is growing interest in optimizing postoperative outcomes for older persons [7].

The traditional clinical approach, focusing on a single disease, is often insufficient in geriatric patients, for many reasons including multimorbidity and frailty, both of which are independent predictors of adverse outcomes [8].

F. P. Prete (✉) · A. Gurrado · S. Malerba · M. Testini
General Surgery, Department of Precision and Regenerative Medicine and Jonian Area (DiMePRe-J), University of Bari, Bari, Italy

Academic Unit of General Surgery "Bonomo", Policlinico di Bari School of Medicine, Bari, Italy
e-mail: francesco.prete@uniba.it; angela.gurrado@uniba.it; mario.testini@uniba.it

V. Boccardi, L. Marano (eds.), *The Frail Surgical Patient*, Practical Issues in Geriatrics, https://doi.org/10.1007/978-3-031-77707-3_8

8.2 The Complexity of the Older Patients

With aging there is a decline in physiological body functions that occurs in multiple body systems with different manifestations: cognitive decline, onset of memory loss and dementia, anxiety, depression; decrease or loss of sensory functions (taste, smell, hearing, and cataracts), atherosclerosis, decreased cardiac output; increase in chest wall stiffness and decline in pulmonary capacity with potential for respiratory failure (e.g., with sedative drugs) and increased risk of aspiration and infections; decrease in gastric mobility, metabolism and absorption of medications, increased risk of malnutrition; renal insufficiency and increased risk of fluid overload; urinary incontinence and increase in urinary tract infections; osteoporosis, increased risk of injuries; chronic pain; decreased hepatic blood flow and microsomal oxidation may increase the half-life of some drugs; lastly, insulin resistance and impaired insulin secretion may drive hyperglycemia. Other peculiarities are low functional performance that commonly translates into reduced mobility and risk of falls, as well as loss of motivation and social isolation [9].

The decline in functioning across multiple physiological systems is associated with reduced homeostatic capacity and generally motivates an age-related decline in physiological reserves in all systems characterized by diminished resilience, loss of adaptive capacity, and increased vulnerability to stressors, which are hallmarks of frailty. Frailty is more frequently encountered in the older persons' cohort, with an estimated prevalence of 10% among older community-dwellers, and more importantly in 18 up to 40% of hospital patients [10]. Objective signs of frailty are unintentional weight loss, self-reported exhaustion, slow walking speed, weak grip strength, and low physical activity levels [11].

In the last 10 years, several studies investigated the impact of frailty on elective surgical activity and it is reported as the main risk factor for morbidity and postoperative mortality [12, 13]. These patients are more likely to experience postoperative complications, of which, the majority occur from postoperative day 3 onwards and imply medical management (for example, delirium, respiratory complications, or acute kidney injury) [8]. This is why, besides aging, physical fitness, as a surrogate for reserve, is considered the most relevant factor for clinical decision-making in the geriatric population.

Frailty is one of the so-called "geriatric giants" that also include malnutrition, cognitive impairment (often undiagnosed at early stages), mobility disorders and falls, visual and auditory disturbances, and incontinence: common, chronic, multiple, and multifactorial age-related health conditions are difficult to treat, reduce social contacts and increase the dependence of older people on caregivers [14–16]. Multimorbidity is also often accompanied by other issues such as polypharmacy, complex medication regimens, adherence, and atypical presentations, where age-related changes are difficult to distinguish from disease, require thorough assessment; iatrogenic disease, often preventable, is common; and reversible conditions are underdiagnosed and undertreated [9, 17].

Therefore, geriatric care of older surgical patients is multifactorial, as they present not only with the index pathology requiring surgery but with concurrent age-related physiological decline, multimorbidity, and geriatric syndromes. And geriatric patients who are particularly at risk of preventable postoperative complications and prolonged admission, or 'high-risk,' are defined by both the surgical procedure (as for cardiac complications in emergency and major vascular procedures, or pulmonary complications in intra-abdominal and thoracic procedures) and patient-level factors [18].

Not the least, in geriatric surgery social support and patient preferences are critical aspects: function and quality of life are important outcomes, and ethical and end-of-life issues guide practice [19].

Specific consideration of the complex multi-faceted aspects of aging, with significant variability in the aging process between individuals, requires a patient-centered approach and justifies the creation of dedicated multidisciplinary programs or functional units aimed at the management of surgical diseases in frail patients [20].

8.3 Shared Multidisciplinary Strategies in Gerosurgery

8.3.1 Perioperative Care

Perioperative care is the practice of *integrated, multidisciplinary, patient*-centered *care*, from the moment surgery is conceived in primary care, through hospital admission, to full recovery [21]. The delivery of quality perioperative care for patients with coexisting multimorbidity and frailty should incorporate assessment, optimization, and management of issues pertaining to the surgical episode, while taking into context assessment and management of underlying chronic disease and geriatric syndromes [22].

To achieve this, patients are seen in multidisciplinary consultative models utilizing Comprehensive Geriatric Assessment (CGA) and optimization methodology, where geriatric deficits are assessed and interventions are prescribed; ongoing patient needs are also fulfilled through a series of interventions [23]. These models of care are increasingly advocated and adopted internationally [24]. High standards in perioperative care will require multidisciplinary collaborative working between all those involved in the perioperative pathway to ensure perioperative care is patient centered rather than specialty centered [25]. This includes geriatricians, anesthesiologists, surgeons, pre-assessment and ward nursing staff, therapists, allied health care professionals, and local managers and commissioning groups. The adoption of a specialized geriatric surgical service promises to prevent the fragmentation of older persons' care by aligning team members to a common goal and fostering ownership, promoting productivity, communication, and attention to detail [26].

8.3.2 The Multidisciplinary Team

Multidisciplinary working, whereby professionals from different specialties and sectors work together to support someone along their journey, is a foundation of perioperative care.

A multidisciplinary team is a group of qualified healthcare professionals, each trained in a different discipline who work together, each one of them providing a different aspect of care based on expertise. They establish common, patient-centered goals, cover the domains of medical problems, provide a more holistic understanding of a patient's condition, and develop personalized treatment strategies for frail patient. The team discusses their recommendations and develops a coordinated, comprehensive, and not overwhelming treatment plan [27].

The team members looking after geriatric surgery patients typically include a wide range of sectors in multidisciplinary care, including primary care, and a wide range of professional roles. Facets of a multidisciplinary team can be highly variable and often consist of physicians (geriatricians, anesthesiologists and intensivists, surgeons, geriatric oncologists, and oncologists) conducting a geriatric assessment in concert with other members of an integrated team composed of specialist nurses, physiotherapists, dieticians, occupational therapists, and family caregivers. Depending on the context, teams may also include other specialist physicians (i.e., cardiologist, nephrologist), pharmacists, medical social workers, and befrienders. It is important to include patients as owners of the care process and informal care as part of the multidisciplinary team approach.

Effective team working requires five core components: team leadership, team orientation, back-up behavior (i.e., mutual support among team members), mutual performance monitoring and adaptability [28]. Roles within a team, e.g., leadership, might vary by the phase of care, setting of care, and the patient's condition [27].

Three mechanisms allow team members to work well together: team members' mutual understanding and trust in the roles of other professionals, shared mental models (of the tasks to be performed and each other's roles), and structures to support communication and follow through of multidisciplinary decisions, as in closed-loop communication [29, 30].

Different levels of collaboration work and team integration have been described, and team integration can assume progressively closer and tight-knitted shapes [31].

Monodisciplinary or intradisciplinary older surgical patients present not only with the index pathology requiring surgery but with concurrent age-related physiological decline, multimorbidity, and geriatric syndromes.

Multidisciplinary: Professionals from multiple disciplines (such as nursing, social work, and medical), communicating via the leader, work independently to assess the patient from multiple angles. Participants may have separate but interrelated roles and maintain their own disciplinary boundaries. The process might be described as additive, not integrative, and patient goals may be conflicting.

Interdisciplinary or interprofessional: Members come together as a whole to discuss their individual assessments to develop a joint service plan for the patient. Practitioners may blur some disciplinary boundaries but still maintain a discipline-specific base for functional assessment, which may be shared across disciplines to coordinate treatment plans. Teams integrate closer to complete a shared goal.

However, maintaining professional boundaries may generate difficulties in multidisciplinary patient care [32]: the team and patient may fail to share a common vision of the final outcome (e.g., in cancer surgery surgeon may be focused on ensuring best long-term survival while an older patients may want to preserve their autonomy and independence from the complications of disease); there may not be sufficient coordination to perform tasks in a timely fashion (the discomfort of monitoring devices, tubes, and postoperative pain may prevent patient from learning perioperative exercises to maintain functional capacity); members of the team may fail to communicate effectively (early signs of cognitive impairment caught by geriatrician, might not be not clearly communicated to the surgeon and anesthesiologist, failing to recognize an increased risk of post-operative cognitive dysfunction and delirium); members of the team may fail to understand other members' roles, and plans may not be followed through from start to finish (e.g., a pain management plan may change in formulation from preoperative to intraoperative to postoperative alternative formulas as anesthesiologist reviews do not coincide).

Transdisciplinary or supra-professional team is composed of professionals from multiple disciplines who join a patient-centered team. They share roles, skills, tasks, and decision-making: in particular, members share responsibility, although there may be a designated leader to oversee a case [31]. They blur professional boundaries, share knowledge and skills, and have an advanced understanding of others' roles. The team integrates elements of assessment and treatment and comes with a unified plan under shared goals. Reported benefits are a dispense of hierarchy; heightened communication; patient-centric design; role enrichment and extension (understanding other disciplines and improving one's own discipline); role expansion (via interdisciplinary education); role release (blurred boundaries); and role support (constant feedback and quality improvement) [32].

While benefits of multidisciplinary team working are not always apparent [33], and more research into the most effective types of multidisciplinary working has been advocated, coordinated and less fragmented care has been documented in a transdisciplinary model of multidisciplinary work [32]. A transdisciplinary geriatric surgery team design has been indicated as ideal to provide multilevel patient risk stratification, identifying the best condition for colorectal surgery [26].

Various implementations of multidisciplinary working have been researched [34], including circumstances where specific support is provided, before or after surgery, from disciplines such as geriatric medicine, nursing, therapists, scientists, or primary care; clinics where patients on the same day visit different professionals to achieve more holistic care; integrated perioperative care pathways effected by multidisciplinary teams; multidisciplinary team meetings where professionals review and plan a patient's care together; and formal integration of services management and funding across sectors.

Local resources, peculiarities of local populations, the available expertise, and specific needs of healthcare centers have contributed to the evolution of different models of care to assess and optimize older persons and/or high-risk surgical patients.

8.4 Assessment and Preoperative Management

8.4.1 Elective Care

The decision to offer major surgery to older persons should also be individualized to their premorbid function, comorbidities, personal wishes, and considerations with regard to postoperative quality of life. The preoperative assessment is a critical opportunity to establish the geriatric patient's baseline functional status and to predict risks of perioperative complications; the high-risk population particularly requires optimization across additional medical, functional, social, and psychological domains.

In the last 10 years, perioperative models of care incorporating CGA and optimization methodology provided by a consultant geriatrician-led multidisciplinary team (MDT) have been implemented for elective surgical procedures [35, 36].

CGA provides a structured, evidence-based methodology for a multidisciplinary diagnostic and treatment process to identify and manage both existing and newly diagnosed medical, functional, and psychosocial issues employing short- and long-term plans for treatment.

CGA review aims to assess:

- Perioperative risk, estimating overall mortality (using, e.g., ASA, P-POSSUM scores [37]) and morbidity and organ-specific risk (e.g., the Lee index of cardiac risk [38], accurate estimation of respiratory capacity, or renal function and nephrotoxic effects of comorbidities such as hypertension or diabetes).
- Risk of functional decline/post-operative cognitive disorders (mild cognitive impairment or dementia, delirium, functional decline through the Clock drawing test, the Mini-Mental State Examination (MMSE), or the Abbreviated Mental Test [39]).
- Medically optimize patients to modify risk (identify and optimize previously unrecognized disease or known comorbidity).
- Provide functional and psychosocial assessment (TUG test for falls [37], predict and modify the risk of hospital-associated deconditioning, and care needs at discharge).
- Promote shared decision-making (assessing capacity and informing discussion of risks and benefits of different treatment options with surgeon, anesthesiologist, and patient) [3].
- Provide an individually tailored perioperative management plan (covering for expected complications, proactively communicating with patients, relatives, surgeons, anesthesiologists, ward teams, primary care, etc.) [3].

Because CGA identifies physical health (including pharmacy and medication assumption), cognition, mental health, functional ability, psychological, and socio-environmental aspects of the older patient, it involves physicians, social workers, nutritionists, physical therapists, occupational therapists, and family in a comprehensive, multi-domain assessment [22]. It is important that anesthesiologists, in their role as perioperative physicians, are formally included in multidisciplinary team models, particularly with regard to preoperative assessment and optimization.

Surgical patients are typically triaged based on the perioperative risk of mortality to the appropriate preoperative assessment clinic: either a nurse-led preoperative assessment or a geriatrician-led dedicated preoperative assessment and optimization clinic (e.g., in the Perioperative Care for Older People undergoing Surgery (POPS) clinic, in the UK [40]), depending on the presence of multimorbidity, geriatric syndromes, or concerns about functional status. This assessment makes use of CGA and optimization harnessing multidisciplinary skills. Higher-risk patients, based on clinical assessment and physiological testing (e.g., cardiopulmonary exercise testing [3]), may attend an anesthesiologist-led clinic, where expert advice and support are provided by a range of healthcare professionals (organ specialists, therapists, and allied healthcare professionals) [41].

The CGA process is iterative, thus allowing the care plan remains responsive to the patient's needs.

Several studies evaluated the CGA impact on postoperative outcomes in geriatric patients undergoing elective abdominal, vascular, spinal, and orthopedic surgery [42–46].

Within the surgical setting, preoperative CGA and optimizing show a positive impact on shorter length of hospital stay (attributed to fewer medical complications), discharge-related issues, and are effective in decreasing mortality after hospital admission, increasing the likelihood that patients will be alive and in their own homes at 3–12 months follow-up [5, 22] and improving the quality of life and reducing caregiver burden [47, 48].

Perioperative CGA implementation was also found to be cost-effective in comparison to standard preoperative care in elective surgery particularly in patients at high risk of complications [6, 44].

The American College of Surgeons National Surgical Quality Improvement Program/American Geriatrics Society (ACSNSQIP/ AGS) 2012 Guidelines for the optimal pre-operative assessment of geriatric surgical patients have identified frailty assessment as a critical component in the pre-operative assessment [49], and CGA-based multidimensional intervention is the accepted gold standard in care for older hospitalized patients with frailty [50]. Multiparametric frailty scales (e.g., Fried Score or Edmonton Frailty Score [51]) are used to identify areas where preoperative optimization is necessary [24].

Different CGA-based models of care have been developed to improve the assessment of older surgical patients in a defined clinical pathway.

8.4.2 Day-Case Surgery

Day-case pathways are well accepted by patients, help to tackle waiting lists, and reduce service costs, [25] they offer shorter waiting times, reduced risk of hospital-acquired infection, and improved outcomes. Effective perioperative care is essential and requires accurate patient selection and the management of comorbidities; pre-emptive standardized analgesia, antiemetics, and hydration regimens to facilitate early discharge; and a proactive management plan for pre-operative issues (e.g., for patients with pre-operative chronic pain needs). Shared multidisciplinary goals of quality improvement to reduce avoidable admission rates are achieved through advancements in less invasive forms of surgical intervention, improved scheduling, enhanced nurse-led discharge protocols, implementation of a postoperative urinary retention policy, improved pain management, and prevention of pre-operative dehydration [25].

8.4.3 Emergency Care

Emergency surgical admissions account for less than 20% of all surgical admissions, yet they have a major impact on the efficient running of elective surgical services. Within the whole cohort, emergency surgery is more common in those aged 85 years or above than any other age group. As the number of pre-existing medical comorbidities and frailty also increases with age, it is not surprising that this cohort has the highest level of postoperative complications, prolonged hospital stays, and elevated mortality rates of all surgical patients [17, 52].

In emergency patients, the process of preoperative assessment and optimization is tailored to the acuity of surgical intervention. A combination of approaches is used to ensure that emergency surgical patients are directed to the appropriate teams and settings in a timely fashion: early warning scores, frailty assessment scores, delirium risk assessments, and mortality scores [48].

In the acute setting, focused and standardized strategies have been developed by emergency departments and their teams to take care of surgical geriatric patients that include prompt diagnosis; realistic risk prediction and identification of frailty; CGA; consideration of patients' wishes and avoidance of futile surgery; consideration of nonsurgical treatments; timely, consultant-delivered surgical intervention; expert perioperative and operative care; careful postoperative management and avoiding "failure to rescue"; management of comorbidities and polypharmacy; trainee and surgeon education; and audit and future research [48, 53]. Reasonable time should be given to address the wishes and concerns of the older and their families while deciding on major surgery.

The geriatric surgical equation in older persons surpasses the mere equation of "time to scan, time to surgery or length of stay." An analysis of the National Emergency Laparotomy Audit (NELA) data focused on patients older than 65 years old who underwent emergency laparotomy between 2014 and 2017 showed that mortality rate reduction correlated with increased implementation of a post-operative geriatrician review, and despite significant variation in short- and long-term outcomes for the emergency surgical population, units employing CGA-based frailty teams for emergency laparotomy patients demonstrate better outcomes [46, 54]. Unfortunately, significant variation also remains in the provision of services, and this figure remains low [55] despite the NELA-reported increase in geriatric medicine team reviews of older patients undergoing laparotomy [54].

8.5 Preoperative Management

The perioperative optimization methodology for elective surgical procedures [34] incorporates behavior change interventions, including smoking cessation, alcohol reduction, and weight management, during an important "teachable moment" before surgery. Functional deficits in activities of daily living are addressed, including medication management and mentation (or the ability of the patient to think preoperatively, which may show postoperative changes); and difficulties with mobility should be referred to an occupational or physical therapist, while appropriate measures should be taken to increase functional reserves where needed.

Examples of preoperative optimization methodology include:

- Prehabilitation, a targeted pre-operative program of physical conditioning (prehabilitation) to address nutrition, physical activity, psychological issues, and pain management, improving postoperative functional outcomes in older surgical patients [56]. Prehabilitation has been shown to be a protective strategy for postoperative complications in high-risk patients undergoing elective abdominal surgery [57], enhancing their capacity to withstand surgical stress and promote postoperative recovery.
- Cardiopulmonary exercise testing [58], to provide an individualized estimate of patient risk and optimize medical comorbidities preoperatively, and direct individualized preoperative exercise programs.
- Patient Blood Management (PBM) strategy to address anemia, including hemoglobin and iron optimization, predeposit autologous blood collection, along with surgical and anesthetic strategies that reduce blood loss [59].
- Prevention of delirium, an acute fluctuating alteration of mental state, reduced awareness, and disturbance of attention which may be triggered by acute medical illness, surgery, trauma, or drugs, by adapting surgical and anesthetic techniques, using opioid-free or low-dose opioid anesthesia and specific monitoring [23, 60]; delirium is independently linked with poor postoperative outcomes, including medical complications, falls, prolonged hospitalization; and addressing visual or hearing impairment through functional aids can significantly reduce the prevalence and duration of delirium in geriatric patients [23].

8.6 Intraoperative Management

Strategies shared between surgeons, anesthesiologists, theatre nursing, and support staff to support geriatric patients intraoperatively will include accurate patient positioning, to reduce the risk of peripheral nerve damage and pressure injuries resulting from malposition, which is increased by skin atrophy and decreased skin integrity in the older persons; individualized type and dosage of anesthesia to reduce the incidence of postoperative delirium and facilitate recovery [23]; depth of anesthesia and residual neuromuscular block monitoring, as complications related to postoperative residual curarization are more frequent in older patients than in younger patients [61]; temperature control; "near zero" fluid balance, to avoid postoperative fluid retention while preventing dehydration; and a restrictive regime for blood transfusion based on intraoperative hypoxia/lactic acidosis.

The adoption of minimally invasive surgery is encouraged whenever possible to reduce endocrine or metabolic response to stress, to promote quicker wound healing, and earlier return of bowel function and mobilization [62], though laparoscopy may also impose physical demands on older patients [63].

8.7 Postoperative Management

The process of recovery for the older patient is conceived as commencing at the time of diagnosis and proceeding as a continuum until the patient has regained a functional capacity comparable to their premorbid state and has integrated into society [64]. In fact, the possibility of postoperative debilitation and loss of independence in older persons are not obviated by lowered surgical mortality risk per se.

A consultant geriatrician-led multidisciplinary team provides ongoing care for elective patients and proactively manages emergency patients with a focus on medical complications and functional deterioration. Postoperative delirium, nausea and vomiting, pain, pulmonary and cardiovascular complications, acute kidney injury and urinary tract infection, nutrition and liquid balance, pressure ulcers, and surgical site infections are managed through shared decision-making and planning of the perioperative period including attention to treatment escalation and advanced care planning [65].

Shared multidisciplinary team care strategies include [22] joint ward rounds led by a consultant geriatrician and surgeon to promote shared clinical working and decision-making; proactive recognition of postoperative medical complications and functional decline; standardized management of medical complications; setting appropriate ceilings for escalation of care; proactive good communication between patient, caregivers, and health care professionals; weekly, geriatrician-led ward based multidisciplinary team meeting; setting of realistic patient-centered goals; promote timely discharge planning and onward referral to appropriate services after hospital discharge; re-evaluate and adjust drug therapy according to home therapy, the surgery performed, comorbidities, and any new pathological changes; and provide the patient and caregiver with resources to deal with problems that may arise at home.

Moreover, the evidence demonstrated that older patients had fewer complications and shorter hospital stays when managed within an enhanced recovery after-surgery program as compared to conventional care [66].

Enhanced recovery program (ERPs) or enhanced recovery after surgery (ERAS) initiatives, designed to expedite surgical recovery, promote optimal outcomes, and prevent prolonged postoperative hospital admissions have been adopted as part of standard care by many surgical specialties and combine organization of care and clinical management throughout the surgical patient pathway, with the aim of improving postoperative outcomes [67]. ERAS appears to be particularly effective in reducing complications and supporting recovery in older and frail patients [68]. This multidisciplinary approach provides the integration of preoperative, intraoperative, and postoperative care, and education to enable patients and families to participate in care.

Components of ERP include a focus on preoperative consent, planning and nutrition; intraoperative management including close fluid balance, maintenance of normothermia, and use of minimally invasive approaches where possible; and postoperative initiatives such as early mobilization, better postoperative pain and nausea control, prompt resumption of normal diet, innovative analgesic techniques, and proactive discharge planning [69].

8.8 Geriatrician-Led Services and MDT Meeting

Multidisciplinary team meetings are often used to review patients throughout the surgical pathway. Core elements of the geriatric MDT meeting will classically include an assimilation of information across key domains such as medical, psychiatric, cognitive, social, and functional [27]. Staff who understand their roles in the team meeting and will take responsibility for aspects of assessment or treatment [42].

Generally, a goal will be established for a patient, that might vary from simple treatment finalities (such as mobilizing independently) to complex discharge planning arrangements or longer-term functional outcomes. There should be agreed plans for short-term management to achieve these goals (such as dressing practice or cognitive assessments) and such plans should be recorded and revisited to assess progress, establish setbacks, and revisit goals. Crucially, though there needs to be interaction with the patient and their family to establish a patient's wishes and to feedback progress or manage expectations.

The MDT meeting may occur in various forms depending on settings, such as the acute admitting Geriatric Surgery wards for emergency contexts [41]. These are typically shorter and more focused and usually delivered standing up—huddled around a ward whiteboard.

Other settings such as community hospitals or community meetings may involve larger teams meeting weekly to discuss more complex cases, perhaps including general practitioners, social workers, and community rehabilitation teams.

Despite their differences in style and context, effective MDT working is underpinned by principles of skills (e.g., good leadership), processes (e.g., good governance in documenting action plans), and critical values (e.g., centrality of the patient's needs and respect for colleagues) [27]. Behavioral evidence from cancer MDTs suggests that if one of the three elements is missing, then the MDT is likely to be ineffective or dysfunctional [70].

Research suggests that such meetings need to be appropriately planned, coordinated, attended, and focus on the cases that may benefit most from multidisciplinary input, as they may help to coordinate care planning and discharge, but can be costly in terms of staff time.

8.9 Current Standards of Care

In 2016, a UK survey showed that only one-third of hospitals had medical support services for older or frail surgical patients and that the model of care in the postoperative period was made up of reactive measures, or committed after the appearance of medical problems, rather than proactive measures throughout the treatment process [22].

In many countries, there have been nationwide initiatives with published actionable plans to provide proactive multidisciplinary care to older persons. Some of the most recent, such as the "proactive care of older people undergoing surgery" [22] in the UK, the "perioperative management of older patients in Italy" [3], and the multiple implementations of the "Geriatric Surgery Quality Improvement Initiative from American College of Surgeons" [49] have all aimed at creating standards; delineating suitable infrastructure; accumulating data and validating outcomes; facilitating the multidisciplinary management of older surgical patients and enabling collaboration among all involved specialties engaged in their care (anesthesiology, geriatrics, surgical specialties, etc.); and stimulating joint studies among units, disciplines and specialties with a view to improving outcomes.

Although there has been a substantial increase in CGA-based perioperative services over the past 10 years, again there has been variable implementation due to the shortage of expertise, education and training programs, and funding [71].

8.10 Factors that Support Effective Multidisciplinary Team Working Along the Surgical Pathway

These include:

- Culture: adhesion and support from professionals and management and patient acceptance of new ways of working such as not always needing to see a surgeon or doctor for every issue [34].
- Leadership that recognizes the value of multidisciplinary care.
- Resources: system-wide funding mechanisms and resources to support multidisciplinary care [27]; protected staff time to prepare for and attend multidisciplinary team activities; coordinators, to organize multidisciplinary working and liaise between partners; technology supporting team working as online forums, virtual meeting spaces, and record sharing platforms; tools and templates to structure multidisciplinary working (meeting agendas, case presentation templates, and discharge summaries).
- Governance: scheduled joint audit meetings (e.g., morbidity and mortality meetings); joint geriatric and surgical clinical governance; development of integrated guidelines, pathways, and patient safety initiatives [25]; and routine national data collection to facilitate robust audit initiatives [71].
- Education and training: training for professionals in communication, teamwork, and use of virtual meeting technology (only the US curriculum for Geriatric

Medicine specifically encourages team training and evaluation [72]); development of national curricula and a training program aligned for perioperative medicine for older surgical patients across anesthetics, surgery and medicine; and promote joint sessions at national and international conferences [27].

8.10.1 Research

Reporting standards and accurate definitions are necessary to adequately compare the efficacy and outcomes of multidisciplinary intervention strategies: difference in aspects of the implementation of interventions limits the comparability of outcomes and estimation of efficacy of intervention: for instance, in the combination of possible interventions of prehabilitation (e.g., exercise, nutrition, psychosocial, and medical optimization), there may be no precise definition of the type of intervention or optimal dose or duration required; moreover implementation may be unimodal (addressing only one domain such as physical fitness) or multimodal (addressing additional domains such as anemia, malnutrition, smoking behavior, and psychological support) [73].

Research is also needed to assess which infrastructure and resources are needed to strengthen and sustain multidisciplinary care around the time of surgery [34].

Research studies should ensure that older people are included, with priorities clearly identified in clinical and health services research. The use of appropriate methodology including quality improvement has been encouraged, along with multi-site, cross-specialty research to address gaps in the literature pertinent to older surgical patients [34].

References

1. Alvarez P. Charted: the world's aging population from 1950 to 2100. Visual Capitalist; 2023.
2. Gaigbe-Togbe V, Bassarsky L, Gu D, et al. World population prospects 2022. New York: Department of Economic Social Affairs, Population Division, UN; 2022.
3. Aceto P, Antonelli Incalzi R, Bettelli G, et al. Perioperative Management of Elderly patients (PriME): recommendations from an Italian intersociety consensus. Aging Clin Exp Res. 2020;32:1647–73.
4. Veering BT. Management of anaesthesia in elderly patients. Curr Opin Anesthesiol. 1999;12(3):333–6.
5. Tsiachristas A, Langhorne P, Burke O, et al. Comprehensive geriatric assessment for older adults admitted to hospital. Cochrane Database Syst Rev. 2017;9:CD006211.
6. Partridge JS, Healey A, Modarai B, et al. Preoperative comprehensive geriatric assessment and optimisation prior to elective arterial vascular surgery: a health economic analysis. Age Ageing. 2021;50(5):1770–7.
7. Thillainadesan J, Yumol MF, Hilmer S, et al. Interventions to improve clinical outcomes in older adults admitted to a surgical service: a systematic review and meta-analysis. J Am Med Dir Assoc. 2020;21(12):1833–43. e20
8. Marano L, Carbone L, Poto GE, et al. Handgrip strength predicts length of hospital stay in an abdominal surgical setting: the role of frailty beyond age. Aging Clin Exp Res. 2022;34(4):811–7.

9. Preston J, Biddell B. The physiology of ageing and how these changes affect older people. Medicine. 2021;49(1):1–5.
10. Fried LP, Tangen CM, Walston J, et al. Frailty in older adults: evidence for a phenotype. J Gerontol A Biol Sci Med Sci. 2001;56(3):M146–57.
11. Hoogendijk EO, Afilalo J, Ensrud KE, et al. Frailty: implications for clinical practice and public health. Lancet. 2019;394(10206):1365–75.
12. Cunha AIL, Veronese N, de Melo BS, et al. Frailty as a predictor of adverse outcomes in hospitalized older adults: a systematic review and meta-analysis. Ageing Res Rev. 2019;56:100960.
13. Panayi A, Orkaby A, Sakthivel D, et al. Impact of frailty on outcomes in surgical patients: a systematic review and meta-analysis. Am J Surg. 2019;218(2):393–400.
14. Boccardi V, Marano L. The geriatric surgery: the importance of frailty identification beyond chronological age. Geriatrics (Basel). 2020;5(1):12.
15. Morley JE. Frailty and sarcopenia: the new geriatric giants. Rev Invest Clin. 2016;68(2):59–67.
16. Aital S. Comprehensive care for geriatric giants: multidisciplinary approaches to elderly health. J Age Geriat Psych. 2023;7(3):150.
17. Barnett K, Mercer SW, Norbury M, et al. Epidemiology of multimorbidity and implications for health care, research, and medical education: a cross-sectional study. Lancet. 2012;380(9836):37–43.
18. Martin P, Team PP. Perioperative quality improvement programme report 3: August 2019–July 2021; 2021.
19. Partridge JS, Ryan J, Dhesi JK. New guidelines for the perioperative care of people living with frailty undergoing elective and emergency surgery—a commentary. Age Ageing. 2022;51(11):afac237.
20. Parés D, Fernandez-Llamazares J. Multidisciplinary unit for the surgical management of geriatric patient. Cir Esp. 2018;96(3):129–30.
21. Grocott MP, Mythen MG. Perioperative medicine: the value proposition for anesthesia?: a UK perspective on delivering value from anesthesiology. Anesthesiol Clin. 2015;33(4):617–28.
22. Partridge J, Sbai M, Dhesi J. Proactive care of older people undergoing surgery. Aging Clin Exp Res. 2018;30(3):253–7.
23. Mohanty S, Rosenthal R, Russell M, et al. Optimal perioperative management of the geriatric patient: best practices guideline from ACS NSQIP®/American Geriatrics Society. J Am Coll Surg. 2016;222(5):930–47.
24. Chow W, Rosenthal R, Merkow R, et al. American College of Surgeons National Surgical Quality Improvement Program; American Geriatrics Society. Optimal preoperative assessment of the geriatric surgical patient: a best practices guideline from the American College of Surgeons National Surgical Quality Improvement Program and the American Geriatrics Society. J Am Coll Surg. 2012;215(4):453–66.
25. Boccardi V, Marano L. Improving geriatric outcomes through nutritional and immunonutritional strategies: focus on surgical setting by a comprehensive evidence review. Ageing Res Rev. 2024;96:102272.
26. Tan K-Y, Tan P, Tan L. A collaborative transdisciplinary "geriatric surgery service" ensures consistent successful outcomes in elderly colorectal surgery patients. World J Surg. 2011;35:1608–14.
27. Ellis G, Sevdalis N. Understanding and improving multidisciplinary team working in geriatric medicine. Age Ageing. 2019;48(4):498–505.
28. Salas E, Sims DE, Burke CS. Is there a "big five" in teamwork? Small Group Res. 2005;36(5):555–99.
29. Maynard MT, Gilson LL. The role of shared mental model development in understanding virtual team effectiveness. Group Org Manag. 2014;39(1):3–32.
30. Johnsen BH, Espevik R, Eid J, et al. Coordinating mechanisms are more important than team processes for geographically dispersed emergency dispatch and paramedic teams. Front Psychol. 2022;13:754855.
31. Martin AK, Green TL, McCarthy AL, et al. Healthcare teams: terminology, confusion, and ramifications. J Multidiscip Healthc. 2022;15:765–72.

32. Tan K-Y. Integrative transdisciplinary care of elderly surgical patients. In: Transdisciplinary perioperative care in colorectal surgery: an integrative approach. Springer; 2014. p. 13–27.
33. Schoenfeld AJ, Sturgeon DJ, Blucher JA, et al. Alterations in 90-day morbidity, mortality, and readmission rates following spine surgery in Medicare accountable care organizations (2009–2014). Spine J. 2019;19(1):8–14.
34. Selwyn D, Multidisciplinary working in perioperative care, Care CfP, Editor. 2020, CPOC.
35. Aggarwal P, Woolford SJ, Patel HP. Multi-morbidity and polypharmacy in older people: challenges and opportunities for clinical practice. Geriatrics. 2020;5(4):85.
36. Saripella A, Wasef S, Nagappa M, et al. Effects of comprehensive geriatric care models on postoperative outcomes in geriatric surgical patients: a systematic review and meta-analysis. BMC Anesthesiol. 2021;21:1–11.
37. Society AG. Summary of the updated American Geriatrics Society/British geriatrics society clinical practice guideline for prevention of falls in older persons. J Am Geriatr Soc. 2011;59(1):148.
38. Lee TH, Marcantonio ER, Mangione CM, et al. Derivation and prospective validation of a simple index for prediction of cardiac risk of major noncardiac surgery. Circulation. 1999;100(10):1043–9.
39. Claus CC, Staekenborg SS, Verweij KH, et al. The clock drawing test is an important contribution to the Mini Mental State Examination in screening for cognitive impairment. Int J Geriatr Psychiatry. 2023;38(4):e5914.
40. UK NGC. Evidence review for preoperative optimisation clinics in older adults; 2020.
41. Marano L, Marmorino F, Desideri I, et al. Clinical nutrition in surgical oncology: young AIOM-AIRO-SICO multidisciplinary national survey on behalf of NutriOnc research group. Front Nutr. 2023;10:1045022.
42. Stuck AE, Siu AL, Wieland GD, et al. Comprehensive geriatric assessment: a meta-analysis of controlled trials. Lancet. 1993;342(8878):1032–6.
43. Partridge JSL, Harari D, Martin F, et al. The impact of pre-operative comprehensive geriatric assessment on postoperative outcomes in older patients undergoing scheduled surgery: a systematic review. Anaesthesia. 2014;69:8–16.
44. Partridge J, Harari D, Martin F, et al. Randomized clinical trial of comprehensive geriatric assessment and optimization in vascular surgery. J Br Surg. 2017;104(6):679–87.
45. McIsaac DI, Huang A, Wong CA, et al. Effect of preoperative geriatric evaluation on outcomes after elective surgery: a population-based study. J Am Geriatr Soc. 2017;65(12):2665–72.
46. Eamer G, Taheri A, Chen SS, et al. Comprehensive geriatric assessment for older people admitted to a surgical service. Cochrane Database Syst Rev. 2018;1:CD012485.
47. Chen Z, Ding Z, Chen C, et al. Effectiveness of comprehensive geriatric assessment intervention on quality of life, caregiver burden and length of hospital stay: a systematic review and meta-analysis of randomised controlled trials. BMC Geriatr. 2021;21:1–14.
48. De Simone B, Dhesi JK, Hoffman MR, et al. Geriatric surgical patients: is it possible to implement the comprehensive geriatric assessment in the emergency setting? Discov Health Sys. 2023;2(1):13.
49. Chow WB, Rosenthal RA, Merkow RP, et al. Optimal preoperative assessment of the geriatric surgical patient: a best practices guideline from the American College of Surgeons National Surgical Quality Improvement Program and the American Geriatrics Society. J Am Coll Surg. 2012;215(4):453–66.
50. Parker SG, McCue P, Phelps K, et al. What is comprehensive geriatric assessment (CGA)? An umbrella review. Age Ageing. 2018;47(1):149–55.
51. Rolfson DB, Majumdar SR, Tsuyuki RT, et al. Validity and reliability of the Edmonton frail scale. Age Ageing. 2006;35(5):526–9.
52. De Felice F, Cattaneo CG, Poto GE, et al. Mapping the landscape of immunonutrition and cancer research: a comprehensive bibliometric analysis on behalf of NutriOnc research group. Int J Surg. 2024;110(1):395–405.
53. Torrance AD, Powell SL, Griffiths EA. Emergency surgery in the elderly: challenges and solutions. Open Access Emerg Med. 2015;7:55–68.

54. Aitken RM, Partridge JS, Oliver CM, et al. Older patients undergoing emergency laparotomy: observations from the National Emergency Laparotomy Audit (NELA) years 1–4. Age Ageing. 2020;49(4):656–63.
55. NHS England Ss, Schedule 2–the services. NHS England, Service specifications; 2021. Available online: https://www.england.nhs.uk/wp-content/uploads//07/thoracic-surgery-servicespecification.pdf.
56. Thomas G, Tahir MR, Bongers BC, et al. Prehabilitation before major intra-abdominal cancer surgery: a systematic review of randomised controlled trials. Eur J Anaesthesiol. 2019;36(12):933–45.
57. Souwer E, Bastiaannet E, de Bruijn S, et al. Comprehensive multidisciplinary care program for elderly colorectal cancer patients: "From Prehabilitation to Independence". Eur J Surg Oncol. 2019;45(2):e21.
58. Levett D, Jack S, Swart M, et al. Perioperative cardiopulmonary exercise testing (CPET): consensus clinical guidelines on indications, organization, conduct, and physiological interpretation. Br J Anaesth. 2018;120(3):484–500.
59. Franchini M, Marano G, Veropalumbo E, et al. Patient blood management: a revolutionary approach to transfusion medicine. Blood Transfus. 2019;17(3):191.
60. Association AP. Diagnostic and statistical manual of mental disorders. Text revision; 2000.
61. Aceto P, Lai C, Perilli V, et al. Stress-related biomarkers of dream recall and implicit memory under anaesthesia. Anaesthesia. 2013;68(11):1141–7.
62. Zhou S, Wang X, Zhao C, et al. Laparoscopic vs open colorectal cancer surgery in elderly patients: short-and long-term outcomes and predictors for overall and disease-free survival. BMC Surg. 2019;19:1–8.
63. Bates AT, Divino C. Laparoscopic surgery in the elderly: a review of the literature. Aging Clin Exp Res. 2015;6(2):149.
64. Tan KY. Geriatric surgery service-our journey piloting in colorectal surgery and future challenges. Ann Acad Med Singap. 2017;46:317–20.
65. Robinson TN, Walston JD, Brummel NE, et al. Frailty for surgeons: review of a national institute on aging conference on frailty for specialists. J Am Coll Surg. 2015;221(6):1083–92.
66. Bagnall N, Malietzis G, Kennedy R, et al. A systematic review of enhanced recovery care after colorectal surgery in elderly patients. Color Dis. 2014;16(12):947–56.
67. Ljungqvist O, Scott M, Fearon KC. Enhanced recovery after surgery: a review. JAMA Surg. 2017;152(3):292–8.
68. Ljungqvist O, Hubner M. Enhanced recovery after surgery—ERAS—principles, practice and feasibility in the elderly. Aging Clin Exp Res. 2018;30:249–52.
69. Dhesi J, Partridge J. Peri-operative care for older patients undergoing surgery. Br Geriatr Soc. 2013;
70. Lamb B, Taylor C, Lamb J, et al. Facilitators and barriers to teamworking and patient centeredness in multidisciplinary cancer teams: findings of a national study. Ann Surg Oncol. 2013;20:1408–16.
71. Joughin AL, Partridge JS, O'Halloran T, et al. Where are we now in perioperative medicine? Results from a repeated UK survey of geriatric medicine delivered services for older people. Age Ageing. 2019;48(3):458–62.
72. Partnership for Health in Aging Workgroup on Interdisciplinary Team Training in Geriatrics. Position statement on interdisciplinary team training in geriatrics: an essential component of quality health care for older adults. J Am Geriatr Soc. 2014;62(5):961–5.
73. Beilstein CM, Krutkyte G, Vetsch T, et al. Multimodal prehabilitation for major surgery in elderly patients to lower complications: protocol of a randomised, prospective, multicentre, multidisciplinary trial (PREHABIL trial). BMJ Open. 2023;13(1):e070253.

Part II

Pre-operative Management

Multidimensional Prognostic Index in Surgery: A Clinical Perspective

9

Luisa Solimando, Wanda Morganti, Nicola Veronese,
Mario Barbagallo, and Alberto Pilotto

9.1 The Comprehensive Geriatric Assessment: The Cornerstone of Geriatric Medicine

The Comprehensive Geriatric Assessment (CGA) is defined as a diagnostic and therapeutic process that identifies the medical, psychosocial, and functional capabilities of older people, in order to develop and carry out a coordinated and integrated management plan. The most important aims of the CGA are to understand the relationship between the various domains typical of older persons, and define a therapeutic and care path that tends toward the correct rehabilitation and maintenance of the older person's self-sufficiency.

To reach this objective, CGA often uses a multidisciplinary team that intercepts the needs of the older person with the use of standardized clinimetric assessment tools, emphasizes the functions of the person, and develops a personalized care plan with the final objective of guaranteeing a good quality of life as much as possible. A recent umbrella review critically examined the most common definitions of CGA, and reported the most frequently explored domains that are included in a standard CGA [1]:

L. Solimando · N. Veronese · M. Barbagallo
Department of Internal Medicine and Geriatrics, University of Palermo, Palermo, Italy
e-mail: nicola.veronese@unipa.it; mario.barbagallo@unipa.it

W. Morganti
Department of Geriatric Care, Neurology and Rehabilitation, Galliera Hospitals, Genoa, Italy
e-mail: wanda.morganti@galliera.it

A. Pilotto (✉)
Department of Geriatric Care, Neurology and Rehabilitation, Galliera Hospitals, Genoa, Italy

Department of Interdisciplinary Medicine, "Aldo Moro" University of Bari, Bari, Italy
e-mail: alberto.pilotto@galliera.it

V. Boccardi, L. Marano (eds.), *The Frail Surgical Patient*, Practical Issues in Geriatrics, https://doi.org/10.1007/978-3-031-77707-3_9

- Medical
- Physical
- Psychological/psychiatric
- Socioeconomic
- Function
- Nutrition

During the last three decades several studies, including randomized clinical trials (RCT), and observational retrospective and longitudinal studies demonstrated a clear and significant efficacy of the CGA in improving several outcomes in different healthcare settings and clinical conditions [2].

A recent umbrella review of 1683 papers, 31 systematic reviews (19 with meta-analysis) including almost 280,000 older subjects confirmed these findings and specifically in the nonorthopedic surgery setting reported that CGA intervention significantly reduced mortality at 12 months, time to surgery, delirium insurgence, and length of hospital stay (in days). Moreover, in older patients with hip fractures who underwent surgical orthopedic treatment, the CGA-based intervention was significantly effective in improving mobility and the Activities of Daily Living (ADL) as well as in reducing delirium and short-term mortality [3] (see Table 9.1).

9.2 The Multidimensional Prognostic Index (MPI): A CGA-Based Prognostic Tool for Clinical Decision-Making

Recently the role of the CGA in defining the individual prognosis as a crucial step for the appropriate clinical decision-making emerged as an important topic in geriatric medicine. Indeed, because of competing chronic conditions and diminished life expectancy, the prognosis is particularly important for clinical decision-making in older patients. For both patients and caregivers, prognostic information, in fact, is needed to inform decisions concerning clinical management, discharge plan, and follow-up.

Many studies reported that the strongest predictors of mortality and other negative outcomes (hospitalization and institutionalization) in older people include comorbidity and functional status. Thus, validated and rigorously assessed for generalizability, accuracy, and potential bias indices that predict mortality for older persons are needed to align the metric to assess the prognosis with the recommendations in clinical guidelines, likely facilitating clinical decision-making [4].

In this context, the Multidimensional Prognostic Index (MPI) [5] is a CGA-based prognostic tool, widely validated in older people, including patients undergoing surgery, highly accurate in predicting several negative events, i.e., mortality, hospitalization, institutionalization, and length of hospital stay [6].

The MPI was initially developed and validated in hospitalized older people. The standard version of the MPI is calculated through a mathematical algorithm that includes information relating to 8 domains [5] as follows:

Table 9.1 Summary of findings of the studies included in the umbrella review pertaining to surgery and orthopedics settings

Participants (Studies)	Study event rates (%)		Relative effect (95% CI)	Anticipated absolute effect		Overall certainty of evidence
	With usual/ standard care	With CGA		Risk with usual/ standard care	Risk difference with CGA	
Surgery setting						
Mortality at 12 months in older adults in surgical ward (emergency surgery)						
4458 (4 RCTs)	523/2932 (17.8%)	206/1526 (13.5%)	RR 0.70 (0.54 to 0.90)	178 per 1000	54 fewer per 1000 (from 82 fewer to 18 fewer)	MODERATE
Reduction in time to surgery in older adults in surgical ward (emergency surgery)						
1107 (3 RCTs)	252/536 (47.0%)	390/571 (68.3%)	RR 0.60 (0.50 to 0.73)	470 per 1000	188 fewer per 1000 (from 235 fewer to 127 fewer)	LOW
Delirium in older adults hospitalized under nonorthopedic surgical teams for operative or nonoperative management						
1139 (5 RCTs)	90/536 (16.8%)	49/603 (8.1%)	RR 0.52 (0.37 to 0.92)	168 per 1000	81 fewer per 1000 (from 106 fewer to 13 fewer)	MODERATE
Length of stay (days) in older adults hospitalized under nonorthopedic surgical teams for operative or nonoperative management						
617 (3 RCTs)	264	353	–	–	MD 1.98 days lower (3.09 lower to 0.88 lower)	MODERATE
Orthopedics setting						
Mobility in older adults with hip fracture trauma						
982 (6 RCTs)	495	487	–	–	SMD 0.32 SD higher (0.12 higher to 0.52 higher)	MODERATE
Delirium in older adults with hip fracture trauma						
1443 (6 RCTs)	313/667 (46.9%)	283/776 (36.5%)	OR 0.71 (0.54 to 0.92)	469 per 1000	84 fewer per 1000 (from 146 fewer to 21 fewer)	HIGH
ADL in older adults with hip fracture trauma						

(continued)

Table 9.1 (continued)

Participants (Studies)	Study event rates (%)		Relative effect (95% CI)	Anticipated absolute effect		Overall certainty of evidence
	With usual/ standard care	With CGA		Risk with usual/ standard care	Risk difference with CGA	
1291 (5 RCTs)	648	643	–	–	SMD 0.26 SD higher (0.04 higher to 0.49 higher)	VERY LOW
Mortality in older adults with hip fracture trauma						
2088 (8 RCTs)	125/1047 (11.9%)	91/1041 (8.7%)	OR 0.73 (0.54 to 0.98)	119 per 1000	29 fewer per 1000 (from 51 fewer to 2 fewer)	LOW

Note: *CI* confidence interval, *RR* risk ratio, *MD* mean difference, *SMD* standardized mean difference, *OR* odds ratio

1. Activities of Daily Living (ADL)
2. Instrumental Activities of Daily Living (IADL)
3. Short Portable Mental Status Questionnaire (SPMSQ)
4. Mini-Nutritional Assessment—Short Form (MNA-SF)
5. Exton-Smith Scale (ESS)
6. Cumulative Illness Rating Scale—Comorbidity Index (CIRS-CI)
7. Number of drugs
8. Co-habitation status: in family, in institution, and alone

The risk category scores associated with each domain must be summed and then divided by the number of completed domains (at least 6) obtaining an MPI total value between 0 and 1: higher scores reflect a higher risk of mortality (see Table 9.2). For clinical reasons, three grades of MPI are identified: low risk, 0.0–0.33; moderate risk, 0.34–0.66; and severe risk, 0.67–1.0 [5]. In hospitalized older patients affected by the most frequent diseases, the MPI proved to be an accurate predictor of in-hospital mortality as well as mortality likelihood after 1 month, 6 months, and 12 months from the hospital discharge. Moreover, the MPI was able to predict the length of hospital stays [7]. The MPI also has clinimetric properties, i.e., it could be expressed using a number that is sensitive to clinical interventions or clinically relevant changes. Other important characteristics of the MPI are [8]:

- Accuracy/calibration: internal validity [5].
- Generalizability: multicenter validation including different geriatrics settings [9, 10].
- Comparability with other mortality (frailty) indices [11].
- Sensitivity to variation of subjects during time (clinimetric property) [12].
- Reliability and feasibility in clinical practice [13].

Table 9.2 Multidimensional prognostic index: composition and scores computation

Questionnaires	Low risk (Score = 0)	Medium risk (Score = 0.5)	High risk (Score = 1)
ADL	6–5	4–3	2–0
IADL	8–6	5–4	3–0
SPMSQ	0–3	4–7	8–10
MNA-SF	12–14	8–11	0–7
ESS	16–20	10–15	5–9
CIRS-CI	0	1–2	≥3
Number of drugs	0–3	4–6	≥7
Co-habitation	Living with family	Institutionalized	Living alone
Add up the scores assigned to each domain, and then divide by the number of completed domains (≥6)		**Total score MPI**	

RISK	Mild (MPI 1)	Moderate (MPI 2)	Severe (MPI 3)
RANGE	0.00–0.33	0.34–0.66	0.67–1.00

- It can be used as an outcome measure in RCT of older patients [14].
- Plasticity: several versions of MPI have been developed and validated for being used in different clinical settings, i.e., (a) the SVaMA-MPI, for older people who undergo a CGA for admission to nursing home or homecare services [15]; (b) the brief-MPI, a short version used in general practice/primary care [16] as well as in emergency departments; and (c) the Selfy-MPI, a self-administered version of the MPI as a screening tool at the population level and in primary care [17]; the TELE-MPI is a useful tool for clinical telemedicine visits [18], etc. (see Table 9.3).

Finally, the MPI showed potential usefulness in clinical decision-making [8]. Indeed, different studies explored the role of the MPI as a prognostic tool and its role in clinical decision-making especially in "undefined" topics of pharmacological treatments of older frail people such as the use of statins in secondary prevention of diabetes mellitus and coronary artery disease, or antidementia drugs in older patients with Alzheimer Disease, the use of anticoagulants in atrial fibrillation or the enteral nutrition in malnourished hospitalized older patients and many other clinical conditions [19, 20].

9.3 CGA and MPI in Surgical Older Patients

Risk scores commonly used for surgical patients (i.e., ASA, APACHE, P-POSSUM) have substantial limitations when applied to older patients. Indeed, most of the risk scores have been standardized on adult target populations; and frequently they consider one single organ function at a time and not the overall functional reserve of the older people according to a multidimensional comprehensive clinical approach [2].

The growing interest in the topic of the multidimensional approach to the older surgical patient is obviously given by the increase in the mean age of the population,

Table 9.3 Multidimensional prognostic index versions

MPI Version	Contexts of administration	Variables	Reference
MPI—Hospital version	Hospitalized older people	ADL, IADL, SPMSQ, MNA-SF, ESS, CIRS-CI, number of drugs, and co-habitation	Pilotto et al., 2008 [5]
MPI—Outpatient version	Outpatient older people (general practice or specialists' clinics)	ADL, IADL, SPMSQ,, MNA-SF, Barthel MOB, CIRS-CI, number of drugs, and co-habitation	Gallucci et al., 2013 [61]
Selfy-MPI	Self-administered version for community-dwelling older people	ADL, Barthel MOB, IADL, TYM, MNA-SF, number of drugs, CIRS-CI, and Gijon social-familial evaluation scale (SFES)	Pilotto et al., 2019 [17]
Selfy-MPI-SF	Self-administered shorter version for community-dwelling older people	Modified versions of: Barthel ADL, IADL, Barthel MOB, TYM test, MNA-SF, CIRS-CI, number of drugs, and co-habitation	Cella et al., 2020 [62]
Brief-MPI	Shorter version for emergency contexts and general practice/primary care	ADL, IADL, SPMSQ, Barthel MOB, MNA-SF, CIRS-CI, number of drugs, and co-habitation	Cella et al., 2022 [16]
Selfy-brief-MPI	Self-administered screening at population level	ADL, IADL, mobility based on MPI InChianti, CCI, MNA-SF, CIRS-CI, number of drugs, and co-habitation	Morganti et al., 2023 [63]
TELE-MPI	Remote administration to older people	ADL, IADL, Barthel MOB, SPMSQ, MNA-SF, CIRS-CI, number of drugs, and co-habitation	Custodero et al., 2021 [18]
MPI—SvaMA standardized multidimensional assessment schedule	Community-dwelling older people's evaluation for admission to nursing home or homecare services	Age, sex, main diagnosis, nursing care needs, SPMSQ, ESS, ADL, Barthel MOB, and social support	Pilotto et al., 2013 [15]
ONCO-MPI	Oncological settings	Age, sex, ADL, IADL, ECOG performance status, MMSE, BMI, CIRS-CI, number of drugs, the presence of caregiver, cancer sites, and cancer stages	Brunello et al., 2016 [46]

ADL Activities of Daily Living, *IADL* Instrumental Activities of Daily Living, *SPMSQ* Short Portable Mental State Questionnaire, *MNA-SF* Mini Nutritional Assessment—Short Form, *ESS* Exton Smith Scale, *CIRS-CI* Cumulative Illness Rating Scale—Comorbidity Index, *Barthel MOB* Barthel Mobility Index, *TYM test* Test Your Memory test, *CCI* Cognitive Change Index, *ECOG* Eastern Cooperative Oncology Group performance status, *MMSE* Mini-Mental State Examination, *BMI* Body Mass Index with consequently an increasing number of multimorbid older people who are candidates for a surgical operation. It is recognized that aging is a risk factor for functional decline and chronic conditions and consequently older adults who undergo surgical interventions are at higher risk for postoperative complications, prolonged hospitalization, increased dependency or institutionalization, and finally mortality after surgery than young or adult subjects [21, 22]. However, the great heterogeneity of the older population suggests that a CGA approach could be very useful to discriminate the specific individual risk independently from a chronological age view. For example, a 90-year-old patient with an active lifestyle could be fitter than a younger, overweight, sedentary, and multimorbid patient [23].

9.3.1 Orthogeriatrics

A high proportion of patients with osteoporotic fractures, mainly hip fractures, have a variable degree of comorbidities and dependence on ADL [24]. In recent years, this topic has become so popular that many researchers focused on finding prognostic scores capable of determining outcomes like mortality and rehospitalization in patients with hip fractures.

Specifically, frailty, which appears widespread in patients with hip fractures, can raise the risk of mortality and morbidity post-surgery [25, 26]. For the purpose of predicting various clinical outcomes in elderly patients with hip fractures, numerous multidimensional frailty indices, including the MPI, have recently been studied and validated [26, 27].

A recent study [27] demonstrates that MPI is associated with short- and long-term mortality and hospital readmission rates in a large cohort of older patients undergoing surgery for hip fracture. Moreover, the MPI was an excellent predictor of other clinical negative events such as respiratory failure, exacerbation of heart failure, and transfusions both in the pre-operative phase and after surgery. These findings are particularly relevant since older patients undergoing surgery for hip fracture are at very high risk for post-surgery complications like infections, malnutrition, bedsores, and loss of muscle mass [27].

Another critical point in older patients with hip fractures is the management of both pre- and postoperative delirium [28]. A recent study showed that the CGA-based MPI, carried out at hospital admission, was a sensitive tool to identify subjects at risk of developing pre-operative delirium; this finding suggests that an early CGA with the calculation of the MPI could represent a crucial step toward individualized decision-making [29].

9.3.2 Cardio-Surgery: The Case of Trans-Catheter Valve Implantation

Another field of application of the CGA-based MPI is clinical decision-making in older patients with aortic and/or mitral valve diseases who are candidates for a valve replacement through a traditional surgical operation or a Transcatheter Aortic Valve Implantation (TAVI).

According to two multicenter investigations, older patients' chances of dying or of a composite risk of mortality and/or nonfatal stroke 1 year after TAVI could be predicted with the MPI [30, 31].

A study from Germany [32] demonstrated that the MPI was useful in predicting the likelihood of procedural success and risk of all-cause mortality at 30-day and 6 months after intervention in 226 people (129 males; median age = 78 years), undergoing percutaneous mitral or tricuspid valve repair procedures (87% using edge-to-edge clips). The MPI was assessed 1-day pre-procedure and 47% of the sample was classified in the moderate (MPI class 2) and high-risk (MPI class 3) categories. Procedural success was 86% and complication rates were low irrespective of frailty status, although frailer patients spent an average of 2.5 more days in hospital post-intervention. Surprisingly, 1.5-month changes in 6-minute walk distance and health-related quality of life were modest and also not influenced by frailty status, with trends actually favoring greater improvements in frailer patients. Finally, the primary outcome of 6-month mortality was 7% in the MPI-2 and MPI-3 classes versus 1% in the low-risk MPI-1 category, corresponding to a multivariable-adjusted hazard ratio of 2.05 (1.40–2.99) per 1-SD increase in MPI score when represented as a continuous variable.

Another study from the Netherlands [33] explored the effectiveness of the MPI in predicting negative outcomes in 376 older patients who underwent a TAVI: 143 (38.0%) patients belonged to the MPI-1 group and 233 (61.9%) patients to the MPI-2–3 group. After 3 years of follow-up, 15% of the patients in the MPI-1 group and 31% of the patients in the MPI-2–3 group died ($p = 0.001$). Patients in MPI-1 had increased chances of overall survival in comparison with patients in MPI groups 2–3 (hazard ratio 0.57, 95% confidence interval 0.33–0.98). These results corroborate the idea that the MPI tool can be used to identify which patients are more likely to benefit long term from a TAVI operation and to evaluate frailty.

The key takeaway is that positive patient-centered outcomes are determined by much more than just the technical success of the procedure, notably the geriatric profile of the patient is to be considered as well. As shown in this study, the first step forward is to assess frailty using objective multidimensional tools and to discourage the binary frail/nonfrail labels in favor of a granular spectrum of frailty severity and treatable domains [34].

9.3.3 Onco-MPI

The use of CGA became clinically useful also in oncological settings. Indeed, CGA can help clinicians, patients, and their caregivers in the choice of the best personalized treatment (e.g., chemotherapy versus surgical intervention). Recent guidelines by the American Society of Clinical Oncology (ASCO) strongly recommend a minimum core of geriatric assessment based on the evaluation of function, comorbidity, falls, depression, cognition, and nutrition in all patients who are candidates for oncological treatments [35].

The CGA may help the management of older individuals with cancer in at least three areas: a) detection of frailty; b) facilitating the choice of the personalized treatment strategy; and c) removal of social barriers to treatment [36].

Recently several studies reported the usefulness of CGA in improving the appropriateness and efficacy of treatments in oncological patients [37–40]. Most of the oncological and hematological treatments are established on the basis of the performance status (PS) evaluation, according to the World Health Organization (WHO) scale or to the Eastern Cooperative Oncology Group (ECOG), this approach may not be enough to correctly evaluate an elderly patient, as the severity of co-morbidities and frailty may not directly correlate with PS alteration [41].

The MPI based on a CGA has been validated in independent cohorts of older patients with cancer demonstrating very good accuracy in predicting one-year mortality and other negative outcomes [42–45]. Interestingly, a cancer-specific modified MPI (Onco-MPI) for mortality prediction of older cancer patients has been developed and validated, including cancer site and staging in the algorithm to calculate the total index [46]. Onco-MPI appears to be a highly accurate and well-calibrated predictive tool for one-year mortality in older cancer patients [10, 47].

9.3.4 Gastrointestinal and Liver Diseases

Another application in surgery could be the prognostic evaluation of patients with upper gastrointestinal bleedings in which the Blatchford score and Rockall score are commonly used. These scores are useful for establishing the need to surgically treat bleeding and estimating the severity of these pathologies, however, these scales exclude some other relevant information regarding older people's general health status and preserved abilities. In fact, upper gastrointestinal bleedings are frequently associated with a wide range of other illnesses and age-related disorders which further complicate the possibilities for a diagnosis and care options and underscore the importance of the comprehensive assessment approach [48]. The MPI demonstrated highly significant predictive efficacy in predicting mortality over a 24-month follow-up period in elderly patients with upper gastrointestinal bleeding [48]. Moreover, the MPI has been demonstrated to be a more reliable predictive tool of mortality than organ-specific measures in older patients with upper gastrointestinal bleeding undergoing acute surgery [49].

The prognosis of older patients with liver disease also may be influenced by a combination of biological, functional, pathological, and environmental factors. Indeed, several tools that effectively identify high-risk patients have been described, but none of these used a multidimensional approach.

For example, the Child-Pugh score is widely accepted and validated as a grading system for determining the prognosis of patients with cirrhosis and esophageal varices [50] and, although it was originally used to predict mortality during surgery, it is now used to determine the prognosis, as well as the required strength of treatment and the necessity of liver transplantation. The score employs five clinical measures of liver disease (encephalopathy, ascites, bilirubin, albumin, and INR).

In order to evaluate the prognostic usefulness of the CGA-based MPI, a study of older patients (mean age of 75.6 ± 6.4 years, ranging from 65 to 92 years) discharged from the hospital with a diagnosis of liver cirrhosis reported that higher MPI grades were significantly associated with progressively higher mortality rates both after 1-month ($p < 0.0001$) and 1-year (MPI $p = 0.002$) of follow-up. Adjusting for age and sex, the prognostic value of the MPI for mortality was confirmed and was highly significant both at 1 month (OR = 10.561, 95% CI = 2.56–43.6, $p < 0.001$) and 1 year (OR = 1.904 95% CI = 1.16–3.12, $p < 0.01$).

Interestingly, in this study the prognostic accuracy of the Child-Pugh score and the MPI was compared revealing that the MPI's area under the ROC curve was significantly higher than the area under the ROC curve for the Child-Pugh score (respectively, AUC = 0.90, 95% CI 0.85–0.96 vs AUC = 0.70, 95% CI 0.52–0.88, $p = 0.03$) suggesting that in this population of older patients, MPI had a significant greater discriminatory power than the Child-Pugh score [51].

Another example of a single-domain prognostic tool is represented by the Model for End- Stage Liver Disease (MELD) score [52] which was initially developed to predict survival in patients with complications of portal hypertension; now, it is the standard on which most decisions regarding liver transplantations are made. Very recently, in the population of older adults waiting for liver transplants, the MPI has proven to be a reliable prognostic tool, specifically identifying appropriate nutritional status and male sex as protective factors and BMI scores and functional impairments as risk factors [53].

9.4 The Impact of CGA in the Perioperative Period: Changes in Tailoring the Pre-operative and Post-operative Paths

A systematic review showed that the activation of a CGA-based pro-active care of older people undergoing surgery (POPS) team that consisted of a consultant geriatrician, clinical nurse specialist, occupational therapist, physiotherapist, and social worker was more effective in reducing medical complications (i.e., pneumonia, delirium, pressure sores, inadequate analgesia, delay to mobilization, and inappropriate catheter use) compared with a classic preoperative care group [54].

Assessment can be carried out during a consultation, or in a day hospital separate from surgical intervention, to avoid the impact of an operation on the patient's basic condition [55]. The goals of this assessment are multiple: to detect anomalies or other comorbidities not identified in clinical history, to predict severe toxicities associated with treatments, and to help determine their type and intensity [56]. Indeed, the CGA helps to identify patient profiles, paving the way for appropriate treatment.

For example, the FRAGIS study [44], an Italian multicentric cohort study, evaluated the usefulness of carrying out the MPI before the intervention and the impact of multidimensional frailty in predicting the main adverse outcomes.

Categorizing "frail" individuals in MPI-2 and 3 categories, and "fit" those in MPI-1, no significant differences were found in the surgical approach, but several peri- and post-operative outcomes appeared to be influenced by frailty:

- The hospital stay after surgery was significantly longer among frail patients (13 vs. 8.5 days).
- Postoperative mortality was significantly higher among frail patients.
- A sixfold higher risk of complications can be observed in frail patients (MPI class 2–3).

In conclusion, CGA in surgical settings could be usefully carried out at different time points. Before surgery, CGA can identify potential risk factors for poor outcomes and aid clinical decision-making on both pre-habilitation interventions and on preventively establishing the most appropriate treatment for the patient (i.e., for frailer patients less invasive surgery or a conservative treatment should be preferred over demolition surgery). Moreover, this preliminary evaluation could have a positive impact on different outcomes such as delirium, mortality, and length of hospital stay. In fact, delirium, which is a syndrome of acute change in cognition and alertness, frequently associated with psychotic behavior, often occurs in surgical settings as a complication in hospitalized older adults [57]. Higher MPI grade (MPI-3) was independently associated with a higher risk of pre-operative delirium (OR 2.45, CI 1.21–4.96) [29], making the MPI a helpful tool for preventing the negative outcomes associated with delirium such as greater need for care, a longer hospital stay, and a greater probability of institutionalization and death [58].

In peri-operative settings, a CGA approach is crucial for the implementation of a tailored treatment program focusing on the defective detected domains. Using CGA-based tools like the MPI, the probable improvement can also be gauged and measured thanks to its clinimetric property. Finally, the follow-up monitoring can be easily carried out relying on instruments like the MPI which offers comparable scores among the different assessments made and can show the treatment trends in the main patients' life domains.

9.5 The Italian Guideline on the Comprehensive Geriatric Assessment of the Older Person

Recently, the Italian General Practitioners/Primary Care (SIMG) and Geriatrics Hospital-Community (SIGOT) Societies together with the Italian National Health Institute and a panel of experts belonging to 25 Scientific Societies have drawn the first Guideline on the CGA of older persons [59, 60]. The main aim of the guideline was to develop clinical and research recommendations on the efficacy of CGA and the utility of CGA-based prognostic tools, based on an extensive review of the literature. More than 20.000 records were retrieved to issue 16 recommendations on the efficacy of CGA and 9 on CGA-based prognostic tools. The recommendations are divided according to the different clinical settings considered: general practice and primary care, medical and surgical clinics, emergency departments, hospital medical and surgical wards, long-term care facilities and nursing homes, hospices, and palliative care networks. Ultimately, a CGA approach can reduce a series of outcomes like hospitalization, mortality, and institutionalization. Regarding CGA-based tools, the MPI appears the more widely applicable tool to predict negative outcomes across different settings.

The following clinical recommendations for surgical settings were drawn:

(i) Using comprehensive geriatric assessment is suggested to reduce the length of stay in older people referred to specialist surgical outpatient clinics.
(ii) Using comprehensive geriatric assessment is suggested to reduce the incidence of post-operative delirium in older people referred to specialist surgical outpatient clinics.
(iii) Using comprehensive geriatric assessment is recommended to reduce the incidence of delirium in older people admitted to orthogeriatric wards and referred to surgical wards.
(iv) Using comprehensive geriatric assessment is not recommended for the sole purpose of reducing mortality or institutionalization rates in nursing homes or re-hospitalization rate in older people admitted to orthogeriatric and in surgical hospital wards.

    Furthermore, for the CGA-based prognostic tools in surgical setting, an important recommendation was made:
(v) Using comprehensive geriatric assessment, through the Multidimensional Prognostic Index (MPI), is suggested to predict post-operative complications in older people with colorectal cancer referred to specialist surgical outpatient clinics.

This work [60] represents a groundbreaking milestone for the specific assessment of older adults; however, it needs more time for dissemination and implementation together with the conduction of further studies to cover the unexplored areas (such as the palliative care network).

9.6 Conclusions

The CGA is a comprehensive strategy that can be used to reduce unfavorable health outcomes in surgical settings, provide tailored, interdisciplinary care plans, and address the needs of older patients having surgery.

Despite the benefits of performing a CGA, this procedure seems to be underutilized, for instance, only 6.4% of patients undergoing cancer surgery have a CGA performed [44].

Prognostic tools that are based on this methodology can be used to carry out more easily a CGA, for example, the MPI can be applied to heterogeneous settings, meeting various organizational and practical needs while maintaining accuracy and reliability for predictions of complications, mortality, and re-hospitalization.

Furthermore, as previously pointed out, there is ample evidence in several surgical contexts, including gastrointestinal, cardio-surgery, orthopedic, and oncological, that MPI is more beneficial than specific investigations that evaluate the function of a single organ.

Throughout the surgical path, the CGA can be advantageously applied to various phases. It can direct clinical decision-making in the pre-operative (pre-habilitation and treatment identification), peri-operative (treatment program planning), and post-operative (follow-up monitoring) phases.

Implementing this strategy in surgical settings and throughout clinical practice should be guided by the landmark Italian Guideline on the CGA for Older Persons and its accompanying recommendations. This work also serves as a recommendation for the CGA's future and for additional research to fill in the gaps that have been identified.

The key takeaway, then, is that using an easy-to-use, reliable, comprehensive tool—like the MPI, which is based on the CGA multidimensional approach—can help clinicians manage older patients more effectively.

References

1. Parker SG, et al. What is comprehensive geriatric assessment (CGA)? An umbrella review. Age Ageing. 2018;47(1):149–55. https://doi.org/10.1093/ageing/afx166.
2. Pilotto A, et al. Three decades of comprehensive geriatric assessment: evidence coming from different healthcare settings and specific clinical conditions. J Am Med Dir Assoc. 2017;18(2):192.e1–192.e11. https://doi.org/10.1016/j.jamda.2016.11.004.
3. Veronese N, et al. Comprehensive geriatric assessment in older people: an umbrella review of health outcomes. Age Ageing. 2022;51(5):afac104. https://doi.org/10.1093/ageing/afac104.
4. Gill TM. The central role of prognosis in clinical decision making. JAMA. 2012;307(2):199. https://doi.org/10.1001/jama.2011.1992.
5. Pilotto A, et al. Development and validation of a multidimensional prognostic index for one-year mortality from comprehensive geriatric assessment in hospitalized older patients. Rejuvenation Res. 2008;11(1):151–61. https://doi.org/10.1089/rej.2007.0569.
6. Pilotto A, et al. Using the multidimensional prognostic index to predict clinical outcomes of hospitalized older persons: a prospective, multicenter, international study. J Gerontol A Biol Sci Med Sci. 2019;74(10):1643–9. https://doi.org/10.1093/gerona/gly239.
7. Pilotto A, et al. The multidimensional prognostic index predicts in-hospital length of stay in older patients: a multicentre prospective study. Age Ageing. 2016;45(1):90–6. https://doi.org/10.1093/ageing/afv167.
8. Cruz-Jentoft AJ, et al. Using the multidimensional prognostic index (MPI) to improve cost-effectiveness of interventions in multimorbid frail older persons: results and final recommendations from the MPI_AGE European project. Aging Clin Exp Res. 2020;32(5):861–8. https://doi.org/10.1007/s40520-020-01516-0.
9. Custodero C, et al. The role of multidimensional prognostic index to identify hospitalized older adults with COVID-19 who can benefit from Remdesivir treatment: an observational, prospective, multicenter study. Drugs Aging. 2023;40(7):643–51. https://doi.org/10.1007/s40266-023-01036-2.
10. Shenoy R, et al. Validation of the Onco-MPI in predicting short-term mortality in older Indian patients with cancer. J Geriatr Oncol. 2023;14(6):101550. https://doi.org/10.1016/j.jgo.2023.101550.

11. Di Prazza A, et al. The importance of prognosis in geriatric patients attending the emergency department: a comparison between two common short geriatric assessment tools. Aging Clin Exp Res. 2023;35(12):3041–6. https://doi.org/10.1007/s40520-023-02603-8.
12. Meyer AM, et al. A tailored discharge program improves frailty and mood in patients undergoing usual rehabilitative care: a randomized controlled trial. J Am Med Dir Assoc. 2022;23(12):1962.e1–1962.e13. https://doi.org/10.1016/j.jamda.2022.09.003.
13. Bonnekoh SI, et al. The multidimensional prognostic index in hospitalized older adults: practicability with regard to time needs. Age Clin Exp Res. 2023;35:711. https://doi.org/10.1007/s40520-022-02311-9.
14. Panza F, et al. Different models of frailty in predementia and dementia syndromes. J Nutr Health Age. 2011;15(8):711–9. https://doi.org/10.1007/s12603-011-0126-1.
15. Pilotto A, et al. Development and validation of a multidimensional prognostic index for mortality based on a standardized multidimensional assessment schedule (MPI-SVaMA) in community-dwelling older subjects. J Am Med Dir Assoc. 2013;14(4):287–92. https://doi.org/10.1016/j.jamda.2013.01.005.
16. Cella A, et al. Validation of abbreviated form of the multidimensional prognostic index (MPI): the BRIEF-MPI project. CIA. 2022;17:789–96. https://doi.org/10.2147/CIA.S355801.
17. Pilotto A, et al. Development and validation of a self-administered multidimensional prognostic index to predict negative health outcomes in community-dwelling persons. Rejuvenation Res. 2019;22(4):299–305. https://doi.org/10.1089/rej.2018.2103.
18. Custodero C, et al. Validation and implementation of telephone-administered version of the multidimensional prognostic index (TELE-MPI) for remote monitoring of community-dwelling older adults. Aging Clin Exp Res. 2021;33(12):3363–9. https://doi.org/10.1007/s40520-021-01871-6.
19. Mattace-Raso F, et al. The challenge of the multifaceted prognosis in the older people and the multidimensional prognostic index. Eur Geriatr Med. 2021;12(2):223–6. https://doi.org/10.1007/s41999-021-00457-9.
20. Zampino M, et al. Biomarkers of aging in real life: three questions on aging and the comprehensive geriatric assessment. GeroScience. 2022;44(6):2611–22. https://doi.org/10.1007/s11357-022-00613-4.
21. Lees M, et al. Perioperative factors predicting poor outcome in elderly patients following emergency general surgery: a multivariate regression analysis. Can J Surg. 2015;58(5):312–7. https://doi.org/10.1503/cjs.011614.
22. Negm A, et al. Cochrane in CORR®: comprehensive geriatric assessment for older people admitted to a surgical service. Clin Orthop Relat Res. 2020;478(7):1409–15. https://doi.org/10.1097/CORR.0000000000001326.
23. Tian BWCA, et al. Assessing and managing frailty in emergency laparotomy: a WSES position paper. World J Emerg Surg. 2023;18(1):38. https://doi.org/10.1186/s13017-023-00506-7.
24. Lawton MP, et al. Assessment of older people: self-maintaining and instrumental activities of daily living. The Gerontologist. 1969;9(3 Part 1):179–86. https://doi.org/10.1093/geront/9.3_Part_1.179.
25. Pioli G, et al. Orthogeriatric co-management—managing frailty as well as fragility. Injury. 2018;49(8):1398–402. https://doi.org/10.1016/j.injury.2018.04.014.
26. Salis F, et al. Orthogeriatric assessment of the elderly patient with fragility hip fracture: preliminary results of a prospective study. JPM. 2023;13(7):1138. https://doi.org/10.3390/jpm13071138.
27. Zanetti M, et al. Multidimensional prognostic index predicts short- and long-term mortality and rehospitalizations in older patients with hip fracture. Aging Clin Exp Res. 2023;35(7):1487–95. https://doi.org/10.1007/s40520-023-02433-8.
28. Rizk P, et al. Review of postoperative delirium in geriatric patients undergoing hip surgery. Geriatr Orthop Surg Rehabil. 2016;7(2):100–5. https://doi.org/10.1177/2151458516641162.
29. Musacchio C, et al. Association between multidimensional prognostic index (MPI) and preoperative delirium in older patients with hip fracture. Sci Rep. 2022;12(1):16920. https://doi.org/10.1038/s41598-022-20734-2.

30. Ungar A, et al. Comprehensive geriatric assessment in patients undergoing transcatheter aortic valve implantation—results from the CGA-TAVI multicentre registry. BMC Cardiovasc Disord. 2018;18(1):1. https://doi.org/10.1186/s12872-017-0740-x.
31. van Mourik MS, et al. Value of a comprehensive geriatric assessment for predicting one-year outcomes in patients undergoing transcatheter aortic valve implantation: results from the CGA-TAVI multicentre registry. J Geriatr Cardiol. 2019;16(6):468–77. https://doi.org/10.11909/j.issn.1671-5411.2019.06.001.
32. Schäfer M, et al. Risk stratification of patients undergoing percutaneous repair of mitral and tricuspid valves using a multidimensional geriatric assessment. Circ Cardiovasc Qual Outcomes. 2021;14(8):e007624. https://doi.org/10.1161/CIRCOUTCOMES.120.007624.
33. Goudzwaard JA, et al. Multidimensional prognostic index and outcomes in older patients undergoing Transcatheter aortic valve implantation: survival of the fittest. JCM. 2021;10(16):3529. https://doi.org/10.3390/jcm10163529.
34. Chetrit J, et al. Frailty: as simple as possible, but no simpler. Circ Cardiovasc Qual Outcomes. 2021;14(10):e008227. https://doi.org/10.1161/CIRCOUTCOMES.121.008227.
35. Mohile SG, et al. Practical assessment and Management of Vulnerabilities in older patients receiving chemotherapy: ASCO guideline for geriatric oncology. JCO. 2018;36(22):2326–47. https://doi.org/10.1200/JCO.2018.78.8687.
36. Balducci L, et al. The application of the principles of geriatrics to the management of the older person with cancer. Crit Rev Oncol Hematol. 2000;35(3):147–54. https://doi.org/10.1016/S1040-8428(00)00089-5.
37. Li D, et al. Geriatric Assessment–Driven Intervention (GAIN) on chemotherapy-related toxic effects in older adults with cancer: a randomized clinical trial. JAMA Oncologia. 2021;7(11):e214158. https://doi.org/10.1001/jamaoncol.2021.4158.
38. Mahmoud AM, et al. A randomized clinical study on the impact of comprehensive geriatric assessment (CGA) based interventions on the quality of life of elderly, frail, onco-hematologic patients candidate to anticancer therapy: protocol of the ONCO-aging study. BMC Geriatr. 2021;21(1):320. https://doi.org/10.1186/s12877-021-02237-3.
39. Mohile SG, et al. Evaluation of geriatric assessment and management on the toxic effects of cancer treatment (GAP70+): a cluster-randomised study. Lancet. 2021;398(10314):1894–904. https://doi.org/10.1016/S0140-6736(21)01789-X.
40. Soo WK, et al. Integrated geriatric assessment and treatment effectiveness (INTEGERATE) in older people with cancer starting systemic anticancer treatment in Australia: a multicentre, open-label, randomised controlled trial. Lancet Healthy Longev. 2022;3(9):e617–27. https://doi.org/10.1016/S2666-7568(22)00169-6.
41. Colloca G, et al. Treating cancer in older and oldest old patients. CPD. 2015;21(13):1699–705. https://doi.org/10.2174/1381612821666150130122536.
42. Giantin V, et al. Does the multidimensional prognostic index (MPI), based on a comprehensive geriatric assessment (CGA), predict mortality in cancer patients? Results of a prospective observational trial. J Geriatr Oncol. 2013;4(3):208–17. https://doi.org/10.1016/j.jgo.2013.04.008.
43. Giantin V, et al. Performance of the multidimensional geriatric assessment and multidimensional prognostic index in predicting negative outcomes in older adults with cancer. Eur J Cancer Care. 2018;27(1):e12585. https://doi.org/10.1111/ecc.12585.
44. Pata G, et al. Multidimensional prognostic index (MPI) score has the major impact on outcome prediction in elderly surgical patients with colorectal cancer: the FRAGIS study. J Surg Oncol. 2021;123(2):667–75. https://doi.org/10.1002/jso.26314.
45. Sbrana A, et al. Effectiveness of multi-prognostic index in older patients with advanced malignancies treated with immunotherapy. J Geriatr Oncol. 2020;11(3):503–7. https://doi.org/10.1016/j.jgo.2019.09.010.
46. Brunello A, et al. Development of an oncological-multidimensional prognostic index (Onco-MPI) for mortality prediction in older cancer patients. J Cancer Res Clin Oncol. 2016;142(5):1069–77. https://doi.org/10.1007/s00432-015-2088-x.

47. Procaccio L, et al. The oncological multidimensional prognostic index is a promising decision-making tool: a real-world analysis in older patients with metastatic colorectal cancer. Eur J Cancer. 2022;177:112–9. https://doi.org/10.1016/j.ejca.2022.09.023.
48. Pilotto A, et al. Usefulness of the comprehensive geriatric assessment in older patients with upper gastrointestinal bleeding: a two-year follow-up study. Dig Dis. 2007;25(2):124–8. https://doi.org/10.1159/000099476.
49. Pilotto A, et al. Upper gastrointestinal disorders. In: Halter JB, Ouslander JG, Studenski S, High KP, Asthana S, Supiano MA, Ritchie CS, Schmader K, editors. Hazzard's geriatric medicine and gerontology. 8th ed. New York: McGraw-Hill Education; 2022. Consultato: 27 febbraio 2024. [Online]. Disponibile su: http://accessmedicine.mhmedical.com/content.aspx?aid=1190912200.
50. Pugh RNH, et al. Transection of the oesophagus for bleeding oesophageal varices. Br J Surg. 2005;60(8):646–9. https://doi.org/10.1002/bjs.1800600817.
51. Pilotto A, et al. The comprehensive geriatric assessment and the multidimensional approach. A new look at the older patient with gastroenterological disorders. Best Pract Res Clin Gastroenterol. 2009;23(6):829–37. https://doi.org/10.1016/j.bpg.2009.10.001.
52. Malinchoc M, et al. A model to predict poor survival in patients undergoing transjugular intrahepatic portosystemic shunts. Hepatology. 2000;31(4):864–71. https://doi.org/10.1053/he.2000.5852.
53. Vogliotti E, et al. Can the multidimensional prognostic index (MPI) be a predictive instrument for mortality in older adult liver transplant candidates? Eur Geriatr Med. 2023;14(4):851–9. https://doi.org/10.1007/s41999-023-00826-6.
54. Partridge JSL, et al. The impact of pre-operative comprehensive geriatric assessment on postoperative outcomes in older patients undergoing scheduled surgery: a systematic review. Anaesthesia. 2014;69(s1):8–16. https://doi.org/10.1111/anae.12494.
55. Feng MA, et al. Geriatric assessment in surgical oncology: a systematic review. J Surg Res. 2015;193(1):265–72. https://doi.org/10.1016/j.jss.2014.07.004.
56. Wildiers H, et al. International Society of Geriatric Oncology Consensus on geriatric assessment in older patients with cancer. JCO. 2014;32(24):2595–603. https://doi.org/10.1200/JCO.2013.54.8347.
57. Fong TG, et al. Delirium in elderly adults: diagnosis, prevention and treatment. Nat Rev Neurol. 2009;5(4):210–20. https://doi.org/10.1038/nrneurol.2009.24.
58. Agrawal S, et al. The association of preoperative delirium with postoperative outcomes following hip surgery in the elderly. J Clin Anesth. 2020;60:28–33. https://doi.org/10.1016/j.jclinane.2019.08.015.
59. Istituto Superiore di Sanità et al., «Linea Guida: La valutazione multidimensionale della persona anziana.» 16 novembre 2023. [Online]. Disponibile su: https://www.iss.it/documents/20126/8331678/LG-C009-SIGOT-SIMG_VMD_persona_anziana.pdf/a7dc753f-01e1-f208-c7cc-d5011f347f95?t=1700574003103.
60. Pilotto A, et al. The Italian guideline on comprehensive geriatric assessment (CGA) for the older persons: a collaborative work of 25 Italian scientific societies and the National Institute of Health. Aging Clin Exp Res. 2024;36(1):121. https://doi.org/10.1007/s40520-024-02772-0.
61. Gallucci M, et al. Multidimensional prognostic index (MPI) in an outpatient setting: mortality and hospitalizations. Eur Geriatr Med. 2013;4(1):S47. https://doi.org/10.1016/j.eurger.2013.07.154.
62. Cella A, et al. Agreement of a short form of the self-administered multidimensional prognostic index (SELFY-MPI-SF): a useful tool for the self-assessment of frailty in community-dwelling older people. Clin Interv Aging. 2020;15:493–9. https://doi.org/10.2147/CIA.S241721.
63. Morganti W, et al. «validation of a brief form of the self-administered multidimensional prognostic index: the SELFY-BRIEF-MPI project», journal of. Clin Med. 2023;12(18):6026. https://doi.org/10.3390/jcm12186026.

Decision Making of Surgical Strategy in Older and/or Frail Persons

10

Carlo Vallicelli, Bruno Amato, Nicola Avenia, Stefania Brozzetti, Paolo Carcoforo, Alessandro Coppola, Chiara D'Alterio, Francesco Menegon Tasselli, Alessandro Puzziello, Aldo Rocca, Sergio Sandrucci, Guido Sciaudone, Brian Tian, Andrea Vicinanza, and Fausto Catena

C. Vallicelli (✉) · F. Catena
General Emergency and Trauma Surgery Department, Maurizio Bufalini Hospital, Cesena, Italy
e-mail: carlo.vallicelli@auslromagna.it

B. Amato
Department of Clinical Medicine and Surgery, University of Naples "Federico II", Naples, Italy
e-mail: bruno.amato@unina.it

N. Avenia
Medical School, Department of General Surgery and Surgical Specialties Unit, S. Maria University Hospital University of Perugia, Terni, Italy
e-mail: nicola.avenia@unipg.it

S. Brozzetti · A. Coppola · C. D'Alterio
Department of Surgery, Sapienza University, Rome, Italy
e-mail: stefania.brozzetti@uniroma1.it; aless.coppola@uniroma1.it; chiara.dalterio@uniroma1.it

P. Carcoforo
Department of Surgery, S. Anna University Hospital and University of Ferrara, Ferrara, Italy
e-mail: ccf@unife.it

F. M. Tasselli
Department of Advanced Medical and Surgical Sciences, University of Campania 'L. Vanvitelli', Naples, Italy

A. Puzziello
General Surgery Unit, AOU San Giovanni di Dio e Ruggi d'Aragona, Dipartimento di Medicina Chirurgia ed Odontoiatria "Scuola Medica Salernitana", Università di Salerno, Fisciano, Italy
e-mail: a.puzziello@unisa.it

A. Rocca · G. Sciaudone
Department of Medicine and Health Science 'V. Tiberio', University of Molise, Campobasso, Italy
e-mail: guido.sciaudone@unimol.it

V. Boccardi, L. Marano (eds.), *The Frail Surgical Patient*, Practical Issues in Geriatrics, https://doi.org/10.1007/978-3-031-77707-3_10

10.1 Introduction

Many countries are facing an aging population. As people live longer, surgeons face the prospect of operating on increasingly older patients. As an example, in England, 2.5 million people above 75 years old, underwent surgery between 2014 and 2015, as opposed to just 1.5 million between 2006–2007 [1, 2]. Nearly 30% of these 2.5 million were over 85 years old [1]. Similarly, women aged 85 years and over now represent the largest proportion of emergency surgical admissions in Australia, compared with all other age and sex groups [3]. In Europe, it is projected that the number of patients above 65 years old, will account for 30% of the population by 2060. In Italy, the average life span now according to data from the World Health Organisation [WHO] is 82.7 years (80.5 for males, 84.8 for females). Recognition of the incoming silver epidemic and preparation of health services for this is of utmost urgency. It is vital that the medical profession be equipped with specific knowledge and experience in managing the elderly patients. Traditional teaching was that with older age, these patients face an increased risk of mortality and morbidity, even to a level deemed too prohibitive for surgery. However, in today's modern world, that is no longer true. An active 90-year-old patient can be much fitter than an overweight, sedentary 65-year-old patient with comorbidities. It is important that today's modern surgeon be equipped with new tools and knowledge to learn how to approach surgery in these patients. In the past, many surgeons used the 'eye-ball test' to determine if an elderly patient is fit for surgery. This imprecise tool has been proven to be subjective and inconsistent between different observers [4], and thus can no longer be applied in today's context. There is a growing body of evidence that shows that frailty—an age-related cumulative decline in multiple physiological systems, is much better predictor of mortality and morbidity than chronological age alone [5, 6]. A detailed analysis will be provided for all the major chapters of abdominal surgery in older and frail patients.

10.2 Emergency General Surgery

Emergency surgery is a special scenario. It has wide-ranging presentations, from a perforated appendix, to an obstructed and perforated colon. Each patient will also present in varying degrees of sepsis and shock. It is difficult to approach each and

S. Sandrucci
Chirurgia Oncologica, Università degli studi di Torino, Turin, Italy
e-mail: sergio.sandrucci@unito.it

B. Tian
Department of General Surgery, Singapore General Hospital, Singapore, Singapore

A. Vicinanza
Scuola di Specializzazione in Chirurgia Generale, Università degli studi di Verona, Verona, Italy

every scenario specifically. Therefore, this book will aim to manage this group as a whole, under the umbrella of 'emergency laparotomy'.

The way to approach this group of patients would be:

1. Stratification of the patient's baseline condition and of the present emergency.
2. Counselling and decision making in surgery—sometimes conservative management is kinder and more appropriate.
3. Preparing the hospital and its appropriate facilities to receive the postoperative patient.
4. Maintaining a multidisciplinary team with a geriatrician, to ensure holistic care.
5. Early discharge planning.

1. *Stratification of the patient's baseline condition and of the present emergency.*

All patients coming in with an acute abdomen should have their histories taken and a physical examination performed. A measurement of the vitals would tell us about the patients' stability and shock status. A full panel of blood taking would be required, including acid base and lactate status. The relevant scans [x-rays and CT scans] would be performed and the relevant diagnosis achieved. Some conditions have their own attendant risk scores and outcomes that cannot be mitigated by further measures. For example, Boey's Index for perforated gastric ulcer; in which case, if a patient presents in an absolute moribund state, the attendant mortality is almost 100%. Another example would be acute biliary pancreatitis with concomitant cholangitis or cholecystitis, whereby there is an associated Ransons', Glasgow or Modified Marshall Score. To that effect, other scores such as APACHE II score, ASA and Mannheim Peritonitis Index scores are also relevant scoring indices that give an indication to the severity of sickness of the patient and possible outcomes. In addition to disease-specific outcomes, all patients being considered for, or undergoing emergency laparotomy aged 65 years or more, should undergo a routine frailty screening, e.g., Clinical Frailty Scale. Vulnerable patients identified via the screening should receive a Comprehensive Geriatric Assessment (CGA) ideally upon admission, if not within 72 h of admission to a ward or step down from critical care to a ward. It is not practical to always stratify frailty properly, especially in sick patients where time is of the essence [7]. In its place, a good screening tool is needed. To that effect, the Clinical Frailty Scale [8] is recommended as it has been validated for use in patients. In the area of surgery, frailty is an independent risk factor for mortality, morbidity, length of stay, and postoperative complications [9, 10]. The Guidelines from the American College of Surgeons for Surgery and the National Institute for Health and Care Excellence have emphasized frailty assessment in acute care settings or preoperative periods as a new screening criterion for fitness [10]. The 15-variable Emergency general surgery specific frailty index (EGSFI) was validated in a prospective cohort [11]. The EGSFI-based frailty status significantly predicted postoperative complications (odd ratio, 7.3; 95% confidence interval, 1.7–19.8), but age was not a relevant factor. Similarly, the Emergency Laparotomy and Frailty [ELF] study showed an association between frailty and 90-day mortality (clinical frailty scale 5, OR 3.18, 95% CI 1.24–8.14), increased risk of complications and length of hospital stay in older emergency laparotomy patients [12]. One of the most important studies in the field of emergency laparotomy and frailty is the NELA audit [13]. The audit adopted the Clinical Frailty Score and found it to be prevalent in 11% of people over 65 years, rising to 50% in those over 85 years of age [13]. This score can also be applied to the younger surgical populations [14]. Therefore the NELA proposed that that the Clinical Frailty Score was the most appropriate screening tool for patients undergoing emergency laparotomy. After screening the patients, the NELA audit utilized a cut-off for Clinical Frailty Score of ≥5 (or aged ≥80 years with any frailty score), to identify patients who should receive geriatrician-led multidisciplinary comprehensive geriatric assessment (CGA) ideally upon admission, if not within 72 h of admission to a ward or step down from critical care to a ward [13]. The CGA has emerging evidence when applied to both elective and emergency older surgical populations [15–17]. Older emergency general surgical patients have been shown to benefit from perioperative CGA in terms of reduced mortality [18], LOS [17] and additional diagnoses and/or interventions made [19]. The CGA [20] is considered the benchmark for frailty assessment and generally includes follow-up care such as geriatric-specific optimization interventions [21]. The CGA addresses multidisciplinary components related to the patients' physical, mental, and psychosocial well-being and functional capabilities. However, it may be time-consuming to administer, and a geriatric assessment composed of questionnaires assessing different domains of well-being can often be used instead [22, 23]. Although most CGA studies for abdominal surgery have been performed for the elective setting and in oncology. There are no known nomograms or actuarial tools that can adequately give a risk score as a composite of the patients' underlying disease, clinical presentation and frailty. However, with the various tools at the clinicians' disposal, the clinician should be able to have a sense of the possible morbidity and mortality outcomes for the patient at presentation.

2. *Counselling and decision making on surgery – sometimes conservative management is kinder and more appropriate.*

Unlike young and fit patients, where 'going all out' aggressively is never disputed, we must be more considerate when approaching elderly patients. Any decisions regarding surgery must consider the patients' degree of frailty, as surgery may at times, result in poor outcomes. Even when outcomes are good, there is a limit to life expectancy. No one—neither surgeons nor patients—can have a true understanding about what their likely outcome is after emergency laparotomy surgery. Especially patients and their families who are likely to be overly optimistic and hopeful, with at times unrealistic expectations. The recent Emergency Laparotomy in the Frail (or ELF) study had highlighted the deleterious effect of frailty on those who require an emergency laparotomy [23]. In nearly 1000 consecutive patients aged over 65 years in 49 sites across England, Scotland and Wales, the ELF study showed that the presence of frailty was associated with greater risks of postoperative mortality. Their findings also demonstrated that as the degree of frailty increased, there was a linear increase in mortality. The NELA audit [13] demonstrated that patients aged 65 years or over have worse clinical outcomes compared to their younger counterparts. These include longer length of hospital stay (median 15.2 days vs. 11.3 days) and higher 30-day and 90-day mortality (15.3% vs. 4.9% and 20.4% vs. 7.2%). In addition, there is an association between frailty, which is known to increase with age, and increased 90-day mortality following emergency laparotomy (aOR for patients who were mildly frail and moderately/severely frail was 3.18 and 6.10), 1-year hospital visits (7.2 vs. 2.0) and care level (aOR for an increase in care level was 4·48 for vulnerable patients, 5·94 for those mildly frail and 7·88 for those moderately or severely frail, compared with patients who were fit). In NELA year 4, 6.7% of older patients compared with 1.9% ($P < 0.001$) of younger patients were discharged to care-home accommodation. In general for patients who survived surgery, frailty is associated with worse surgical outcomes: increased mortality, prolonged hospital stay, complications and an increased level of social care provision on discharge from hospital [24]. Over 30% of older patients don't return to their own homes after emergency laparotomy surgery [25]. However, data highlighting long-term quality of life following emergency surgery are lacking, and epidemiological studies addressing this neglected area are desperately needed. The research community is working hard to gather the evidence for the best interventions for this frail group of patients. The recent EPOCH study, a large-scale and well-designed step-wedged randomized controlled study of the implementation of a care pathway, in emergency abdominal surgery, showed no benefit of the intervention [26]. It is critical therefore that any treatment plans for frail older adults should align with patients' goals of care and should be based on a discussion regarding realistic outcomes. When contemplating the care plan for a frail patient, the goals of care should be discussed with the patient, engaged family, caregivers or advocates, and other members of the multidisciplinary team that may include representatives from surgery, geriatrics, palliative care, primary care, oncology, radiation oncology, and so on [27]. Typically, these discussions address domains such as anticipated longevity, functional status, independence, and comfort [28, 29]. In circumstances involving potential surgical intervention, deliberating whether to proceed with surgery should consider the likely treatment outcomes (including curative vs. palliative objectives) and patient and family preferences. A realistic picture should be presented based on the anticipated risks of morbidity, mortality, and cognitive decline for each of the proposed treatment options taking into consideration the patient's unique presentation, degree of frailty, and functional status [30]. Specifically, patients may value their functional performance and cognitive status more than other treatment-related considerations and, as a result, patients may base their decisions on the likelihood of maintaining a certain level of performance. On an individual patient basis, it is important to clarify what matters most to patients, and online resources are available to facilitate these discussions (e.g., the American Geriatrics Society's Health in Aging Foundation website, https://www.

healthinaging.org/age-friendly-healthcareyou/care-what-matters-most). In practice, it may be helpful to include a geriatrician and/or the patient's primary care physician in treatment planning discussions. When planning operative treatment, it is helpful to clarify patients' current living situation and existing support, to communicate goals for postoperative disposition as well as code status, and to have patients designate a surrogate decision-maker. Importantly, clinicians should recognize that patients' goals of care may change during the perioperative period [26]. In the emergency setting, it may be difficult to have comprehensive goals of care discussions with patients, particularly if they are septic or unstable, have cognitive impairment, or are otherwise unable to have a meaningful discussion. An interdisciplinary, 23-member expert panel recommended a structured communication framework addressing nine key elements to facilitate decision-making among seriously ill older patients with emergency surgical conditions [31]. The difficulties with having discussions in the setting of emergency circumstances highlight the importance of taking the opportunity to engage patients and their families in early goals of care discussions, especially when patients have multiple comorbidities or a condition that may result in a subsequent emergency (e.g., obstructing colorectal cancer) [32, 33]. Special consideration should be given to patients above 90 years old, where morbidity and mortality rates may be high and natural life span is limited. Even in individuals with relatively few comorbidities, these patients still have a relatively limited life expectancy. For example, a 90-year-old woman in England expected to live a further 4.50 years and a man 3.94 years [34]. The decision to operate on anyone aged over 90 years should take this into account.

3. *Preparing the family, the hospital and its appropriate facilities to receive the postoperative patient.*

Postoperative care is vital to the outcome of the patient. In the geriatric group, recovery can be a prolonged, painful and expensive process. And even if the patient survives, function can be severely impaired. Not only should the patients and their families be aware; they must also equipped to handle the postoperative sequelae.

Unique outcomes that the post-op geriatric patient might experience:

(i) *Decline in Cognitive Function.*

The prevalence of dementia is estimated to be 5% among 70- to 79-year-olds, 24% among 80- to 89-year-olds, and nearly 40% among people older than 90 years [35]. Meanwhile, mild cognitive impairment (MCI) is distinguished from dementia in that the impairment is not severe enough to interfere with independent function. MCI is common among older adults, even those living independently, and affects up to 50% of patients older than 65 years [36]. Although the American College of Surgeons and the American Geriatrics Society recommend routinely assessing preoperative cognitive function and advocate using cognitive assessment tools such as the Mini-Cog preoperatively to detect MCI [37], the results of studies evaluating an association between MCI and postoperative outcomes such as complications, length of stay, and mortality are mixed and studies have been underpowered [38, 39]. Nonetheless, the most compelling reason to evaluate for cognitive impairment preoperatively is to predict and prepare patients and caregivers for the likelihood of postoperative decline. The degree of cognitive decline associated with an individual surgery or anesthetic exposure is unknown. The Mayo Clinic performed a 5-year longitudinal study of 1819 patients aged ≥70 years and showed that exposure to general anesthesia and surgery was associated with subtle accelerated cognitive decline. Moreover, decision-making capacity may be diminished in patients with cognitive impairment or dementia, and family members, healthcare surrogates, and primary care physicians should be included in the decision-making process in appropriately selected patients [40]. Upon returning home postoperatively, patients with cognitive or memory impairment may benefit from close surveillance from caregivers or home care services.

(ii) *Postoperative Delirium.*

Delirium is associated with functional and cognitive decline, increased morbidity and mortality, longer lengths of stay, higher rates of nursing home placement, and increased healthcare costs [41–47]. Moreover, as complications may present atypically in older adults, clinicians should recognize that postoperative delirium may be an indicator or manifestation of an underlying complication.

Maintaining an appropriate index of suspicion in frail older adults experiencing postoperative delirium and initiating a broad clinical workup under these circumstances may be advised (e.g., evaluating for infections, electrolyte abnormalities, and drug side effects) [48]. The Confusion Assessment Method screens for delirium by evaluating for (1) mental status changes with acute onset and fluctuating severity, (2) inattention, (3) disorganized thinking, and (4) an altered level of consciousness. Using the Confusion Assessment Method, the presence of 1, 2, and either 3 or 4 confirms the diagnosis of delirium [49]. Patients experiencing delirium may benefit from early geriatric or neuropsychiatric specialist consultation to assist with perioperative management as well as multimodal, nonpharmacologic interventions such as cognitive stimulation, early mobilization, preservation of the sleep-wake cycle, and ensuring adequate hydration. Importantly, delirium can be prevented in up to 50% of patients by using a delirium prevention bundle [50]. Watt et al. performed a meta-analysis of 8557 patients older than 60 years who underwent elective orthopedic, cardiac, or abdominal surgery and found a pooled postoperative delirium incidence rate of 18.4% (95% CI, 14.3–23.3). In this study, the strongest predictors of postoperative delirium were a personal history of delirium (OR 6.4; 95% CI, 2.2–17.9), frailty (OR 4.1; 95% CI, 1.4–11.7), and cognitive impairment (OR 2.7; 95% CI, 1.9–3.8). In this study, prognostic factors that could potentially be modified to reduce the incidence of delirium included decreasing the use of psychotropic medications, smoking cessation, and increasing caregiver support [51]. Another intervention shown to decrease the incidence of delirium is avoiding or reducing the use of specific medications such as opioids, benzodiazepines, antihistamines, atropine, sedative hypnotics, and corticosteroids [52]. In 2019, in an effort to reduce adverse drug events in older patients and to decrease the incidence of delirium, the American Geriatric Society updated the Beers Criteria describing potentially inappropriate medication use in patients aged ≥65 years and specifically highlighted the detrimental effects related to antipsychotics, benzodiazepines, H2 receptor antagonists, anticholinergics, and meperidine [53].

(iii) *Need for Social Support.*

Social frailty, an incompletely explored concept, has been defined as a continuum of being at risk of losing or having lost resources that are needed to fulfill one or more basic social needs. Increasing age and lower levels of education are significant risk factors for developing social frailty [54, 55]. Considering that older adults rely on their social relationships and environment to effectively participate in multimodality care pathways, the concept of social frailty has become increasingly relevant to this vulnerable patient population [56]. Although this topic has been widely discussed, large prospective studies evaluating this concept especially in post laparotomies, have not been reported. In an observational study, Hawkins et al. [57] evaluated 63 patients undergoing lower extremity amputation and showed that increased social integration (i.e., the number of contacts and interactions in a patient's social network) was associated with improved postoperative function and quality of life (QoL). Another prospective study of 972 consecutive patients undergoing colorectal cancer resection showed that increased social support and decreased psychological distress improved health-related QoL 1 year after surgery [58]. A systematic review of 19 randomized trials by Gardner et al. [59] showed that providing practical social support was effective in enabling home-based health behavior change in frail older adults. In this study, patients with social support were more likely to have been instructed regarding positive behavioral changes and to have experienced appropriate changes in their environment; instituting positive behaviors such as using social services and following an individualized care path led to improvement in social functioning and general health.

4. *Maintaining a Multidisciplinary Team With a Geriatrician, to Ensure Holistic Care.*

Geriatricians and practitioners with geriatrics expertise have specialized training and experience in assessing and managing geriatric syndromes (e.g., dementia, delirium, propensity for falling, comorbidity, and polypharmacy) and frailty and can improve the perioperative care of patients with these conditions. However, multidisciplinary approaches engaging these providers are commonly underused due to practice patterns and the limited number of available specialists [60]. Additionally, as previously mentioned, access to resources and support may limit the individual practitioner's ability to engage a multidisciplinary team for the care of these patients. To supplement the work of geriatricians, practices can use other specialists, such as adult/geriatric nurse practitioners, social workers, nurse navigators, pharmacists, dieticians, rehabilitative medicine physicians, physical and occupational therapists, psychologists, and psychiatrists, to complete portions of the geriatric assessment and provide geriatric-related optimization [61]. The NELA audit [13] showed that preoperative geriatrician review was recorded in 5.2% of older patients in year 4 of audit. Patients aged ≥85 years were more likely to receive geriatrician review; 20% postoperatively and 9.7% preoperatively. Preoperative geriatrician review in patients aged ≥65 years was associated with increased mortality (22.2 vs. 13.3%, $P < 0.001$ 30-day mortality; 27.9 vs. 17.6%, $P < 0.001$ 90-day mortality), whereas postoperative review was associated with reduced mortality (9.2 vs. 16.1%, $P < 0.001$ 30-day mortality; 17.2 vs. 20.9% for 90-day mortality). All had a longer median time to theater (95.9 vs. 32.2 h, $P < 0.001$ for preoperative review; 96.0 vs. 37.3 h, $P < 0.001$ for postoperative review). This subgroup had no observed difference between baseline physiological and biochemical measures; however were more likely to have predicted mortality risk ≥5% using all methods of risk assessment, be ASA grade 4 and have been admitted from a care home. Preoperative and postoperative geriatrician review was associated with increased LOS of 2.4 and 9.3 days, respectively, compared with older patients who did not receive geriatrician review. Covariates associated with discharge to care home included admission from care home (OR 11.113), age ≥85 years (OR 2.481) and postoperative geriatrician review (OR 2.329) [13]. Although geriatrician review is associated with reduced mortality in this cohort, only 24% of patients aged 70 years or over were assessed by a geriatrician following emergency laparotomy between December 2017 and November 2018 [62]. This low level of involvement of geriatricians reflect systemic issues, chiefly, the difficulty in recruiting geriatric medicine consultants [63].

The United Kingdom has acted on the results of the NELA audit and is attempting to make systematic changes to improve this statistic. It is recognized that one of the drivers to improve the care of emergency laparotomy patients include an enhanced best practice tariff (BPT) for delivery of specific care criteria known to be associated with improved outcome. In comparison, for hip fractures, UK national outcomes have improved following introduction of a BPT incentivizing geriatrician review, amongst other measures [64]. However, the current emergency laparotomy BPT criteria does not require geriatrician review.

Therefore, the British Geriatrics Society and Age Anaesthesia Association have established new standards of care for older people undergoing emergency laparotomy [65, 66]. Perhaps, the NHS England may implement these recommendations into the next iteration of the emergency laparotomy BPT as a driver to deliver evidence-based care for this high-risk group. This could be a good example for the rest of the world to learn and follow.

5. *Early discharge planning.*

Outcomes after surgery have been measured by several indicators such as length of stay, morbidity, mortality, overall survival, disease-free survival, as well as time to first flatus or time to first oral intake. However, many of these metrics may have limited relevance to frail older adults who may be more concerned about anticipated disability and dependence than even a cancer diagnosis or limitation in life expectancy. Banks et al. [67] analyzed data from a survey of 89,574 Australians (age >45 years) and found that, although 7.5% of all respondents suffered from high levels of psychological distress, those with cancer and disability attributed stress much more strongly to their level of disability than to their cancer diagnosis. Another study published by a social research institute was based on surveys, found that although longevity may be the most important priority for most patients, this notion changes for older, retired patients who rank continued independence as important as maintaining health [68]. Functional recovery may incorporate organ-specific post-operative outcomes and patients' ability to regain preoperative functional status. Loss of independence, or an increase in support required by patients after hospital discharge, is an example of a relevant functional recovery metric used to evaluate frail older patients. Regaining independence, typically measured as a composite outcome, includes an assessment of cognition and nutritional status and the ability to perform routine ADLs and to walk proficiently. Although a variety of instruments have been proposed to evaluate these kinds of domains, the most compelling literature uses the ADL, Mini-Cog, and Timed Up and Go/6-min walk distance scores [69–74]. De Roo et al., in a retrospective matched cohort study, highlighted the importance of analyzing less conventional outcomes like functional decline, which was defined as an increase in the number of ADLs requiring assistance after surgery. In this study, 289 patients who underwent colorectal surgery and were older than 65 years were compared to 867 control patients who did not undergo surgery [173]. De Roo et al. found that patients who underwent surgery and had a complication (90 patients, 31% of the surgical cohort) had a higher likelihood of functional decline (OR 2.96; 95% CI, 1.70–5.14) compared to controls and those who did not have a surgical complication (OR 1.82; 95% CI, 1.22–2.71) [75]. Patient-reported outcomes (PROs), despite their complexity, can be captured by integrating smart devices into electronic medical record systems and using a variety of programs to collect data [76, 77]. The University of California, Los Angeles 3-Item Loneliness Scale, evaluating how often patients feel they lack companionship or feel left out or isolated from others, was also reported to be useful in assessing PROs in frail individuals.

To conclude, major abdominal surgery in an emergency setting carries with it a high morbidity. Patient selection and identification of those who will likely benefit from surgery is difficult in the frail and elderly owing to the combination of multiple comorbidities and the general decreased physiological reserve associated with aging. As highlighted in the National Confidential Enquiry into Patient Outcome and Death report on surgery in the elderly, identification of frailty is a key factor in case selection. Frailty should be considered an independent risk factor for poor surgical outcomes. However, assessment of frailty is in itself difficult. Clear and frank information about the significant risks associated with surgery in elderly patients must be discussed with patients and their families to help set realistic expectations.

10.3 Hepatic Surgery

Liver resections (LRs) are the treatment of choice for a range of primary malignancies and for an expanded histotype of liver metastases. Especially with the recent increase in experience and advances in technical and instrumental development, LRs are increasingly being performed safely in elderly patients. Large and qualified multicentric studies have shown that LRs are widely applied in current practice among elderly patients, providing good short- and long-term results [78, 79]. Maintaining the quality of life and functional independence of older patients with cancer involves appropriate cancer treatment. Therapeutic indications to improve the safety and efficiency of treatment of liver malignancies requires a multidisciplinary approach made up of hepato-biliary surgeons, interventional radiologists, gastroenterologists, hepatologists, and oncologists. Considering the availability of several evidence-based treatments, therapeutic indication shall keep into account oncological principles and liver function on one side, and performance status, tolerability of treatment, comorbidities and actual life expectancy on the other.

Frail and older patients may benefit with curative liver resections from an oncological standpoint as much as their younger ones. However, age alone is not a good outcome predictor: fit elderly patients may tolerate radical and invasive approaches while unfit patients may not [80]. Physiological age is a new fundamental concept to assess an advance in age patient's performance status beyond his chronological age, which is still today too often used as a threshold to exclude or include a patient into specific treatment protocols. A careful anesthesiological and geriatric assessment is required in the strategies decision making process. The physical frailty and comorbidities are disadvantages for postoperative complications tolerance in old and frail patients, affecting patient selection [81]. Recent developments in surgical technique, surgical equipment, interventional radiology and radiotherapy allow us to use different techniques and approaches in order to treat these cancers in different older patients.

In all cases, the treatment decision has to be hierarchically dictated by the efficacy of each therapy, according to evidence endorsed by the clinical practice of expert centers [82]. Extension and complexity of LRs are associated with different outcomes. Potential predictive surgical risk factors, like difficult LRs for deep tumors centrally localized, in proximity of major vessels, prolonged surgical time and increased blood loss, are associated with higher complication rates [83].

Several comorbidities, functional or cognitive decline, require specific less invasive therapeutic approaches, however, achieving satisfactory results, disease-free survival or long-term survival. Minor surgery combined with interventional radiology makes the treatment safer for unfit patients.

Radiofrequency or microwave thermal ablation is considered the best chance of care for small lesions in patients unfit for resection, due to their mini-invasive nature, high effectiveness, low rates of adverse events, short hospitalization times, and relatively few contraindications. Oncological outcomes are similar to surgery when performed for very small hepatocellular carcinoma [84] and recently, promising results in terms of overall survival have also been reported for other lesions such as colorectal liver metastases [85]. Ablation combined with surgery is a precious strategy for managing older patients that are not enabled for extended surgery.

Patients advanced in age are especially in need of a tailored therapy, where benefits are well weighted against invasiveness of treatment and its side effects, in spite of assuring the best quality of life and survival.

10.4 Colorectal Surgery

Colorectal cancer (CRC) is a disease that predominantly affects older adults, with a median age at diagnosis of 70 years, with peak incidence between the eighth and ninth decades of life [86]; despite a better prognosis of CRC in recent decades [87], there is evidence demonstrating inequalities in treatment and worse survival in older patients. In fact, patients over 70 years old are less likely to receive guideline-recommended care [88] due to a number of complex factors related both to the patient, i.e., inadequate representation in clinical trials, and to medical and/or logistical factors, i.e., difficulty in accessing geriatric examination in a timely manner, which is critical in assessing conditions such as frailty and/or complex comorbidities [89]. Indeed, studies show that of older patients with colorectal cancer, 31.4% undergo surgery and chemotherapy, 53.2% undergo surgery alone, and 15.4% of patients access palliative care alone, never having surgery. There is also a difference in treatment in the <70 versus ≥ 70 years old age groups with regard to combination surgery/chemotherapy (51.3% vs. 8.7%) or surgery alone (30.3% vs. 73.8%) [90]. In frail and older patients or those with comorbidities, under and/or overtreatment is often performed, resulting in reduced survival or functional status [91]. Fundamental, therefore, is the distinction between "fit" patients who have maintained physiologic reserve and can benefit from standard treatments, from "frail" patients who must undergo tailored interventions and prehabilitation if not exclusive palliative strategies. However, in the population over 75 years of age, age is only one of the criteria in the decision-making process: in fact, other existing factors need to be considered, which may be medical such as increased frailty and comorbidity, or social such as movement limitations and the need for caregiver assistance [92]. To meet this need, multidisciplinary teams (MDTs) have emerged that specialize in the evaluation of such patients [93], going on to objectively determine the benefits and risks of one treatment over another.

Regarding the surgery of older patient with CCR, the most common tools that can predict the rate of postoperative complications have several limitations, as they are often based on a single organ system without considering the patient's physiological reserve. For this reason, it is necessary to identify patients who will benefit from a comprehensive geriatric assessment (CGA) [94], also provided for in the joint guidelines of the American Geriatrics Society and the American College of Surgeons National Surgical Quality Improvement Program [95], by employing the G8 screening tool, an essential tool in assessing the general health status of the elderly patient with cancer [96], exploited, however, in only 6. Four percent of cancer surgery cases [97], and the Multidimensional Frailty Score (MFS) which can predict mortality and postoperative complications in older patients undergoing surgery [98]. However, there is no agreement among the various tools which one is better than the others, making it difficult for individual clinicians to establish an optimal treatment plan as multiple domains have to be considered in older patients with colorectal cancer. An MDT and specifically a Geriatric Multidisciplinary Oncology Clinic (GMOC), which includes in addition to surgeons, specialists such as radiation oncologists, medical oncologists, radiologists, geriatricians, nurses, etc., is able to establish appropriate treatment plans "tailored" to the frail and older patients [99] with CCR, remembering that survival is not the primary aim, as the ability to remain independent is often the goal to be achieved [100]. GMOC can reduce the percentage of incomplete decisions made by individual physicians, with a change in therapeutic management demonstrated in more than 10% of cases, a reduction in postoperative complications and hospital stay, and an improvement in CCR patient outcomes. Indeed, there is ample evidence that frail patients with CCR in the postoperative period may have a longer hospital stay and higher rates of complications (up to 60%) including delirium, pneumonia, and urinary infections, i.e., higher mortality than younger patients [101]. Finally, because modern treatment protocols are standardized for patients with high-performance status, the evaluation of older patient with CCR within the GMOC allows discernment between more or less aggressive treatments identified on the individual patient's characteristics.

Regarding surgical treatment in the older patients with CCR, both endoscopic and open, laparoscopic, or robotic interventions are possible. In the former case, the approach for adenomas and early-stage tumors is endoscopic submucosal dissection (ESD), which although less invasive than surgery, still involves risk of perforation (6%) and bleeding (1%), so caution should be exercised in using it in elderly patients because of the risk of exacerbations of comorbidities that may exacerbate post-ESD complications. In case of T1 CRC, where revision surgical colic resection would be indicated, there is no consensus on the real efficacy and reasonableness of additional surgery in the frail and older patient [102]. In contrast in the case of the patient with preserved functional reserve, surgical resection is feasible, and randomized controlled trials have shown that laparoscopic surgery for CRC has an equivalent oncologic outcome and better short-term outcomes than open surgery, even in the over-70-year-old population [103]. Indeed, laparoscopic colectomy compared with open surgery provides advantages, including less invasiveness, lower mortality rates, shorter hospital stay and lower costs, with comparable oncologic outcomes.

In conclusion, future research should focus on facilitating access to a GMOC with specific geriatric expertise to identify elderly patients who are more likely to benefit from CRC treatment, giving importance rather than chronological age alone to the use and cost-effectiveness of specific screening tools [104]. In the future, better access to specific GMOC for older patients diagnosed with CRC will enable more appropriate treatment decisions that can improve the overall survival of these patients.

10.5 Pancreatic Surgery

According to the constant increase in the population's average age and above all considering that pancreatic ductal adenocarcinoma (PDAC) is a strictly age-related disease, it seems clear that there is a doubt regarding the need to extend the surgical indication for this pathology also to aging patients. However, it is also necessary to reflect not only on the resectability of the pancreatic lesion which is only an anatomical and biological concept but also on the operability of the patient and the possibility of guaranteeing the latter access to a treatment that combines surgical resection and systemic therapy. A combination that to date guarantees the best results in terms of median survival at 5 years, configuring itself as the standard of care for a resectable disease [105, 106].

The evidence regarding the applicability of the standard treatment in all patients regardless of age is conflicting, especially if we consider how the most recent studies increasingly show that polychemotherapy regimens based on fluoro folates, irinotecan, and combined platinum derivatives succeed to guarantee better results in terms of survival than gemcitabine monotherapy, whether used in an adjuvant or neoadjuvant setting or metastatic disease [107]. However, in the majority of cases, oncology teams reserve this type of treatment only for patients under 70–75 years of age, for whom either mono-chemotherapy regimens or schemes based on gemcitabine and nab-paclitaxel are generally preferred [108]. Therefore, there are still not enough data about the applicability of these regimens in elderly patients.

Some retrospective studies show that among patients undergoing surgical resection for pancreatic adenocarcinoma, there is a substantial age difference between those who can access polychemotherapy adjuvant therapy regimens compared to those who receive therapies with single chemotherapy agents which tend to be older people. Therefore, age is configured as a prognostic factor regarding the accessibility to valid adjuvant therapy post-pancreatectomy.

Due to the lack of uniformity of data on which is the best treatment for this category of patients, some authors have studied the difference in outcome between geriatric patients who have undergone surgery versus chemotherapy as monotherapy [109]. The majority of these conclude that the standard of care can be offered to this geriatric population, provided that the patient is adequately studied to highlight any specific pre-treatment age-related frailties [110, 111].

On the other hand, there are some recent cases, albeit from retrospective and single-center studies, which elicit that age "per se" is not configured as a factor statistically associated with survival. Therefore, it is not a limiting criterion for proposing a standard treatment to these patients and the effect of surgery is independent of age [112, 113].

Moreover, in light of the ever so common tendency to adopt less and less invasive approaches, it is important to highlight how regardless of the scarcity of evidence, it appears that the laparoscopic and robotic approach in patients over 70 years old not only it is not associated with high rates of complications, but in some cases, it seems to reduce complications slightly [114].

Ultimately, in decision-making for geriatric patients suffering from resectable pancreatic neoplasm, although the evidence is conflicting, it emerges more and more that, using adequate evaluation scales such as Lawton's Instrumental Activities of Daily Living (IADL) impairment (IADLb4) and the Cumulative Index Rating Scale-Geriatric (CIRS-G), it is possible to adequately frame the patient, take into account comorbidities, and be able to calibrate the choice of treatment on the patient, not only taking into account age as a limiting best medical treatment.

10.6 Gastric Cancer Surgery

More than one-third of patients are diagnosed of gastric cancer at age 75 or older. While age alone is not a contraindication for surgery, it is important to assess the overall health status and comorbidities of the elderly patient before making a decision. Older patients are at an increased risk of frailty, vulnerable to stressors and with a limited ability to adapt to change. Besides survival, addressing quality of life (QoL) and functional outcomes is especially important for this patient group.

A number of studies have reported conflicting outcomes for patients ≥80 years old with gastric cancer who undergo surgery. The postoperative morbidity and mortality of older patients after gastrectomy were reported to be higher than in younger patients [115, 116] although some reports found no significant differences in the incidence of morbidity or mortality between older patients and control groups [117, 118] These results may be influenced by selection bias among patients who undergo surgery.

Older patients often have a longer recovery period after surgery: postoperative care should include early mobilization, nutritional support, pain management, and close monitoring for any complications. Rehabilitation programs may be beneficial to optimize functional recovery.

Frailty and sarcopenia are being used increasingly frequently to evaluate older patients and seem to have significant adverse impacts on the occurrence of postoperative outcomes [119]. Recently, the comprehensive geriatric assessment (CGA), including the Barthel Index, the Mini-Mental State Examination, Instrumental Activities of Daily Living, the Vitality Index, and the Geriatric Depression Score, was reported to be an independent predictor of the OS in older patients with gastrointestinal cancer [120]. In addition, the Geriatric Prognostic Score (GPS), which is calculated by age, sex, cancer type, clinical cancer stage, PS, BMI, and CGA, has been developed [121]. It will be necessary to consider the surgical indications of elderly patients, especially those ≥90 years old and those with PS ≥ 3, using CGA and GPS.

The POSSUM scoring system has been also developed for surgical risk assessment of older patients. The POSSUM can reportedly help identify high-risk octogenarians undergoing curative gastrectomy [122]. Onodera's Prognostic Nutritional Index, originally developed as a predictor of the surgical risk of resection and anastomosis for advanced gastrointestinal cancer in Japan, also appears to be useful for predicting long-term outcomes of older patients with gastric cancer [123].

The optimal surgical treatment strategy for gastric cancer in older patients remains a matter of debate. The treatment goals should be discussed thoroughly with the patient and their family, taking into account their wishes, quality of life considerations, and expectations.

Some patients may suffer from malnutrition after gastrectomy, whereas gastrectomy may relieve symptoms due to gastric outlet obstruction or bleeding. Treatment choices that balance the survival and quality of life are important, especially for elderly patients.

The surgical treatment options for gastric cancer vary with regard to invasiveness of surgery and the extent of lymphadenectomy performed. Studies are ongoing to investigate which kind of surgery is most suitable for older patients, considering the balance of the curability of cancer and the quality of life after surgery. Currently, minimally invasive gastrectomy (MIG) is gaining ground over open gastrectomy (OG) as it is associated with better short- and long-term outcomes, including improved QoL. A meta-analysis conducted in older Asian populations has shown that laparoscopic surgery is feasible and safe for patients 65 years and older [124].

In a review of Argillander et al. [125], they found low-quality evidence that older patients (>75 years) may gain a survival benefit from undergoing gastrectomy compared to conservative treatment. The results of their meta-analyses support MIG as the preferred treatment option compared to the more traditional OG in older patients. The effect of extended lymphadenectomy on survival outcomes in older patients remains unclear and studies addressing QoL are absent. Baseline frailty assessment of older patients were lacking in all studies.

Frailty, as defined by the Modified Frailty Index, is an independent predictor of non-home discharge [126] and postoperative pulmonary infection [127] in older patients with gastric cancer who underwent gastrectomy. In patients with gastric cancer above the age of 80 years, frailty can independently predict the recurrence-free survival.

Wang et al. [128] focused on the impact of preoperative frailty on adverse clinical outcomes in patients with gastric cancer undergoing gastrectomy. Their meta-analysis confirmed that frailty is associated with a reduced overall survival and disease-specific survival among these patients. Patients with gastric cancer undergoing gastrectomy having frailty conferred a 2.08-fold and 84% poor in-hospital and long-term follow-up overall survival. Frailty is also associated with 94% poor disease-specific survival. In addition, patients with gastric cancer having frailty has a 3.63-fold higher risk of readmission within 1 year of follow-up.

In some cases, palliative procedures or non-surgical treatment options may be considered instead of curative surgery. A study by Endo et al. [129] included patients ≥80 years old who underwent any surgical procedure or best supportive care (BSC) and showed that such patients lived significantly longer after surgery than after BSC. The patients who underwent surgery were in better condition with a younger age, better PS, higher hemoglobin level, better physiological scores, and better PNIs than those who did not undergo surgery. The prognoses of patients with surgery were significantly better than those of patients without surgery, even after

PSM. However, subgroup analyses showed that patients ≥90 years old and those with PS 3 enjoyed no survival benefit with surgery.

10.7 Conclusions

The geriatric characteristics make the patient fragile and vulnerable, with an increased risk of comorbidity and loss of autonomy, as well as a reduction in life expectancy. Geriatric age does not necessarily correlate with frailty and a tailored preoperative evaluation is required for every single geriatric patient. Conversely, frailty is associated with an increased risk of all complications and death, after both elective surgery and emergency surgery. For this reason, several fragility scores have been developed over the years to perform a preoperative assessment of the geriatric surgical patient, in order to estimate the risk of morbidity and mortality and to direct the surgeon toward the most appropriate therapeutic or palliative act and reduce the risk of complications in the postoperative period through the adoption of measures tailored to the specific patient. This is an area that certainly gives space to further evaluation and interpretation, given the constant aging of the general population and the increase in life expectancy even in the frail patient.

References

1. Health & Social Care Information Centre. Hospital Episode Statistics, Admitted Patient Care—England, 2014–15: Procedures and interventions.
2. Health & Social Care Information Centre. Hospital Episode Statistics, Admitted Patient Care—England, 2006–07: Main operations summaries.
3. Australian Institute of Health and Welfare. Australian hospital statistics 2012–13. In: Health services series; no 54. Canberra: Australian Institute of Health and Welfare; 2014.
4. Hubbard RE, Story DA. Does frailty lie in the eyes of the beholder? Heart Lung Circ. 2015;24(6):525–6.
5. Rockwood K, Howlett SE, MacKnight C, Beattie BL, Bergman H, Hebert R, et al. Prevalence, attributes, and outcomes of fitness and frailty in community-dwelling older adults: report from the Canadian study of health and aging. J Gerontol A Biol Sci Med Sci. 2004;59(12):1310–7.
6. Song X. Prevalence and 10-year outcomes of frailty in older adults in relation to deficit accumulation. J Am Geriatr Soc. 2010;58(4):681–7.
7. Lee H, Lee E, Jang IY. Frailty and comprehensive geriatric assessment. J Korean Med Sci. 2020;35(3):e16. https://doi.org/10.3346/jkms.2020.35.e16. PMID: 31950775; PMCID: PMC6970074.
8. Rockwood K, Song X, MacKnight C, Bergman H, Hogan DB, McDowell I, et al. A global clinical measure of fitness and frailty in elderly people. CMAJ. 2005;173(5):489–95.
9. Robinson TN, Walston JD, Brummel NE, Deiner S, Brown CH 4th, Kennedy M, et al. Frailty for surgeons: review of a National Institute on Aging conference on frailty for specialists. J Am Coll Surg. 2015;221(6):1083–92.
10. Makary MA, Segev DL, Pronovost PJ, Syin D, Bandeen-Roche K, Patel P, et al. Frailty as a predictor of surgical outcomes in older patients. J Am Coll Surg. 2010;210(6):901–8.
11. Orouji Jokar T, Ibraheem K, Rhee P, Kulavatunyou N, Haider A, Phelan HA, et al. Emergency general surgery specific frailty index: a validation study. J Trauma Acute Care Surg. 2016;81(2):254–60.

12. Parmar KL, Law J, Carter B. Frailty in older patients undergoing emergency laparotomy: results from the UK observational emergency laparotomy and frailty (ELF) study. Ann Surg. 2019;273:709.
13. Aitken RM, Partridge JSL, Oliver CM, Murray D, Hare S, Lockwood S, Beckley-Hoelscher N, Dhesi JK. Older patients undergoing emergency laparotomy: observations from the National Emergency Laparotomy Audit (NELA) years 1–4. Age Ageing. 2020;49(4):656–63.
14. Smart R, Carter B, McGovern J, et al. Frailty exists in younger adults admitted as surgical emergency leading to adverse outcomes. J Frailty Aging. 2017;6:219–23.
15. The Royal College of Surgeons of England and Department of Health. The high-risk general surgical patient: raising the standard. In: Updated recommendations on the perioperative Care of the High-Risk General Surgical Patient. London: The Royal College of Surgeons of England; 2018.
16. Partridge JS, Harari D, Martin FC, et al. Randomized clinical trial of comprehensive geriatric assessment and optimization in vascular surgery. Br J Surg. 2017;104:679–87.
17. Vilches-Moraga A, Fox J. Geriatricians and the older emergency surgical patient: proactive assessment and patient centred interventions. Salford-POP-GS Aging Clin Exp Res. 2018;30:277–31.
18. Partridge JSL, Harari D, Martin FC, et al. The impact of preoperative comprehensive geriatric assessment on postoperative outcomes in older patients undergoing scheduled surgery: a systematic review. Anaesthesia. 2014;69:8–16.
19. Shipway D, Koizia L, Winterkorn N, Fertleman M, Ziprin P, Moorthy K. Embedded geriatric surgical liaison is associated with reduced inpatient length of stay in older patients admitted for gastrointestinal surgery. Future Healthcare J. 2018;5:108–16.
20. Oliver CM, Bassett MG, Poulton TE, et al. Organisational factors and mortality after an emergency laparotomy: multilevel analysis of 39 903 National Emergency Laparotomy Audit patients. Br J Anesth. 2018;121:1346–56.
21. Mason MC, Crees AL, Dean MR, et al. Establishing a proactive geriatrician led comprehensive assessment in older emergency surgery patients: outcomes of a pilot study. Int J Clin Pract. 2018;72:e13096.
22. Brown AS, Brummel-Smith K, Burgess L, et al. National Institutes of Health consensus development conference statement: geriatric assessment methods for clinical decisionmaking. J Am Geriatr Soc. 1988;36:342–7.
23. Puts MTE, Alibhai SMH. Fighting back against the dilution of the comprehensive geriatric assessment. J Geriatr Oncol. 2018;9:3–5.
24. Hewitt J, Long S, Carter B, Bach S, McCarthy K, Clegg A. The prevalence of frailty and its association with clinical outcomes in general surgery: a systematic review and metaanalysis. Age Ageing. 2018;47:793–800.
25. Carter B, Law J, Hewitt J, et al. Association between preadmission frailty and care level at discharge in older adults undergoing emergency laparotomy. Br J Surg. 2020;107:218.
26. Peden CJ, Stephens T, Martin G, et al. Effectiveness of a national quality improvement programme to improve survival after emergency abdominal surgery (EPOCH): a stepped-wedge cluster-randomised trial. Lancet. 2019;393:2213–21.
27. Payton P, Shook JE. Perioperative understanding of geriatric patients. Clin Podiatr Med Surg. 2019;36:131–40.
28. Kumar C, Salzman B, Colburn JL. Preoperative assessment in older adults: a comprehensive approach. Am Fam Physician. 2018;98:214–20.
29. Schamp R, Tenkku L. Managed death in a PACE: pathways in present and advance directives. J Am Med Dir Assoc. 2006;7:339–44.
30. Fried TR, Bradley EH, Towle VR, Allore H. Understanding the treatment preferences of seriously ill patients. N Engl J Med. 2002;346:1061–6.
31. Cooper Z, Koritsanszky LA, Cauley CE, et al. Recommendations for best communication practices to facilitate goal-concordant care for seriously ill older patients with emergency surgical conditions. Ann Surg. 2016;263:1–6.

32. Vilches-Moraga A, Fox J. Geriatricians and the older emergency general surgical patient: proactive assessment and patient centred interventions. Salford-POP-GS Aging Clin Exp Res. 2018;30:277–82.
33. Desserud KF, Veen T, Søreide K. Emergency general surgery in the geriatric patient. Br J Surg. 2016;103:e52–61.
34. Office for National Statistics England. National life table; 2015.
35. Plassman BL, Langa KM, Fisher GG, et al. Prevalence of dementia in the United States: the aging, demographics, and memory study. Neuroepidemiology. 2007;29:125–32.
36. Plassman BL, Langa KM, Fisher GG, et al. Prevalence of cognitive impairment without dementia in the United States. Ann Intern Med. 2008;148:427–34.
37. Chow WB, Rosenthal RA, Merkow RP, Ko CY, Esnaola NF. American College of Surgeons National Surgical Quality Improvement Program; American Geriatrics Society. Optimal preoperative assessment of the geriatric surgical patient: a best practices guideline from the American College of Surgeons National Surgical Quality Improvement Program and the American Geriatrics Society. J Am Coll Surg. 2012;215:453–66.
38. Borson S, Scanlan JM, Chen P, Ganguli M. The mini-cog as a screen for dementia: validation in a population-based sample. J Am Geriatr Soc. 2003;51:1451–4.
39. Luan Erfe BM, Erfe JM, Brovman EY, Boehme J, Bader AM, Urman RD. Postoperative outcomes in SAVR/TAVR patients with cognitive impairment: a systematic review. Semin Thorac Cardiovasc Surg. 2019;31:370–80.
40. Fields LM, Calvert JD. Informed consent procedures with cognitively impaired patients: a review of ethics and best practices. Psychiatry Clin Neurosci. 2015;69:462–71.
41. Leslie DL, Marcantonio ER, Zhang Y, Leo-Summers L, Inouye SK. One-year health care costs associated with delirium in the elderly population. Arch Intern Med. 2008;168:27–32.
42. McCusker J, Cole M, Dendukuri N, Belzile E, Primeau F. Delirium in older medical inpatients and subsequent cognitive and functional status: a prospective study. CMAJ. 2001;165:575–83.
43. Inouye SK, Rushing JT, Foreman MD, Palmer RM, Pompei P. Does delirium contribute to poor hospital outcomes? A threesite epidemiologic study. J Gen Intern Med. 1998;13:234–42.
44. O'Keeffe S, Lavan J. The prognostic significance of delirium in older hospital patients. J Am Geriatr Soc. 1997;45:174–8.
45. Hshieh TT, Yue J, Oh E, et al. Effectiveness of multicomponent nonpharmacological delirium interventions: a meta-analysis. JAMA Intern Med. 2015;175:512–20.
46. Robinson TN, Raeburn CD, Tran ZV, Angles EM, Brenner LA, Moss M. Postoperative delirium in the elderly: risk factors and outcomes. Ann Surg. 2009;249:173–8.
47. Marcantonio ER, Goldman L, Mangione CM, et al. A clinical prediction rule for delirium after elective noncardiac surgery. JAMA. 1994;271:134–9.
48. Rostoft S, Hamaker ME. Basic geriatric principles for colorectal surgeons: how to optimize assessment and care of older patients in the perioperative period. Eur J Surg Oncol. 2020;46:310–5.
49. Neufeld KJ, Thomas C. Delirium: definition, epidemiology, and diagnosis. J Clin Neurophysiol. 2013;30:438–42.
50. Siddiqi NHJ, Clegg A, Teale EA, Young J, Taylor J, Simpkins SA. Interventions for preventing delirium in hospitalised non-ICU patients. Cochrane Database Syst Rev. 2016;3:CD005563.
51. Watt J, Tricco AC, Talbot-Hamon C, et al. Identifying older adults at risk of delirium following elective surgery: a systematic review and meta-analysis. J Gen Intern Med. 2018;33:500–9.
52. Shi C, Jin J, Qiao L, Li T, Ma J, Ma Z. Effect of perioperative administration of dexmedetomidine on delirium after cardiac surgery in elderly patients: a double-blinded, multi-center, randomized study. Clin Interv Aging. 2019;14:571–5.
53. By the 2019 American Geriatrics Society Beers Criteria® Update Expert Panel. American Geriatrics Society 2019 Updated AGS beers criteria® for potentially inappropriate medication use in older adults. J Am Geriatr Soc. 2019;67:674–94.
54. Gale CR, Westbury L, Cooper C. Social isolation and loneliness as risk factors for the progression of frailty: the English longitudinal study of ageing. Age Ageing. 2018;47:392–7.

55. Bunt S, Steverink N, Olthof J, van der Schans CP, Hobbelen JSM. Social frailty in older adults: a scoping review. Eur J Ageing. 2017;14:323–34.
56. Dent E, Morley JE, Cruz-Jentoft AJ, et al. Physical frailty: ICFSR international clinical practice guidelines for identification and management. J Nutr Health Aging. 2019;23:771–87.
57. Hawkins AT, Pallangyo AJ, Herman AM, et al. The effect of social integration on outcomes after major lower extremity amputation. J Vasc Surg. 2016;63:154–62.
58. Gonzalez-Saenz de Tejada M, Bilbao A, Baré M, et al. Association of social support, functional status, and psychological variables with changes in health-related quality of life outcomes in patients with colorectal cancer. Psychooncology. 2016;25:891–7.
59. Gardner B, Jovicic A, Belk C, et al. Specifying the content of home-based health behaviour change interventions for older people with frailty or at risk of frailty: an exploratory systematic review. BMJ Open. 2017;7:e014127.
60. Ghignone F, van Leeuwen BL, Montroni I, et al. International Society of Geriatric Oncology (SIOG) surgical task force. The assessment and management of older cancer patients: a SIOG surgical task force survey on surgeons' attitudes. Eur J Surg Oncol. 2016;42:297–302.
61. Williams GR, Weaver KE, Lesser GJ, et al. Capacity to provide geriatric specialty care for older adults in community oncology practices. Oncologist. 2020;25:1032–8.
62. Fifth Patient Report of the National Emergency Laparotomy Audit. December 2017 to November 2018. Royal College of Anaesthetists, December 2019. Retrieved June 2020, from National Emergency Laparotomy Audit.
63. Royal College of Physicians. Focus on physicians: 2018–19 census (UK consultants and higher specialty trainees); 2020. Retrieved June 2020.
64. Oakley B, Nightingale J, Moran C, Moppett IK. Does achieving the best practice tariff improve outcomes in hip fracture patients? An observational cohort study. BMJ Open. 2017;7:e014190.
65. McCarthy K, Hewitt J. Special needs of frail people undergoing emergency laparotomy surgery. Age Ageing. 2020;49:540–3.
66. British Geriatrics Society. BGS position statement: older patients undergoing emergency laparotomy; 2020. Retrieved June 2020, from British Geriatrics Society.
67. Banks E, Byles JE, Gibson RE, et al. Is psychological distress in people living with cancer related to the fact of diagnosis, current treatment or level of disability? Findings from a large Australian study. Med J Aust. 2010;193(S5):S62–7.
68. IPSOS MORI. Exploring the attitudes and behaviours of older people living with cancer. https://www.ipsos.com/ipsos-mori/en-uk/exploring-attitudes-and-behavioursolder-people-living-cancer. Published 2015.
69. Huisman MG, Audisio RA, Ugolini G, et al. Screening for predictors of adverse outcome in onco-geriatric surgical patients: a multicenter prospective cohort study. Eur J Surg Oncol. 2015;41:844–51.
70. Huisman MG, van Leeuwen BL, Ugolini G, et al. "Timed up & go": a screening tool for predicting 30-day morbidity in oncogeriatric surgical patients? A multicenter cohort study. PLoS One. 2014;9:e86863.
71. Pédziwiatr M, Pisarska M, Major P, et al. Laparoscopic colorectal cancer surgery combined with enhanced recovery after surgery protocol (ERAS) reduces the negative impact of sarcopenia on short-term outcomes. Eur J Surg Oncol. 2016;42:779–87.
72. Calle A, Onder G, Morandi A, et al. Frailty related factors as predictors of functional recovery in geriatric rehabilitation: the sarcopenia and function in aging rehabilitation (SAFARI) multi-centric study. J Nutr Health Aging. 2018;22:1099–106.
73. Katz S, Akpom CA. A measure of primary sociobiological functions. Int J Health Serv. 1976;6:493–508.
74. Ketelaars L, Pottel L, Lycke M, et al. Use of the Freund clock drawing test within the mini-cog as a screening tool for cognitive impairment in elderly patients with or without cancer. J Geriatr Oncol. 2013;4:174–82.

75. De Roo AC, Li Y, Abrahamse PH, Regenbogen SE, Suwanabol PA. Long-term functional decline after high-risk elective colorectal surgery in older adults. Dis Colon Rectum. 2020;63:75–83.
76. Shahrokni A, Alexander K. What will perioperative geriatric assessment for older cancer patients look like in 2025? Advantages and limitations of new technologies in geriatric assessment. Eur J Surg Oncol. 2020;46:305–9.
77. Gensheimer SG, Wu AW, Snyder CF. PRO-EHR users' guide steering group; PRO-EHR users' guide working group. Oh, the places we'll go: patient-reported outcomes and electronic health records. Patient. 2018;11:591–8.
78. Ghanie A, Formica MK, Dhir M. Systematic review and meta-analysis of 90-day and 30-day mortality after liver resection in the elderly. Surgery. 2022 Oct;172(4):1164–73. https://doi.org/10.1016/j.surg.2022.05.032.
79. Notarnicola M, Felli E, Roselli S, Altomare DF, De Fazio M, de'Angelis N, Piardi T, Acquafredda S, Ammendola M, Verbo A, Pessaux P, Memeo R. Laparoscopic liver resection in elderly patients: systematic review and meta-analysis. Surg Endosc. 2019 Sep;33(9):2763–73. https://doi.org/10.1007/s00464-019-06840-9.
80. Yamamoto H, Kaibori M, Matsushima H, Kosaka H, Matsui K, Sekimoto M. Efficacy and safety of liver resection in super elderly patients with hepatocellular carcinoma. Asian Pac J Cancer Prev. 2023;24(3):1089–94. https://doi.org/10.31557/APJCP.2023.24.3.1089.
81. Schiergens TS, Stielow C, Schreiber S, Hornuss C, Jauch KW, Rentsch M, Thasler WE. Liver resection in the elderly: significance of comorbidities and blood loss. J Gastrointest Surg. 2014 Jun;18(6):1161–70. https://doi.org/10.1007/s11605-014-2516-2.
82. Vitale A, Trevisani F, Farinati F, Cillo U. Treatment of hepatocellular carcinoma in the precision medicine era: from treatment stage migration to therapeutic hierarchy. Hepatology. 2020 Dec;72(6):2206–18. https://doi.org/10.1002/hep.31187.
83. Ban D, Tanabe M, Ito H, Otsuka Y, Nitta H, Abe Y, Hasegawa Y, Katagiri T, Takagi C, Itano O, Kaneko H, Wakabayashi G. A novel difficulty scoring system for laparoscopic liver resection. J Hepatobiliary Pancreat Sci. 2014;21(10):745–53. https://doi.org/10.1002/jhbp.166.
84. Filippo R, Conticchio M, Ratti F, Inchingolo R, Gelli M, Anelli FM, Laurent A, Vitali GC, Magistri P, Assirati G, Felli E, Wakabayashi T, Pessaux P, Piardi T, Di Benedetto F, de'Angelis N, DFJ B, Rampoldi AG, Adam R, Cherqui D, Aldrighetti L, Memeo R. Liver resection versus radiofrequency ablation in octogenarian patients for hepatocellular carcinoma: a propensity score multicenter analysis. Surg Endosc. 2023;37(4):3029–36. https://doi.org/10.1007/s00464-022-09826-2.
85. Dijkstra M, Nieuwenhuizen S, Puijk RS, Timmer FEF, Geboers B, Schouten EAC, Opperman J, Scheffer HJ, Vries JJJ, Swijnenburg RJ, Versteeg KS, Lissenberg-Witte BI, van den Tol MP, Meijerink MR. Thermal ablation compared to partial hepatectomy for recurrent colorectal liver metastases: an Amsterdam Colorectal Liver Met Registry (AmCORE) based study. Cancers (Basel). 2021;13(11):2769. https://doi.org/10.3390/cancers13112769. PMID: 34199556; PMCID: PMC8199651.
86. Wang SJ, Hathout L, Malhotra U, Maloney-Patel N, Kilic S, Poplin E, Jabbour SK. Decision-making strategy for rectal cancer management using radiation therapy for elderly or comorbid patients. Int J Radiat Oncol Biol Phys. 2018;100(4):926–44.
87. Allemani C, Matsuda T, Di Carlo V, Harewood R, Matz M, Nikšić M, Bonaventure A, Valkov M, Johnson CJ, Estève J, Ogunbiyi OJ, Azevedo E, Silva G, Chen WQ, Eser S, Engholm G, Stiller CA, Monnereau A, Woods RR, Visser O, Lim GH, Aitken J, Weir HK, Coleman MP, CONCORD Working Group. Global surveillance of trends in cancer survival 2000-14 (CONCORD-3): analysis of individual records for 37 513 025 patients diagnosed with one of 18 cancers from 322 population-based registries in 71 countries. Lancet. 2018;391(10125):1023–75.
88. Adelson P, Fusco K, Karapetis C, Wattchow D, Joshi R, Price T, Sharplin G, Roder D. Use of guideline-recommended adjuvant therapies and survival outcomes for people with colorectal cancer at tertiary referral hospitals in South Australia. J Eval Clin Pract. 2018;24(1):135–44.

89. Chen RC, Royce TJ, Extermann M, Reeve BB. Impact of age and comorbidity on treatment and outcomes in elderly cancer patients. Semin Radiat Oncol. 2012;22(4):265–71.
90. Koroukian SM, Xu F, Bakaki PM, Diaz-Insua M, Towe TP, Owusu C. Comorbidities, functional limitations, and geriatric syndromes in relation to treatment and survival patterns among elders with colorectal cancer. J Gerontol A Biol Sci Med Sci. 2010;65(3):322–9.
91. Janssen-Heijnen ML, Houterman S, Lemmens VE, Louwman MW, Maas HA, Coebergh JW. Prognostic impact of increasing age and co-morbidity in cancer patients: a population-based approach. Crit Rev Oncol Hematol. 2005;55(3):231–40.
92. Buntinx F, Campbell C, van den Akker M. Cancer in the elderly. J Cancer Epidemiol. 2014;2014:872029. https://doi.org/10.1155/2014/872029. Epub 2014 Apr 30. PMID: 24876840; PMCID: PMC4021674.
93. Papamichael D, Audisio RA, Glimelius B, de Gramont A, Glynne-Jones R, Haller D, Köhne CH, Rostoft S, Lemmens V, Mitry E, Rutten H, Sargent D, Sastre J, Seymour M, Starling N, Van Cutsem E, Aapro M. Treatment of colorectal cancer in older patients: International Society of Geriatric Oncology (SIOG) consensus recommendations 2013. Ann Oncol. 2015;26(3):463–76.
94. Hamaker ME, Wildes TM, Rostoft S. Time to stop saying geriatric assessment is too time consuming. J Clin Oncol. 2017;35(25):2871–4.
95. Mohanty S, Rosenthal RA, Russell MM, Neuman MD, Ko CY, Esnaola NF. Optimal Perioperative Management of the Geriatric Patient: a Best Practices Guideline from the American College of Surgeons NSQIP and the American Geriatrics Society. J Am Coll Surg. 2016;222(5):930–47.
96. Bellera CA, Rainfray M, Mathoulin-Pélissier S, Mertens C, Delva F, Fonck M, Soubeyran PL. Screening older cancer patients: first evaluation of the G-8 geriatric screening tool. Ann Oncol. 2012;23(8):2166–72.
97. Ghignone F, van Leeuwen BL, Montroni I, Huisman MG, Somasundar P, Cheung KL, Audisio RA, Ugolini G, International Society of Geriatric Oncology (SIOG) Surgical Task Force. The assessment and management of older cancer patients: A SIOG surgical task force survey on surgeons' attitudes. Eur J Surg Oncol. 2016;42(2):297–302.
98. Kim SW, Han HS, Jung HW, Kim KI, Hwang DW, Kang SB, Kim CH. Multidimensional frailty score for the prediction of postoperative mortality risk. JAMA Surg. 2014;149(7):633–40.
99. Presley CJ, Krok-Schoen JL, Wall SA, Noonan AM, Jones DC, Folefac E, Williams N, Overcash J, Rosko AE. Implementing a multidisciplinary approach for older adults with cancer: geriatric oncology in practice. BMC Geriatr. 2020;20(1):231.
100. Stegmann ME, Festen S, Brandenbarg D, Schuling J, van Leeuwen B, de Graeff P, Berendsen AJ. Using the Outcome Prioritization Tool (OPT) to assess the preferences of older patients in clinical decision-making: a review. Maturitas. 2019;128:49–52.
101. Couwenberg AM, de Beer FSA, Intven MPW, Burbach JPM, Smits AB, Consten ECJ, Schiphorst AHW, Wijffels NAT, de Roos MAJ, Hamaker ME, van Grevenstein WMU, Verkooijen HM. The impact of postoperative complications on health-related quality of life in older patients with rectal cancer; a prospective cohort study. J Geriatr Oncol. 2018;9(2):102–9.
102. Itatani Y, Kawada K, Sakai Y. Treatment of elderly patients with colorectal cancer. Biomed Res Int. 2018;11(2018):2176056.
103. Devoto L, Celentano V, Cohen R, Khan J, Chand M. Colorectal cancer surgery in the very elderly patient: a systematic review of laparoscopic versus open colorectal resection. Int J Color Dis. 2017;32(9):1237–42.
104. Decoster L, Van Puyvelde K, Mohile S, Wedding U, Basso U, Colloca G, Rostoft S, Overcash J, Wildiers H, Steer C, Kimmick G, Kanesvaran R, Luciani A, Terret C, Hurria A, Kenis C, Audisio R, Extermann M. Screening tools for multidimensional health problems warranting a geriatric assessment in older cancer patients: an update on SIOG recommendations. Ann Oncol. 2015;26(2):288–300.
105. Sinn M, Bahra M, Denecke T, et al. Perioperative treatment options in resectable pancreatic cancer—how to improve long-term survival. World J Gastrointest Oncol. 2016;8:248–57.

106. Eubanks A, et al. Age as a prognostic indicator for adjuvant therapy in patients who underwent pancreatic resections for cancer. J Geriatr Oncol. 2018;9:362. https://doi.org/10.1016/j.jgo.2017.12.004.
107. Conroy T, Desseigne F, Ychou M, Bouché O, Guimbaud R, Bécouarn Y, et al. FOLFIRINOX versus gemcitabine for metastatic pancreatic cancer. N Engl J Med. 2011;364:1817–25.
108. Von Hoff DD, Ervin T, Arena FP, Chiorean EG, Infante J, Moore M, et al. Increased survival in pancreatic cancer with nab-paclitaxel plus gemcitabine. N Engl J Med. 2013;369:1691–703.
109. Audisio RA, Pope D, Ramesh HS, Gennari R, Van Leeuwen BL, West C, et al. Shall we operate? Preoperative assessment in elderly patients (PACE) can help. A SIOG surgical task force prospective study. Crit Rev Oncol Hematol. 2008;65:156–63.
110. Oliveira-Cunha M, Malde DJ, Aldouri A, Morris-Stiff G, Menon KV, Malvern SA. Result of pancreatic surgery in the elderly: is age a barrier? HBP (Oxf). 2013;15:24–30.
111. Nagrial AM, Chang DK, Nguyen NQ, Johns AL, Chantrill LA, Humphris JL, et al. Adjuvant chemotherapy in elderly patients with pancreatic cancer. Br J Cancer. 2014;110:313–9.
112. Castel-Kremer E, et al. An onco-geriatric approach to select older patients for optimal treatments of pancreatic adenocarcinoma. J Geriatr Oncol. 2018;9:373. https://doi.org/10.1016/j.jgo.2018.03.007.
113. Tan E, et al. Postoperative outcomes in elderly patients undergoing pancreatic resection for pancreatic adenocarcinoma: a systematic review and meta-analysis. Int J Surg. 2019;72:59–68.
114. van der Heijde N, Balduzzi A, Alseidi A, Dokmak S, Polanco PM, Sandford D, Shrikhande SV, Vollmer C, Wang SE, Besselink MG, Asbun H, Abu Hilal M. The role of older age and obesity in minimally invasive and open pancreatic surgery: a systematic review and meta-analysis. Pancreatology. 2020;20(6):1234–42. https://doi.org/10.1016/j.pan.2020.06.013. ISSN 1424-3903.
115. Fujiwara Y, Fukuda S, Tsujie M, Ishikawa H, Kitani K, Inoue K, et al. Effects of age on survival and morbidity in gastric cancer patients undergoing gastrectomy. World J Gastrointest Oncol. 2017;9:257–62.
116. Xu Y, Wang Y, Xi C, Ye N, Xu X. Is it safe to perform gastrectomy in gastric cancer patients aged 80 or older?: A metaanalysis and systematic review. Medicine (Baltimore). 2019;98(24):e16092. https://doi.org/10.1097/MD.0000000000016092.
117. Mita K, Ito H, Hashimoto M, Murabayashi R, Asakawa H, Nabetani M, et al. Postoperative complications and survival after gastric cancer surgery in patients older than 80 years of age. J Gastrointest Surg. 2013;17:2067–73.
118. Sakurai K, Muguruma K, Nagahara H, Kimura K, Toyokawa T, Amano R, et al. The outcome of surgical treatment for elderly patients with gastric carcinoma. J Surg Oncol. 2015;111:848–54.
119. Shen Y, Hao Q, Zhou J, Dong B. The impact of frailty and sarcopenia on postoperative outcomes in older patients undergoing gastrectomy surgery: a systematic review and meta-analysis. BMC Geriatr. 2017;17:188.
120. Xue DD, Cheng Y, Wu M, Zhang Y. Comprehensive geriatric assessment prediction of postoperative complications in gastrointestinal cancer patients: a meta-analysis. Clin Interv Aging. 2018;24(13):723–36.
121. Yamasaki M, Maekawa Y, Sugimoto K, Mizushima T, Eguchi H, Ogihara T, et al. Development of a geriatric prognostic scoring system for predicting survival after surgery for elderly patients with gastrointestinal cancer. Ann Surg Oncol. 2019;26:3644–51.
122. Kim SY, Kim JH, Chin H, Jun KH. Prediction of postoperative mortality and morbidity in octogenarians with gastric cancer—comparison of P-POSSUM, O-POSSUM, and E-POSSUM: a retrospective single-center cohort study. Int J Surg. 2020;77:64–8.
123. Sakurai K, Tamura T, Toyokawa T, Amano R, Kubo N, Tanaka H, et al. Low preoperative prognostic nutritional index predicts poor survival post-gastrectomy in elderly patients with gastric cancer. Ann Surg Oncol. 2016;23:3669–76.
124. Lou S, Yin X, Wang Y, Zhang Y, Xue Y. Laparoscopic versus open gastrectomy for gastric cancer: a systematic review and meta-analysis of randomized controlled trials. Int J Surg.

2022;102:106678. https://doi.org/10.1016/j.ijsu.2022.106678. Epub 2022 May 16. PMID: 35589049.

125. Argillander TE, Festen S, van der Zaag-Loonen HJ, de Graeff P, van der Zaag ES, van Leeuwen BL, Nagengast WB, Verhage RJJ, Ruurda JP, van Munster BC, van Duijvendijk P. Outcomes of surgical treatment of non-metastatic gastric cancer in patients aged 70 and older: a systematic review and meta-analysis. Eur J Surg Oncol. 2022;48(9):1882–94.
126. Osaki T, Saito H, Shimizu S, Murakami Y, Miyatani K, Matsunaga T, et al. Modified frailty index is useful in predicting non-home discharge in elderly patients with gastric cancer who undergo gastrectomy. World J Surg. 2020;44(11):3837–44.
127. Meng Y, Zhao P, Yong R. Modified frailty index independently predicts postoperative pulmonary infection in elderly patients undergoing radical gastrectomy for gastric cancer. Cancer Manag Res. 2021;13:9117–26.
128. Wang X, Sun Y, Wang P, Jie Y, Liu G, Gong D, Fan Y. Impact of frailty on survival and readmission in patients with gastric cancer undergoing gastrectomy: a meta-analysis. Front Oncol. 2022;31(12):972287. https://doi.org/10.3389/fonc.2022.972287. PMID: 36387139; PMCID: PMC9659614.
129. Endo S, Fujiwara Y, Higashida M, et al. Survival analyses of elderly gastric cancer patients with or without surgery. Surg Today. 2022;52(1):75–83.

The Nurse: Perioperative Care and Management

11

Luca Cordelio Dimonte Camicia, Alessia Barcaroli, and Dalila Carioti

11.1 Introduction

The perioperative phase is a critical period that requires thorough assessment, preparation, and coordination of care to optimize patient outcomes. This chapter focuses on the role of nursing in providing assistance and highlights key aspects such as risk assessment, patient preparation, and the implementation of ERAS and Fast Track Surgery protocols.

11.1.1 Preoperative Risk Assessment

Before surgery, patients need to follow recommendations provided by the orthopedic surgeon to prepare themselves physically. This may involve weight loss to facilitate postoperative recovery, muscle strengthening to enhance rehabilitation, smoking cessation to reduce pulmonary and vascular complications, and discontinuation of certain medications like anticoagulants. Additionally, assessments such as imaging diagnostics, laboratory tests, electrocardiogram, urine culture, and anesthesia evaluations are conducted to evaluate the patient's health status and identify any risks associated with the surgery.

11.1.2 Patient Preparation

Patient preparation plays a crucial role in ensuring a smooth surgical experience. The day before the procedure, patients are advised to follow a light diet in the evening,

L. C. D. Camicia (✉) · A. Barcaroli · D. Carioti
Institute of Orthopedics and Traumatology, Santa Maria della Misericordia Hospital, Perugia, Italy
e-mail: luca.camicia@ospedale.perugia.it

V. Boccardi, L. Marano (eds.), *The Frail Surgical Patient*, Practical Issues in Geriatrics, https://doi.org/10.1007/978-3-031-77707-3_11

abstain from clear liquids for a few hours before surgery, and avoid food intake for 6–8 h prior to the operation. The carbohydrate-rich drink (CHD) treatment before surgery increases patient comfort by reducing preoperative discomfort (such as hunger, thirst, dry mouth, fatigue and headache) and early postoperative complications (vomiting and pain) [1]. Various preoperative measures, including trichotomy, oral hygiene, showering with bactericidal solutions, and application of antiseptics to the incision site, are performed. Nurses are responsible for administering prescribed therapies, premedication, thromboprophylaxis, antibiotic prophylaxis, and, if necessary, placing a urinary catheter.

11.1.3 ERAS and Fast Track Surgery Protocols

The ERAS protocol is a multidisciplinary approach involving surgeons, anesthesiologists, nurses, physiotherapists, and nutritionists. Its primary objectives are to reduce surgical stress, enhance the body's response to surgical insults, and decrease hospitalization duration. The protocol includes interventions such as preoperative carbohydrate beverages, minimally invasive surgery, optimized fluid management, early mobilization, early oral intake, and effective pain management. Fast Track Surgery, developed by Henrik Kehlet [2], complements the ERAS approach and aims to minimize blood loss, improve postoperative pain management, enable early rehabilitation, and facilitate rapid discharge.

11.1.4 Nursing Care and Model Application

Nurses play a central role in guiding patients throughout the preoperative journey. By utilizing theoretical models such as Majory Gordon's theoretical model, nurses can assess the functional and dysfunctional areas of individuals and formulate appropriate nursing diagnoses using the NANDA taxonomy. Based on these diagnoses, nurses establish patient-centered goals (NOC) and choose suitable nursing interventions (NIC) to meet the patient's needs. The nursing process involves evaluating outcomes and comparing them against predetermined goals.

Preoperative nursing assistance is essential for ensuring the well-being and safety of patients before surgery. This article highlighted the importance of risk assessment, patient preparation, and the implementation of ERAS and Fast Track Surgery protocols. A key mechanism behind the effectiveness of ERAS is the dampening of the stress responses to the surgical insult combined with the use of treatments that support return of functions that delay recovery in traditional care [3]. By following a comprehensive approach and collaborating with other healthcare professionals, nurses can contribute significantly to positive patient outcomes.

11.2 Intraoperative Phase: Nursing Care and Patient Management

This part focuses on the intraoperative phase of surgical care, specifically highlighting the role of nursing in providing comprehensive assistance during this crucial period. It discusses the responsibilities of the intraoperative nursing team, including the operating room nurse, instrument nurse, anesthesia technician, and other healthcare professionals. This part also addresses patient preparation, positioning, anesthesia induction, surgical procedures, and postoperative transfer to the recovery room.

11.2.1 Intraoperative Nursing Care

During the intraoperative phase, the patient is attended by a multidisciplinary team, including the operating room nurse, instrument nurse, surgeon, anesthesiologist, anesthesia technician, healthcare assistants, and other supporting staff. Each member of the team plays a vital role in ensuring the smooth progress of the surgery.

11.2.2 The Role of the Operating Room Nurse

The operating room nurse assumes various responsibilities, including:

Patient care and management: Assisting the patient in the operating room, ensuring the functionality of medical equipment, collect vital signs and connect monitoring devices before sedation, establishing peripheral venous access, and maintaining accurate nursing documentation.

Monitoring and coordination: Verifying the proper functioning of electromedical equipment and collaborating with other team members to ensure a sterile environment.

Intraoperative documentation: Compiling the necessary nursing records during the surgical procedure.

11.2.3 The Role of the Instrument Nurse

The instrument nurse is responsible for:

Aseptic preparation: Ensuring the sterile preparation of surgical materials and instruments.

Instrument count: Conducting an accurate count of surgical instruments at the beginning and end of each procedure.

Sterility maintenance: Maintaining the sterility of the surgical field and actively collaborating with the surgical team.

11.2.4 The Role of the Anesthesia Technician

The anesthesia technician assists the anesthesiologist during various activities in the operating room, including:

Preparation of anesthesia materials: Setting up the anesthesia cart with all necessary materials, such as needles, cannulas, tourniquets, sterile dressings, and disposable central venous catheter kits.

Equipment management: Ensuring the proper functioning, cleaning, disinfection, and sterilization of anesthesia equipment.

Monitoring responsibilities: Regularly surveilling anesthesia equipment during the procedure and monitoring vital signs such as blood pressure, body temperature, respiration, and anesthetic gas pressure using specialized monitors.

11.2.5 Intraoperative Procedures and Patient Management

The patient is transported to the reception area of the operating room, where preoperative checks and documentation take place. The operating room nurse welcomes the patient, provides explanations of the procedure, and addresses any questions or concerns. Preoperative education may represent a useful adjunct, with low risk of undesirable effects, particularly in certain patients, for example people with depression, anxiety or unrealistic expectations, who may respond well to preoperative education that is stratified according to their physical, psychological and social need [4, 5].

Following this, the patient is transferred to the operating room and positioned appropriately on the operating table. Correct positioning is crucial for optimal surgical exposure, joint stress reduction, prevention of pressure injuries, and maintenance of cardiorespiratory function and airway patency. The specific positioning (supine or lateral) and the use of supportive padding depend on the surgical approach determined by the surgeon.

Once the patient is prepared and connected to monitoring devices, the anesthesiologist induces anesthesia, leading to the loss of consciousness. The surgeon then proceeds, after which the patient is transferred to the recovery room, where they regain consciousness post-anesthesia. In the recovery room, the patient is placed on a stretcher or bed, covered and warmed, and their vital signs and overall condition are regularly assessed. The recovery room nurse closely monitors the patient for potential complications, such as hematoma, hypoxia, shock, arrhythmias, respiratory distress, nausea, vomiting, or hypothermia.

The recovery room nurse utilizes assessment tools like the Aldrete Score (Fig. 11.1) or the White and Song Scale (Fig. 11.2) to evaluate the patient's readiness for discharge from the recovery area. Additionally, the nurse provides emotional support, informs the patient and their family about the surgery outcome, and facilitates their return to the assigned unit.

	Original 1970 version	Modified by author in 1995	Additional criteria by Marshall and Chang in 1999 for ambulatory surgery
Activity	Able to move 4 extremities voluntarily or on command (2 Points) Able to move 2 extremities voluntarily or on command (1 Point) Unable to move extremities voluntarily or on command (0 Points)		Steady gait without dizziness or meets pre-anaethetic level (2 Points) Requires Assistance (1 Point) Unable to ambulate (0 Points)
Respiration	Able to breathe deeply and cough freely (2 Points) Dyspnoea or limited breathing (1 Point) Apnoeic (0 Points)		Not included
Circulation	BP ±20% of pre-anaesthetic level (2 Points) BP ±20-49% of pre-anaesthetic level (1 Point) BP ±50% of pre-anaesthetic level (0 Points)	Sometimes heart rate is included (but was not in the author's second paper) Heart rate ±20bpm pre-anaethetic level (2 points) Heart rate ±20-35bpm pre-anaesthetic level Heart rate ±35-50bpm pre-anaesthetic level Patients ±50bpm or >110bpm or with a change in ECG rhythm must be evaluated by an anaesthesiologist. These additional points change the overall target score.	BP ±20% of pre-anaesthetic level (2 Points) BP ±20-40% of pre-anaesthetic level (1 Point) BP ±40% of pre-anaesthetic level (0 Points)
Consciousness	Fully awake (2 Points) Arousable on calling (1 Point) Not responding (0 Points)		Not included
Colour or O_2 Saturation	Normal (2 Points) Pale, dusky, blotchy, jaundiced, or other (1 Point) Cyanotic (0 Points)	Able to maintain SpO_2 >92% on room Air (2 Points) Needs supplementary O_2 to maintain SpO_2 >90% (1 Point) SpO_2 <90% despite supplementary O2 (0 Points)	Not Included
Pain			Minimal to no pain, controllable with oral analgesics (2 Points) This target not met (1 Point)
Surgical Bleeding (as expected for procedure)			Minimal/Does not require dressing change (2 Points) Moderate/Up to two dressing changes required (1 Point) Severe/More than three dressing changes required (0 Points)
Nausea and Vomiting			None to minimal (2 Points) Moderate (1 Point) Severe (0 Points)
Interpretation of score	"Score of 9 or greater allows patient to leave Post Anaesthetic Care Unit"		"Patients who score 9 or greater and have an appropriate escort can go home."

Fig. 11.1 Aldrete score

White and Song scale:

(a) **Level of consciousness:**	
- awake and oriented	Points 2
- arousable with minimal stimulation	Points 1
- responsive only to tactile stimulation	Points 0
(b) **Physical activity:**	
- moves all extremities on command	Points 2
- weakness in moving extremities	Points 1
- unable to move extremities voluntarily.	Points 0
(c) **Hemodynamic stability:**	
- P.A.± 15% of preoperative values	Points 2
- P.A.± 30 of preoperative values	Points 1
- P.A > 30% of preoperative values	Points 0
(d) **Respiratory stability:**	
- Able to breathe deeply	Points 2
-shallow breathing (tachypnea) with good ability to cough	Points 1
-dyspnea with weak ability to cough	Points 0
(e) **Oxygen saturation:**	
>90% in room air	Points 2
- requires supplemental oxygen	Points 1
- <90% with supplemental oxygen	Points 0
(f) **Postoperative pain:**	
- Absent or mild	Points 2
- Moderate or severe, controlled with e.v. analgesics.	Points 1
- Persistent severe	Points 0
(g) **Postoperative vomiting:**	
- Absent or mild nausea	Points 2
- Transient vomiting or retching	Points 1
- Moderate/severe persistent vomiting or nausea	Points 0

Fig. 11.2 White and song scale

During patient transfer, the nurse ensures the continuity of care by summarizing the intraoperative progress, including vital signs, diuresis, drains, infusions, blood loss, transfusions, ongoing therapies, critical events, and necessary postoperative interventions. The patient's transfer is performed safely and efficiently by qualified personnel, following designated clean routes with prompt access, and avoiding pauses or interruptions. In cases of complex patients or transfers to the intensive care unit (ICU), the nurse, sometimes accompanied by an anesthesiologist, ensures continuous care during the transport process.

Intraoperative nursing care is vital for ensuring patient safety and optimal surgical outcomes. This article outlined the responsibilities of the intraoperative nursing team, patient preparation, positioning, anesthesia induction, surgical procedures, and postoperative transfer to the recovery room. By implementing comprehensive nursing practices, healthcare professionals contribute to the well-being and successful recovery of patients during the intraoperative phase.

11.3 Postoperative Phase: Nursing Care and Patient Management

This part focuses on the postoperative phase of surgical care and emphasizes the role of nursing in restoring physiological balance, managing postoperative pain, preventing complications, and educating patients to enhance their level of autonomy. The article discusses the importance of documentation review upon the patient's return to the assigned unit and highlights nursing interventions related to patient positioning, wound care, drainage management, prevention of pressure injuries, prevention and recognition of complications, delirium management, thromboembolism prophylaxis and pain management. The significance of interdisciplinary collaboration and patient education is also emphasized.

11.3.1 Postoperative Nursing Care

Postoperative nursing care aims to restore physiological balance, manage postoperative pain, prevent complications, and educate patients to enhance their level of independence. Upon the patient's return to the assigned unit, it is essential to review documentation, including the anesthesiology report and surgical procedure description, as they provide important information about the type of anesthesia, administered medications, blood loss, fluid infusions, wound extension, and any postoperative instructions or prescriptions from the surgeon.

The nursing staff takes the necessary measures to position the patient appropriately, elevate the limb to promote venous return, administer intravenous infusions, monitor vital signs, and assess the surgical wound for potential dressing changes. The patient may have a spacer between their legs, compressive bandaging to reduce the risk of hematoma, and wound drainage tubes to collect postoperative blood loss.

In the 4 h following the surgery, the drained blood can be reinfused if there are no contraindications and proper equipment is available for collection, centrifugation, washing, and reinfusion. The only contraindication to this procedure is doubtful sterility due to contamination of the surgical field with microorganisms or neoplastic cells. Risks associated with this procedure include disseminated intravascular coagulation (DIC) and mechanical hemolysis of red blood cells, as the red blood cell membrane is more sensitive to mechanical stress.

11.3.2 Recognize Complication

An important aspect of postoperative care is the nurse's ability to recognize and manage potential postoperative complications, such as surgical site infection, thromboembolism, pressure injuries, delirium (more common in older individuals), management of surgical drains, nausea and vomiting.

The control of the surgical wound is crucial for the assessment of potential infection, which manifests as pain, temperature rise above 38 °C after the fifth postoperative day, and limited range of motion. According to the World Health Organization (WHO), the adult BMI threshold is 25 for overweight and 30 for obesity.

Surgical drains are used to allow the drainage of fluids that accumulate at the surgical site and facilitate the early detection of complications by assessing the aspirated content (hemorrhage, air presence, serosanguinous material). Drains should be closed and unidirectional to prevent the return of drained material into the cavity and potential contamination by external microorganisms. The content should be assessed regularly, documenting both quantity and quality.

Thromboembolic complications necessitate the nurse's ability to recognize signs and symptoms of deep vein thrombosis (DVT), such as excessive swelling of the calf or foot, edema, pale or shiny skin, redness, positive Homans sign (dorsiflexion of the foot), and pulmonary embolism (PE) symptoms, including tachycardia, dyspnea, tachypnea, and sharp chest pain. Due to the high risk of thromboembolic events, in addition to anticoagulant therapy, the use of antithrombotic stockings for the first 30 days or until full weight-bearing during rehabilitation is indicated.

A review of current guidelines for thromboembolic prophylaxis suggests that a multimodal approach combining chemical and mechanical prophylaxis yields positive clinical outcomes with minimal negative consequences. It is recommended to develop individual protocols based on patient needs and to move away from a general protocol for thromboembolism prevention [6].

Prevention of pressure injuries requires special attention, particularly for patients who are very thin. Nurses use assessment scales like the Braden Scale (Fig. 11.3) and implement interventions such as early mobilization, adequate nutrition, and the use of dressings like alginates, hydrocolloid dressings and hydrogels.

11.3.3 Pain and Delirium

Delirium, an acute and reversible disturbance of attention, cognition, and level of consciousness, should be prevented. Causes of delirium include dehydration, pain, stress, recent anesthesia, and the use of opioid analgesics. Nurses assess the patient's mental state using assessment scales like the Confusion Assessment Method (CAM). The CAM is a score that evaluates altered levels of consciousness, acute onset, disorganized thinking, and attention deficits. Delirium can be diagnosed with the presence of the first two criteria, with the addition of the third or fourth criterion. Preventive measures should focus on avoiding triggering factors.

A cornerstone of postoperative care is effective pain management. Pain varies depending on the patient's tolerance, emotional response to surgery, surgical access, and type of intervention. Proper pain management leads to faster recovery, reduced costs, shorter hospital stays, and early initiation of rehabilitation programs. Pain assessment is performed using scales such as the Visual Analog Scale (VAS,

BRADEN SCALE FOR PREDICTING PRESSURE SORE RISK

Patient's Name ______________ Evaluator's Name ______________ Date of Assessment

SENSORY PERCEPTION ability to respond meaning-fully to pressure-related discomfort	**1. Completely Limited** Unresponsive (does not moan, flinch, or grasp) to painful stimuli, due to diminished level of con-sciousness or sedation. OR limited ability to feel pain over most of body	**2. Very Limited** Responds only to painful stimuli. Cannot communicate discomfort except by moaning or restlessness OR has a sensory impairment which limits the ability to feel pain or discomfort over ½ of body.	**3. Slightly Limited** Responds to verbal com-mands, but cannot always communicate discomfort or the need to be turned. OR has some sensory impairment which limits ability to feel pain or discomfort in 1 or 2 extremities.	**4. No Impairment** Responds to verbal commands. Has no sensory deficit which would limit ability to feel or voice pain or discomfort..				
MOISTURE degree to which skin is exposed to moisture	**1. Constantly Moist** Skin is kept moist almost constantly by perspiration, urine, etc. Dampness is detected every time patient is moved or turned.	**2. Very Moist** Skin is often, but not always moist. Linen must be changed at least once a shift.	**3. Occasionally Moist:** Skin is occasionally moist, requiring an extra linen change approximately once a day.	**4. Rarely Moist** Skin is usually dry, linen only requires changing at routine intervals.				
ACTIVITY degree of physical activity	**1. Bedfast** Confined to bed.	**2. Chairfast** Ability to walk severely limited or non-existent. Cannot bear own weight and/or must be assisted into chair or wheelchair.	**3. Walks Occasionally** Walks occasionally during day, but for very short distances, with or without assistance. Spends majority of each shift in bed or chair	**4. Walks Frequently** Walks outside room at least twice a day and inside room at least once every two hours during waking hours				
MOBILITY ability to change and control body position	**1. Completely Immobile** Does not make even slight changes in body or extremity position without assistance	**2. Very Limited** Makes occasional slight changes in body or extremity position but unable to make frequent or significant changes independently.	**3. Slightly Limited** Makes frequent though slight changes in body or extremity position independently.	**4. No Limitation** Makes major and frequent changes in position without assistance.				
NUTRITION usual food intake pattern	**1. Very Poor** Never eats a complete meal. Rarely eats more than ⅓ of any food offered. Eats 2 servings or less of protein (meat or dairy products) per day. Takes fluids poorly. Does not take a liquid dietary supplement OR is NPO and/or maintained on clear liquids or IV's for more than 5 days.	**2. Probably Inadequate** Rarely eats a complete meal and generally eats only about ½ of any food offered. Protein intake includes only 3 servings of meat or dairy products per day. Occasionally will take a dietary supplement. OR receives less than optimum amount of liquid diet or tube feeding	**3. Adequate** Eats over half of most meals. Eats a total of 4 servings of protein (meat, dairy products per day. Occasionally will refuse a meal, but will usually take a supplement when offered OR is on a tube feeding or TPN regimen which probably meets most of nutritional needs	**4. Excellent** Eats most of every meal. Never refuses a meal. Usually eats a total of 4 or more servings of meat and dairy products. Occasionally eats between meals. Does not require supplementation.				
FRICTION & SHEAR	**1. Problem** Requires moderate to maximum assistance in moving. Complete lifting without sliding against sheets is impossible. Frequently slides down in bed or chair, requiring frequent repositioning with maximum assistance. Spasticity, contractures or agitation leads to almost constant friction	**2. Potential Problem** Moves feebly or requires minimum assistance. During a move skin probably slides to some extent against sheets, chair, restraints or other devices. Maintains relatively good position in chair or bed most of the time but occasionally slides down.	**3. No Apparent Problem** Moves in bed and in chair independently and has sufficient muscle strength to lift up completely during move. Maintains good position in bed or chair.					
				Total Score				

Fig. 11.3 Braden scale

Fig. 11.4), Numerical Rating Scale (NRS, Fig. 11.5) or Verbal Rating Scale (VRS, Fig. 11.6). Pain levels should be monitored every 2 h for the first 6 h and every 8 h for the subsequent 48 h after surgery.

A study aimed to evaluate the factors influencing nurses' decision-making regarding the administration of opioid analgesics when the prescription is based on "as needed" for postoperative pain. The results revealed a knowledge deficit as the main reason why nurses were unable to administer adequate analgesics for postoperative pain. Integrating enabling and reinforcing factors can help nurses develop decision-making skills to improve pain management and patient outcomes [7].

Pain management may involve the use of elastomeric pumps, Patient-Controlled Analgesia (PCA) devices, or, in the case of epidural anesthesia, continuous infusion

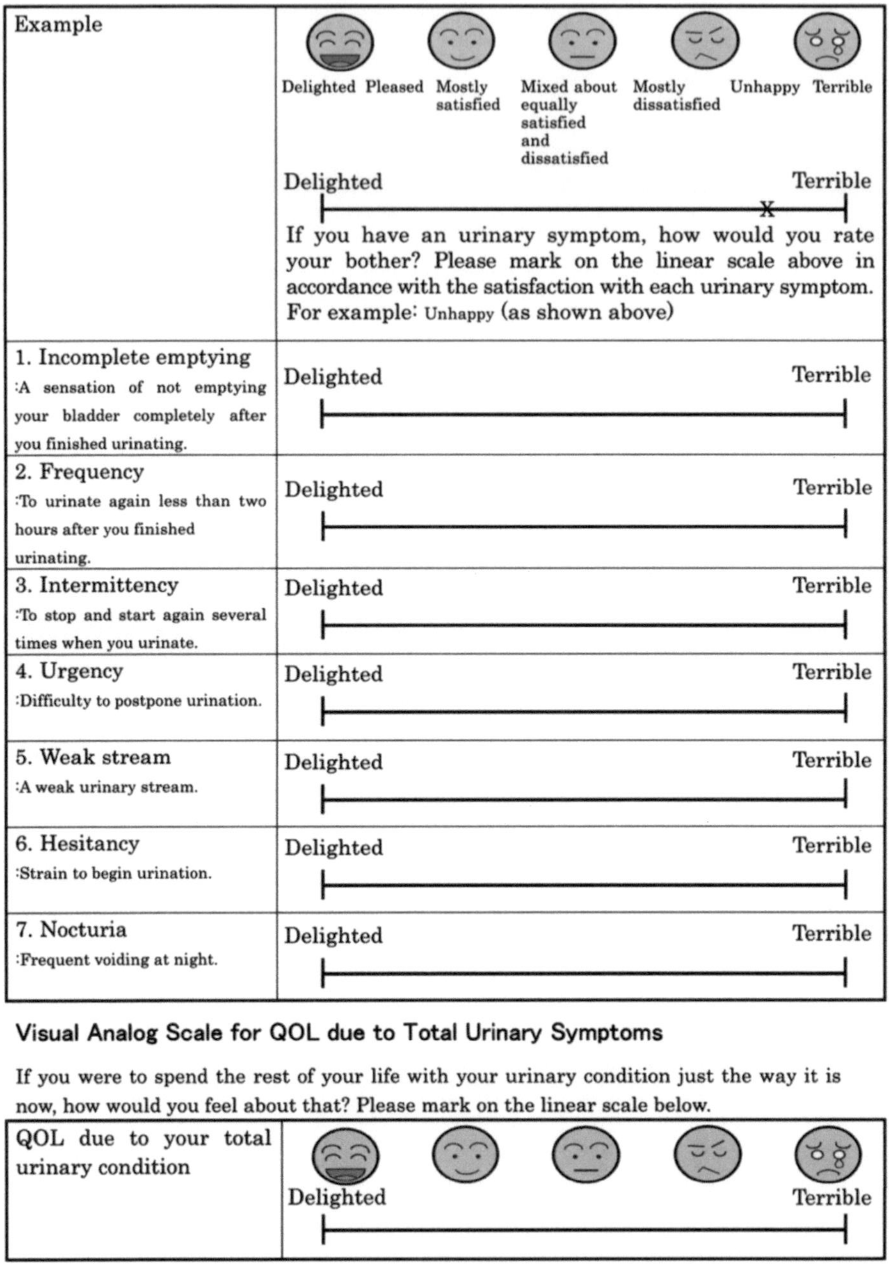

Example	Delighted / Pleased / Mostly satisfied / Mixed about equally satisfied and dissatisfied / Mostly dissatisfied / Unhappy / Terrible Delighted ——X— Terrible If you have an urinary symptom, how would you rate your bother? Please mark on the linear scale above in accordance with the satisfaction with each urinary symptom. For example: Unhappy (as shown above)
1. Incomplete emptying :A sensation of not emptying your bladder completely after you finished urinating.	Delighted —— Terrible
2. Frequency :To urinate again less than two hours after you finished urinating.	Delighted —— Terrible
3. Intermittency :To stop and start again several times when you urinate.	Delighted —— Terrible
4. Urgency :Difficulty to postpone urination.	Delighted —— Terrible
5. Weak stream :A weak urinary stream.	Delighted —— Terrible
6. Hesitancy :Strain to begin urination.	Delighted —— Terrible
7. Nocturia :Frequent voiding at night.	Delighted —— Terrible

Visual Analog Scale for QOL due to Total Urinary Symptoms

If you were to spend the rest of your life with your urinary condition just the way it is now, how would you feel about that? Please mark on the linear scale below.

QOL due to your total urinary condition	Delighted —— Terrible

Fig. 11.4 Vas scale

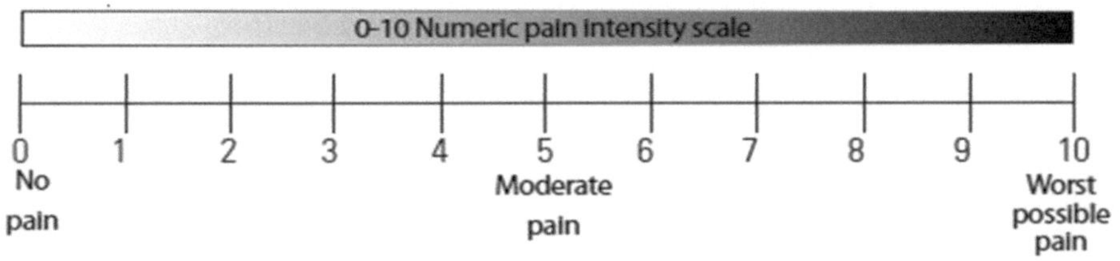

Fig. 11.5 Numeric pain scale

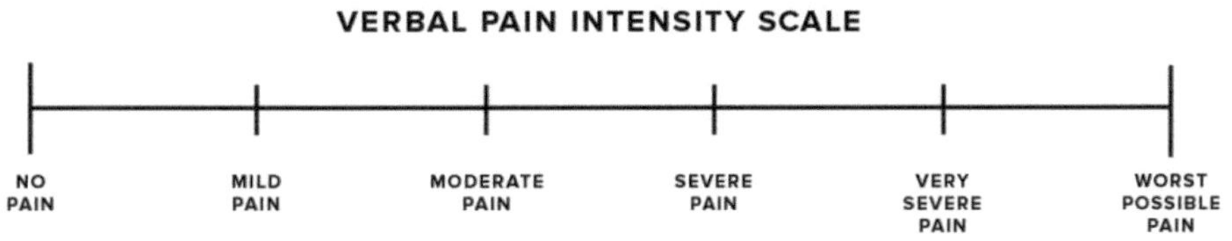

Fig. 11.6 Verbal pain scale

via a catheter in the spine for the first 24–48 h. However, with the implementation of fast-track approaches and Enhanced Recovery After Surgery (ERAS) protocols, intra-articular drains and various catheters are avoided to prevent patients from being restricted to their beds.

PCA allows patients to self-administer a predetermined dosage of analgesics by pressing a button. The device is controlled by a small computer that monitors the frequency of use and prevents exceeding a certain dosage. Nurses play a crucial role in providing patient education on the proper use of opioids.

A study conducted in 2015 assessed nurses' knowledge and attitudes regarding opioid use. The results revealed a knowledge gap in pain management among nurses caring for patients receiving opioid analgesics. The study highlighted the need for additional education and sufficient information for nurses to improve opioid management and patient outcomes [8].

Another study aimed to compare patient-reported responses regarding postoperative in the pain management interventions received after hip replacement surgery with documented interventions in their nursing records. Interviews were conducted to patients on the third postoperative day, and interventions were measured and compared using the Quality of Diagnoses, Interventions, and Outcomes (Q-DIO) tool. The study found that the most frequently reported pain level was "no pain" (NRS 0–10 points). However, 17–50% of patients reported pain levels of three or higher, and 11–22% reported pain levels of five or higher during movement or ambulation. The study also revealed that interviews with patients and nurses revealed more pain management interventions than were documented [9]. Pain assessments and effective pain interventions should be improved and properly documented.

11.3.4 Mobilization: Evidence from Orthopedic Setting

Mobilization in the fast-track and ERAS protocols typically begins 4 h after surgery, with passive mobilization performed by nurses in collaboration with physiotherapists or orthopedic specialists, depending on the patient's needs. After passive and active mobilization, the patient may engage in short walks, using assistive devices such as canes, walkers, ergonomic belts (for hemiplegic patients with prostheses), or lifts (only used with a "spoon stretcher" to avoid joint dislocation).

Certain fundamental rules must be followed, such as using a spreader to maintain abduction of the limb, avoiding flexion beyond 90°, not turning the patient predominantly toward the operated side, not rotating the leg inward, avoiding leg crossing, and assisting the operated limb during bed-to-chair transfers.

On the second and third postoperative days, in addition to passive mobilization, active mobilization, and ambulation, if the patient's clinical condition allows, exercises involving stair climbing and descending are initiated. Once it is verified that the patient has been able to complete the rehabilitation program and their clinical condition is suitable, they can be discharged. The typical length of hospital stay days was higher before, but with the implementation of ERAS protocols, it has been reduced to 3.9 days with a high level of postoperative satisfaction [10].

A randomized study explored the influence of rehabilitative nursing care using the Health Action Process Approach (HAPA) model on preoperative nursing effects, evaluating the impact on quality of life and postoperative rehabilitation. Two groups of patients were assessed and compared based on nursing satisfaction, pain scores, Harris Hip Function Score, stand-up-walk test time, Modified Barthel Index (MBI), and quality of life score. The study concluded that the nursing rehabilitation program using the HAPA model, compared to routine nursing rehabilitation, effectively improved functional recovery of the hip joint, helped promote patients' ability to perform activities of daily living, alleviated pain and anxiety, and achieved gait stability in the early postoperative phase [11].

Overall, postoperative nursing care plays a crucial role in promoting patient recovery, optimizing pain management, preventing complications, and facilitating the patient's transition to a higher level of autonomy. It requires a comprehensive understanding of the surgical procedure, vigilant assessment skills, effective interdisciplinary collaboration, and patient education. By providing holistic and individualized care, nurses contribute significantly to positive postoperative outcomes.

References

1. Ertural F. The effect of preoperative oral carbohydrate solutions on patient comfort and anxiety. J Perianesth Nurs. 2023;38(1):e30–6.
2. Kehlet H. Fast-track hip and knee arthroplasty: clinical and organizational aspects. Acta Orthop. 2012;83(346):1–39.
3. Ljungqvist O. ERAS—enhanced recovery after surgery: moving evidence-based perioperative care to practice. J Parenter Enter Nutr. 2017;41(5):632–6.

4. McDonald S. Preoperative nursing assessment and preparation. Br J Perioper Nurs. 2004;14(5):202–8.
5. McDonald S, et al. Pre-operative education for hip or knee replacement. Cochrane Database Syst Rev. 2004;2014(5):CD003526.
6. Khatkar H, Elahi Z, See A, McDonald S, Neal-Smith G. Preventing Venous Thromboembolism after elective total hip arthroplasty surgery - are the current guidelines appropriate? Venous thromboembolism prophylaxis in elective total hip arthroplasty surgery. J Clin Orthop Trauma. 2022;26:101782. https://doi.org/10.1016/j.jcot.2022.101782. PMID: 35145851; PMCID: PMC8814685.
7. Yin HH, Tse MM, Wong FK. Systematic review of the predisposing, enabling, and reinforcing factors which influence nursing administration of opioids in the postoperative period. Jpn J Nurs Sci. 2015;12(4):259–75. https://doi.org/10.1111/jjns.12075. Epub 2015 Mar 17. PMID: 25781037.
8. Costello M, Thompson S. Preventing Opioid Misuse and Potential Abuse: The Nurse's Role in Patient Education. Pain Manag Nurs. 2015;16(4):515–9. https://doi.org/10.1016/j.pmn.2014.09.008. Epub 2014 Dec 8. PMID: 25497402.
9. Zanon DC, Gralher D, Müller-Staub M. Interventionen zur Pflegediagnose "Akute Schmerzen" – Evaluation der schmerzlindernden Pflege bei hospitalisierten Patientinnen und Patienten nach Hüftendoprothesenversorgung im Vergleich zur Pflegedokumentation mittels Q-DIO-Pain: eine Mixed Methods Studie [Interventions of the nursing diagnosis "Acute Pain" – Evaluation of patients' experiences after total hip arthroplasty compared with the nursing record by using Q-DIO-Pain: a mixed methods study]. Pflege. 2017;30(3):129–38. German. https://doi.org/10.1024/1012-5302/a000533. Epub 2017 Mar 22. PMID: 28326887.
10. Frassanito L, Vergari A, Nestorini R, Cerulli G, Placella G, Pace V, Rossi M. Enhanced recovery after surgery (ERAS) in hip and knee replacement surgery: description of a multidisciplinary program to improve management of the patients undergoing major orthopedic surgery. Musculoskelet Surg. 2020;104(1):87–92. https://doi.org/10.1007/s12306-019-00603-4. Epub 2019 May 3. PMID: 31054080.
11. Meng X, Yu Y. Effect of rehabilitation nursing under the guidance of the health action process approach model on perioperative nursing effect of artificial hip arthroplasty: effect on promoting quality of life and postoperative rehabilitation. Comput Math Methods Med. 2022;2022:1247002.

12 The Nutritionist: Malnutrition Risk Assessment and Management

Ilenia Grandone

12.1 Introduction

12.1.1 Malnutrition in Surgery Settings

Experts define malnutrition as "an acute, subacute, or chronic state of nutrition in which varying degrees of overnutrition or undernutrition, with or without inflammatory activity, have led to a change in body composition and diminished function." Recently, ESPEN defined diagnostic criteria for malnutrition based on two options: body mass index (BMI) <18.5 kg/m^2; combined weight loss >10% or >5% over 3 months and reduced BMI, or a low fat-free mass index (FFMI) [1].

In order to detect and treat malnutrition in older patients undergoing surgery, it is necessary to understand how the surgical event impacts metabolism and nutritional status. Impaired nutritional status has significant effects on the outcome of the surgical intervention itself and the potential occurrence of short- and long-term complications. Malnutrition is indeed associated with a high incidence of perioperative complications, sepsis, prolonged hospitalization, morbidity, and mortality.

The first aspect that influences the nutritional status of older patients undergoing surgery during hospitalization is the more or less prolonged fasting associated with most procedures, coupled with bed rest, which quickly affects muscle trophism. Furthermore, patients undergoing surgery may suffer from low-grade chronic inflammation, such as in the case of tumors, diabetes, renal and hepatic insufficiency. Surgery is associated with an increased inflammatory response to stress, depending on the type and extent of the damaged tissue, resulting in increased catabolism and the need for an adequate organ response, which may be compromised in the case of pre-existing malnutrition [2].

I. Grandone (✉)
Diabetology Dietetics and Clinical Nutrition Unit, Santa Maria Hospital, Terni, Italy

V. Boccardi, L. Marano (eds.), *The Frail Surgical Patient*, Practical Issues in Geriatrics, https://doi.org/10.1007/978-3-031-77707-3_12

Acute inflammatory response requires a high consumption of energy substrates normally used as nutrients, leading to an extremely rapid depletion of lean mass. Therefore, nutritional support during acute events becomes essential but insufficient to counteract catabolism and the impact on muscle mass. It is necessary to act, whenever possible, prior to the surgical procedure. Preoperative nutritional intervention is not always able to restore the deficit of lean mass in terms of intensity and duration but can always improve the acute stress response by accelerating functional recovery.

These considerations have made nutritional screening and supplementation indispensable within the multimodal approach of 'Enhanced Recovery After Surgery' (ERAS) protocols, which will be discussed later in this book. Adequate preparation and tailored therapy require adequate knowledge of the typical changes in body composition in elderly patients and a screening of nutritional status, which should be performed using validated and feasible tests [3].

12.1.2 Aging and Sarcopenia

Aging is a natural biological process that involves physiological changes in organs and systems, as well as in body composition, basal metabolism, and distribution of fat and muscle. Specifically, adipose mass increases while plasma volume, body water, and lean mass—in terms of function and strength—decrease, leading to the typical condition known as sarcopenia. This physiological reduction, which is approximately 30-40% compared to a young adult, is caused by the progressive decline in physical activity and the sedentary lifestyle typically associated with aging. Furthermore, it is important to emphasize that sarcopenia is not necessarily associated with a low body mass index but is often correlated with conditions of malnutrition due to excess, and in this context, it is defined as sarcopenic obesity.

In 2019, the European Working Group on Sarcopenia in Older People (EWGSOP) published a revision of the European consensus, defining sarcopenia as "a progressive and generalized skeletal muscle disorder that is associated with an increased likelihood of adverse outcomes, including falls, fractures, physical disability, and mortality." Sarcopenia is considered a major cause of frailty and disability in older population 'Fig. 12.1.'

12.2 Nutritional Screening and Assessment

Nutrition screening has been defined by the American Society for Parenteral and Enteral Nutrition (ASPEN) as "a process to identify an individual who is malnourished or who is at risk for malnutrition to determine if a detailed nutrition assessment is indicated". It involves a multidimensional evaluation of the geriatric patient, which requires a multidisciplinary team including a geriatrician, a nutritionist, a dietitian, and other healthcare professionals as needed for a comprehensive diagnostic and therapeutic approach. The nutritional screening process involves several key

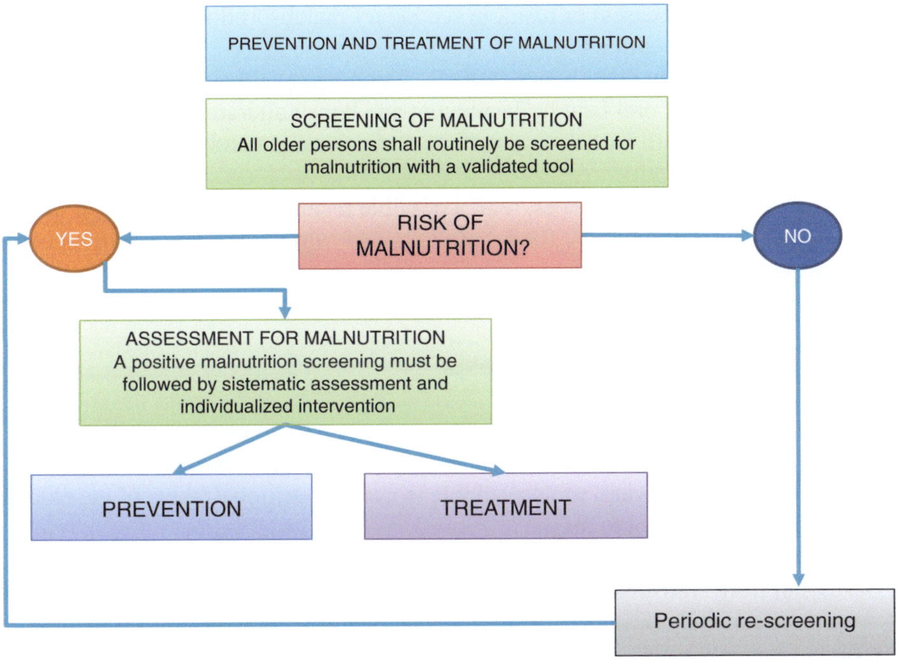

Fig. 12.1 Prevention and treatment of malnutrition, adapted from Clinical Nutrition 2022 41,958-989. (https://doi.org/10.1016/j.clnu.2022.01.024)

steps, including medical history, screening tests, anthropometric assessment, biochemical tests, instrumental exams, and evaluation of body composition and function in a nutritional context [4].

12.2.1 Medical History

When collecting data, it is important to consider the following checkpoints [5]:

- Social context of the patient, including access to food and preparation, autonomy in meal management, and the presence of any functional dependency conditions; in such cases, the presence and collaboration of a caregiver are necessary.
- Presence of psychological and cognitive comorbidities that may affect eating behavior.
- Evaluation of activities of daily living (ADLs), presence of disabilities, immobilization syndrome, and history of pressure ulcers.
- Polypharmacy and comorbidities that may affect nutritional status (renal insufficiency, liver disease, cardiovascular diseases, neurological and neurodegenerative disorders, endocrine and autoimmune diseases, cancer, diabetes mellitus,

gastrointestinal diseases) or result in secondary malabsorption conditions, previous surgical interventions.
- Presence of sensory disturbances (smell, vision, taste) either primary or secondary to medication; oral health; dysphagia; and bowel alterations.
- Weight history, with particular attention to usual weight and any recent changes in the last 3–6 months.
- Dietary habits and preferences, with a possible recall of the last 24 h or, if necessary, the administration of a food diary to assess caloric intake and nutrient composition of the diet.

12.2.2 Nutritional Screening Tests

Regardless of the specific diagnosis and in overweight and obese individuals, malnutrition and its risks should be systematically and routinely screened using a validated tool. There are several tools available to assess nutritional status of the elderly [6]; the most common ones are:

- MNA or Mini Nutritional Assessment, which has been validated for over 20 years and is specifically designed for individuals over 65, allowing for the identification of patients at risk of malnutrition. The "MNA-short form" can be completed in just 5 min by the patient or caregiver and includes five simple questions.
- Malnutrition Screening Tool (MUST) is suitable for all patients, not just the elderly, particularly in a hospital care setting. It requires the evaluation of a few parameters and can be easily delegated even to personnel with limited nutritional expertise.
- Subjective Global Assessment (SGA) is a test that correlates weight changes, nutritional intake, and gastrointestinal symptoms of the patient.
- Additionally, the SARC-f test may be useful, which considers all pathognomonic aspects of sarcopenia through its five components: muscle strength (Strength), walking (Assistance with walking), rising from a chair (Rise from chair), climbing stairs (Climb stairs), and number of falls in the last year (Falls).

12.2.3 Biochemical Markers

In addition to routinely collected parameters (blood count, renal and liver function, lipid profile, electrolytes, serum iron, and ferritin) that can provide an indirect assessment of nutritional status, there are specific biochemical markers that can be useful in the diagnosis and monitoring of patients at risk or affected by protein-energy malnutrition, in the context of nutritional, medical history. These include in particular:

- Serum albumin and protein electrophoresis
- Transferrin

- Vitamins D, B12, A, and E, and folic acid
- Serum prealbumin (with a half-life of about 48 hours, to estimate short-term changes in nutritional status) and retinol-binding protein
- Serum pseudocholinesterase

During a presurgical evaluation, biochemical parameters can have prognostic and predictive significance: decreased synthesis of negative acute-phase proteins will result in reduced serum albumin, transferrin, prealbumin, and retinol-binding protein concentrations that are potent indicators of poor outcome. In particular, as indicated in the guidelines, preoperative serum albumin is a prognostic factor for complications after surgery and is also associated with impaired nutritional status. Albumin may also be considered to define surgical patients at severe nutritional risk by the presence of at least one of the following criteria [7]:

- Weight loss >10–15% within 6 months
- BMI <18.5 kg/m^2
- Subjective Global Assessment (SGA) Grade C
- preoperative serum albumin <30 g/l (with no evidence of hepatic or renal dysfunction)

However, serum concentrations of albumin and prealbumin decline in the presence of inflammation, regardless of underlying nutrition status; therefore, experts have advised that albumin and prealbumin not be used in isolation to assess nutritional status because they are fundamentally markers of inflammatory metabolism.

12.2.4 Anthropometric Values

It is important to note that the most commonly used anthropometric assessment measures may not be accurate or feasible for use in the elderly. Physical and metabolic changes that occur with aging can lead to inaccurate results. For instance, measuring height accurately may be difficult due to vertebral compression, inability to stand up straight in patients, being bed bound, and osteoporosis. Among the main clinical markers of malnutrition, simply measuring weight and assessing unintentional weight loss would represent an important diagnostic parameter. Lack of body weight recording has been associated with increased mortality and hospitalization. Regarding body mass index, it is considered that the reference values for adults are not suitable for the elderly, and a normal range value of weight/height^2 ratio between 27 and 32 is suggested. The distribution of body fat also has prognostic significance, and estimating body fat mass and muscle trophism, in addition to second-level instrumental tests, can also be deduced from skinfold thickness measurements. Measuring mid-arm circumference or knee height may provide more accurate measurements, especially when integrated with other body composition measurement methods.

12.2.5 Evaluation of Body Composition

Handgrip Strength (HGS) Assessing muscle strength is a complex procedure that requires choosing accurate and simple tests for daily clinical practice. Measuring handgrip strength is a simple and inexpensive method. To obtain accurate measurements, a calibrated handheld dynamometer should be used under well-defined test conditions, with interpretive data from reference populations. Handgrip strength correlates moderately with strength in other body compartments, making it a reliable surrogate for assessing arm and leg strength. Low handgrip strength (cutoff points: <27 kg for men and < 16 kg for women) is a strong predictor of negative patient outcomes, including longer hospital stays, increased functional limitations, poor health-related quality of life, and mortality [8]. Standardized and accurately executed handgrip strength testing can be a valuable tool not only for evaluating nutritional status but also for assessing frailty, disability, and monitoring the effectiveness of therapeutic interventions.

Bioelectrical Impedance Analysis (BIA) and Dual-Energy X-Ray Absorptiometry (DXA) The most accurate methods for assessing muscle mass in clinical settings are bioelectrical impedance analysis (BIA) and dual-energy X-ray absorptiometry (DXA). BIA is the most commonly used method for evaluating body composition. BIA equipment indirectly estimates muscle mass based on whole-body electrical conductivity. BIA measurements are advantageous due to their affordability, portability, speed, simplicity, and non-invasiveness. However, BIA data can be influenced by the patient's hydration status, and further studies are needed to validate prediction equations for specific populations. Additionally, bioimpedance assessment allows the measurement of phase angle, which has a normal range of 5° to 9° and can provide an estimate of health status and adequacy of body composition. It is also a predictive value for mortality and postoperative complications, particularly in oncologic patients.

Dual-energy X-ray absorptiometry (DXA) is considered the gold standard for measuring body composition and bone mineral density. It is highly accurate, widely available, non-invasive, and rapid. DXA is the only radiological tool with accepted cutoff values for diagnosing sarcopenia. However, one disadvantage is that DXA instruments are not yet portable, they are expensive, and measurements can be influenced by the patient's hydration status.

Lumbar Third Vertebra Imaging by Computed Tomography Computed tomography (CT) has been used for imaging tumors and monitoring their response to treatment in cancer patients. This technique can also provide practical and precise measurements of body composition, including the detection of low muscle mass. CT images of the specific lumbar vertebral landmark (L3) show a significant correlation with whole-body muscle mass and can predict prognosis. One of the main advantages is that this method does not require additional diagnostic tests for oncology patients.

12.3 Nutritional Management and Intervention

A positive malnutrition screening should be followed by a systematic assessment, individualized intervention, monitoring, and corresponding adjustment of interventions (Fig. 12.2). Nutrition support intervention in patients identified by screening and assessment at risk for malnutrition or malnourished can improve clinical outcomes. Nutrition is one of the few modifiable risk factors for frailty, and it should be a target for both prevention and treatment of this syndrome. To establish appropriate nutritional intervention, it is necessary to estimate the patient's caloric requirements and compare them with the investigated caloric intake obtained during the dietary anamnesis [9]. This will help to decide on the most suitable dietary therapy and possible caloric and protein supplementation.

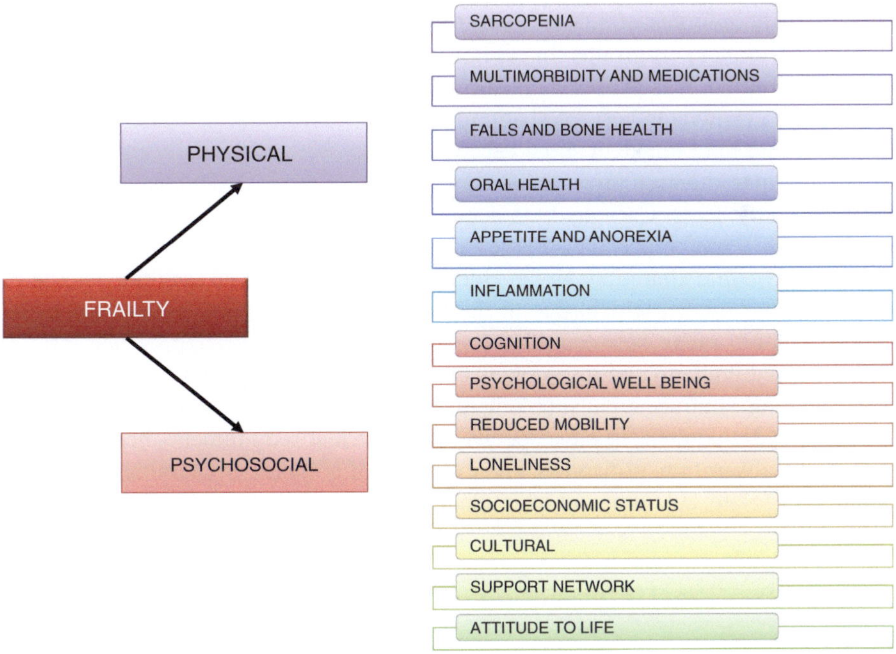

Fig. 12.2 Frailty. Adapted from Nutrients 2021, 13, 2349. https://doi.org/10.3390/nu13072349

12.3.1 Estimation of Caloric and Nutritional Requirements in Elderly Patients

Energy expenditure, which is the caloric intake needed to cover energy needs, physiologically decreases with age, primarily due to the progressive loss of lean body mass, which represents the metabolically active component of our body. Additionally, with age, the level of physical activity also decreases, increasing the time spent at rest. Daily energy requirements should be estimated through indirect calorimetry, but in clinical practice, formulas considering age, weight, height, and sex are often used. Generally, caloric needs range between 25 and 35 kcal/kg/day, but they should be adjusted based on activity and stress coefficients. For older underweight individuals (BMI < 21 kg/m^2), energy requirements between 32 and 38 kcal/kg are assumed. Minimal requirements for ill older persons are estimated to be between 27 and 30 kcal/kg. In general, it can be stated that the guiding value for energy intake in older persons is 30 kcal per kg of body weight per day, and this value should be individually adjusted based on nutritional status, physical activity level, disease status, and tolerance.

Protein needs usually do not change with age, despite the reduction in lean body mass. Protein intake in older persons should be at least 1 g of protein per kg per day. Growing evidence suggests that older people might need higher amounts of protein than younger adults for optimal preservation of lean body mass, body functions, and health. Daily amounts of 1.0–1.2 g/kg have been suggested for healthy older persons by several expert groups. In case of illness, protein requirements may even be further increased. It is necessary to stimulate the consumption of foods containing high-quality protein and essential amino acids.

Regarding lipid intake, it should account for 25–30% of the daily caloric intake, with particular attention given to the consumption of monounsaturated and polyunsaturated fatty acids. Carbohydrate needs should constitute 50–60% of the energy intake, with a preference for complex carbohydrates, considering the high prevalence of glycemic alterations in the elderly population. Special attention should be given to fiber intake, which, due to the high frequency of bowel disorders in the elderly, should range between 20 and 30 g/day, choosing an appropriate ratio of soluble (predominant) and insoluble fiber and avoiding excesses. It is advisable and possible to use nutraceutical supplements to achieve the desired goals.

Many older adults also have special micronutrient requirements because aging affects the absorption, utilization, and excretion of complex B vitamins, vitamin D, vitamin E, folate, calcium, and other electrolytes.

12.3.2 Nutritional Intervention

In order to improve oral intake, it is necessary to document food intake and nutritional counseling should be provided as needed. The first step is dietary adjustment with possible modification of meals according to the patient's needs and concomitant conditions. Older persons with malnutrition or at risk of malnutrition with chronic conditions should be offered oral nutritional supplements (ONS) when dietary counseling and food fortification are not sufficient to increase dietary intake and reach nutritional goals. ONS are specific nutritional formulas for oral consumption, with different consistencies and compositions of micronutrients and macronutrients specific to each condition. They offer the possibility to increase or ensure nutrient intake in case of insufficient oral food intake.

In addition to oral nutritional balanced supplements, increasing the quantity and quality of dietary protein stimulates muscle protein synthesis in the elderly. Since older adults are at risk of having a low intake of high-quality protein, to counteract protein catabolism, they should increase the anabolic stimulus by consuming 30 g of protein per meal. For this purpose, it could be useful to supplement with whey protein and essential amino acids, particularly leucine (Leu). Whey protein increases postprandial plasma amino acid availability and contains a high concentration of leucine, which specifically stimulates skeletal muscle protein synthesis. Therefore, whey protein and essential amino acids containing leucine are recommended interventions for sarcopenia. Nutrition intervention in malnourished patients has been associated with improved physical function, quality of life, and a reduction in hospital readmissions. It should always be encouraged and implemented through the collaboration of various actors in the multidisciplinary team.

References

1. Mueller C, Compher C, Druyan M, the American Society for Parenteral and Enteral Nutrition (A.S.P.E.N.) Board of Directors. A.S.P.E.N. Clinical guidelines nutrition screening, assessment, and intervention in adults. J Parenter Enter Nutr. 2011;35:1.
2. American Society for Parenteral and Enteral Nutrition (A.S.P.E.N.) Board of Directors and Clinical Practice Committee: Definition of terms, style, and conventions used in A.S.P.E.N. Board of Directors–approved documents American Society for Parenteral and Enteral Nutrition http://www.nutritioncare.org/Library.aspx. July 8, 2010.
3. Volkert D, Beck A, Cederholm T, Cruz-Jentoft A, Hooper L, Kiesswetter E, Maggio M, Raynaud-Simon A, Sieber C, Sobotka L, van Asselt D, Wirth R, Bischoff S. ESPEN practical guideline: clinical nutrition and hydration in geriatrics. Clin Nutr. 2022;41:958–89.
4. Weimann A, Braga M, Carli F, Higashiguchi T, Hübner M, Klek S, Laviano A, Ljungqvist O, Lobo D, Martindale R, Waitzberg D, Bischoff S, Singer P. ESPEN guideline: clinical nutrition in surgery. Clin Nutr. 2017;36:623–50.
5. Papadopoulou S. Sarcopenia: a contemporary health problem among older adult populations. Nutrients. 2020;12:1293. https://doi.org/10.3390/nu12051293.
6. Lochlainn M, Cox N, Wilson T, Hayhoe R, Ramsay S, Granic A, Isanejad M, Roberts H, Wilson D, Welch C, Hurst C, Atkins J, Mendonça N, Horner K, Tuttiett E, Morgan Y, Heslop P, Williams E, Steves C, Greig C, Draper J, Corish C, Welch A, Witham M, Sayer A, Robinson S. Nutrition and frailty: opportunities for prevention and treatment. Nutrients. 2021;13(7):2349. https://doi.org/10.3390/nu13072349.
7. Cruz-Jentoft A, Bahat G, Bauer J, Boirie Y, Bruyère O, Cederholm T, Cooper C, Landi F, Rolland Y, Sayer A, Schneider S, Sieber C, Topinkova E, Vandewoude M, Visser M, Zamboni M, Writing Group For The European Working Group On Sarcopenia In Older People 2 (Ewgsop2), and the Extended Group for Ewgsop2. Sarcopenia: revised European consensus on definition and diagnosis. Age Ageing. 2019;48:16–31. https://doi.org/10.1093/ageing/afy169.
8. Rondanelli M. Alimentazione e nutrizione nell'anziano. Il Pensiero Scientifico Editore; 2015.

9. Rondanelli M, Klersy C, Terracol G, Talluri J, Maugeri R, Guido D, Faliva M, Solerte B, Fioravanti M, Lukaski H, Perna S. Whey protein, amino acids, and vitamin D supplementation with physical activity increases fat-free mass and strength, functionality, and quality of life and decreases inflammation in sarcopenic elderly. AJCN. First published ahead of print February 10. 2016; https://doi.org/10.3945/ajcn.115.113357.

The Importance of Hydration and Nutritional Support 13

Massimiliano Cavallo

13.1 Malnutrition and Dehydration as Risk Factors for Complication in Geriatric Surgery

Geriatric people are more prone to be malnourished and/or dehydrated due to a lot of factors such as dysgeusia, dysphagia and reduced sense of thirst. Surgery represents one of the major stresses for individuals, especially for elderly people. In fact, surgery exposes people to a catabolic cascade of events that leads to a quick and deep consumption of energetical substrates. Due to the activation of stress hormones (catecholamines and glucagon) and of pro-inflammatory cytokines, surgery determines an insulin-resistant state with rapid consumption of glycogen stores and consequent stimulation of gluconeogenesis processes that need amino acids and their direct precursors. The insulin-resistant state reflects itself in hyperglycemia that could worsen a prior condition of diabetes or altered glycemic metabolism and that could last for a few hours to 2–4 weeks. Hyperglycemia leads to an immune dysfunction increasing the risk of infections and mortality. Protein catabolism enhanced by gluconeogenesis affects skeletal muscle health with consequent sarcopenia, would healing alteration and immune system dysfunction (Fig. 13.1).

According to these considerations, being malnourished represents a risk factor to develop major complications of surgery like dehiscence and generally to worsen prognosis and mortality. On the other side, also the importance of hydration is well known. In fact, a state of dehydration is one of the main risk factors not only of surgery complications but also of geriatric syndromes like delirium.

M. Cavallo (✉)
Internal Medicine Unit, "Santa Maria" Hospital Terni, Terni, Italy
e-mail: m.cavallo@aospterni.it

V. Boccardi, L. Marano (eds.), *The Frail Surgical Patient*, Practical Issues in Geriatrics, https://doi.org/10.1007/978-3-031-77707-3_13

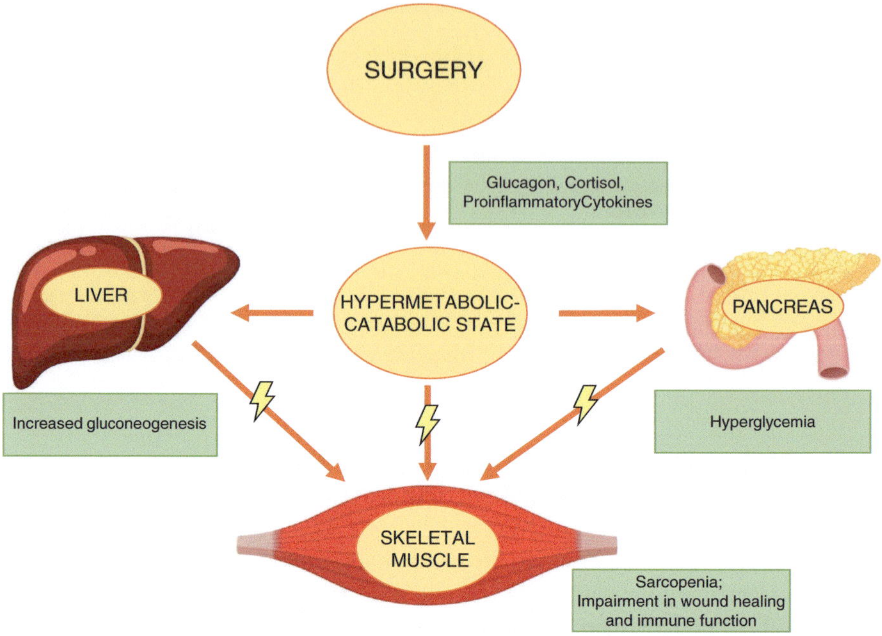

Fig. 13.1

13.2 How to Evaluate Malnutrition and Dehydration in Older People

A comprehensive multidisciplinary assessment of the state of nutrition and hydration of older people is a seminal element of geriatric care. The most recent scientific guidelines underline with a high level of evidence this statement. Independently from the setting of care of older people, everyone must receive at least a first visit to assess the risk of malnutrition and dehydration. All figures involved in geriatric care must know the basic elements of correct management of nutrition and hydration in older and often people. A first work of screening should be followed by a series of revaluation planned in a specific timeline to better understand the real benefit of the prescribed intervention to counterbalance worsening of malnutrition and dehydration. It's important to ensure both at home and in geriatric institutions and, as better as possible, in hospital a dining setting that allow older people to safely consume their meals and to let them to have a free access to water and other liquids. The screening of malnutrition could be assessed with specific questionnaires validated by literature; in particular, it is possible to use MUST, MNA-SF and GNRI. MUST (Malnutrition Universal Screening Tool) consists of a five-step evaluation of malnutrition risk. First, BMI is calculated or estimated if not available data of weight and height; then, the amount of unplanned weight loss in the past 3 or 6 months could be estimated. Considering the effect of the current acute disease and summing all the scores of this first three steps, the derived score (0 = low risk; 1 = medium risk; 2 = high risk) indicates the grade of malnutrition letting health care professionals to develop a specific nutritional plan.

The short form of MNA (Mini Nutritional Assessment) consists in five simple questions that examinates a reduction in appetite or food intake in the last 3 months; the grade of weight loss in the same period; problems of motion; presence of acute illness or psychological distress and the presence of neuropsychological problems: the score obtained from these answers together with the quartile of BMI (or calf circumference in centimeters) let to know the risk of malnutrition (0–7 points = malnourished, 8–11 points = at risk of malnutrition; 12–14 points = no problems of nutrition.

Finally, GNRI (Geriatric Nutritional Risk Index) score is the result of a specific equation considering serum albumin, actual weight, and ideal weight (<82 high risk of malnutrition; 82–91 moderate risk; 92–98 low risk; >98 no risk).

Older people are at increased risk of dehydration due to many causes. A certain grade of kidney dysfunction occurs very frequently in the geriatric population with a consequent reduced capability to manage water and solutes such as sodium. The hormonal control of fluid omeostasis is altered in older people, leading to a reduction in thirst sensation. This last condition is worsened by polypharmacotherapy and cognitive or physical impairment. Dehydration is often present at the time of hospital admission representing a seminal risk factor to clinical complications. On the other hand, it is possible to identify a certain group of elderly people at risk or affected by overhydration due to heart failure, kidney impairment, or protein deficiency. Clinical assessment of the state of hydration in geriatric people represents a difficult clinical challenge. Various are the developed methods: from clinical signs (systolic blood pressure, heart rate, and capillary refill) to biochemical assays (serum osmolarity, creatinine, urea, and electrolytes) to ultrasonographical measurement of inferior vena cava to bioimpedance analyses. All of them present limits in older people. To date, calculated plasma osmolarity derived with the specifical formula [osmolarity = 1.86(Na + K) + 1.15(Glucose/18) + (Urea/6) + 14] with a cut-off >295 indicating dehydration, still represents the better method to evaluate hydration state in older people.

Once assessed the grade of malnutrition and dehydration, a pivotal role for geriatric team is to establish an individualized plan to ameliorate the actual situation to minimize the possible effects of surgery in older people.

13.3 How to Manage Preoperative Nutritional Care in Older People

The most recent ESPEN guidelines suggest 30 kcal per kg body weight as a sufficient caloric intake for older people. Almost 1 g of protein per kg body weight is recommended but in specific conditions as infections, wounds or inflammatory diseases protein intake could reach up to 2 per kg body weight. As regards liquids, women could drink almost 1.6 l of water daily while men up to 2 l not considering water contained in other foods like fruit, vegetables, and others. Due to the difficulties to ensure these levels of liquid intake in older people, a range of appropriate drinks could be offered to them according to their preferences. In a residential care setting, drinking could be promoted by offering various sources of drinks, encouraging elderly people to drink, and helping them if necessary. A nasogastric or intravenous administration could become compulsory if calculated osmolarity overcomes 295 mmol/l and considering plasma levels of sodium.

Ensuring these recommended levels in older people represents a difficult clinical challenge. Prior to surgery, especially planned, it is compulsory, as above described, a comprehensive assessment of the grade of nutrition and hydration. Several days before surgery, it is, in fact, possible to elaborate a specific nutrition plan to counterbalance the possible dangerous effects of surgery.

A personalized diet elaborated by a professional team of geriatricians, nutritionists, and dietitians represent the first step for the management of older people prior to surgery. When only diet, even if enriched by fortified foods, could not ensure adequate caloric intake in qualitative and quantitative terms, oral nutrition supplements (ONS) could be prescribed containing at least 400 kcal with 30 g of proteins. Older people with known or newly diagnosed problems of dysphagia could be referred to a speech and language therapist receiving specific care like texture-modified enriched foods. Finally, if it is not possible to treat malnutrition neither with diet nor with ONS, enteral nutrition (EN) represents the first choice. In fact, only when a digestive tube could not be used (gastrointestinal problems or surgery) parenteral nutrition (PN) could be considered. EN and PN are considered specific care, so they could be encouraged when they represent a real therapeutical chance for ameliorating clinical conditions and quality of life of patients not being recommended in the end of life or not being possible requesting sedation or immobilization of patients. On the other side, also geriatric surgery's guidelines have been deeply modified in the last decades. For years, in fact, due to the hypothetical risk of aspiration during anesthesia, long fasting from midnight before surgery has been suggested. The most recent guidelines on geriatric surgery, instead, declare that a prolonged fasting before surgery is unnecessary in most patients. A lot of specific protocols encourage patients to assume 2 hours before the intervention, a specific amount of carbohydrates to counterbalance the insulin-resistant state caused by the surgery itself and to generally ameliorate well-being. Older people who are expected to not consume an adequate caloric intake in the 5 days before surgery could be absolutely treated with a specific nutritional plan following best clinical practice in terms of compositions of meals and, if not applicable, EN and/or PN. Some studies suggest that not only are carbohydrates seminal to contrast surgical resistant state due to the incapability of glucose alone to stop gluconeogenesis, but also encourage the use of a protein source, especially essential amino acids, with a higher bioavailability. Resuming, a specific tailored, multidisciplinary assessment of nutrition and hydration state is compulsory for all elderly people planned for surgery, especially for those who are expected to not consume an adequate quantity of macronutrients in the 5 days before surgery. The consumption of 1.5–2 g per kg body weight of proteins could be encouraged in the days before the intervention. The 6 h before surgery meal could be complete with all macronutrients with special regards to high-quality proteins and carbohydrates. Even if current guidelines emphasize the chance to assume a certain quantity of carbohydrates 2 h before surgery, it could be considered to add also essential amino acids to have a synergic action to counteract surgical insulin-resistant state and reduce possible muscle wasting that represents one of the main determinants of complications. The role of the nutritional team is fundamental to take care of older people undergoing surgery.

Perioperative management of fluids represents a difficult clinical challenge. To date, oral fluid intake up to 2 h before surgery is highly recommended to reduce the need for intravenous administration and the risk of a fluid overload. Experimental data establish that the perioperative fluid turnover (diuresis, insensible perspiration, evaporation from the wound) does not exceed 1–1.5 ml/kg/h. In elective surgery, a zero-balance fluid (restrictive) approach monitoring intraoperative fluid loss and postoperative weight has been demonstrated to reduce major and minor complications. A "goal-directed fluid therapy" requiring continuous monitoring of circulatory status is a recent dynamic way to evaluate the real fluid requirement of people during surgery and could ameliorate prognosis in high-risk surgery in multimorbid patients. Fluids also postoperative nausea and vomiting. In conclusion, hydration state clinical management represents a seminal element of care in older people undergoing surgery.

References

1. Volkert D, Beck AM, Cederholm T, Cruz-Jentoft A, Hooper L, Kiesswetter E, Maggio M, Raynaud-Simon A, Sieber C, Sobotka L, van Asselt D, Wirth R, Bischoff S. ESPEN practical guideline: clinical nutrition and hydration in geriatric. Clin Nutr. 2022;41:958–89. https://doi.org/10.1016/j.clnu.2022.01.024.
2. Weimann A, Braga M, Carli F, Higashiguchi T, Hubner M, Klek S, Laviano A, Ljungqvist O, Lobo DN, Martindale RG, Waitzberg D, Bischoff SC, Singer P. ESPEN practical guideline: clinical nutrition in surgery. Clin Nutr. 2021;40:4745–61. https://doi.org/10.1016/j.clnu.2021.03.031.
3. Hirsh KR, Wolfe RR, Ferrando AA. Pre- and post-surgical nutrition for preservation of muscle mass, strenght, and functionality following orthopedic surgery. Nutrients. 2021;13:1675. https://doi.org/10.3390/nu13051675.
4. Voldby AW, Brandstrup B. Fluid therapy in the perioperative setting—a clinical review. J Intensive Care. 2016;4:27. https://doi.org/10.1186/s40560-016-0154-3. PMID: 27087980; PMCID: PMC4833950
5. Boccardi V, Caponi C, Bianco AR, Tagliavento M, Croce MF, Scamosci M, Ruggiero C, Mecocci P. Dealing with dehydration in hospitalized oldest persons: accuracy of the calculated serum osmolarity. Aging Clin Exp Res. 2022;34(10):2547–52. https://doi.org/10.1007/s40520-022-02185-x. Epub 2022 Jul 6
6. Li S, Xiao X, Zhang X. Hydration status in older adults: current knowledge and future challenges. Nutrients. 2023;15(11):2609. https://doi.org/10.3390/nu15112609. PMID: 37299572; PMCID: PMC10255140

The Geriatrician: From Patient-Centered Perioperative Care to Geriatric Syndromes Management

14

Arianna Sala, Caterina Trevisan, Amedeo Zurlo, and Stefano Volpato

An increasing number of older patients is undergoing both emergency and elective surgery worldwide as a consequence of (a) the demographic transition, with a relevant growth of people older than 75 years especially in developed countries; (b) the advances in surgical and anesthetic techniques, which are associated with less perioperative risks; and (c) the shift in patient expectation of healthcare [1]. For these reasons, it is essential to plan new surgery care pathways that can adapt to the needs of this large population and face the challenges related to the management of older adults in clinical practice.

14.1 Establishing Goals of Care and Surgery

The assessment of middle-aged and adult patients undergoing surgery is traditionally focused on identifying the surgical problem and the most appropriate surgical approach. The ultimate goal of surgery in these patients is complete recovery and disease resolution. This disease-centered approach is hard to be applied when managing older patients since they usually present not only the disease requiring surgery but also the consequences of age-related dysfunctions in multiple organs and systems, other comorbidities, and geriatric syndromes. These additional conditions increase the risk of peri- and postoperative complications, particularly when multimorbidity and geriatric syndromes are not properly assessed and treated in the perioperative period. Besides cardiovascular, respiratory, and renal complications, other specific age-related conditions such as malnutrition, cognitive decline, and impaired functional status often coexist in older surgical patients during hospital stays. However, despite being more prone to adverse outcomes, older patients may benefit

A. Sala · C. Trevisan · A. Zurlo · S. Volpato (✉)
Università di Ferrara, Ferrara, Italy
e-mail: arianna.sala@unife.it; caterina.trevisan@unife.it; amedeo.zurlo@unife.it; stefano.volpato@unife.it

V. Boccardi, L. Marano (eds.), *The Frail Surgical Patient*, Practical Issues in Geriatrics, https://doi.org/10.1007/978-3-031-77707-3_14

from surgical intervention in terms of clinical resolution, symptom relief (palliative surgery), and improved survival compared to younger people [2]. In this context, the most challenging task concerns, therefore, the preoperative assessment, which should lead to clearly identifying patients' overall healthcare goals and carefully evaluating their health and functional status. In order to establish a patient-centered care plan for older candidates for surgery, the patient, the surgeon, and the anesthesiologist should first discuss the target of the surgical procedure, ask about the patient's health priorities and expectations, and evaluate if the potential benefits of surgery really outweigh the risks. Health professionals taking care of older surgical patients should advise patients and caregivers on the potential impact of surgical procedures on symptoms, functional status, unbalances of coexistent conditions, and, eventually, survival. From this point of view, the concepts of quality of life and healthspan, the preoperative risk profile, the availability of healthcare assistance after surgery, and the social context should be assessed. Healthspan is defined as the time during which an individual maintains health and well-being, which allows him/her to live independently despite the coexistence of one or more chronic conditions [3, 4]. Indeed, major surgeries can certainly increase lifespan; however, at the same time, some procedures and especially their complications can dramatically decrease quality of life and healthspan [5]. To limit as much as possible negative outcomes, surgeons, anesthesiologists, and geriatricians should always discuss the most appropriate surgical procedure based on the disease and the patient's general conditions. Where possible, laparoscopic surgery should be the standard treatment in older patients. Its benefits include less severe neuroendocrine/metabolic response to stress, avoiding general anesthesia, more limited blood losses, decreased postoperative pain, shorter hospital stay, and faster return to previous mobility.

Finally, it is necessary to establish which secondary strategies should be adopted in case of postsurgical complications. In this regard, the multidisciplinary team members should observe the patient's advance instructions, such as "do not resuscitate" orders, and the patient's decision-making capability should always be respected to avoid a paternalistic approach.

14.2 Preoperative Assessment

14.2.1 Risk Stratification

The preoperative assessment evaluates the geriatric surgical patient's health status to estimate his/her surgical risk, manage vulnerability, and prevent possible complications [6].

This evaluation requires a multi-professional team-based approach involving a geriatrician, surgeon, anesthetist, and nurse. The Comprehensive Geriatric Assessment (CGA) is a multimodal, multidisciplinary, and multi-professional process aimed at identifying the clinical profile and risk of older individuals, helping to define a tailored therapeutic and care plan, and improving clinical and functional outcomes [7]. CGA provides detailed data on clinical, functional, and cognitive domains of older patients and information on non-medical domains, including economic and socioenvironmental factors. Most of CGA include measurable dimensions grouped into four main domains:

- Physical health (clinical history, medications chronically used, physical examination, laboratory data, disease-specific severity indicators, and preventive health practice).
- Functional status (basic and instrumental activities of daily living, mobility level, balance, and fall risk).
- Neuropsychological health (cognitive and affective status);
- Socioenvironmental status (social interactions, social support, environmental safety, and economic level).

These points will be better explored later in this chapter.

Frailty is an age-related decline in physiological reserves due to the aging-related accumulation of chronic diseases and functional deficits. This process results in diminished resilience, loss of adaptive capacity, and increased vulnerability to stressors [8]. Therefore, frailty is both a risk factor for adverse postoperative outcomes (medical complications, prolonged hospitalization, institutionalization, hospital readmission, and short- and long-term mortality) and a useful tool for perioperative surgical risk stratification. Since the CGA is time-consuming and requires trained personnel to perform and interpret the various assessments, in the last decades, several simpler frailty screening tools have been proposed and introduced in clinical practice. These include the Clinical Frailty Scale (a clinically oriented adaptation of the Frailty Index, which considers the number of deficits of an individual) and the Edmonton Frail Scale (a reduced version of the Frailty Index with clinical and functional domains). In addition, other approaches more focused on identifying physical frailty use physical performance tests, such as the walking speed at the usual pace for 6 m, the Short Physical Performance Battery (SPPB), and the 6-min walk test [6] (Fig. 14.1).

14.2.2 Physical Health

The preoperative evaluation of the older individual's health status usually starts with a physical examination and the revision of medical records to derive the presence of chronic conditions and the medications chronically used. Below are described the main aspects assessed preoperatively concerning this health domain.

Nutritional Status Increasing age is often associated with malnutrition, a pivotal factor in surgery as it is frequently a cause and a consequence of postoperative complications. In general surgery, 20–50% of patients are at risk of malnutrition. In older and frail patients, the causes of malnutrition are multifactorial, including physiological problems (poor dentition, decreased salivation, taste impairment), comorbidities (chronic disease, dysphagia, atrophic gastritis, cancer), psychological

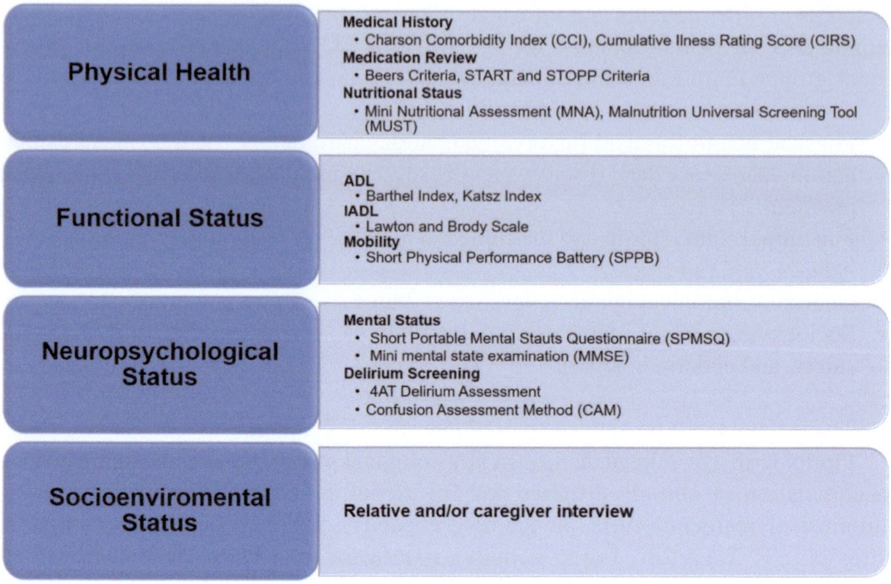

Fig. 14.1 Preoperative assessment in geriatric patients

impairments (depression, dementia) and social factors (isolation, inability in preparing meals, poverty) [9]. Nutritional assessment is, therefore, essential in these patients, and the most used tools for preoperative evaluation are the Mini Nutritional Assessment and the Malnutrition Universal Screening Tool. The European Society for Clinical Nutrition and Metabolism guidelines recommend routine screening for malnutrition on hospital admission, investigation of food intake, regular assessment of weight and nutritional counseling [10]. A preoperative serum albumin concentration of 3 g/dl may be considered indicative of severe nutritional risk, as well as a weight loss >10–15% in the previous 6 months or a BMI < 20 kg/m^2. Patients at high nutritional risk before surgery should be managed with evidence-based interventions to improve nutritional status. Nutritional support includes offering individualized nutritional advice and counseling; correction of any deficiency; oral nutritional support; fortified diets, and, when necessary, enteral, and parenteral nutrition.

Multimorbidity Multimorbidity is defined as the coexistence of two or more chronic conditions and is often associated with the need for multiple drugs [11] and impaired resistance to stressors, disability, functional decline, and frailty. The prevalence of multimorbidity in older people is very high, with more than 60% of geriatric patients presenting with multiple diseases.

The assessment tools available estimate the impact of these coexistent conditions on the biological systems in terms either of their cumulative effect, including but not limited to the Charlson Comorbidity Index and Cumulative Illness Rating Scale, or of their interactive effect, such as the Geriatric Index of Comorbidity.

The most common chronic disease in older patients is hypertension, affecting 45–50% of patients over 70 years of age, followed by coronary artery disease (35%), diabetes (12–15%), chronic kidney diseases (20–30%), chronic obstructive pulmonary disease (9%), dementia (7%) and sensory impairment (20%). Chronic diseases are strongly associated with increased surgical and postoperative complications and higher healthcare costs [12].

Cardiovascular Diseases Cardiovascular diseases most frequently observed among older patients include hypertension, a history of coronary artery disease, congestive heart failure, conduction and rhythm disorders, and valvulopathy (especially aortic stenosis). According to the guidelines for the evaluation of cardiac risk published by the American College of Cardiology and the American Heart Association, the preoperative risk assessment should focus on three main points: the surgical risk for postoperative cardiac events, the patient's functional capacity, and the risk indices [13].

The type of surgery is a determinant of the cardiac complications' risk, ranging between <1% for low-risk surgery, including endoscopy and ophthalmic, to 1–5% for intermediate-risk procedures such as orthopedic or thoracic surgery, and >5% for those at high risk, mainly vascular and cardiac surgery. In patients with good health status undergoing non-cardiac surgery, cardiopulmonary fitness is generally defined in terms of metabolic equivalents, and has demonstrated to predict perioperative and long-term cardiac risk [14]. The picture may change in older people, whose preoperative cardiopulmonary fitness is often impaired already before surgery, making it necessary to use measures different than metabolic equivalents to assess functional capacity and obtain some prognostic estimations.

In older people, heart failure has been reported as the main risk index of perioperative mortality. Besides the Goldman risk index and the Lee index, the ACS-NSQIP Surgical Risk Calculator has been validated explicitly in geriatric patients' preoperative assessment, showing high specificity and sensitivity in the prediction of heart complications and mortality, particularly if combined with cardiac biomarkers [15].

The risk of postoperative venous thromboembolism is associated with increased age, immobilization, and comorbidities such as cardiovascular disorders or cancer. Therefore, risk stratification through validated scores such as the Padua Prediction Score for Risk of Venous Thromboembolism [16] and correction of modifiable risk factors with sustained perioperative thromboprophylaxis is essential.

Respiratory Function Respiratory comorbidities, particularly chronic obstructive pulmonary disease (COPD), are common in geriatric patients and contribute to perioperative and postoperative morbidity and mortality. Overall risk factors for postoperative pulmonary complications include the surgical site, hypoalbuminemia <3 g/dl, COPD, recent smoking, poor general health status, and functional dependency [17]. Therefore, the perioperative evaluation is based on clinical examination and medical history, including smoking habits, occupational exposures, respiratory symptoms, limited exercise capacity, pre-existent lung disease, and infections. A seven-variable risk assessment tool has been prospectively validated by the Assess Respiratory Risk in Surgical Patients in Catalonia Group [18]. Routine preoperative spirometry is not recommended before high-risk surgery except for resectional thoracic surgery, where poor preoperative lung function contraindicates surgery. Preoperative preventive strategies for reducing the risk of postoperative pulmonary complications in older surgical patients should include risk factor reduction and optimization of COPD or asthma treatment [19].

Renal Function In older patients, Chronic Kidney Disease (CKD), comorbidities (hypertension, diabetes, heart failure), polypharmacy and surgery are major risk factors for acute kidney injury (AKI), and both CKD and AKI are independently associated with poor surgical outcomes. In addition, anesthetic pharmacokinetics and pharmacodynamics could be modified by renal impairment. The optimal perioperative approach in preventing AKI in older surgical patients includes maintaining fluid balance, avoidance of nephrotoxic drugs with regard to non-steroidal anti-inflammatory drugs, angiotensin-converting enzyme inhibitors and contrast agents, and appropriate adjustment dosage of drugs excreted by the renal system [20].

Hematological Disorders Anemia is common in older patients and should always be assessed before every surgical procedure with moderate-to-high anticipated blood loss (>500 ml) because of its association with increased morbidity and mortality in surgical patients. Patient Blood Management is a multimodal, multidisciplinary strategy designed to minimize the use of blood transfusion and to improve patients' outcomes. This strategy improves hemoglobin levels through intravenous iron and vitamin supplements, limiting perioperative blood loss, and using a restrictive transfusion threshold [21]. Patient Blood Management should be started before surgery, especially in elective surgery, and continued throughout the perioperative period [22].

Medication Use According to the American College of Surgeons/ American Geriatrics Society Best Practices Guidelines, a comprehensive medication review should be part of the preoperative assessment of older surgical patients to collect the patient's medication history (including over-the-counter drugs, vitamins, and nutritional supplements), to identify drugs or other substances that should be continued during the perioperative period and to deprescribe those harmful, inappropriate or contraindicated [23].

It is well known that older patients are the most medicaments consumers (3.9 medications/day for ages 65–80 years; 4.4 medications/day for ages over 80 years). Cardiovascular drugs (65%), followed by those acting on the central nervous system (41%) are the more commonly prescribed medications. Polypharmacy, which is defined as the use of 5 or more medications, is associated with negative outcomes, including adverse drug reactions, cognitive impairment, delirium, and prolonged postoperative length of stay in older surgical patients. Due to age-related changes in pharmacodynamics and pharmacokinetics, geriatric patients are vulnerable to the effects of drugs, especially those given during the perioperative period, when neuroendocrine and fluid balance modifications occur. Moreover, polypharmacy increases the risk of negative drug interactions and of receiving potentially inappropriate medications, defined as drugs that should be avoided in older patients due to the high risk of adverse reactions and/or insufficient evidence of their benefits [24]. In a review by Johnson S., 55% of surgical patients aged ≥65 years received a potentially inappropriate medication in hospital [25, 26].

Validated tools are available to identify potentially inappropriate medications among older patients. The updated Beers criteria include a list of medications that should always be avoided in older adults or only in specific circumstances, such as in the presence of certain diseases or conditions. The Screening Tool of Older Persons' Prescriptions (STOPP) and Screening Tool to Alert to Right Treatment (START) criteria identify, respectively, a list of medications to be discontinued in older adults due to incorrect dosage regimen or duration of treatment (STOPP) and a list of appropriate drugs for prevention and treatment of specific diseases (START) [26].

Inappropriate use of drugs acting on the central nervous system (such as benzodiazepines) is frequent in older patients and increases the risk of falls, delirium, and cognitive deterioration. Anticholinergic medications (antiemetics, antispasmodics, antihistamines, and antiparkinsonian agents), in particular, are commonly prescribed to older patients without considering their association with cognitive dysfunction, urinary retention, and constipation, which may themself precipitate or worsen delirium. The optimal perioperative management of antihypertensive agents in older people has not been well established since perioperative hypotension, and hypertension are both associated with adverse outcomes, but it is acceptable to continue these medications in the absence of hypotension. Moreover, current recommendations suggest maintaining beta-blocker treatment in patients already receiving these drugs. The perioperative period could be an opportune window to assess cardiovascular risk and to review the indication and overall appropriateness for antiplatelet therapy and statins, often overprescribed in older people. Proton pump inhibitors, by reducing gastric acidity, expose geriatric patients to the risk of *Clostridium difficile* colitis and should be therefore deprescribed if not indicated. Non-steroidal anti-inflammatory drugs should be prescribed at the lowest possible dose and for the shortest possible period for the risk of gastric and renal injury and only if paracetamol is ineffective as a first-line pain therapy. Older patients are more susceptible to opioids' adverse events (nausea, vomiting, and constipation);

therefore, starting doses should be generally lower than younger patients. In addition, they are associated with an increased risk of perioperative delirium [27].

14.2.3 Functional Status

Functional status is defined as the ability to perform daily activities and maintain a social role. Its impairment is associated with poor surgical outcomes in older patients; therefore, it should be assessed during the preoperative period. The Basic Activities of Daily Living (BADL), including own self-care, can be easily evaluated by the Katsz Index or the Bartel Index, while the instrumental activities (IADL), including shopping, managing money, cooking, household maintenance, and using the telephone can be investigated by Lawton and Brody scale..

Assessment of mobility overlaps with functional assessment, and the Short Physical Performance Battery (SPPB) has been identified as one of the leading tools to assess surgical patients' physical performance. The SPPB evaluates three elements of physical function: balance, assessed through three levels of difficulty; lower limb strength (indirectly estimated from repeated chair standing) and gait speed, thus allowing a complete evaluation of lower extremity function, essential to maintain autonomy [28].

14.2.4 Neuropsychological Health

The prevalence of minor or major neurocognitive disorders in people older than 65 years is 35–50% [29]. Postoperative delirium and cognitive impairment affect 20–80% and 12–15%, respectively, of geriatric surgical patients and are associated with adverse long-term outcomes, longer hospital stays, increased health costs, and a high risk of institutionalization after discharge. A preoperative mental status examination (such as the Mini-Mental State Examination) and preoperative delirium screening using validated tools such as The Arousal, Attention, Abbreviated Mental Test 4, and Acute change Test (4AT) and The Confusion Assessment Method (CAM) together with the investigation of risk factors for postoperative delirium, (better explored later), should be considered for all geriatric surgical patients [30].

14.2.5 Social Status

During the preoperative assessment, it is recommended to investigate the availability of family support in order to eventually plan substitutive support measures using appropriate risk assessment tools for difficult discharge (better explored later).

14.3 Postoperative Care and Prevention of Geriatric Complications

The main goals of postoperative care in older surgical patients are the prevention of geriatric complications, including but not limited to function and mobility impairment, delirium, malnutrition, and infections, as well as the definition of a personalized hospital discharge plan (Fig. 14.2).

14.3.1 Enhanced Recovery after Surgery Protocols

Enhanced Recovery After Surgery Protocols (ERAS) consist of multimodal perioperative management with the goal to minimize loss of functional capacity and enhance the postoperative recovery process after elective surgery. These protocols include the whole perioperative period and reduce post-surgery complications, length of hospital stay, and costs associated with hospitalization [31]. According to previous studies, factors associated with enhanced recovery after surgery, shorter hospitalization, and lower morbidity are prehabilitation, the absence of a nasogastric tube, early mobilization, oral nutrition, urinary catheter removal, and use of nonopioid analgesia [32]. Older patients are more often at risk of nutritional disorders, mobilization difficulties, and impaired cognitive status. In addition, comorbidities are more prevalent in these patients. Therefore, modulation in stress response after surgery through ERAS is highly effective in reducing complications and helping recovery in older and frail patients. Prehabilitation improve the

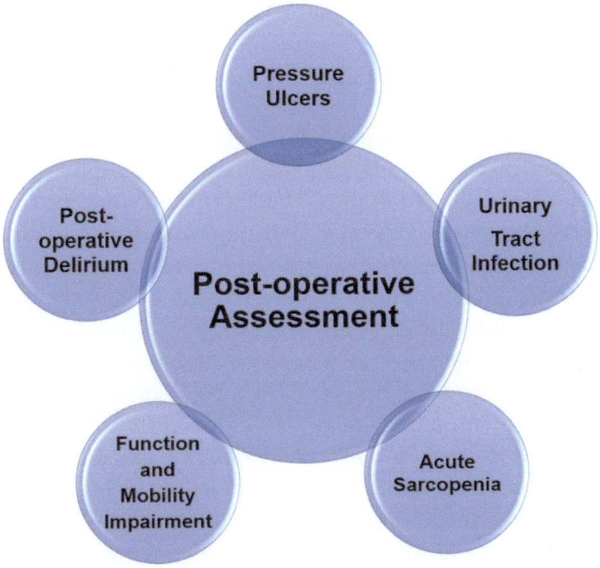

Fig. 14.2 Postoperative assessment in geriatric patients

functional and physiological capacity of the individuals to enable them to tolerate surgical stress and promote postoperative recovery. Multimodal prehabilitation including home aerobic training, strength training and respiratory exercises together with nutrition assessment and pain management, improves both preoperative fitness and postoperative functional outcomes in geriatric surgical patients. The median duration of this process is 4 weeks with a frequency of 5 sessions per week of moderate to high intensity, generally fitted to the patient's tolerance. This concept of prehabilitation a few weeks before surgery is equally beneficial compared to enhancing operative procedures and postsurgical care [33].

14.3.2 Function and Mobility Preservation

In older patients, one of the most important endpoints after surgery is the recovery of pre-morbid functional status, particularly walking ability. It is well known that hospitalization in older people is associated with functional decline, new disability, risk of longer hospital stay, and mortality [34]. Considering surgical patients, up to 50% do not recover baseline functional status [35]. This negative effect is mainly due to the prolonged bed rest, which increased the risk of incident motor disability and several complications, including loss of muscle mass and strength (acute sarcopenia), pulmonary infections, deep vein thrombosis, reduced peristalsis with subsequent loss of appetite and constipation, urinary incontinence, altered cognitive status and increased risk of pressure ulcers. ERAS protocols recommend early mobilization and walking as essential interventions to prevent these complications. Patients with more severe physical impairment might benefit from early physiotherapeutic interventions to reinforce muscle function and recover mobility.

14.3.3 Acute Sarcopenia

Sarcopenia, a condition defined by the loss of muscle mass, strength, and function, is associated with adverse outcomes such as frailty, falls, disability, decreased quality of life, and mortality. The European Working Group on Sarcopenia in Older People criteria (EWGSOP2) distinguishes three sarcopenia states, i.e., probable sarcopenia (the presence of isolated low muscle strength), confirmed sarcopenia (low muscle strength plus low muscle mass or muscle quality), and severe sarcopenia (low muscle strength, low muscle quantity/quality, and low physical performance) [36]. Acute sarcopenia, whose duration is less than 6 months, is usually the consequence of an acute disease. Low muscle strength can be assessed by measuring grip strength with a dynamometer, with a cutoff for sarcopenia of <27 kg in men and <16 kg in women. Dual-energy X-ray absorptiometry (DEXA) scan is the gold standard for estimating muscle mass, but alternative and more accessible methods are represented by the bioelectrical impedance analysis (BIA) and anthropometric parameters, such as calf circumference (considering a cutoff of <31 cm to define low muscle mass). Concerning low physical performance, the EWGSOP2 recommends using a gait speed of ≤0.8 m/s [37].

Concerning the pathophysiology of sarcopenia in older patients undergoing surgery, evidence suggests that surgery leads to an inflammatory reaction and prolonged immobilization responsible for loss of muscle mass and strength. Malnutrition, anemia, and polypharmacy are, as well, essential contributors to the loss of muscle mass, strength, and physical performance. Deficiencies in protein intake (most surgeries require a period of preoperative fasting) or malabsorptive states can directly cause muscle wasting, since proteins are crucial component of muscle maintenance. A meta-analysis by Shrestha A and colleagues shows that resistance-based training improves muscle strength, mass, and performance in older surgical patients [38].

14.3.4 Delirium

Delirium is defined by the Diagnostic and Statistical manual of Mental disorders (DSM-V) as an acute change of mental state, characterized by decreased consciousness and disturbance of attention, that may be triggered by acute disease, surgery, pain, or medications (precipitating factors) [39]. Age, comorbidities, and preexisting cognitive impairment are the major predisposing factors. Different clinical forms of delirium are described according to psychomotor features: hyperactive, hypoactive, and mixed.

Postoperative delirium (POD) affects 20–80% of geriatric surgical patients and typically occurs postoperatively between days 1 and 7. It is associated with poor outcomes, including medical complications, falls, permanent cognitive impairment, prolonged hospital stay, institutionalization, and death, and can cause patient and caregiver distress [40].

Since prevention remains the best treatment for delirium, perioperative delirium assessment should be performed and repeated over at least 5 days after surgery. Well-validated screening tools, such as the 4AT and the CAM facilitate recognition of POD and should be used both in the pre- and postoperative period. The CAM may be useful in screening for delirium. Still, the sensitivity and specificity of this scale vary considerably due to the need of specific training for users [41], whereas the 4AT is fast and easier to use. In addition, the latter instrument offers good sensitivity and has wide applicability in different clinical settings allowing assessment of patients who cannot complete cognitive tests because of drowsiness or agitation [42]. The Richmond Agitation Sedation Scale, which evaluates the level of consciousness's alteration, may be an alternative screening scale for delirium. It is rapid to perform by simply monitoring the patient during routine clinical care. All patients with delirium should receive a personalized treatment plan, including recognition of underlying acute medical illness and other clinical conditions that may cause delirium. Effective interventions to prevent delirium and to promote its resolution when present include preoperative medication review, early mobilization, adequate analgesia, promotion of physiologic sleep–wake rhythm, maintenance of adequate nutrition and hydration, and the provision of visual and auditory aids.

Inadequate analgesia for older surgical patients contributes to postoperative morbidity, including delirium. Pain should be assessed using the numerical rating scale, visual analogic scale, or verbal rating scale in patients with mild-to-moderate cognitive impairment, while specific scales (PAINAD, NOPPAIN, and Doloplus-2) are recommended for those with severe cognitive disorders. Since opioid medication for treating postoperative pain can cause delirium, analgesic plans for older adults should consider multimodal strategies (including non-pharmacological methods) and reducing the use of opioids.

Oral nutritional intake in the postoperative period is often insufficient in older frail patients; therefore, oral nutritional support should be continued from the preoperative period or started early after surgery. Oral feeding should always be preferred to enteral or parenteral nutrition. In addition, fluid status should be assessed daily for at least the first 5 postoperative days, and oral fluid intake should be started as soon as possible. In order to reduce the prevalence and duration of postoperative delirium, functional aids for visual and hearing impairment should be available to the patient after surgery, and the patient's level of comprehension should be systematically tested at critical steps of the care process. Cognitive changes after anesthesia include postoperative neurocognitive dysfunction, and avoiding episodes of deep anesthesia during surgery lasting more than 1 h can considerably reduce the risk of postoperative delirium. In addition, the invasive devices, such as the intravenous lines and the urinary catheter, should be removed early. It is also important to highlight the role of family and caregivers in supporting the patient that, in this situation, needs psychological reassurance. The flexibility of hospital visiting schedules should be encouraged. These interventions require a multidisciplinary approach, coordinated where possible by the geriatrician.

A systematic review and meta-analysis [43] demonstrated that multicomponent nonpharmacological interventions for delirium prevention decrease the incidence of both delirium and falls during hospitalization in older individuals. The effect of these interventions on delirium prevention is considerable and showed a risk reduction of more than 50% (OR 0.47; 95% CI: 0.38–0.58).

14.3.5 Pressure Ulcers

A pressure ulcer is defined by the National Pressure Ulcer Advisory Panel (NPUAP) as impaired integrity of the skin or underlying tissue caused by the compression of the skin between the bone and an outside surface, resulting in altered tissue perfusion. Four stages of severity of a pressure ulcer has been defined by the NPUAP: from stage 1, consisting of a redness that does not disappear by pressing, to a stage 4 ulcer involving the destruction and necrosis of the skin together with the muscles, bones, and tendons. The prevalence of postoperative pressure ulcers is 20%, and they are associated with delayed hospital discharge, increased health care costs, and severe impact on patient's prognosis. According to a systematic review and meta-analysis by Shafipour V et al., risk factors for developing pressure ulcers in older surgery patients are limited mobility, cognitive impairment, comorbidities such as diabetes, heart failure, and musculoskeletal disorders, lower Braden Scores at hospital admission, prolonged duration of surgery, postoperative urinary tract infection and malnutrition [44]. Health care teams should, therefore, assess the risk of pressure ulcers in all surgical patients and should apply multimodal measures to prevent and treat pressure ulcers since hospital admission, according to local guidelines [45]. Main interventions should include daily monitoring of the skin status, frequent patient's postural change, early start of rehabilitation, use of dynamic anti-decubitus mattresses which can change pressure points by a motorized mechanism and early removal of eventual urinary catheters.

14.3.6 Urinary Tract Infection

Geriatric patients are at high risk for urinary tract infections, mainly if bedridden, incontinent, and with urinary catheters (approximately 80% of urinary tract infections). According to guidelines for the prevention and management of catheter-associated urinary tract infections [46], the main indications for the use of catheters are urinary retention, perioperative use for specific surgical procedures, and daily assessment of urine output in acutely ill patients. Other appropriate uses include sacral or perineal wound healing in incontinent patients, patient comfort at the end of life, and prolonged immobilization of patients with spine or pelvic fractures.

In addition, guidelines recommend limited use of the urinary catheter and aseptic insertion. Early removal of urinary catheters, preferably within 48 hours, is associated with a lower risk of urinary tract infection, lower occurrence of delirium, and faster hospital discharge as suggested by clinical evidences [46].

14.4 Hospital Discharge and Continuity of Care

After surgery, older surgical patients often need prolonged hospitalization in non-surgical wards, or a period of care in intermediate care facilities, before returning home. For some patients, worsening health and functional status resulting from the negative effects of the disease and surgery make a return to home impossible. From this point of view, it is essential to establish a hospital discharge plan based on an organizational framework that considers (1) appropriate assessment of the patient's clinical, social, and care status; recognition of the expectations of the patient and their relatives; (2) formalization of institutional roles or teams dedicated to the planning and coordination of discharge; (3) good knowledge of transitional management programs; and (4) strong communication beatene hospital, home care services, residential facilities and nursing homes, including the primary care physician. Therefore, throughout the perioperative period, attention should be paid to how the patient can be discharged into the most appropriate setting to guarantee continuity of care and adequate support. Anticipating which elderly patients will require discharge to an additional care facility rather than their home is important for preoperative counseling of expected outcomes and preoperative care planning for both the patient and their family. The lack of an appropriate and patient-centered discharge plan and transition program increases the risk of early hospital re-admission and may negatively affect the functional status of the patients and the quality of life of both patients and caregivers [47].

The available evidences shows that a Comprehensive Geriatric Assessment of older patients in community settings can reduce the risk of readmission in those recently discharged [48]. Key elements of CGA for discharge planning include targeting criteria to identify vulnerable patients, a program of multidimensional assessment including rating scales for the risk of difficult discharge, such as the Blaylock Risk Assessment Screening Score (BRASS) [49] and home follow-up.

There is evidence that some frail patients may develop a transient period of health vulnerability following hospitalization for an acute surgical illness, known as Post-Hospital Syndrome [50]. This syndrome is characterized by the risk of early re-hospitalization due to physiologic stressors resulting from the initial admission, including disruption in sleep-wake cycles, inadequate pain control, deconditioning, and changes in nutritional status. Patients hospitalized within 90 days of elective surgery are at increased risk of postoperative adverse events characteristic of post-hospital syndrome [51].

14.5 Conclusions

Surgery is a stressful event for older patients. Recognized goals of multidimensional and multidisciplinary perioperative geriatric assessment are the evaluation of the patient's health status to delineate the surgical risk that may condition the outcomes of the intervention. Data obtained by Comprehensive Geriatric Assessment and frailty evaluation are useful in establishing patients' and caregivers' surgical goals and preferences and identifying the most appropriate treatment, the surgery invasiveness and duration, and the best perioperative strategy. These data should be used not only in perioperative surgical risk assessment but also in prevention and management of postoperative geriatric syndromes and complications (including functional decline, delirium, malnutrition, sarcopenia, and infections) as well as in delineating a personalized hospital discharge plan.

References

1. Aucoin S, McIsaac DI. Emergency general surgery in older adults. Anesthesiol Clin. 2019;37:493–505.
2. Partridge J, Sbai M, Dhesi J. Proactive care of older people undergoing surgery. Aging Clin Exp Res. 2018;30:253–7.
3. Jones TS, Moore JT, Robinson TN. Perioperative care strategy for older adults. Med Clin North Am. 2020;104:895–908.
4. Tinetti ME, Fried T. The end of the disease era. Am J Med. 2004;116:179–85.

5. Crimmins EM. Lifespan and healthspan: past, present, and promise. Gerontologist. 2015;55:901–11.
6. Makary MA, et al. Frailty as a predictor of surgical outcomes in older patients. J Am Coll Surg. 2010;210:901–8.
7. Rubenstein LZ, Joseph T. Freeman award lecture: comprehensive geriatric assessment: from miracle to reality. J Gerontol A Biol Sci Med Sci. 2004;59:M473–7.
8. Clegg A, Young J, Iliffe S, Rikkert MO, Rockwood K. Frailty in elderly people. Lancet. 2013;381:752–62.
9. Venianaki M, et al. Factors associated with malnutrition and its impact on postoperative outcomes in older patients. J Clin Med. 2021;10:2550.
10. Weimann A, et al. ESPEN guideline: clinical nutrition in surgery. Clin Nutr. 2017;36:623–50.
11. Hewitt J, et al. Prevalence of multimorbidity and its association with outcomes in older emergency general surgical patients: an observational study. BMJ Open. 2016;6:e010126.
12. Bettelli G. Preoperative evaluation in geriatric surgery: comorbidity, functional status and pharmacological history. Minerva Anestesiol. 2011;77:637–46.
13. Poldermans D, et al. Guidelines for pre-operative cardiac risk assessment and perioperative cardiac management in non-cardiac surgery. Eur J Anaesthesiol. 2010;27:92–137.
14. Freeman WK, Gibbons RJ. Perioperative cardiovascular assessment of patients undergoing noncardiac surgery. Mayo Clin Proc. 2009;84:79–90.
15. Marković DZ, et al. Addition of biomarker panel improves prediction performance of American College of Surgeons National Surgical Quality Improvement Program (ACS NSQIP) calculator for cardiac risk assessment of elderly patients preparing for major non-cardiac surgery: a pilot study. Aging Clin Exp Res. 2018;30:419–31.
16. Barbar S, et al. A risk assessment model for the identification of hospitalized medical patients at risk for venous thromboembolism: the Padua Prediction Score. J Thromb Haemost. 2010;8:2450–7.
17. Epidemiology, practice of ventilation and outcome for patients at increased risk of postoperative pulmonary complications. Eur J Anaesthesiol. 2017;34:492–507.
18. Mazo V, et al. Prospective external validation of a predictive score for postoperative pulmonary complications. Anesthesiology. 2014;121:219–31.
19. Smetana GW. Preoperative pulmonary assessment of the older adult. Clin Geriatr Med. 2003;19:35–55.
20. Aceto P, et al. Perioperative Management of Elderly patients (PriME): recommendations from an Italian intersociety consensus. Aging Clin Exp Res. 2020;32:1647–73.
21. Musallam KM, et al. Preoperative anaemia and postoperative outcomes in non-cardiac surgery: a retrospective cohort study. Lancet. 2011;378:1396–407.
22. Franchini M, et al. Patient blood management: a revolutionary approach to transfusion medicine. Blood Transfus. 2019;17:191–5.
23. Mohanty S, et al. Optimal perioperative Management of the Geriatric Patient: a best practices guideline from the American College of Surgeons NSQIP and the American Geriatrics Society. J Am Coll Surg. 2016;222:930–47.
24. Zhang X, et al. Potentially inappropriate medications in hospitalized older patients: a cross-sectional study using the beers 2015 criteria versus the 2012 criteria. Clin Interv Aging. 2017;12:1697–703.
25. Finlayson E, et al. Inappropriate medication use in older adults undergoing surgery: a National Study. J Am Geriatr Soc. 2011;59:2139–44.
26. O'Mahony D, et al. STOPP/START criteria for potentially inappropriate prescribing in older people: version 2. Age Ageing. 2014;44:213–8.
27. Johnson S, Haywood C. Perioperative medication management for older people. J Pharm Pract Res. 2022;52:391–401.
28. Baldasseroni S, et al. Pre-operative physical performance as a predictor of in-hospital outcomes in older patients undergoing elective cardiac surgery. Eur J Intern Med. 2021;84:80–7.

29. Bacigalupo I, et al. A systematic review and meta-analysis on the prevalence of dementia in Europe: estimates from the highest-quality studies adopting the DSM IV diagnostic criteria. J Alzheimers Dis. 2018;66:1471–81.
30. Crosby G, Culley DJ, Hyman BT. Preoperative cognitive assessment of the elderly surgical patient. Anesthesiology. 2011;114:1265–8.
31. Ljungqvist O, Scott M, Fearon KC. Enhanced recovery after surgery. JAMA Surg. 2017;152:292.
32. Parks L, Routt M, De Villiers A. Enhanced recovery after surgery. J Adv Pract Oncol. 2018;9:511–9.
33. Gillis C, Ljungqvist O, Carli F. Prehabilitation, enhanced recovery after surgery, or both? A narrative review. Br J Anaesth. 2022;128:434–48.
34. Volpato S, et al. Characteristics of nondisabled older patients developing new disability associated with medical illnesses and hospitalization. J Gen Intern Med. 2007;22:668–74.
35. Lawrence VA, et al. Functional independence after major abdominal surgery in the elderly. J Am Coll Surg. 2004;199:762–72.
36. Cruz-Jentoft AJ, et al. Sarcopenia: revised European consensus on definition and diagnosis. Age Ageing. 2019;48:16–31.
37. Volpato S, et al. Prevalence and clinical correlates of sarcopenia in community-dwelling older people: application of the EWGSOP definition and diagnostic algorithm. J Gerontol A Biol Sci Med Sci. 2014;69:438–46.
38. Shrestha A, Dani M, Kemp P, Fertleman M. Acute sarcopenia after elective and emergency surgery. Aging Dis. 2022;13:1759.
39. Association AP, T. F. D. Diagnostic and statistical manual of mental disorders: DSM-5™. 5th ed. Arlington: American Psychiatric Publishing; 2013.
40. Robinson TN, Wu DS, Pointer LF, Dunn CL, Moss M. Preoperative cognitive dysfunction is related to adverse postoperative outcomes in the elderly. J Am Coll Surg. 2012;215:12–7.
41. Inouye SK. Clarifying confusion: the confusion assessment method. Ann Intern Med. 1990;113:941.
42. Bellelli G, et al. Validation of the 4AT, a new instrument for rapid delirium screening: a study in 234 hospitalised older people. Age Ageing. 2014;43:496–502.
43. Hshieh TT, et al. Effectiveness of multicomponent nonpharmacological delirium interventions. JAMA Intern Med. 2015;175:512.
44. Shafipour V, Ramezanpour E, Heidari Gorji MA, Moosazadeh M. Prevalence of postoperative pressure ulcer: a systematic meta-analytic review. Electron Physician. 2016;8:3170–6.
45. Chiari P, et al. Predictive factors for pressure ulcers in an older adult population hospitalized for hip fractures: a prognostic cohort study. PLoS One. 2017;12:e0169909.
46. Conway LJ, Larson EL. Guidelines to prevent catheter-associated urinary tract infection: 1980 to 2010. Heart Lung. 2012;41:271–83.
47. Gonçalves-Bradley DC, Lannin NA, Clemson LM, Cameron ID, Shepperd S. Discharge planning from hospital. Cochrane Database Syst Rev. 2016; https://doi.org/10.1002/14651858.CD000313.pub5.
48. Briggs R, et al. Comprehensive geriatric assessment for community-dwelling, high-risk, frail, older people. Cochrane Database Syst Rev. 2022;2022; https://doi.org/10.1002/14651858.CD012705.pub2.
49. Blaylock A, Cason CL. DISCHARGE PLANNING: predicting patients' needs. J Gerontol Nurs. 1992;18:5–9.
50. Krumholz HM. Post-hospital syndrome—an acquired, transient condition of generalized risk. N Engl J Med. 2013;368:100–2.
51. Zurlo A, Zuliani G. Management of care transition and hospital discharge. Aging Clin Exp Res. 2018;30:263–70.

Open Surgery: What, Why, When, and Whom

15

Andrea Polistena, Giovanni Domenico Tebala, Roberto Cirocchi, Stefano Avenia, Giuseppe Cavallaro, Francesca Duro, Roberta Lucchini, Maria Chiara Ranucci, Alessandro Sanguinetti, and Nicola Avenia

15.1 Introduction

The increasing age of the population is an inevitable phenomenon, observed in the world [1]. It is believed that the number of people older than 65 will be higher than those of children under 5 within a few years. The number of octogenarians has risen

A. Polistena (✉)
Department of Surgery, Policlinico Umberto I, Sapienza University of Rome, Rome, Italy
e-mail: andrea.polistena@uniroma1.it

G. D. Tebala
Department of Digestive and Emergency Surgery, General Surgery Unit, S. Maria Hospital, Terni, Italy
e-mail: g.tebala@aospterni.it

R. Cirocchi · M. C. Ranucci
Department of Digestive and Emergency Surgery, S. Maria Hospital, Terni, University of Perugia, Terni, Italy
e-mail: roberto.cirocchi@unipg.it

S. Avenia · F. Duro
General and Emergency Surgery, Ospedale Santa Maria della Miseriricordia, University of Perugia, Perugia, Italy

G. Cavallaro
Department of Medico-Surgical Sciences and Biotechnologies, ICOT Hospital, Sapienza University of Rome, Latina, Italy
e-mail: giuseppe.cavallaro@uniroma1.it

R. Lucchini · A. Sanguinetti
Department of General Surgery and Surgical Specialties, S. Maria Hospital, Terni, Italy
e-mail: r.lucchini@aospterni.it; a.sanguinetti@aospterni.it

N. Avenia
Medical School, Department of General Surgery and Surgical Specialties Unit, S. Maria University Hospital University of Perugia, Terni, Italy
e-mail: nicola.avenia@unipg.it

V. Boccardi, L. Marano (eds.), *The Frail Surgical Patient*, Practical Issues in Geriatrics, https://doi.org/10.1007/978-3-031-77707-3_15

by more than 50% over the last 15 years. People aged 85 and older will increase from 2.8% in 2011 to 7.8% in 2050, with an average life expectancy of 85.3 years for males and 90.5 years for females [1], with obvious implications, both for the health policies and from the clinical point of view. Though it is now accepted that the chronological age determines the clinical choices less than the so-called biological age [2]. Several urgent mortality prediction models have been developed that can be used in both urgent and elective surgery in frail patients. The most important ones are the Physiological and Operative Severity Score for the Enumeration of Mortality (POSSUM) [3], the Portsmouth- Physiological and Operative Severity Score for the Enumeration of Mortality (P-POSSUM) [4], the Acute Physiology And Chronic Health Evaluation II (APACHE II) [5]. In the common clinical practice of the last 30 years there was a shift from conventional surgical laparotomic approach to laparoscopic access. This trend is also reported in the United States and Western Europe in which the share of older adults is increasing. Nowadays, minimally invasive surgery is the gold standard surgical approach in older and frail patients disproportionately affected by conditions, such as gastrointestinal cancer, acute cholecystitis, and colonic complicated diverticulitis. The advantages of minimally invasive surgery have been reported and are associated with a reduction of postoperative pain, hospital length of stay and a quicker return to regular quality of life. Conversely, a minimally invasive approach may be a challenge for surgeons, especially when the laparoscopic skill is not higher, and for small hospitals. When the laparoscopic skill is not higher, the operative time is longer, and it is associated with the increased risk of cardiovascular complications (asystolia, myocardial infarction, and arrhythmia) that are commonly consequent to hypercapnia and acidosis. The hypercapnia is usually associated with a long laparoscopic operative time, although the intra-abdominal pressure can be less than 10 mm Hg. A long-time of Trendelenburg's position is associated with congestive heart failure and decreased lung compliance. When treating older patients, surgeons face these specific challenges and complications, which increase the perioperative risk, mostly in frail individuals. Approximately half of all patients presenting for elective surgery are frail. While there is some disagreement about the exact definition of frailty, it is broadly defined as diminished physiological reserve in multiple organ systems, resulting in an increased vulnerability to stressors. Generally, there are two major approaches to diagnosing frailty. First, a frailty phenotype may exist based solely on physiological factors, such as resilience and strength. Alternatively, frailty may be defined more broadly, considering physiological and social factors, comorbidities, and measures of disabilities. For the above reasons, an accurate patient selection is required, and a critical evaluation of the most appropriate approach (open vs. minimally invasive) has to be taken into account. In small hospitals (spoke or rural), there are usually few multidisciplinary resources to perform low postoperative support care in easy laparoscopic surgical treatment (cholecystectomy, small incisional or umbilical hernia repair), when the laparoscopic operative time is longer can be needed an adequate intensive area to understand of the pathophysiological changes that occur perioperatively in frail persons. These lower hospitals' resources (nurse staffing, poor specialist multidisciplinary evaluation, absence of intensive care unit) are associated with a higher surgical rescue failure for the more quickly deterioration of the elderly associated with complications. Nowadays, relative surgical contraindications to minimally invasive surgery in older people can be the same as for young people: intestinal obstruction, huge tumor changes in the abdominal cavity, generalized peritonitis, and irreducible hernia. In this chapter, we focused on some of the most common surgical treatments performed in older people, as previously reported in the seminal article published by Bates in 2015 [6], aiming to define the current indications and clinical evidence in supporting an open approach instead of minimally invasive procedures:

- cholecystectomy and hepatobiliopancreatic surgery,
- inguinal hernia repair,
- ventral hernia repair,
- colon-rectal surgery,
- gastric surgery,
- adrenal surgery.

15.2 Cholecystectomy

Gallstones overall prevalence in the general population is 10–15%, and between 20 and 40% of patients will develop gallstone-related complications. Acute calculus cholecystitis is the first clinical presentation with an incidence of 10–15%. Cholecystectomy is considered the standard treatment for gallstone disease and is the most common definitive therapeutic approach for acute calculus cholecystitis [7].

Several recommendations, consensus, and guidelines were published in recent years to define diagnostic criteria, severity classification, and therapeutic indications [8–10]. One of the most relevant issues in this clinical setting is the optimal management of the subgroup of frail patients for whom surgery would be considered a 'very high risk' procedure. A logical consequence of this is to define whether the older people can be considered or not a specific risk for surgery in this setting mostly compared to antibiotic treatment only with or without percutaneous catheter drainage [11]. When common bile duct stones are suspected, preoperative magnetic resonance cholangiopancreatography is recommended as second-line assessment. Either preoperative endoscopic ultrasound, intraoperative cholangiography, or laparoscopic ultrasound can be used based on local expertise and availability. Removal of common bile duct stones is recommended either preoperatively, intraoperatively, or postoperatively based on institutional experience. According to current guidelines for elective surgery, laparoscopic cholecystectomy is recommended as the first-line treatment for patients with acute calculous cholecystitis [7]. Open cholecystectomy is indicated in septic shock or for anaesthesiology contraindications due to increased risk of bile duct injuries, blood loss, and operative time, with an increased morbidity and mortality rates observed in laparoscopic approach when local inflammation induces gangrenous and emphysematous changes [12]. The technical limitation in this setting is overcome by improved expertise and technological innovation within the laparoscopic approach, allowing at least an initial minimally invasive exploration to decide if the procedure is feasible or if it is recommended to convert to open surgery. Anyway, the current evidence confirms the feasibility and safety of laparoscopic cholecystectomy over open cholecystectomy in the treatment of patients with acute cholecystitis [13].

Another important issue is the timing of surgery in the acute setting. When comparing early cholecystectomy with delayed surgery, no differences were observed in mortality, bile duct injury, bile leakage, overall complications, and conversion to open surgery were seen, but an early approach was associated with a significant reduction in wound infection, hospitalization, duration of surgery and quality of life [14].

Although with low evidence, a weak recommendation is provided to offer laparoscopic cholecystectomy as the first option, even in patients older than 80 years old [7]. This approach is supported by several publications, such as the retrospective analysis based on the American College of Surgeons National Surgical Quality Improvement Program database, performed on very older patients who underwent laparoscopic and open cholecystectomy between 2005 and 2012. The mortality rate after cholecystectomy in very older patients did not differ significantly compared to the younger counterpart. The mortality and morbidity for laparoscopic and elective procedures were significantly lower than for open procedures and emergent procedures, respectively [15]. Nevertheless, a recent systematic review and meta-analysis on 326,517 patients showed increased overall and major complications in older individuals following laparoscopic cholecystectomy with an associated sevenfold increase in perioperative mortality, which increases to tenfold in patients $\geq$ 80 years old group. This study confirms the evidence of higher risks in such patients undergoing cholecystectomy, requiring adequate selection with geriatric assessment and specific intervention in this group of individuals [16]. Age is therefore confirmed as a general risk factor for cholecystectomy. Frailty beyond chronological age might further increase this risk, and it implies the necessity of a specific geriatric intervention to select those individuals with the highest surgical risk or with absolute contraindications to surgery. In conclusion, open cholecystectomy cannot be recommended as a first approach both in elective and emergency surgery for gallbladder stones and acute calculous cholecystitis. Meticulous patient selection and geriatric assessment are strongly recommended before surgery. Open direct approach or conversion from laparoscopy must be reserved in older patients similarly as in the younger counterpart to severe local inflammation with risk of bile duct injuries, massive blood loss, and prolonged operative time. Although early laparoscopic cholecystectomy was shown as superior to percutaneous transhepatic gallbladder drainage in high-risk patients with acute cholecystitis, nonoperative management with antibiotic treatment and percutaneous drainage must always be considered for frail, very older patients not fit for surgery especially because drainage potentially converts a septic patient with cholecystitis into a non-septic patient [7].

15.3 Hepatobiliopancreatic Surgery

15.3.1 Hepatocellular Carcinoma

Hepatocellular carcinoma (HCC) showed an increasing incidence in the last decades with a parallel increase in the percentage of older patients affected. The treatment of this group of subjects represents an important clinical issue. The leading criteria of treatment still refer to the Milan criteria [17]. Accordingly, liver transplantation represents one of the treatment options together with liver resection and other percutaneous treatments according to stage and Child-Pugh classification. Although there is a higher risk of graft failure in the older recipient population, age alone should not be a contraindication for liver transplantation. Careful selection of donors and recipients along with optimal management of risk factors during the postoperative period is necessary to maximize the transplant outcomes in this population [18]. Consequently, due to the shortage of organ donors and to the defined age limits (70 years) usually, older and frail patients are usually excluded from transplantation and referred for surgical resection when surgical fit or for alternative treatments. There is some robust evidence to support the choice of hepatectomy for older patients with HCC within Milan criteria. In fact, age was shown in multivariate analysis as an independent risk factor for non-cancer-related death, but not similarly for recurrence and cancer-related death, confirming surgical resection as a safe and effective treatment for patients with HCC, although an increased incidence of perioperative morbidity which requires a strict selection of surgical cases [19].

When considering the optimal approach for liver resection, minimally invasive techniques were shown to be superior in the postoperative outcomes to open liver resection with comparable survival outcomes [20].

On the other hand, advanced age, severe comorbidity, and frailty may not recommend a surgical indication. Therefore, it is not uncommon that this group of patients is referred to percutaneous approaches. When analyzing the efficacy of ablation versus resection, recent studies showed similar outcomes. This is mostly since a higher liver cancer or other cause-related death rate in very older patients may shorten the life expectancy, which may lead to the same OS regardless of whether resection or ablation is chosen [21].

15.3.2 Liver Metastases

The treatment of liver metastases in older patients may follow the same criteria reported above regarding liver resection for HCC.

Older patients usually are less referred to curative-intent liver resection, and especially if comorbidities and frailty are present, ablative treatment is preferred. When surgery is possible, excellent survival and good quality of life are gained even in older adults [22].

Always, the key to the treatment choice is a preliminary multidimensional assessment and a multidisciplinary evaluation to offer surgical or local ablative treatment whenever possible. Evidence supports that liver resection for colorectal liver metastases should not be excluded a priori in older patients, since similar operative and postoperative outcomes as younger patients were shown. However, elderly patients are usually associated with an increased risk of postoperative mortality and have worse overall survival, thus, comorbidities and frailty must be always considered [23].

15.3.3 Intrahepatic Cholangiocarcinoma

The general consideration above expressed for hepatocarcinoma and liver metastasis regarding liver resection are similarly related to intrahepatic cholangiocarcinoma. The incidence rate of intrahepatic cholangiocarcinoma has been increasing worldwide during the last decades, showing a prevalence in the sixth decade of life, for this reason, this highly malignant entity is of great interest [24]. Surgery still represents in the general population the most effective curative therapy for cholangiocarcinoma even with limited 5-year survival ranging from 10% to 40%. To improve surgical resection containing tumor relapse and for those patients with unresectable tumors, many options are available including chemotherapy, radiation therapy, immunotherapy, and targeted therapy. When considering older patients with intrahepatic cholangiocarcinoma a specific evaluation must be considered to balance the potential benefit of liver resection with the potential morbidity associated with a major surgical procedure. Feasibility and safety of major hepatic resection in the older patients was proven [25] while strong evidence on survival benefit in this group of patients is lacking. As a matter of fact, surgical complications are increased in older population, especially when extensive demolition is required to gain free margins, which are usually larger than what is normally recommended when treating hepatocarcinoma and metastases, considering the high aggressiveness of this tumor [26]. Therefore, an appropriate selection of patients is strictly recommended mostly focused on frailty and type of surgery required. A Propensity Scores Matching Analysis from the SEER database on older patients with intrahepatic cholangiocarcinoma showed an OS and CSS benefit for surgical treatment in non-metastatic stage vs non-surgical treatment. Limited nodal involvement (N0-N1) is again associated with a prognostic advantage in those patients fit for surgery. Therefore, surgery must be offered after complete staging and multidimensional assessment. More advanced stages and frails must be referred to chemotherapy or palliative treatment options [24].

15.3.4 Perihilar Cholangiocarcinoma

A recent multicentric study showed that minimally invasive surgery, although the complexity of the surgical procedures, generally seems to be safe and feasible for experienced surgeons with no significant differences compared to open surgery in terms of major postoperative complications and with the advantage of shorter hospital stay [27]. Either in terms of long-term prognosis or short-term outcomes, both approaches seem to be equivalent [28]. The main point to debate on the minimally invasive approach to perihilar cholangiocarcinoma is to define an effective superiority over open surgery and to consider the level of technical expertise required.

For the first point, feasibility and safety and an advantage in shorter hospital stays were proven, although the counterpart is represented by longer surgical duration, which must be a challenge when examining older and fragile patients. For the second point we must consider that minimally invasive hepatobiliary surgery so far is maintained in an exploratory phase with the biliary-enteric anastomosis performed through the service incision and that the technique is extremely demanding and must be reserved to high volume specialized institutions [29].

15.3.5 Pancreatic Cancer

Pancreatic cancer is typically observed in advanced age, with an incidence of approximately 50-fold higher in octogenarians than in patients in their early 40 s [30]. Current expertise in pancreatic surgery in high-volume centers offers a prognostic advantage in primary resectable or in borderline resectable tumors after neoadjuvant treatment. Pancreaticoduodenectomy has become accepted as a safe and effective procedure, with acceptable morbidity and mortality rates even in elderly patients aged 70 or 75 years or older as it is in younger patients [31, 32]. The efficacy of surgery for pancreatic cancer for patients 80 years of age and older is controversial. Again, careful selection is strongly recommended because pancreaticoduodenectomy is associated with a higher incidence of severe postoperative complications and a small change of long-term survival [33]. Generally, for pancreatic cancer patients, minimally invasive procedures including laparoscopic and robotic surgery were shown as feasible and safe based mostly on retrospective series although comparative long-term is lacking to date. Based on the existing evidence, current observed benefits of minimally invasive pancreatoduodenectomy over open pancreatoduodenectomy seem scarce, but incoming results from several ongoing randomized controlled trials will present a clarification on short- and long-term outcomes between these two approaches [34, 35].

In patients with left-sided pancreatic tumors confined to the pancreas, a minimally invasive approach showed in a recent clinical trial advantages over the open approach in terms of functional recovery, less delayed gastric emptying, and better quality of life without increasing costs. No significant difference in the overall complication rate was observed between the two approaches [34]. A very recent meta-analysis detected evidence of advantages for minimally invasive pancreatic surgery compared to the open approach in terms of reduced length of hospital stay and intraoperative blood loss. Again, the morbidity rate and mortality rate were not significantly different. The above study included patients over 18 years of age with no specific focus on older individuals but as a consequent consideration on these results is that longer duration of surgery in minimally invasive approach might be challenging especially for these patients and that an even more accurate selection of surgical candidates must be carried out when frailty is present [35]. In summary, chronological age independently predicted morbidity and mortality after pancreaticoduodenectomy. Advanced age also may have a role in failure to rescue because the mortality in those who have complications is higher in the older than in younger patients.

Benefit of surgery in this setting is confirmed unless the patient is frail as well as older, considering in this group palliative treatment and supportive nonoperative management. Surgical indication must be balanced with the evidence that advanced age is independently associated with morbidity and death following pancreaticoduodenectomy, suggesting that advanced age may have a role in the failure to rescue in complicated patients. In those patients fit for surgery, the choice between minimally invasive or open access is still under investigation. Laparoscopic and robotic pancreatoduodenectomy was shown as feasible and safe even in older people despite missing definitive results on short- and long-term outcomes between these two approaches. The choice for open surgery must be considered based on life expectancy, center experience, locoregional features of the tumor, and general contraindication to long anesthesia related to the minimally invasive procedure always after a preoperative geriatric assessment, mostly for fragile patients.

15.4 Inguinal Hernia Repair

Inguinal and femoral hernias are very common clinical situations worldwide, and its incidence is higher in older people. In current practice, geriatric patients presenting with asymptomatic groin hernia are often managed conservatively to avoid the surgery-related risk of complications. A watchful waiting is recognized as an acceptable option for patients with asymptomatic or minimally symptomatic inguinal hernias. In these patients, the treatment of inguinal hernia is commonly performed through conventional open access (inguinal incision) as suggested by international guidelines [36]. In uncomplicated inguinal hernia, a lot of surgeons suggested performing an ambulatory treatment in regional anesthesia; in effect, this type of anesthesia is associated with a lower rate of complications [37]. In case of recurrent hernia, the laparoscopic repair is safe in fit patients without cardiovascular or respiratory comorbidities [38].

15.5 Ventral Hernia

Ventral hernias are among the most encountered surgical diseases, older patients are particularly at risk of developing ventral hernias because of the loss of strength of the abdominal wall with age, and the development of comorbidities that increase intra-abdominal pressure, such as chronic constipation, bladder outlet obstruction and chronic cough. Laparoscopic incisional hernia repair is associated with some advantages (decreased wound complications, length of hospital stay) [39], but in real life, open access is the most common surgical treatment (71.1%) [40].

15.6 Colorectal Surgery

In the last decade, systematic review and meta-analysis (15 studies: 1436 laparoscopic surgeries and 1810 open surgeries) have reported that robotic and laparoscopic surgery is feasible and safe in older patients [41, 42], furthermore laparoscopic colorectal resection has some advantages in short-term outcomes compared with open surgery [43]: blood loss, overall morbidity (OR = 0.5427, 95%CI: 0.4425–0.6655, $P < 0.0001$), incisional surgical site infection (OR = 0.6262, 95%CI: 0.4310–0.9097, $P = 0.0140$), bowel obstruction (OR = 0.6248, 95%CI: 0.4519–0.8638, $P = 0.0044$), and cardiovascular complications (OR = 0.4767, 95%CI: 0.2805–0.8101, $P = 0.0062$). Moreover, some surgeons reported a decrease in postoperative pulmonary complications following laparoscopic colorectal resection in the older patients [44]. In real life, the surgeons performed a selection between older patients who underwent open versus laparoscopic surgery: the open colectomy is most frequently performed in stage II tumors and III; differently, the MIS is commonly performed in stage 0/I tumors [45, 46]. Nowadays, Keller performed the analysis of a national inpatient database that reported a slow adoption of laparoscopy for colorectal cancer surgery in the older patients. Probably, laparoscopic surgery is performed in fit persons associated with a lower tumor stage (short operative time); conversely, in unfit patients (comorbidities, frailty, malnutrition, impaired functional and cognitive status), the conventional laparotomic access is the preferred surgical approach [47, 48]. The open access in colorectal surgery is the best strategy to treat complications (obstruction, perforation, and hemorrhage) [49], as reported in the statement of WSES guidelines on colon and rectal cancer emergencies: obstruction and perforation reported: "The use of laparoscopy in the emergency treatment of Occlusive Left Colonic Cancer" (OLCC) cannot be recommended and should be reserved to selected favorable cases and in specialized centers [50]. Open surgical access is associated with higher sensitivity for direct visual inspection and for surgeons' hands; this can be extremely important during complex resection for locally advanced cancer, that are still commonly associated with a high laparotomic conversion rate [51]. Furthermore, the risk of laparotomic conversion is higher in older patients (75 +), male, ASA III+, and had a high frequency of Charlson's comorbidity score 3 + [52]. Differently, the treatment of complicated diverticulitis is mostly performed through laparotomic access. Mbadiwe reported that patients between 80 and 89 years of age underwent a laparoscopic approach in 2.1% of non-complicated diverticulitis and 11.4% of complicated diverticulitis, while, respectively, 35.4% and 42.5% in patients between 60 and 79 years and 53% and 38.4% between 40 and 59 years [53].

15.7 Gastric Surgery

Together with the increased proportion of the olders in the general population, the number of surgical procedures for older patients with gastric cancer has been increasing. Nowadays, laparoscopic gastric surgery appears to be superior to open surgery in improving patient survival and quality of life, but some contraindications are still reported for patients with multiple prior laparotomies, those with locally invasive or very large tumors. Additionally, patients with neoadjuvant treatment sometimes have intense peritumoral fibrosis that prompts an open approach [54].

15.8 Open Adrenalectomy

Open Adrenalectomy still plays a fundamental role in the treatment of malignant neoplastic disease of the adrenal gland, with radiologic evidence of infiltration of near structures, and large tumours. In all other cases, this approach represents a second choice dictated by the experience of the surgeon [55]. Open adrenalectomy can be performed using several approaches: the most used is the abdominal approach, through a median or subcostal laparotomy. This approach allows a peritoneal exploration, looking for possible metastases. A lateral approach with an incision in the ipsilateral flank below the last rib, especially for en-bloc nephro-surrenectomies, may also be used.

In conclusion, nowadays, open access is still important in the modern armamentarium of the surgical operating theatre; in effect, the skills of open surgery will remain indispensable in visceral surgery.

References

1. Luo Y, Su B, Zheng X. Trends and challenges for population and health during population aging—China, 2015-2050. China CDC Wkly. 2021;3:593–8. https://doi.org/10.46234/ccdcw2021.158.
2. Rudnicka E, Napierała P, Podfigurna A, et al. The World Health Organization (WHO) approach to healthy ageing. Maturitas. 2020;139:6–11. https://doi.org/10.1016/j.maturitas.2020.05.018.
3. Copeland GP, Jones D, Walters M. POSSUM: a scoring system for surgical audit. Br J Surg. 1991;78:355–60. https://doi.org/10.1002/bjs.1800780327.
4. Prytherch DR, Whiteley MS, Higgins B, et al. POSSUM and Portsmouth POSSUM for predicting mortality. Physiological and operative severity score for the enumeration of mortality and morbidity. Br J Surg. 1998;85:1217–20. https://doi.org/10.1046/j.1365-2168.1998.00840.x.
5. Jones DR, Copeland GP, De Cossart L. Comparison of POSSUM with APACHE II for prediction of outcome from a surgical high-dependency unit. Br J Surg. 1992;79:1293–6. https://doi.org/10.1002/bjs.1800791216.
6. Bates AT, Divino C. Laparoscopic surgery in the elderly: a review of the literature. Aging Dis. 2015;6:149–55. https://doi.org/10.14336/AD.2014.0429.
7. Pisano M, Allievi N, Gurusamy K, et al. 2020 World Society of Emergency Surgery updated guidelines for the diagnosis and treatment of acute calculus cholecystitis. World J Emerg Surg. 2020;15:61. https://doi.org/10.1186/s13017-020-00336-x.

8. Ansaloni L, Pisano M, Coccolini F, et al. 2016 WSES guidelines on acute calculous cholecystitis. World J Emerg Surg. 2016;11:1–23.
9. Yokoe M, Takada T, Strasberg SM, et al. TG13 diagnostic criteria and severity grading of acute cholecystitis (with videos). J Hepatobiliary Pancreat Sci. 2013;20:35–46.
10. Pisano M, Ceresoli M, Cimbanassi S, et al. 2017 WSES and SICG guidelines on acute calcolous cholecystitis in elderly population. World J Emerg Surg. 2017;14:1–16.
11. Loozen CS, Van Santvoort HC, Van Duijvendijk P, et al. Laparoscopic cholecystectomy versus percutaneous catheter drainage for acute cholecystitis in high risk patients (CHOCOLATE): multicentre randomised clinical trial. BMJ. 2018;363:k3965.
12. Borzellino G, Sauerland S, Minicozzi AM, et al. Laparoscopic cholecystectomy for severe acute cholecystitis. A meta-analysis of results. Surg Endosc Other Interv Tech. 2008;22:8–15.
13. Coccolini F, Catena F, Pisano M, et al. Open versus laparoscopiccholecystectomy in acute cholecystitis. Systematic review and meta-analysis. Int J Surg. 2015;18:196–204.
14. Song G-M, Wei Bian X-TZ, et al. Laparoscopic cholecystectomy for acute cholecystitis: early or delayed? Evidence from a systematic review of discordant meta-analyses. Medicine (Baltimore). 2016;95:e3835.
15. Irojah B, Bell T, Grim R, et al. Are they too old for surgery? Safety of cholecystectomy in superelderly patients (≥ age 90). Perm J. 2017;21:16–013. https://doi.org/10.7812/TPP/16-013.
16. Kamarajah SK, Karri S, Bundred JR, et al. Perioperative outcomes after laparoscopic cholecystectomy in elderly patients: a systematic review and meta-analysis. Surg Endosc. 2020;34:4727–40. https://doi.org/10.1007/s00464-020-07805-z.
17. Mazzaferro V, Regalia E, Doci R, et al. Liver transplantation for the treatment of small hepatocellular carcinomas in patients with cirrhosis. N Engl J Med. 1996;334:693–9.
18. Okumura K, Lee JS, Dhand A, Sogawa H, et al. Trends and outcomes of liver transplantation among older recipients in the United States. World J Transplant. 2022;12:259–67. https://doi.org/10.5500/wjt.v12.i8.259.
19. Lu Y, Liang L, Lu WF, et al. The prognosis of elderly patients with hepatocellular carcinoma after curative hepatectomy a multicenter competing risk analysis. Clin Res Hepatol Gastroenterol. 2023;47:102147. https://doi.org/10.1016/j.clinre.2023.102147.
20. Jiang S, Yu D, He H, et al. Short- and long-term outcomes in laparoscopic versus open hepatectomy for hepatocellular carcinoma in elderly patients: a systematic review and meta-analysis. J Laparoendosc Adv Surg Tech A. 2023;33:321–34. https://doi.org/10.1089/lap.2022.0524.
21. Zou HL, Tang H, An C, et al. Overall survival rates become similar between percutaneous ablation and hepatic resection with increasing age among elderly patients with early hepatocellular carcinoma. World J Oncol. 2023;14:125–34. https://doi.org/10.14740/wjon1479.
22. Lehtomäki K, Soveri LM, Osterlund E, et al. Resectability, resections, survival outcomes, and quality of life in older adult patients with metastatic colorectal cancer (the RAXO-study). J Clin Med. 2023;18(12):3541. https://doi.org/10.3390/jcm12103541.
23. Amato B, Aprea G, De Rosa D, et al. Laparoscopic hepatectomy for HCC in elderly patients: risks and feasibility. Aging Clin Exp Res. 2017;29:179–83. https://doi.org/10.1007/s40520-016-0675-6.
24. Chen K, Yu H, Yang J, et al. Survival benefit of surgical treatment for elderly patients with intrahepatic cholangiocarcinoma: a retrospective cohort study in the SEER database by propensity score matching analysis. Curr Oncol. 2023;30:2642–52. https://doi.org/10.3390/curroncol30030201.
25. Oishi K, Itamoto T, Kohashi T, et al. Safety of hepatectomy for elderly patients with hepatocellular carcinoma. World J Gastroenterol. 2014;20:15028–36.
26. Vitale A, Spolverato G, Bagante, et al. A multi-institutional analysis of elderly patients undergoing a liver resection for intrahepatic cholangiocarcinoma. J Surg Oncol. 2016;113:420–6.
27. Wang M, Qin T, Zhang H, et al. Laparoscopic versus open surgery for perihilar cholangiocarcinoma: a multicenter propensity score analysis of short-term outcomes. BMC Cancer. 2023;23:394. https://doi.org/10.1186/s12885-023-10783-9.
28. Qin T, Wang M, Zhang H, Minimally Invasive Pancreas Treatment Group in the Pancreatic Disease Branch of China's International Exchange and Promotion Association for Medicine

and Healthcare, et al. The long-term outcome of laparoscopic resection for perihilar cholangiocarcinoma compared with the open approach: a real-world multicentric analysis. Ann Surg Oncol. 2023;30:1366–78. https://doi.org/10.1245/s10434-022-12647-1.
29. Ratti F, Fiorentini G, Cipriani F, et al. Perihilar cholangiocarcinoma: are we ready to step towards minimally invasiveness? Updat Surg. 2020;72:423–33. https://doi.org/10.1007/s13304-020-00752-3.
30. Aprea G, De Rosa D, Milone M, et al. Laparoscopic distal pancreatectomy in elderly patients: is it safe? Aging Clin Exp Res. 2017;29:41–5. https://doi.org/10.1007/s40520-016-0677-4.
31. Oguro S, Shimada K, Kishi Y, et al. Perioperative and long-term outcomes after pancreaticoduodenectomy in elderly patients 80 years of age and older. Langenbeck's Arch Surg. 2013;398:531–8. https://doi.org/10.1007/s00423-013-1072-7.
32. Park HM, Park SJ, Han SS, et al. Surgery for elderly patients with resectable pancreatic cancer, a comparison with non-surgical treatments: a retrospective study outcomes of resectable pancreatic cancer. BMC Cancer. 2019;19:1090. https://doi.org/10.1186/s12885-019-6255-3.
33. Kim JS, Choi M, Kim SH, et al. Safety and feasibility of laparoscopic pancreaticoduodenectomy in octogenarians. Asian J Surg. 2022;45:837–43. https://doi.org/10.1016/j.asjsur.2021.09.021.
34. de Rooij T, van Hilst J, Bosscha K, et al. Dutch Pancreatic Cancer Group. Minimally invasive versus open pancreatoduodenectomy (LEOPARD-2): study protocol for a randomized controlled trial. Trials. 2018;19:1. https://doi.org/10.1186/s13063-017-2423-4.
35. Jin J, Shi Y, Chen M, et al. Robotic versus open pancreatoduodenectomy for pancreatic and periampullary tumors (PORTAL): a study protocol for a multicenter phase III non-inferiority randomized controlled trial. Trials. 2021;22:954. https://doi.org/10.1186/s13063-021-05939-6.
36. HerniaSurge Group. International guidelines for groin hernia management. Hernia. 2018;22:1–165. https://doi.org/10.1007/s10029-017-1668-x.
37. Chlebny T, Zelga P, Pryt M, Zelga M, Dziki A. Safe and uncomplicated inguinal hernia surgery in the elderly—message from anesthesiologists to general surgeons. Pol Przegl Chir. 2017;89(2):5–10. https://doi.org/10.5604/01.3001.0009.9149. PMID: 28537570
38. He Z, Hao X, Li J, et al. Laparoscopic inguinal hernia repair in elderly patients: single center experience in 12 years. Ann Laparosc Endosc Surg. 2017;2:88.
39. Elhage SA, Shao JM, Deerenberg EB, et al. Laparoscopic ventral hernia repair in the geriatric population: an assessment of long-term outcomes and quality of life. Am Surg. 2020;86:1015–21. https://doi.org/10.1177/0003134820942149.
40. Aly S, de Geus SWL, Carter CO, et al. Laparoscopic versus open ventral hernia repair in the elderly: a propensity score-matched analysis. Hernia. 2021;25:673–7. https://doi.org/10.1007/s10029-020-02243-1.
41. Devoto L, Celentano V, Cohen R, et al. Colorectal cancer surgery in the very elderly patient: a systematic review of laparoscopic versus open colorectal resection. Int J Color Dis. 2017;32:1237–42. https://doi.org/10.1007/s00384-017-2848-y.
42. Li Y, Wang S, Gao S, et al. Laparoscopic colorectal resection versus open colorectal resection in octogenarians: a systematic review and meta-analysis of safety and efficacy. Tech Coloproctol. 2016;20:153–62. https://doi.org/10.1007/s10151-015-1419-x.
43. Fujii S, Tsukamoto M, Fukushima Y, et al. Systematic review of laparoscopic vs open surgery for colorectal cancer in elderly patients. World J Gastrointest Oncol. 2016;8:573–82. https://doi.org/10.4251/wjgo.v8.i7.573.
44. Chern YJ, You JF, Cheng CC, et al. Decreasing postoperative pulmonary complication following laparoscopic surgery in elderly individuals with colorectal cancer: a competing risk analysis in a propensity score-weighted cohort study. Cancers (Basel). 2021;14:131. https://doi.org/10.3390/cancers14010131.
45. Thompson HM, Williams H, Omer DM, Yuval JB, Verheij FS, Fiasconaro M, Widmar M, Wei IH, Pappou EP, Smith JJ, Nash GM, Weiser MR, Paty P, et al. Comparison of short-term outcomes and survival between minimally invasive colectomy and open colectomy in patients 80 years of age and older. J Robot Surg. 2023; https://doi.org/10.1007/s11701-023-01575-1. Epub ahead of print

46. Boselli C, Cirocchi R, Gemini A, et al. Surgery for colorectal cancer in elderly: a comparative analysis of risk factor in elective and urgency surgery. Aging Clin Exp Res. 2016;29:65–71. https://doi.org/10.1007/s40520-016-0642-2.
47. Keller DS, Qiu J, Kiran RPA. National study on the adoption of laparoscopic colorectal surgery in the elderly population: current state and value proposition. Tech Coloproctol. 2019;23:965–72. https://doi.org/10.1007/s10151-019-02082-y.
48. Keller DS, de Paula TR, Qiu J, Kiran RP, et al. The trends in adoption, outcomes, and costs of laparoscopic surgery for colorectal cancer in the elderly population. J Gastrointest Surg. 2021;25:766–74. https://doi.org/10.1007/s11605-020-04517-6.
49. Vilsan J, Maddineni S, Ahsan N, et al. Open, laparoscopic, and robotic approaches to treat colorectal cancer: a comprehensive review of literature. Cureus. 2023;15:e38956. https://doi.org/10.7759/cureus.38956.
50. Pisano M, Zorcolo L, Merli C, et al. 2017 WSES guidelines on colon and rectal cancer emergencies: obstruction and perforation. World J Emerg Surg. 2018;13:36. https://doi.org/10.1186/s13017-018-0192-3.
51. Ptok H, Kube R, Schmidt U, et al. "Colon/Rectum Carcinoma (Primary Tumor)" Study Group. Conversion from laparoscopic to open colonic cancer resection—associated factors and their influence on long-term oncological outcome. Eur J Surg Oncol. 2009;35:1273–9. https://doi.org/10.1016/j.ejso.2009.06.006.
52. de Neree Tot Babberich MPM, van Groningen JT, et al. Dutch surgical colorectal audit. Laparoscopic conversion in colorectal cancer surgery; is there any improvement over time at a population level? Surg Endosc. 2018;32:3234–46. https://doi.org/10.1007/s00464-018-6042-2.
53. Mbadiwe T, Obirieze AC, Cornwell EE 3rd, Turner P, Fullum TM. Surgical management of complicated diverticulitis: a comparison of the laparoscopic and open approaches. J Am Coll Surg. 2013;216(4):782–8.; discussion 788-90. https://doi.org/10.1016/j.jamcollsurg.2013.02.003.
54. Okumura N, Son T, Kim YM, et al. Robotic gastrectomy for elderly gastric cancer patients: comparisons with robotic gastrectomy in younger patients and laparoscopic gastrectomy in the elderly. Gastric Cancer. 2016;19:1125–34. https://doi.org/10.1007/s10120-015-0560-6.
55. Yip L, Duh QY, Wachtel H, et al. American Association of Endocrine Surgeons Guidelines for adrenalectomy: executive summary. JAMA Surg. 2022;157:870–7. https://doi.org/10.1001/jamasurg.2022.3544.

Minimally Invasive Surgery Choice: What, Why, When, and Whom

16

Paolo Sapienza, Daniele Crocetti, Giovanni Docimo, Michelangelo Miccini, Immacolata Iannone, Alessandro Puzziello, Bruno Amato, and Enrico Fiori

The answers to these questions might be complex but, in this chapter, we will try to highlight the intriguing aspects of the literature to direct the surgeons to choose the optimal treatment for frail older patients. From a general point of view, minimally invasive surgery has the advantage to be better tolerated by these patients [1]; thus, we may come to the erroneous conclusion that, when technically feasible, these patients should always be treated with a minimally invasive approach; unfortunately, this is not always possible.

The first question we are going to answer presents an initial dichotomy regarding the target organs and the best approach between laparoscopic and robotic to treat older and frail patients.

Current scientific literature seems to demonstrate the superiority of laparoscopic gastrectomy either total or subtotal compared to traditional surgery for the treatment of gastric neoplasms at an early stage (early gastric cancer). Nevertheless, the spread of laparoscopic surgery is limited by the technical difficulties related to the total D2 gastrectomy that includes the dissection of the lymph nodes at the level of the celiac

P. Sapienza · D. Crocetti · M. Miccini · I. Iannone · E. Fiori (✉)
Department of Surgery, "Sapienza" University of Rome, Rome, Italy
e-mail: paolo.sapienza@uniroma1.it; daniele.crocetti@uniroma1.it; michelangelo.miccini@uniroma1.it; immacolata.iannone@uniroma1.it; enrico.fiori@uniroma1.it

G. Docimo
Department of Medical and Advance Surgical Science, University of Campania "Luigi Vanvitelli", Naples, Italy
e-mail: giovanni.docimo@unicampania.it

A. Puzziello
Department of Medicine, Surgery and Dentistry, University of Salerno, Fisciano, Italy
e-mail: alessandro.puzziello@unisa.it

B. Amato
Department of Public Health, University of Naples Federico II, Naples, Italy
e-mail: bruno.amato@unina.it

V. Boccardi, L. Marano (eds.), *The Frail Surgical Patient*, Practical Issues in Geriatrics, https://doi.org/10.1007/978-3-031-77707-3_16

trunk, the left gastric artery, and the hepatic peduncle. Thus, laparoscopic D2 gastrectomy with spleen preservation is reserved to high-volume centers. In a recent randomized multicentric study [2], laparoscopic gastrectomy in Western countries showed that postoperative hospitalization does not decrease, and the percentage of complications and oncological efficacy does not differ from traditional surgery. A recent umbrella review [3] compared the results of gastrectomy performed robotically or laparoscopically. No differences were observed in complications' rate, morbidity, mortality, anastomotic dehiscence, anastomotic stenosis, intestinal obstruction, and conversion to traditional surgery. The effectiveness and safety of the robotic gastrectomy is not supported by clear evidence, and therefore, data reported in the current meta-analyses must be cautiously interpreted especially in the presence of great samples' heterogeneity. Some points are certain, namely, robotic gastrectomy is associated with earlier re-feeding, lower intraoperative bleeding, and longer operative time.

In frail patients, the current literature has not yet come to final conclusions, results need to be evaluated very carefully, and there are no prospective randomized studies that address both the potential advantage of one of the minimally invasive approaches and the long-term oncological results [4, 5]. Today, we can recommend, in frail patients, both the laparoscopic and robotic approaches in gastric subtotal resections at an early stage of the disease within prospective randomized trials.

Surgical treatment of primary or secondary liver neoplasms (hepatocarcinoma, cholangiocarcinoma, and colorectal cancer metastases) is considered to be an effective treatment, and it should be theoretically proposed to frail older patients. A systematic review and meta-analysis [6] published in 2021 demonstrated that the laparoscopic approach is superior to traditional surgery in terms of short-term results (blood loss and postoperative hospitalization) and, at the same time, it is not inferior to traditional surgery at mid-term interval. This study has some biases, among which the lack of description of the type of hepatectomy performed and the indications for hepatic resection. Two other recent systematic reviews of the literature and meta-analyses [7, 8] combined with the propensity score method demonstrated that laparoscopic treatment of hepatocarcinoma, including major and minor hepatectomy, in frail patients, has a considerable advantage over traditional liver resections, in terms of short-term postoperative outcomes and it has not affected the mid- and long-term oncological results. The rate of complications and postoperative length of stay was significantly lower in the group of older patients treated with laparoscopic liver resection than those treated with an open approach.

Synthetically, we can say that liver resections in frail older patients can be performed laparoscopically with the same oncological results as traditional surgery associated with all the well-known advantages of minimally invasive approaches. The complexity of liver resections is still a challenge for the surgeon, and the data reported in the literature are anecdotal.

Recently, the laparoscopic approach for liver resections has been added to the robotic one. The latter offers several advantages mainly linked to an improvement of dexterity and precision in movements, a better and magnified vision, and an absence of tremors and fatigue. A recent study [9] showed that major hepatectomies performed using robotic technology are as effective as those performed with laparoscopic technique in terms of intraoperative results (blood loss) and short-term postoperative results. These results are, however, offset by longer operative times.

We can, therefore, put forward the hypothesis that robot can be used for various types of liver resection even if there are no randomized trials comparing the laparoscopic with the robotic approach and there are no studies on frail patients [10].

The minimally invasive approach to neoplastic diseases of pancreatic origin is a substantial innovation. A randomized multicentric study [11] showed that, in expert hands, laparoscopic pancreaticoduodenectomy is associated with lower hospitalization and morbidity and mortality similar to those of traditional surgery. Nevertheless, the authors conclude that the clinical benefits of this laparoscopic surgery are margina,l also considering the necessary, yet far from simple, procedural learning curve.

Laparoscopic body-tail pancreas resections for neoplastic pathology, on the other hand, appear to have an advantage over traditional surgery in terms of complications, blood loss, and postoperative hospitalization [12], although no studies are specifically focused on frail older patients. With the introduction of robotics for the treatment of body-tail resections of the pancreas, the choice between the two approaches is mainly linked to the long learning curve of the robot. Moreover, although it seems that the percentage of major complications is equivalent to these two approaches, a robotic procedure decreases the percentage of conversions, and it allows a better preservation of the spleen but has a longer operative time and postoperative length of stay [13].

Currently, there are no randomized prospective studies comparing the robotic or laparoscopic approach with conventional surgery, but only observational studies have compared the different approaches to neoplasms of the head or tail body of the pancreas in the frail patient. A retrospective study [14] demonstrated a reduction in operating time, blood loss, and postoperative length of stay. Furthermore, the postoperative complications, the 90-day mortality, and the percentage of re-interventions were superimposed.

In conclusion, we can say that both laparoscopic and robotic pancreatic resections can be performed in frail older patients but require a long learning curve and results, currently optimistic, should be supported by prospective and randomized trials including this subset of patients.

The surgical treatment of colon cancer currently provides a preferential minimally invasive approach. The international and national guidelines propose, in fact, a laparoscopic approach in colon cancer as preferable to open surgery, if performed by surgeons with adequate training, as the oncological outcomes are equivalent to the laparotomy technique. Robotic surgery could be included in this context, proposing objective advantages over laparoscopic surgery but, at the present, it must be demonstrated by randomized trials and meta-analysis. Robotic surgery has an advantage in the right hemicolectomy for an easier performance of an intracorporeal ileocolic anastomosis, and it allows, in addition, a reduction in operative time and blood loss when compared to laparoscopy [15–18]. Another point in favor of colorectal resections by robot is the possibility to perform a total mesorectal excision (TME) in rectal tumors as demonstrated by the REAL study [19] where it has been shown that robotic surgery allows better results in terms of oncological radicality. The Authors report a greater number of macroscopically complete resections associated with an earlier discharge, a lower use of demolitive interventions (Miles intervention) for cancers of the lower rectum, fewer complications, and intraoperative blood loss in the group of patients treated with robotic surgery.

As for the frail patient, the current literature demonstrated that laparoscopic rectal surgery represents, also in this subgroup of patients, preferable to traditional surgery as shown by a recent meta-analysis [19, 20]. This study demonstrated the superiority of laparoscopic surgery in terms of mortality, postoperative complications, blood loss, reduced hospitalization times, and a faster functional recovery of the intestine. A recent study [21] showed that robotic surgery can also be used to treat rectal cancer with surgical and oncological results similar to laparoscopic surgery although operating times are significantly higher. There are no randomized trials demonstrating the non-inferiority, the clinical and oncological superiority, or the cost/benefit ratio of the robotic approach in colorectal surgery for frail older patienst.

The second question regarding the reason why we should choose noninvasive surgery in frail older patients is briefly herein described.

Smaller Incisions: Minimally invasive surgery requires smaller incisions, which means less pain and smaller scars for the patient.

Faster Recovery: Since minimally invasive surgery is less invasive, the patient recovers faster and returns to their normal activities faster.

Shorter Hospital Stays: Patients might be discharged earlier from the hospital, thus reducing the risk of hospital-acquired infections and other complications.

Bleeding Reduction: Minimally invasive surgery permits to reduce the amount of blood loss during surgery, useful in older persons who might be at higher risk for bleeding.

Reduced Risk of Infections: Because minimally invasive surgery requires smaller incisions, the risk of infections is lower than that of traditional open surgery.

Reduced Risk of Hernias: Traditional open surgery might predispose to the risk of hernias, which it requires additional surgery.

Finally, the majority of frail older patients can undergo minimally invasive surgery, since age per se does not affect the choice of procedure. Specifically, cardiovascular comorbidities do not represent an absolute contraindication, but it should be noted that contraindications to laparoscopy are instead represented by major coagulation alterations, severe respiratory insufficiency, severe chronic obstructive pulmonary disease, severe coronary heart disease and heart valve disease, and intracranial hypertension. Previous abdominal or thoracic surgery is considered a relative contraindication due to possible visceral-parietal or visceral adhesions that can make minimally invasive surgery risky or difficult, with a high risk of conversion to open surgery. During laparoscopy or robotic surgery, it is also recommended to avoid, in frail older patients, extreme or prolonged Trendelenburg or anti-Trendelenburg positions, as well as it is advisable to speed up surgical times and keep the intraperitoneal insufflation as low as possible, compatibly with adequate surgical maneuverability.

In the selection of the frail and older patients, biochemical markers are crucial, especially the blood count. Since the frequent risk of bleeding in the frail older patients, due to concomitant presence of several pathologies needing different drug therapies, it is recommended to implement the “Patient Blood Management” strategy in the pre- and postoperative period: i.e., optimization of hemoglobin values and iron, conservation of autologous blood heritage (blood conservation), and surgical and anaesthetic strategies that reduce blood loss. Careful routine screening (RBC, Hb, ferritin) of all patients undergoing surgery with an expected blood loss greater than 500 mL is also recommended. Correction of serum iron values is recommended in patients with iron deficiency anemia. The use of minimally invasive techniques, reducing the endocrine-metabolic response to stress and improving the postoperative outcome, is substantially indicated and validated also in frail older patients: This is mainly valid in elective surgery, i.e., when the patient has the possibility and the times to reach the operating table in the best possible clinical conditions. Otherwise, in an emergency setting, the choice between open surgery versus minimally invasive approaches remains strongly linked to the hemodynamic and clinical stability of the patients, as can happen in patients with multiple traumas, with blunt abdominal trauma, or with suspicion of active bleeding from intra-abdominal organs.

16.1 Conclusions

Theoretically, mini-invasive approaches should be always preferred in frail older patients whenever it is possible, indicated, and when oncological results are comparable with an open approach. Furthermore, the choice between a robotic or laparoscopic approach for upper gastrointestinal, hepatobiliopancreatic, and colorectal tumors is not yet well-standardized. Therefore, this choice should be tailored on the patient conditions’ and tumor stage. At present, no conclusive data support the superiority of a robotic approach over a laparoscopic one.

References

1. Bàllesta López C, Cid JA, Poves I, Bettónica C, Villegas L, Memon MA. Laparoscopic surgery in the elderly patient. Surg Endosc. 2003;17(2):333–7. https://doi.org/10.1007/s00464-002-9056-7. Epub 2002 Oct 8. Erratum in: Surg Endosc. 2002 Dec;16(12):1809.
2. van der Veen A, Brenkman HJF, MFJ S, Haverkamp L, Luyer MDP, Nieuwenhuijzen GAP, Stoot JHMB, Tegels JJW, Wijnhoven BPL, Lagarde SM, de Steur WO, Hartgrink HH, Kouwenhoven EA, Wassenaar EB, Draaisma WA, Gisbertz SS, van der Peet DL, May AM, Ruurda JP, van Hillegersberg R, LOGICA Study Group. Laparoscopic versus open gastrectomy for gastric cancer (LOGICA): a multicenter randomized clinical trial. J Clin Oncol. 2021;39(9):978–89. https://doi.org/10.1200/JCO.20.01540. Epub 2021 Jan 6

3. Marano L, Fusario D, Savelli V, Marrelli D, Roviello F. Robotic versus laparoscopic gastrectomy for gastric cancer: an umbrella review of systematic reviews and meta-analyses. Updat Surg. 2021;73(5):1673–89. https://doi.org/10.1007/s13304-021-01059-7. Epub 2021 May 25. PMID: 34031848; PMCID: PMC8500879
4. Chen WZ, Dong QT, Zhang FM, Cai HY, Yan JY, Zhuang CL, Yu Z, Chen XL. Laparoscopic versus open resection for elderly patients with gastric cancer: a double-center study with propensity score matching method. Langenbeck's Arch Surg. 2021;406(2):449–61. https://doi.org/10.1007/s00423-020-01978-w. Epub 2020 Sep 3
5. Okumura N, Son T, Kim YM, Kim HI, An JY, Noh SH, Hyung WJ. Robotic gastrectomy for elderly gastric cancer patients: comparisons with robotic gastrectomy in younger patients and laparoscopic gastrectomy in the elderly. Gastric Cancer. 2016;19(4):1125–34. https://doi.org/10.1007/s10120-015-0560-6. Epub 2015 Nov 5
6. Hildebrand N, Verkoulen K, Dewulf M, Heise D, Ulmer F, Coolsen M. Short-term outcomes of laparoscopic versus open hepatectomy in the elderly patient: systematic review and meta-analysis. HPB (Oxford). 2021;23(7):984–93. https://doi.org/10.1016/j.hpb.2021.01.016. Epub 2021 Feb 3
7. Wang Q, Li HJ, Dai XM, Xiang ZQ, Zhu Z. Laparoscopic versus open liver resection for hepatocellular carcinoma in elderly patients: systematic review and meta-analysis of propensity-score matched studies. Int J Surg. 2022;105:106821. https://doi.org/10.1016/j.ijsu.2022.106821. Epub 2022 Aug 7
8. Wang S, Ye G, Wang J, Xu S, Ye Q, Ye H. Laparoscopic versus open liver resection for hepatocellular carcinoma in elderly patients: a systematic review and meta-analysis of propensity score-matched studies. Front Oncol. 2022;12:939877. https://doi.org/10.3389/fonc.2022.939877. PMID: 36452485; PMCID: PMC9702063
9. Liu L, Wang Y, Wu T, Lin J, Deng L, Jiang J, An T. Robotic versus laparoscopic major hepatectomy for hepatocellular carcinoma: short-term outcomes from a single institution. BMC Surg. 2022;22(1):432. https://doi.org/10.1186/s12893-022-01882-8. PMID: 36528768; PMCID: PMC9759871
10. Guerra F, Di Marino M, Coratti A. Robotic surgery of the liver and biliary tract. J Laparoendosc Adv Surg Tech A. 2019;29(2):141–6. https://doi.org/10.1089/lap.2017.0628. Epub 2018 Aug 17
11. Wang M, Li D, Chen R, Huang X, Li J, Liu Y, Liu J, Cheng W, Chen X, Zhao W, Li J, Tan Z, Huang H, Li D, Zhu F, Qin T, Ma J, Yu G, Zhou B, Zheng S, Tang Y, Han W, Meng L, Ke J, Feng F, Chen B, Yin X, Chen W, Ma H, Xu J, Liu Y, Lin R, Dong Y, Yu Y, Liu J, Zhang H, Qin R, Minimally Invasive Treatment Group in the Pancreatic Disease Branch of China's international Exchange and Promotion Association for Medicine and Healthcare (MITG-P-CPAM). Laparoscopic versus open pancreatoduodenectomy for pancreatic or periampullary tumours: a multicentre, open-label, randomised controlled trial. Lancet Gastroenterol Hepatol. 2021;6(6):438–47. https://doi.org/10.1016/S2468-1253(21)00054-6. Epub 2021 Apr 27
12. Lyu Y, Cheng Y, Wang B, Zhao S, Chen L. Assessment of laparoscopic versus open distal pancreatectomy: a systematic review and meta-analysis. Minim Invasive Ther Allied Technol. 2022;31(3):350–8. https://doi.org/10.1080/13645706.2020.1812664. Epub 2020 Sep 9
13. Lof S, van der Heijde N, Abuawwad M, Al-Sarireh B, Boggi U, Butturini G, Capretti G, Coratti A, Casadei R, D'Hondt M, Esposito A, Ferrari G, Fusai G, Giardino A, Groot Koerkamp B, Hackert T, Kamarajah S, Kauffmann EF, Keck T, Marudanayagam R, Nickel F, Manzoni A, Pessaux P, Pietrabissa A, Rosso E, Salvia R, Soonawalla Z, White S, Zerbi A, Besselink MG, Abu Hilal M, European Consortium on Minimally Invasive Pancreatic Surgery (E-MIPS). Robotic versus laparoscopic distal pancreatectomy: multicentre analysis. Br J Surg. 2021;108(2):188–95. https://doi.org/10.1093/bjs/znaa039.
14. Liu Q, Jiang N, Tian E, Li M, Zhang H, Zhao G, Tan X, Wang W, Han B, Yuan J, Gan Q, Ma Y, Zhao Z, Liu R. Short-term outcomes of robotic versus open pancreaticoduodenectomy in elderly patients: a multicenter retrospective cohort study. Int J Surg. 2022;104:106819. https://doi.org/10.1016/j.ijsu.2022.106819. Epub 2022 Aug 7

15. Park JS, Kang H, Park SY, Kim HJ, Woo IT, Park IK, Choi GS. Long-term oncologic after robotic versus laparoscopic right colectomy: a prospective randomized study. Surg Endosc. 2019;33(9):2975–81. https://doi.org/10.1007/s00464-018-6563-8. Epub 2018 Nov 19
16. Dohrn N, Oppermann C, Yikilmaz H, Laursen M, Khesrawi F, Clausen FB, Jakobsen HL, Brisling S, Lykke J, Eriksen JR, Klein MF, Gögenur I. The effect of intracorporeal versus extracorporeal anastomosis in robotic right colectomy on perianastomotic perfusion: a substudy to a multicenter RCT. Langenbeck's Arch Surg. 2022;407(8):3577–86. https://doi.org/10.1007/s00423-022-02693-4. Epub 2022 Sep 28
17. Dohrn N, Yikilmaz H, Laursen M, Khesrawi F, Clausen FB, Sørensen F, Jakobsen HL, Brisling S, Lykke J, Eriksen JR, Klein MF, Gögenur I. Intracorporeal versus extracorporeal anastomosis in robotic right colectomy: a multicenter, triple-blind, randomized clinical trial. Ann Surg. 2022;276(5):e294–301. https://doi.org/10.1097/SLA.0000000000005254. Epub 2021 Oct 13
18. Bednarski BK. Minimally invasive rectal surgery: laparoscopy, robotics, and transanal approaches. J Surg Oncol. 2020;122(1):78–84. https://doi.org/10.1002/jso.25925. Epub 2020 Apr 14
19. Feng Q, Yuan W, Li T, Tang B, Jia B, Zhou Y, Zhang W, Zhao R, Zhang C, Cheng L, Zhang X, Liang F, He G, Wei Y, Xu J, REAL Study Group. Robotic versus laparoscopic surgery for middle and low rectal cancer (REAL): short-term outcomes of a multicentre randomised controlled trial. Lancet. Gastroenterol Hepatol. 2022;7(11):991–1004. https://doi.org/10.1016/S2468-1253(22)00248-5. Epub 2022 Sep 8
20. Luo W, Wu M, Chen Y. Laparoscopic versus open surgery for elderly patients with colorectal cancer: a systematic review and meta-analysis of matched studies. ANZ J Surg. 2022;92(9):2003–17. https://doi.org/10.1111/ans.17972. Epub 2022 Aug 15. PMID: 35969025
21. de'Angelis N, Abdalla S, Bianchi G, Memeo R, Charpy C, Petrucciani N, Sobhani I, Brunetti F. Robotic versus laparoscopic colorectal cancer surgery in elderly patients: a propensity score match analysis. J Laparoendosc Adv Surg Tech A. 2018;28(11):1334–45. https://doi.org/10.1089/lap.2018.0115. Epub 2018 May 31

Geriatric Trauma

17

Camilla Cremonini, Dario Tartaglia, Serena Musetti, Chiara Ranucci, Silvia Strambi, Stefano Avenia, Francesca Duro, Massimo Chiarugi, and Federico Coccolini

17.1 Introduction

The modern society is experimenting a demographic shift in distribution toward older age (defined as “population ageing”) due to the fact the people worldwide are living longer. This demographic trend started in high-income countries and now is spreading also in middle- and low-income countries, making older people the age category at more rapid growth. In 2021, in some countries (i.e., Japan, Italy, and others), the older population reached more than 20%, whereas in the United States, it was around 16% [1]. By 2030, the population aged 60 years and over will increase from 1 billion in 2020 to 1.4 billion, and by 2050, the same population will double (2.1 billion). The World Health Organization (WHO) states that “the number of persons aged 80 years or older is expected to triple between 2020 and 2050 to reach 426 million” [2]. Furthermore, the older population itself is becoming increasingly older [3]. This development is likely to have profound implications, not only for individuals, but also for governments and civil society, impacting especially health and social care systems. Countries all over the world are facing the challenge to ensure that their health and social systems are ready to deal with this demographic shift.

The impaired neurological and motor function consequent to aging leads to decreased alertness and response to external stimuli; these changes associated with a more active lifestyle conducted by older people expose them to an higher risk of being victims of traumatic events and serious injuries. Trauma is actually the fifth leading cause of death in all age groups and the eight cause of death in the older population.

C. Cremonini · D. Tartaglia · S. Musetti · S. Strambi · M. Chiarugi · F. Coccolini (✉)
General, Emergency and Trauma Surgery Department, Pisa University Hospital, Pisa, Italy
e-mail: dario.tartaglia@unipi.it; massimo.chiarugi@med.unipi.it

C. Ranucci · S. Avenia · F. Duro
General Surgery, Sapienza University, Rome, Italy

V. Boccardi, L. Marano (eds.), *The Frail Surgical Patient*, Practical Issues in Geriatrics, https://doi.org/10.1007/978-3-031-77707-3_17

Geriatric trauma represents a difficult challenge for trauma teams: Even if mechanism of injury may be similar, older patients (OP) have higher rates of morbidity and mortality when compared to their younger counterpart with similar Injury Severity Score (ISS) [4]. There is a strict correlation between age alone and mortality: some studies suggest that mortality increases for every year beyond age 65 years [5–7]. Several factors contribute to the higher mortality of geriatric trauma patients (GPT), other than frailty and poor physiological reserve [8]. Firstly, anatomic and physiologic senescence-related changes affect stress response and compensatory mechanism, having several repercussions on how the body reacts. Additionally, 80% of GTP have at least one pre-existing comorbid conditions. Chronic diseases and prescribed medications further amplify the alteration of the stress response to traumatic injuries. Lastly, undertriage (defined as failure to correctly triage a trauma patient underestimating the injury burden) and the consequent delayed treatment is another important factor that impacts the mortality rate related to geriatric trauma [9]. Thus, some studies suggest to use age > or =70 years alone as a trauma team activation criterion, although not recommended by the Committee on Trauma [10]. Since OP with severe injuries often do not meet trauma activation criteria, using age as a criteria to activate the trauma team may reduce potentially dangerous undertriage [11].

The literature has proven that geriatric trauma patients cannot be treated as other trauma victims and represent a specific category. Other than trying to avoid undertriage, some therapeutic strategies have to be adopted in order to reduce the risk of mortality and to limit preventable deaths. Acknowledging the different trauma physiology and the worse outcomes related to severe injuries in GTP is the first step to provide a tailored therapeutic approach. Acceptable treatments and outcomes may be provided also with proper identification of the patient at high risk, followed by early aggressive treatment and early admission to the intensive care unit (ICU) [6, 12, 13].

17.2 Age Definition and Mechanism of Injury

Although there is a difference between demographic age and biological age, statistics usually define old people or older people as above a certain age threshold. Usually, a patient is considered "geriatric" when older than 65 years. Age cutoffs differ from series to series when trying to define GTP. Caterino et al., studying a large series of patients, demonstrated a significantly greater mortality in the age group of 70–74 years old when stratified by ISS; the authors concluded with the suggestion to use an age of 70 as an appropriate cutoff to define older trauma patients [14]. Goodmanson and colleagues, on the other hand, showed a significantly increased mortality risk above 57 years [5]. The American College of Surgeons recommends 55 years of age as a special consideration for triage [15], as also stated in the ATLS (Advanced Trauma Life Support) principles that recommend transport of any patient older than 55 years to a Level I Trauma Center. Despite the lack of consensus on the age threshold to adopt, a "geriatric" or "older" trauma patient is usually defined as older than 65 years by the majority of studies [6, 16, 17]; nonetheless, patients older than 55 years are at high risk for mortality following trauma.

Blunt trauma is the predominant mechanism of injury in OP. The most common mechanism is represented by ground-level fall (GLF), reaching up to 70% of cases [18, 19]. Physical impairments (comprehensive of visual, cognitive, and neurological impairments), medication use, dementia, and unsteady walking are all factors that increase the risk of falls in geriatric patients. Severe traumatic brain injury (TBI), hip, femur, and ribs fractures are common injuries after ground-level falls in GTPs. The second most common mechanism of injury is "automobile accidents" that includes: pedestrian struck by a car, passenger, or driver in motor-vehicle crash (MVC). The highest mortality rate among GTPs is reached when they present as pedestrian struck by a vehicle (auto vs pedestrian, AVP) [18, 20]. Spinal injuries and TBI are increasingly common with older age, when considering AVP as mechanism of trauma [7]. Older people are more likely to be pedestrian victims as their reflexes are slower. The same reason why older driver may be victims of MVC: impaired vision and hearing, confusion, and slower reaction times are all adjunctive risk factors. Additionally, older people may be victims of medical problems like stroke, myocardial infarction, or syncopal episodes that may be the cause of the following trauma. Other mechanisms are burns and penetrating trauma. The mortality associated with small to moderate size burns remains high in OP, compared to younger counterparts [21]. Older people are often victims of domestic abuses and assaults, as well as intentional self-harm or suicide attempt, all conditions that must be taken into account when treating a GTP. Penetrating trauma is most commonly due to a suicide attempt, and firearms injuries are primarily characterized by gunshot wounds of the head [22]. The related mortality is extremely high. Social context (urban setting) and comorbidities (depression and chronic pain) may deeply affect OPs quality of life. Geriatric patients may also be victims of assault, and in that case, thorax and abdomen are the most commonly involved area (43%), followed by the extremities (16.9%).

17.3 Effects of Aging

Aging affects cellular metabolic activity leading to progressive organ disfunction and eventually failure. The following declined ability to respond to external stimuli, due to impaired homeostatic mechanism, leads to an increased susceptibility to the insult caused by traumatic injuries. This process is usually described as poor physiologic reserve, which explains why stresses usually tolerated by younger patients may be devastating in GTPs. There is also the adjunctive effect of medications (i.e., betablockers, diuretics, and anticoagulant) and pre-existing comorbidities that impact morbidity and mortality.

The aged cardiovascular system is characterized by decreased responsiveness to endogenous stimulation, mainly due to a reduced receptor's response to catecholamines with a consequent declined sympathetic activity [23]. Furthermore, the heart becomes stiffer as fat and fibrous tissue replace cardiac muscle cells, with a reduced cardiac compliance and myocardial contraction's efficiency. This leads to a limited capability to increase cardiac output, worsened by the assumption of *betablockers medication* that, with the ß-adrenergic blockage, can mask tachycardia as an early indicator of shock. Malnutrition and long-term use of medications like diuretics cause a *chronic hypovolemic status* in GTPs. In addition, *the atherosclerotic vascular occlusive disease* makes several vital organs more sensitive to an even minor reduction in blood flow. All these factors together explain why OP have ***low tolerance to hypotension*** secondary to blood loss, and even a systolic pressure of 100 mmHg may indicate a state of shock. Heffernan et al. found that in GTPs, mortality increased with a systolic blood pressure <110 mmHg (vs. >95 mm Hg in younger patients) and with an heart rate greater than 90 beats/min (vs. >130 beats/min in younger patients) [24]. Since the presence of "normal" initial vital signs is unreliable, early advanced monitoring of vital signs is essential to not underestimate hypoperfusion and to correctly execute fluid resuscitation, avoiding overload. It is also recommended to use base deficit and lactate level as useful predictor of shock.

Respiratory rate and the pulmonary compliance are usually decreased, as a consequence of fibrotic lung tissue, increased chest wall stiffens, and weakness of respiratory muscle. Additionally, gas exchange is impaired and the ability to prevent hypoxia is limited; OP also present impaired muco-ciliary clearance of bacteria and reduced cough effectiveness. Hence, early intubation is recommended in patients with borderline respiratory function [25].

Glomerular and tubular senescence decrease the ability to preserve volume in response to stress hormones. Moreover, the kidney filtration system is less functional and the organ is more susceptible to reduced blood flow: Even a temporary hypotension and hypoperfusion or nephrotoxic drugs represent a trigger for an acute kidney injury [26].

Osteoporosis and arthritis decrease bone density and make GTPs susceptible to fracture, even in low-energy trauma [27]. Lastly, the loss of adequate thermoregulation may drive to hypothermia even after a mild or moderate trauma, resulting in coagulopathy and in consequent raising of mortality risk [28].

Among pre-existing comorbidities associated with higher risk of mortality after trauma in geriatric patients, cirrhosis, coagulopathy, chronic obstructive pulmonary disease (COPD), ischemic heart disease, and diabetes mellitus appear to be the most related to worse outcomes. GTPs with one or more of these conditions are almost two times more likely to die than those without these comorbidities [29].

Aging changes and cornerstones of management in assessing and treating OPs during primary survey are listed in Fig. 17.1.

PRIMARY SURVEY	Ageing changes to consider	Management strategies
Airway	• Mouth changes (dental prosthesis/edentulousness) • Spine arthrosis • Protective airway reflexes impairment	• Consider early intubation • Adequate dose of medications for rapid sequence intubation (reduce doses to 20-40% to minimize risk of cardiovascular collapse)
Breathing	• Reduced pulmonary compliance • Impaired gas exchange • Reduced cough effectiveness • Impaired muco-ciliary clearance • Higher risk of rib fractures (for osteoporosis) • Pre-existing respiratory diseases	• Higher risk of pneumonia and respiratory failure • Consider early intubation • Aggressively treat rib fractures (e.g. analgesia, oxygen support etc) • Provide mechanical ventilation when necessary
Circulation	• Decreased responsiveness to hypovolemia • Reduced cardiac compliance and contractility • Pre-existing cardiovascular diseases • Effect of medications (e.g. betablockers, diuretics) • Low tolerance to hypotension (forces status of hypovolemia and poor physiologic reserve)	• Monitor vital signs often • Remember unreliable vital signs (hypotension at SBP < 110 mmHg) • Recognize signs of hypoperfusion, that may be occult (e.g. INR, ABG) • Early aggressive resuscitation (e.g. transfusion) • Avoid fluid overload • Consider early advance monitoring (e.g. central venous pressure)
Disability	• Cerebral atrophy, cerebrovascular vessel plaque • Pre-existing neurological or psychiatric diseases • Cognitive decline • Medications: anticoagulant, antiplatelet	• Monitor GCS often • Higher risk of ICH • Remember that combination of polypharmacy and injury may lead to delirium • Liberal use of CT scan • Early anticoagulant reversal and coagulopathy correction
Exposure	• Loss of thermoregulation • Nutritional deficiency • Loss of sub-cutaneus fat and skin elasticity	• Higher risk of hypothermia • Administer IV warm fluids, use thermal blanket • Higher risk of pressure injuries • Remove spine boards and cervical collars as soon as possible
ADJUNCTIVE CONSIDERATIONS	• Gather information about clinical history and home-medications as soon as possible • Calculate/estimate ISS	• Consider the effects of: antiplatelet, anticoagulant, betablockers and diuretics • Risk/benefit: balance between conservative management and invasive procedures

SBP: systolic blood pressure; INR: international normalized ratio; ABG: arterial blood gas; GCS: Glasgow Coma Scale; ICH: intracranial hemorrhage

Fig. 17.1 Ageing changes and key points of management during primary survey in Older Patients

17.4 Specific Geriatric Injuries

17.4.1 Traumatic Brain Injury

Traumatic brain injury (TBI) is a major problem in OP being the most common injury of this population [18]. Falls are the leading cause of TBI for GTPs, followed by MVC, with different rates according to the series [20, 30]. Two are the principal mechanisms that put older patient at higher risk of TBI: First, with the aging process, the dura becomes more adherent to the to the skull; second, due to several pre-existing comorbid conditions, older people often take anticoagulant or antiplatelet medications, thus increasing the risk of hemorrhage. Additionally, other mechanisms play a role. Cerebrovascular atherosclerosis and the consequent microenvironmental changes rise the chance of secondary damage [20]. For example, the decreased free radical clearance ability may intensify oxidative damage after TBI. The majority of older adults also presents moderate cerebral atrophy that may determine a normal initial neurological examination despite an underlying brain injury, making the diagnosis more difficult.

TBI is associated with high rates of morbidity and mortality in GTPs, not only for the severity of the injury but especially for the very low chances of recovery [31]. A complete functional recovery is rare and the following impairment of living functions may deeply affect the quality of life [30]. Outcomes after TBI are much worse in OP than in their younger counterpart: Older age itself [32] and severity are known variables related to negative outcomes after TBI, but there are other factors too. According to some studies, low admission Glasgow Coma Scale (GCS) score is associated with poor outcomes in OP with head injury being an independent risk factor for mortality [18, 19, 33]. Despite this finding, the available scientific literature states do not consider the GCS as a reliable tool to assess TBI in GTPs, because of high prevalence of pre-existing comorbid conditions like dementia, cognitive impairment (i.e., Alzheimer disease), or depressive syndrome that may alter it. These neurological conditions are also associated with a slower recovery after TBI [34]. Other studies, looking at specific TBI cohorts of GTPs, indicated "male gender" as a predictive factor for a worse outcome. Women have better outcomes which are likely due to estrogen and progesterone release, which act in the reparation process and play a role in the maintenance of adequate cerebral perfusion [35, 36]. However, data are inconclusive at the moment, since other studies do not agree with this finding [37].

Another factor deeply affecting TBI outcomes is the anticoagulation and/or antiplatelet therapy, that the majority of older people is usually taking. Intracranial hemorrhages are significantly associated even with minor falls in anticoagulated patients [38]. These medications also make the management of GTPs particularly challenging, being related with higher mortality and worse outcome [39]. When warfarin is the medication taken, aggressive and early reversal of anticoagulant therapy may improve outcome. The use of prothrombin complex concentrate (PCC), plasma, and vitamin K may accomplish this task. In treating GTPs with a ICH after a fall, administration of PCC is as effective in short-term outcomes as plasma, being more successful and faster in achieving INR reversal [40]. Over the last decades, new oral anticoagulants (NOACs) like, for example, dabigatran , that inhibits thrombin, and apixaban, that inhibits factor Xa, have gained consent and became available worldwide. NOACs are as effective as warfarin and seem relatively safer, with a minor risk of intracranial hemorrhage when using low doses, as stated by the RE-LY trial [41]. Since the mechanism of NOACs consists in the direct inhibition of the coagulation cascade, these medications have a shorter half-life compared to warfarin (8–16 h vs 1 week, respectively), hence are easier to manage. The major limitation of NOACs is the lack of a specific antidote [30]; there is also a slightly increased risk of late ICH; thus, repeated clinical evaluation is recommended [38].

In TBI, the maintaining of an appropriate blood pressure and, consequently, a correct cerebral oxygenation is crucial. In the literature, there are updated guidelines for the treatment of such trauma [42], that among other strategies suggest:

- carefully avoid hypoperfusion (maintaining systolic blood pressure ≥110 mm Hg or above for patients >70 years old);
- careful use of mannitol to control intracranial pressure (ICP) raise; careful use of anticonvulsant within 7 days of injury;
- avoid prolonged prophylactic hyperventilation, since it is just recommended as a temporizing measure for the reduction of elevated ICP;
- early tracheostomy to reduce mechanical ventilation days.

Other than the general TBI management recommendations, studies have assessed the value of some acute neurosurgical interventions including ICP monitoring, craniotomy, and decompressive craniectomy in OP with moderate-to-severe TBI [43]. While the criteria for surgical evacuation and ICP monitoring are well-established for young patients, there are some controversies regarding OPs. Although some evidences show that ICP monitoring is likely related to improved outcomes in some GPs [44], it is possible that the older population may benefit from the definition of geriatric-specific clinical criteria to determine whether ICP monitor placement is appropriate. Furthermore, OPs who underwent craniotomy for hematoma evacuation show acceptable outcomes, with longer hospitalization and rehabilitation time, compared to the younger counterpart. Decompressive craniectomy, on the other hand, seems associated with worse 6-month Glasgow Outcome Scale (GOS) outcomes compared to those treated with craniotomy [45].

Regarding the venous thromboembolism chemoprophylaxis in GTPs with severe TBI, the literature showed that is safe and that low-molecular-weight heparin (LMWH) was superior to unfractionated heparin, being associated with a decreased risk of overall mortality and reduced risk of pulmonary embolism [46].

17.4.2 Rib Fractures

Older patients present an higher risk of rib fractures (RFs), even after minor thoracic trauma, due to the age-related reduced bone density and osteoporosis that makes bones more fragile. Consequently, ribs fractures are a common injury in GTPs [47]. Ground-level falls are the most common mechanism of injury related to rib fracture in GPs, followed by motor-vehicle accident.

Rib fractures are associated with high mortality and morbidity in the older trauma population [48], and these high rates are mainly associated with pain-induced hypoventilation, pneumonia, and respiratory failure [49]. In the GP, the respiratory performance is already impaired by the aging process that reduces the muco-ciliary clearance of bacteria, the cough effectiveness, and the lung and chest wall compliance. As a consequence, relatively simple rib fractures can easily lead to pneumonia and other pulmonary complications as respiratory failure. In patients older than 65 years old, rib fractures are associated with an average mortality risk of 20% and a pneumonia acquisition risk of 19% [50]. Moreover, it appears to be a linear relationship between the number of rib fractures and these outcomes: for each additional rib fractured, mortality increases by 19% and the risk of pneumonia by 27% [50].

The main goal of management is to provide adequate analgesia to allow respiratory function and to prevent pulmonary complications; additionally, oxygen support and pulmonary toilette play an important role [49]. In fact, early intubation is recommended in patients with borderline respiratory function [25]. Pain control is critical in case of GPs with multiple rib fractures: it is usually recommended to avoid polypharmacy or opioids endo-venous administration, due to their undesirable side effects that include delirium, sedation, and hypotension. Modern regional analgesic techniques, such as epidural anesthesia and paravertebral blocks, may be adopted in the treatment of RFs alleviating the burden of systemic narcotic side effects [49]: Some evidences suggest a decreased risk of delirium using regional anesthesia [51].

The surgical fixation or rib plating is gaining more consent as a valid treatment option, even in OPs, since some recent literature showed benefits in terms of mortality, respiratory complications, and recover [52–54]. Flail chest, severe pain, and chest wall deformity have been proposed as indications for rib fixation, although practice varies considerably between trauma centers. The current role of rib plating still remains unclear, and there are no definitive guidelines regarding technique and timing, but there is growing consensus toward it and larger studies are needed [54].

17.4.3 Pelvic Fractures

Pelvic fractures are common in GTPs for the same anatomical changes in bone density described above. In fact, 64% of pelvis fractures are associated with preexisting osteoporosis and this rate rises to 94% in <60-year-old patients [55]. In OPs, the most common cause of pelvic fracture is low-energy impact (usually ground-level falls) [56]. Mortality from pelvic fractures is four times than in the younger counterpart and is mostly due to massive hemorrhage. Morbidity, on the other hand, is related to incomplete healing and/or nerve damage [57]. Transfusions need and hospital length of stay are high, with fewer patients that return to a normal quality of life. Therefore, prevention of falls is one of the major intervention to achieve in order to reduce mortality.

Pelvic fracture management is standardized, due to defined algorithms and guidelines [58], and the same principles valid for the treatment of adult patients may be translated to GPs. As stated by these guidelines and by ATLS principles, first steps are based on physical examination (mechanism of injury, inspection, determination of pain site, bimanual compression of iliac wings) followed by pelvic X-ray that represents the first radiological modality used. CT scan may be useful in suspected active bleeding in order to define the site of a subsequent angiographic embolization if necessary [59]. When underlying osteoporosis is suspected, an extensive investigation, including of levels of calcium, thyroid function, and sexual hormones in the serum, should be carried out [58]. The main goal of management is the earliest possible mobilization of patients to prevent side effects of immobilization such as osteopenia, pulmonary infections, or thromboembolic events. Some injuries (i.e., isolated anterior pelvic ring fractures) may be treated conservatively, while others (i.e., posterior ring fractures) may require surgical stabilization [58]. In case of bleeding, strategies like pelvic binder positioning, angiography and/or angioembolization, and surgery must be taken into account as for younger patients. In case of mechanical unstable pelvic fractures, the potential risk associated with operative treatment always need to be addressed. Selected geriatric patients with low-energy fractures, especially those with persistent pain, may benefit from surgical stabilization after a period of conservative treatment [60]. Other specific management strategies of OPs include considering comorbidities and home medications: a prompt correction of coagulopathy in patients on anticoagulants is essential.

References

1. The Organization for Economic Cooperation and Development. Older Population [Internet]. Available from: https://data.oecd.org/pop/older-population.htm
2. World Health Organization. Ageing and health. Available from: https://www.who.int/newsroom/fact-sheets/detail/ageing-and-health#:~:text=At this time the share,2050 to reach 426 million.
3. U.S. Department of Health and Human Services A for CL. Projected future growth of older population [Internet]. Available from: https://acl.gov/aging-and-disability-in-america/data-and-research/projected-future-growth-older-population
4. Hashmi A, Ibrahim-Zada I, Rhee P, Aziz H, Fain MJ, Friese RS, et al. Predictors of mortality in geriatric trauma patients: a systematic review and meta-analysis [internet]. J Trauma Acute Care Surg. 2014;76:894–901. [cited 2023 Aug 4] Available from: https://pubmed.ncbi.nlm.nih.gov/24553567/
5. Goodmanson NW, Rosengart MR, Barnato AE, Sperry JL, Peitzman AB, Marshall GT. Defining geriatric trauma: when does age make a difference? Surgery (United States).

2012;152(4):668–75. [cited 2023 Aug 4] [Internet] Available from: https://pubmed.ncbi.nlm.nih.gov/23021136/
6. Wilson MS, Konda SR, Seymour RB, Karunakar MA. Early predictors of mortality in geriatric patients with trauma. J Orthop Trauma. 2016:e299–304. [cited 2023 Aug 5]. Lippincott Williams and Wilkins [Internet] Available from: https://pubmed.ncbi.nlm.nih.gov/27124822/
7. Demetriades D, Murray J, Martin M, Velmahos G, Salim A, Alo K, et al. Pedestrians injured by automobiles: relationship of age to injury type and severity. J Am Coll Surg. 2004;199(3):382–7. [cited 2023 Aug 5] [Internet] Available from: https://pubmed.ncbi.nlm.nih.gov/15325607/
8. Joseph B, Pandit V, Zangbar B, Kulvatunyou N, Hashmi A, Green DJ, et al. Superiority of frailty over age in predicting outcomes among geriatric trauma patients: a prospective analysis. JAMA Surg. 2014;149(8):766–72. [Internet] [cited 2023 Aug 5] Available from: https://pubmed.ncbi.nlm.nih.gov/24920308/
9. Horst MA, Morgan ME, Vernon TM, Bradburn EH, Cook AD, Shtayyeh T, et al. The geriatric trauma patient: a neglected individual in a mature trauma system. J Trauma Acute Care Surg. 2020:192–8. Lippincott Williams and Wilkins [Internet] [cited 2023 Aug 4] Available from: https://pubmed.ncbi.nlm.nih.gov/32118822/
10. Demetriades D, Sava J, Alo K, Newton E, Velmahos GC, Murray JA, et al. Old age as a criterion for trauma team activation. J Trauma. 2001;51(4):754–6. [cited 2023 Aug 2] [Internet] Available from: https://pubmed.ncbi.nlm.nih.gov/11586171/
11. Bardes JM, Benjamin E, Schellenberg M, Inaba K, Demetriades D. Old age with a traumatic mechanism of injury should be a trauma team activation criterion. J Emerg Med. 2019;57(2):151–5. [Internet] Aug 1 [cited 2023 Aug 2] Available from: https://pubmed.ncbi.nlm.nih.gov/31078345/
12. Bonne S, Schuerer DJE. Trauma in the older adult. Epidemiology and evolving geriatric trauma principles. Clin Geriatr Med. 2013;29:137–50. [Internet] [cited 2023 Aug 4] Available from: https://pubmed.ncbi.nlm.nih.gov/23177604/
13. Scalea TM, Simon HM, Duncan AO, Atweh NA, Sclafani SJ, Phillips TFSG. Geriatric blunt multiple trauma: improved survival with early invasive monitoring. J Trauma. 1990;30(2):129–34.
14. Caterino JM, Valasek T, Werman HA. Identification of an age cutoff for increased mortality in patients with older trauma. Am J Emerg Med. 2010;28(2):151–8. [Internet]. [cited 2023 Aug 5] Available from: https://pubmed.ncbi.nlm.nih.gov/20159383/
15. Shafi S, Nathens AB, Cryer HG, Hemmila MR, Pasquale MD, Clark DE, et al. The trauma quality improvement program of the American College of Surgeons Committee on trauma. J Am Coll Surg. 2009;209:4. [Internet] [cited 2023 Aug 5] Available from: https://pubmed.ncbi.nlm.nih.gov/19801325/
16. Grossman MD, Miller D, Scaff DW, Arcona S. When is an older old? Effect of preexisting conditions on mortality in geriatric trauma. J Trauma. 2002;52(2):242–6. [Internet] [cited 2023 Aug 5] Available from: https://pubmed.ncbi.nlm.nih.gov/11834982/
17. Jacobs DG, Plaisier BR, Barie PS, Hammond JS, Holevar MR, Sinclair KE, et al. Practice management guidelines for geriatric trauma: the EAST practice management guidelines work group. J Trauma. 2003;54:391–416. Injury, Infection and Critical Care. Lippincott Williams and Wilkins [Internet] [cited 2023 Aug 5] Available from: https://pubmed.ncbi.nlm.nih.gov/12579072/
18. Labib N, Nouh T, Winocour S, Deckelbaum D, Banici L, Fata P, et al. Severely injured geriatric population: morbidity, mortality, and risk factors. J Trauma. 2011;71:1908–14. Injury, Infection and Critical Care [cited 2023 Aug 16] [Internet] Available from: https://pubmed.ncbi.nlm.nih.gov/21537212/
19. Lalwani S, Gera S, Sawhney C, Mathur P, Lalwani P, Misra M. Mortality profile of geriatric trauma at a level 1 trauma center. J Emerg Trauma Shock. 2020;13(4):269–73. [cited 2023 Aug 4] [Internet] Available from: /pmc/articles/PMC8047951/
20. Thompson HJ, McCormick WC, Kagan SH. Traumatic brain injury in older adults: epidemiology, outcomes, and future implications. J Am Geriatr Soc. 2006;54:1590–5. [cited 2023 Aug 16]. [Internet] Available from: https://pubmed.ncbi.nlm.nih.gov/17038079/

21. Wibbenmeyer LA, Amelon MJ, Morgan LJ, Robinson BK, Chang PX, Lewis R, et al. Predicting survival in an older burn patient population. Burns. 2001;27(6):583–90. [cited 2023 Aug 16] [Internet] Available from: https://pubmed.ncbi.nlm.nih.gov/11525852/
22. Lustenberger T, Inaba K, Schnüriger B, Barmparas G, Eberle BM, Lam L, et al. Gunshot injuries in the older: patterns and outcomes. A national trauma databank analysis. World J Surg. 2011;35(3):528–34. Available from: https://pubmed.ncbi.nlm.nih.gov/21203760/ [Internet] [cited 2023 Sep 20]
23. Haddad F, Hunt SA, Rosenthal DN, Murphy DJ. Right ventricular function in cardiovascular disease, part I: anatomy, physiology, aging, and functional assessment of the right ventricle. Circulation. 2008;117:1436–48. [Internet] [cited 2023 Aug 20].Available from: https://pubmed.ncbi.nlm.nih.gov/18347220/
24. Heffernan DS, Thakkar RK, Monaghan SF, Ravindran R, Adams CA, Kozloff MS, et al. Normal presenting vital signs are unreliable in geriatric blunt trauma victims. J Trauma. 2010;69(4):813–8. [Internet] [cited 2023 Aug 20] Available from: https://pubmed.ncbi.nlm.nih.gov/20938267/
25. Bonomo L, Larici AR, Maggi F, Schiavon F, Berletti R. Aging and the respiratory system. Radiol Clin North Am. 2008;46:685–702. [cited 2023 Aug 20] [Internet] Available from: https://pubmed.ncbi.nlm.nih.gov/18922288/
26. Candela-Toha AM, Recio-Vázquez M, Delgado-Montero A, del Rey JM, Muriel A, Liaño F, et al. El cálculo de la creatinina sérica basal sobrestima el diagnóstico de alteración renal aguda en pacientes operados de cirugía cardíaca. Nefrologia. 2012;32(1):53–8. Available from: https://pubmed.ncbi.nlm.nih.gov/22240879/ [Internet] [cited 2023 Aug 20]
27. Lach HW, Lorenz RA, L'Ecuyer KM. Aging muscles and joints mobilization. Crit Care Nurs Clin North Am. 2014;26:105–13. [Internet] [cited 2023 Aug 20] Available from: https://pubmed.ncbi.nlm.nih.gov/24484927/
28. Newman PC, Vernon TM, Bresz KE, Schwartz JAT. Location of injury and other factors associated with increased survival among severely injured geriatric trauma patients. Am Surg. 2022;88(4):613–7. [Internet] [cited 2023 Aug 20] Available from: https://pubmed.ncbi.nlm.nih.gov/34787509/
29. Min L, Burruss S, Morley E, Mody L, Hiatt JR, Cryer H, et al. A simple clinical risk nomogram to predict mortality-associated geriatric complications in severely injured geriatric patients. J Trauma Acute Care Surg. 2013;74(4):1125–32. Apr [cited 2023 Aug 20] [Internet] Available from: https://pubmed.ncbi.nlm.nih.gov/23511155/
30. Harvey LA, Close JCT. Traumatic brain injury in older adults: characteristics, causes and consequences. Injury. 2012;43(11):1821–6. [Internet] [cited 2023 Aug 20] Available from: https://pubmed.ncbi.nlm.nih.gov/22884759/
31. Lau L, Ajzenberg H, Haas B, Wong CL. Trauma in the aging population: geriatric trauma pearls. Emerg Med Clin North Am. 2023;41:183–203. [cited 2023 Aug 4] W.B. Saunders [Internet] Available from: https://pubmed.ncbi.nlm.nih.gov/36424040/
32. Czosnyka M, Balestreri M, Steiner L, Smielewski P, Hutchinson PJ, Matta B, et al. Age, intracranial pressure, autoregulation, and outcome after brain trauma. J Neurosurg. 2005;102(3):450–4. [Internet] [cited 2023 Aug 20] Available from: https://pubmed.ncbi.nlm.nih.gov/15796378/
33. Knudson MM, Lieberman J, Morris JA, Cushing BM, Stubbs HA. Mortality factors in geriatric blunt trauma patients. Arch Surg. 1994;129(4):448–53. [Internet] [cited 2023 Aug 20] Available from: https://pubmed.ncbi.nlm.nih.gov/8154972/
34. Flanagan SR, Hibbard MR, Gordon WA. The impact of age on traumatic brain injury. Phys Med Rehabil Clin N Am. 2005;16:163–77. [cited 2023 Aug 20] [Internet] Available from: https://pubmed.ncbi.nlm.nih.gov/15561549/
35. Gibson CL, Gray LJ, PMW B, Murphy SP. Progesterone for the treatment of experimental brain injury; a systematic review. Brain. 2008;131:318–28. [Internet]. [cited 2023 Aug 23]. Available from: https://pubmed.ncbi.nlm.nih.gov/17715141/

36. Roof RL, Hall ED. Gender differences in acute CNS trauma and stroke: neuroprotective effects of estrogen and progesterone. J Neurotrauma. 2000;17(5):367–88. [cited 2023 Aug 23] [Internet] Available from: https://pubmed.ncbi.nlm.nih.gov/10833057/
37. Coimbra R, Hoyt DB, Potenza BM, Fortlage D, Hollingsworth-Fridlund P. Does sexual dimorphism influence outcome of traumatic brain injury patients? The answer is no! J Trauma. 2003;54(4):689–700. [Internet] [cited 2023 Aug 23] Available from: https://pubmed.ncbi.nlm.nih.gov/12707530/
38. Cocca AT, Privette A, Leon SM, Crookes BA, Hall G, Lena J, et al. Delayed intracranial hemorrhage in anticoagulated geriatric patients after ground level falls. J Emerg Med. 2019;57(6):812–6. [Internet] [cited 2023 Aug 23] Available from: https://pubmed.ncbi.nlm.nih.gov/31735656/
39. Howard JL, Cipolle MD, Horvat SA, Sabella VM, Reed JF, Fulda G, et al. Preinjury warfarin worsens outcome in older patients who fall from standing. J Trauma. 2009;66(6):1518–22. [Internet] [cited 2023 Aug 23] Available from: https://pubmed.ncbi.nlm.nih.gov/19509609/
40. Paisley MJ, Johnson A, Price S, Chow B, Limon L, Sharma R, et al. Reversal of warfarin anticoagulation in geriatric traumatic brain injury due to ground-level falls. Trauma Surg Acute Care Open. 2019;4:1. [Internet] [cited 2023 Aug 23] Available from: https://pubmed.ncbi.nlm.nih.gov/31897435/
41. Eikelboom JW, Wallentin L, Connolly SJ, Ezekowitz M, Healey JS, Oldgren J, et al. Risk of bleeding with 2 doses of dabigatran compared with warfarin in older and younger patients with atrial fibrillation: an analysis of the randomized evaluation of long-term anticoagulant therapy (RE-LY) trial. Circulation. 2011;123(21):2363–72. [Internet] [cited 2023 Sep 20] Available from: https://pubmed.ncbi.nlm.nih.gov/21576658/
42. Carney N, Totten AM, O'Reilly C, Ullman JS, Hawryluk GWJ, Bell MJ, et al. Guidelines for the management of severe traumatic brain injury, fourth edition. Neurosurgery. 2017;80(1):6–15. [Internet] [cited 2023 Sep 20] Available from: https://pubmed.ncbi.nlm.nih.gov/27654000/
43. Gardner RC, Dams-O'Connor K, Morrissey MR, Manley GT. Geriatric traumatic brain injury: epidemiology, outcomes, knowledge gaps, and future directions. J Neurotrauma. 2018;35:889–906. [cited 2023 Sep 20] Mary Ann Liebert Inc. [Internet] Available from: https://pubmed.ncbi.nlm.nih.gov/29212411/
44. You W, Feng J, Tang Q, Cao J, Wang L, Lei J, et al. Intraventricular intracranial pressure monitoring improves the outcome of older adults with severe traumatic brain injury: an observational, prospective study. BMC Anesthesiol. 2016;16:1. [Internet] [cited 2023 Sep 20] Available from: https://pubmed.ncbi.nlm.nih.gov/27401211/
45. Kinoshita T, Yoshiya K, Fujimoto Y, Kajikawa R, Kiguchi T, Hara M, et al. Decompressive craniectomy in conjunction with evacuation of intracranial hemorrhagic lesions is associated with worse outcomes in older patients with traumatic brain injury: a propensity score analysis. World Neurosurg. 2016;89:187–92. [Internet] [cited 2023 Sep 20]; Available from: https://pubmed.ncbi.nlm.nih.gov/26851740/
46. Condon F, Grigorian A, Russell D, Demetriades D. Venous thromboembolism chemoprophylaxis in geriatric trauma patients with isolated severe traumatic brain injury. Eur J Trauma Emerg Surg. 2023; [Internet] [cited 2023 Sep 20]; Available from: https://pubmed.ncbi.nlm.nih.gov/37306760/
47. Hoepelman RJ, Beeres FJP, Heng M, Knobe M, Link BC, Minervini F, et al. Rib fractures in the older population: a systematic review. Arch Orthop Trauma Surg. 2023;143:887–93. [cited 2023 Sep 20] Springer Science and Business Media Deutschland GmbH [Internet] Available from: https://pubmed.ncbi.nlm.nih.gov/35137253/
48. Barry R, Thompson E. Outcomes after rib fractures in geriatric blunt trauma patients. Am J Surg. 2018;215(6):1020–3. [Internet] [cited 2023 Sep 20] Available from: https://pubmed.ncbi.nlm.nih.gov/29548528/
49. Coary R, Skerritt C, Carey A, Rudd S, Shipway D. New horizons in rib fracture management in the older adult. Age Ageing. 2020;49(2):161–7. Available from: https://pubmed.ncbi.nlm.nih.gov/31858117/ [Internet] [cited 2023 Sep 20]

50. Bulger EM, Arneson MA, Mock CN, Jurkovich GJ. Rib fractures in the older. J Trauma. 2000:1040–6. Lippincott Williams and Wilkins [cited 2023 Sep 20] [Internet] Available from: https://pubmed.ncbi.nlm.nih.gov/10866248/
51. O'Connell KM, Quistberg DA, Tessler R, Robinson BRH, Cuschieri J, Maier RV, et al. Decreased risk of delirium with use of regional analgesia in geriatric trauma patients with multiple rib fractures. Ann Surg. 2018;268(3):534–40. [cited 2023 Sep 20] [Internet] Available from: https://pubmed.ncbi.nlm.nih.gov/30048325/
52. Fitzgerald MT, Ashley DW, Abukhdeir H, Christie DB. Rib fracture fixation in the 65 years and older population: a paradigm shift in management strategy at a level I trauma center. J Trauma Acute Care Surg. 2017:524–7. [Internet]. Lippincott Williams and Wilkins [cited 2023 Sep 20]. Available from: https://pubmed.ncbi.nlm.nih.gov/28030506/
53. Duong W, Grigorian A, Nahmias J, Farzaneh C, Christian A, Dolich M, et al. An increasing trend in geriatric trauma patients undergoing surgical stabilization of rib fractures. Eur J Trauma Emerg Surg. 2022;48(1):205–10. [Internet] [cited 2023 Sep 20] Available from: https://pubmed.ncbi.nlm.nih.gov/33095279/
54. Wasfie T, Sowa M, White H, Nesheiwat Oms-Iv SN, Hille J, Hella J, et al. Rib plating outcomes in older trauma patients with multiple rib fractures: a community hospital experience. Am Surg. 2023;89:7. [Internet] [cited 2023 Sep 20] Available from: https://pubmed.ncbi.nlm.nih.gov/37501312/
55. Krappinger D, Kammerlander C, Hak DJ, Blauth M. Low-energy osteoporotic pelvic fractures. Arch Orthop Trauma Surg. 2010;130:1167–75. [cited 2023 Sep 20] [Internet] Available from: https://pubmed.ncbi.nlm.nih.gov/20521061/
56. Stahel PF, Hammerberg EM. History of pelvic fracture management: a review. World J Emerg Surg. 2016;11:1.
57. Balogh Z, King KL, Mackay P, McDougall D, Mackenzie S, Evans JA, et al. The epidemiology of pelvic ring fractures: a population-based study. J Trauma. 2007;63(5):1066–72. [Internet] Available from: https://pubmed.ncbi.nlm.nih.gov/17993952/ [cited 2023 Sep 20]
58. Coccolini F, Stahel PF, Montori G, Biffl W, Horer TM, Catena F, et al. Pelvic trauma: WSES classification and guidelines. World J Emerg Surg. 2017;12
59. Schicho A, Schmidt SA, Seeber K, Olivier A, Richter PH, Gebhard F. Pelvic X-ray misses out on detecting sacral fractures in the older—importance of CT imaging in blunt pelvic trauma. Injury. 2016;47(3):707–10. [Internet] [cited 2023 Sep 20] Available from: https://pubmed.ncbi.nlm.nih.gov/26861798/
60. Timmer RA, Verhage SM, Krijnen P, Meylaerts SAG, Schipper IB. Indications for surgical fixation of low-energy pelvic ring fractures in older: a systematic review. Arch Orthop Trauma Surg. 2023;143:2417–28. Springer Science and Business Media Deutschland GmbH [cited 2023 Sep 20] [Internet] Available from: https://pubmed.ncbi.nlm.nih.gov/35462589/

Part III

Post-operative Management

Pain Assessment and Management 18

Lucia Muraca and Pietro Maglio

18.1 Introduction

As the general population is aging, the percentage of older people requiring surgery is increasing. Conversely, postoperative pain is underestimated and therefore poorly or ineffectively treated for cultural reasons.

Pain is a very frequent clinical condition in older and frail patient with a prevalence as high as 67% in acute inpatients and 83% in long-term care. In the geriatric patient, pain is associated with disability, emotional disturbance, and difficulty walking with possible falls. Quality of life is particularly affected by the association between pain and anxiety, sleep disturbances, and social withdrawal.

Very common clinical syndromes in geriatric age such as depressive state and "cognitive impairment" are exacerbated by pain, which thus represents a major economic burden for the health care system [1].

Given the gradual increase in the average age of the population, a further increase in the prevalence of chronic pain is expected in the future, which is, however, underestimated because of the difficulty in diagnosis: Considering pain as a natural consequence of age or possible pathology or even as an inevitable consequence of the surgical act is quite common, and its symptoms are minimized.

Another important consideration is that in strongly religious populations, pain is considered cathartic for the purification of the soul leading 8% of the population to accept it without complaint.

L. Muraca (✉)
Pain Medicine, General Practitioner, AISD (Italian Pain Study Association) and SIMG (Italian College of General Practitioners and Primary Care), Calabria and Southern Italy Referent, Catanzaro, Italy

P. Maglio
Department of Anesthesia, Intensive Care and Interventional Pain Management Unit, "Renato Dulbecco" University Hospital, Catanzaro, Italy

V. Boccardi, L. Marano (eds.), *The Frail Surgical Patient*, Practical Issues in Geriatrics, https://doi.org/10.1007/978-3-031-77707-3_18

Pain management in this population is further complicated by the presence of comorbidities that lead the patient to take many medications but especially by inter-individual variability related to pharmacogenetics and gender diversity [2].

Polymorphisms in genes can result in changes in the action of a drug in terms of both pharmacokinetics and pharmacodynamics, causing the occurrence of adverse effects or the absence of clinical response to a given treatment. The genes that determine the response to a given drug, in fact, can be divided into two major classes: genes that code for the primary target such as the receptor, ion channels, or enzymes, and genes that code for transporter proteins involved in the absorption, distribution, and elimination of different drugs.

Thus, pharmacokinetic aspects are essential in the therapeutic response to a given drug therapy and changes in individual parameters on a pharmacogenetic or gender basis aspect; also, interaction with other drugs may be responsible for adverse reactions or therapeutic failures on an individual basis. Thus, the evaluation of pain and the good performance of a therapeutic treatment is difficult because of the lack of a system that is as objective as possible considering all the variables we have here considered [3]. Nevertheless, adequate treatment of pain after surgery is essential for the direct reduction of postoperative-related morbidity and mortality by improving short- and long-term outcomes.

18.2 Pathophysiology of Pain

The new definition of pain, coined by the *International Association for the Study of Pain,* defines it as "An unpleasant sensory and emotional experience caused, or similar to that caused, by ongoing or potential tissue damage" [4]. In the new definition, compared with the previous definition, reference to verbal expression of pain was removed because it was considered to discriminate against those who cannot express themselves, such as the infant and the elderly with cognitive impairment. In fact, verbal description is only one of many behaviors for expressing pain; the inability to communicate does not negate the possibility of a human being or animal feeling pain. The new definition emphasizes that pain is always a personal experience, which is influenced to varying degrees by biological, psychological, and social factors. Under physiological conditions, pain represents an early warning system in order to alert the body that a given algogenic stimulus could lead to a potentially, even lethal, injury. The nociceptive system, which enables the transmission of such a peripheral stimulus to the structures of the "pain matrix" (structures involved in pain perception), not only provides a signal, but is able to give that signal a connotation of adversity, such that a behavioral modification is enacted to avoid a reiteration of the injury.

Acute pain arises from activation of nociceptors at the site of stimulus application; if the stimulus is not capable of causing tissue injury, we perceive pain transiently. If, on the other hand, the stimulus is of such intensity that it causes tissue damage, the pain lasts until there is repair of the injured tissue.

Five physiological processes are involved in the nociceptive pathway.

Transduction: Through specific receptor-channels, nociceptive stimuli hypersensitize peripheral nociceptors; these stimuli are converted into electrical activity generating an action potential representing nerve impulse.

Conduction: The nerve impulse generated travels along nerve fibers and reaches the spinal synapse in the dorsal horns of the spinal cord.

Transmission: is a phenomenon that occurs in the synapse between 1- and 2-order neurons in the dorsal horn of the spinal cord through the release of glutamate (excitatory neuron) and/or modulatory neuropeptides (substance p and CGRP).

Perception: The experience of pain is not a direct mechanical response to noxious stimuli, but rather a cortical reprocessing of a nociceptive impulse, so perception is the conscious experience of pain. For the perceptual process to be a real experience, there must be involvement of the brain areas of the "pain matrix."

Modulation: Not all signals we receive are noxious, but only those that possess an intensity that exceeds the threshold of activation of the nociceptive system. Descending pathways contribute to the modulation of pain transmission at the spinal level through post-synaptic action on the projections of neurons or interneurons in the dorsal horns of the spinal cord. A key region of the encephalon involved in descending modulation is the *periaqueductal gray matter* (PAG), which projects its fibers onto the rostral part of the *ventromedial medulla* (RVM). Many other brain regions project fibers onto the PAG, such as the cortex, limbic system, hypothalamus, and amygdala. Thus thoughts, emotions, and stress can affect the activity of this area. This system uses opioid mediators such as enkephalin, dynorphin, and serotonin and can give endogenous analgesia (pain relief) when activated. The RVM is in connection with the posterior horns and can inhibit or facilitate nociceptive signal transmission.

The crucial and fundamental role of the PAG in the descending system seems now definitely established, attributing to it, in an absolutely well-founded way, the characteristics of a principal and indispensable site in the modulation of pain. It is natural, however, that the PAG is not the only structure involved in pain modulation; in fact, it interacts with other structures in the brainstem such as the noradrenergic locus coeruleus nuclei and the RVM, which includes the serotonergic nuclei (raphe magnus, gigantocellular), and the latter is the main relay in the integration of ascending nociceptive input with descending.

18.3 Classification of Pain

Pain management is critically important to preserve function, reduce patient disability, and minimize patient suffering. Some 42 years after its first definition, the IASP (International Association for the study of pain) has reformulated the "Pain" definition [1]. The current definition describes pain as "unpleasant sensory and emotional experience associated with and similar associated with actual or potential tissue damage," which highlights two fundamental points in the difficulty of coping with pain: subjectivity and the involvement of the emotional sphere; hence, the so-called Biopsychosocial Model.

18.3.1 Acute and Chronic Pain [5]

Pain, starting from a temporal concept (duration), can be classified as acute and chronic.

- It is acute and generally physiological if there is a temporal correlation between the cause and the symptomatology, if it is of short duration and disappears with the elimination of the stimulus that has determined it, as in the case of postoperative pain, trauma pain, or visceral colic.
- In contrast, pain is defined as chronic if it has lasted for at least 3 months, with an intensity that is not always related to the pathogenic noxa, often unresponsive to treatment. In these cases, the pain loses its alarm function, no longer representing a symptom, but a real disease and is no longer physiological.

18.3.2 Primary and Secondary Chronic Pain

Chronic pain, in turn, according to the *International Classification of Disease* (ICD) [6], can be further subdivided into primary chronic pain if it is identified as a pathology; think for example of fibromyalgia, and secondary chronic pain if it can be linked to an organic cause as in the case of chronic inflammation of musculoskeletal or nervous system conditions as in the case of osteoarthritis, multiple sclerosis, neuropathic pain, and cancer pain.

18.3.3 Nociceptive, Neuropathic, and Nociplastic Pain

If, however, we consider the pathogenetic mechanism, pain can be classified into: nociceptive, neuropathic, and nociplastic.

- **Nociceptive pain** is when the stimulus physiologically activates nociceptors, which signal its presence in the area (primary pain) or in a metamerically related location (pain reported), as in the case of right shoulder pain in a gallbladder colic.
- **Neuropathic pain** refers to an injury to the central or peripheral nervous system such as in diabetic or postherpetic neuropathy.
- **Nociplastic pain** is generally an expression of central sensitization. In fact, IASP defines it as "pain resulting from an alteration of the nociceptive system, without any evidence of actual or potential tissue damage or evidence of disease or injury to the system somatosensory nociceptive." Typical example of this category is fibromyalgia.

18.4 Assessment of the Patient in Pain

Pain is a complex phenomenon, and in its assessment, a number of aspects must be investigated that are useful in framing the phenomenon itself and in order to break it down into its different components; a systemic initial assessment of pain is the indispensable starting point for targeted and comprehensive care, just as subsequent reevaluations are essential in order to identify any changes in a timely manner and allow the adjustment of pharmacological and nonpharmacological therapy. The framing of pain is a parallel pathway to the clinical evaluation of the disease that generates it: The diagnosis of the type of pain, its intensity, location, impact on quality of life, and duration differ from the diagnosis of the disease that generates pain, which instead requires its own specific evaluation.

Onset, Duration, and Time Course: It is of paramount importance to investigate anamnestically whether there is a cause-and-effect relationship with any factor (a disease, trauma or event) and how long the pain has been present. On the other hand, symptom frequency, maximum algic intensity (morning, afternoon, or night), and periods of spontaneous remission without medication characterize the time course.

Factors That Aggravate/Alleviate Pain: The presence of such factors is assessed by trying to understand whether the pain is spontaneous or whether it is provoked by movements, food, bodily activities (swallowing, chewing, Valsalva maneuver...). Spontaneous pain is defined as pain that is present on awakening even before the patient makes the first movements or actions. In addition, it is useful to know the possible response to previous treatment even if the patient has taken therapy independently.

Location: During the examination, it is necessary for the patient to tell about his pain and accurately describe its location. The area of pain describes a map that it is useful to draw on the patient's body so as to have topographical references. The distribution of pain reported by the patient that coincides with the innervation of a nerve territory is one of the elements (but not the only one) that can point toward neuropathic pain.

Qualitative Description: Pain semantics (e.g., pain reported by the patient as burning sensation, electric shock, and pinprick) has been considered a highly significant element in directing the diagnosis toward neuropathic pain. In the light of the latest updates, pain semantic has been sharply downgraded in its predictive value for diagnostic guidance and its contribution to diagnosis is now considered to be much lower, not exceeding 20% when used as the only element [7].

As described earlier, nociceptive pain is defined as pain resulting from actual or probable nonneural tissue damage and is due to nociceptor activation. For clinical purposes, the term nociceptive pain can be used when pain is proportional to nociceptive input and is thought of in opposition to neuropathic pain. The latter is defined as pain caused by a primary lesion or disease of the somatosensory nervous system. This first distinction is a key division that differentiates two types of pain:

neuropathic and nociceptive. Excluding or confirming whether the pain presented by the patient has a neuropathic genesis or not is a key step in the pain assessment pathway. In fact, the diagnostic treatment plan for a patient with suspected neuropathic pain involves sharing the same with a specialist center for both diagnostic insights and appropriate therapy. Initially, the integrity of the somatosensory system, e.g., the fibers involved in the transmission of the pain impulse from the site of pain to the spinal cord, is assessed through the three tests with the cotton ball, the tip of one, and the hot water tube. If deficits are found in at least one of the three fibers, the pain is defined as "suspected" neuropathic. If there is no deficit in the somatosensory system, further diagnostic investigation should be made by investigating the presence of primary allodynia, which is assessed by administering appropriate stimuli to the patient. The test is positive (reduced algic threshold) if these stimuli are painful in the area reported as painful by the patient and are not painful in the contralateral symmetrical area (in which the patient does not report pain). In contrast, the test is negative if the stimulus is found to be non-painful. A reduced algic threshold is always indicative of an inflammatory process; otherwise, that is, when the algic threshold is normal, the pain is not generated by an inflammatory process but is a structural mechanical pain. Finally, it is important to conclude the examination with a search for the possible presence of secondary allodynia since, if present and significant, it guides the choice of certain drugs that act at the synaptic level.

18.4.1 The Phenomenon of Spinal Sensitization

Impulses originating from nociceptive C- and A-delta fibers reach the central nervous system, specifically at the level of the posterior horns of the spinal cord (site of the first nociceptive synapse). Spinal sensitization refers to a condition of hyperexcitability of spinal neurons; continuous and persistent nociceptive input from the periphery is necessary for the formation and maintenance of this condition [8]. A kind of "relay center" for nociception is present at the level of the dorsal horns of the spinal cord: The nociceptive impulse modifies the synapse and determines hyperexcitability of the spinal cord dorsal horn neurons. This pathophysiological phenomenon results in two detectable elements: **amplification of the area of pain**, the persistence of the nociceptive stimulus over time results in an amplification of the area of pain reported by the patient; and **secondary allodynia**, if mild stimuli are applied at the skin level within the area of pain (brushing the skin with cotton ball or soft brush), the patient reports perceiving the evoked sensation as unpleasant. This phenomenon reveals that there are spinal neurons in the synapse that have lowered their threshold whereby tactile stimuli that are normally perceived as non-painful/annoying are "caught" by the "overexcited" synapse; thus, the sensation reported by the patient is "unpleasant" unlike, for example, the same stimulus administered counter laterally or outside the pain area.

18.4.2 Intensity, Tolerability, and Problems Performing Daily Activities

The final step in pain assessment is to measure the intensity and its impact on quality of life and disability.

There are mainly three methods for assessing pain intensity:

- *Visual Analog Scale* (VAS);
- *Verbal Rating Scale* (VRS);
- *Numeric Rating Scale* (NRS).

The VAS and VRS are commonly used to assess how much pain affects daily activities.

The most appropriate time frame for measurement varies according to circumstances: For acute pain assessment or postoperative pain in the ward, instantaneous (acute) measurement is most appropriate. For chronic pain (lasting more than 3 months), with its day-to-day fluctuations, an average assessment over the preceding weeks (1–4 weeks) is recommended.

In chronic low back pain, it is not uncommon to ask the patient to report the intensity of instantaneous pain and the most intense pain over the previous weeks by averaging the perceived values. All the rating scales produced the same predictivity and responsiveness coefficients on the patients studied; in addition, the VRS seems suitable for cohorts of patients of different ages both older and young. The most frequent criticism of the VAS assessment method concerns the difficulty of patient comprehension (failure rates ranging from 7% to 16%). The rate may increase in the presence of cognitive difficulties and in frail patients due to problems with verbal comprehension and visuospatial perception.

The VAS method is influenced by the patient's age, while the NRS or VRS methods suffer from approximation in cases where lexical skills are impaired and schooling rate low. The VAS has been shown to be easy to manage clinically and sensitive to changes in pain before and after treatment. In addition to these methods, there is the possibility, in some cases of elderly patients with impaired cognitive function, for preference of facial mimicry scales (The Faces Pain Scale) originally dedicated to the assessment of children and containing faces depicting expressions of increasing pain severity, each with intensity variables from 0 to 6 [9].

The pain that the patient reports is a symptom characterized by a certain intensity and duration. Pain can interfere, in various ways, with the life of the person experiencing it, since, as noted above, it is not only a symptom but is primarily an experience, which is conditioned by psychological factors and the social status in which the patient has lived or is living. Pain intensity has no diagnostic value, simply indicating the extent of pain and suffering experienced at that time. In a study by Ballantyne et al., it is pointed out that the intensity of pain does not at all reflect the clinical situation of the patient with chronic pain (e.g., the amount of impulses coming from the body), as pain is not a simple numerically quantifiable pathophysiological phenomenon, but a "being sick" on the part of the patient with the involvement of life in its physical, psychological, and social aspects. An interesting fact to associate with that of pain intensity is its interference with life or rather with daily activities.

Rating scales such as the Oswestry Disability Index (ODI) and the *Roland Morris Disability Questionnaire* (RMDQ) have been commonly used for decades now to measure a patient's functions and activities. These are rather complex questionnaires that take more time to complete but allow for the exploration of many dimensions of the patient during daily activities. The ODI has 10 domains with a selection of six severity levels each. The RMDQ has 24 yes-no answer questions. Other assessment methods such as the McGill Pain Questionnaire, the Brief Pain Inventory, and the 36-Item Short Form Health Survey stimulate patients (through questions) to narrate their experience by describing qualitative and quantitative aspects of pain [10, 11].

The PAINAD (pain assessment in advanced dementia) is a multidimensional pain assessment scale used for patients with marked cognitive impairment or who are uncooperative [12].

In fact, one of the most important obstacles to pain assessment in dementia concerns the ability to communicate and remember pain. This tool, therefore, consists of observing the patient's behaviors, providing a quantitative analysis of the discomfort observed in his body language. The five basic parameters are as follows: breathing, vocalization, facial expression, body language, and consolation. A score ranging from 0 to 2 is given for each item, in ascending order of observed discomfort. Finally, the sum of the values obtained from each item is performed going to form a score ranging from 0 to 10, divided as follows: 0—absence of pain; 1 to 3—mild pain; 4 to 6—moderate pain; and 7 to 10—severe pain [13].

18.5 The Treatment of Pain

Treating pain in older persons is not easy to manage due to the presence of concomitant diseases that lead patients to take multiple medications: Pain is often undertreated assuming analgesic drugs as need arises.

Analgesic therapy should be as easy as possible to manage at home, possibly administered orally, safe, with few side effects and appropriate for the type of pain that can be expected based on the type of surgery and the patient's characteristics.

Pain management is made, in the elderly, more complex due to the presence of comorbidities that force the patient to take polypharmacy, hence a higher rate of adverse drug reactions from drug interactions.

The most often prescribed and self-prescribed analgesics are acetaminophen and *nonsteroidal anti-inflammatory drugs* (NSAIDs), with little use of opioids.

Recent findings in the field of pain pathophysiology are changing the pharmacological approach to pain. The rational choice of appropriate drugs is dictated by the ability to identify the pain generator (the point where pain originates) and the pathogenetic mechanisms of pain, in order to recognize and typify nociceptive (inflammatory and mechanical-structural), neuropathic, and mixed pain. Clinical examination alone, when properly conducted, already allows rational drug selection. Prescribing multiple drugs simultaneously, aimed at controlling each mechanism identified with the examination, is the basis of so-called combination therapy [14]. The action becomes "synergistic," and thus more effective, by combining drugs that act peripherally on nociceptors (anti-inflammatories and steroids), at the nerve fiber level (sodium channel inhibitors) and at the synaptic level as modulators (acetaminophen, opioids, alpha-2delta ligands, and antidepressants) from time to time. The interest in combination therapy also lies in the fact that this modality allows, in certain cases, to act with lower average drug doses; so, it is possible that the incidence of dose-dependent side effects and interaction-related effects may decrease. In contrast, combining multiple drugs exposes one to certain risks. The first risk is related to possible lower adherence of the population to the prescribed therapy. The *World Health Organization* (WHO) states that medication nonadherence is a serious phenomenon, of vast magnitude and with significant consequences for both individual patients and the community. A further risk of multiple drug administration for pain control relates to the elderly patient on polypharmacy. In this case, an appropriate treatment regimen must be chosen, respecting the delicate balance between the real benefits that pain control might have on quality of life and the risk of drug interactions and/or side effects, often complicated by even serious consequences.

18.5.1 Paracetamol and NSAIDs

In the choice of postoperative therapeutic strategy, paracetamol (a central analgesic) whose mechanism of action, which still is not entirely clear, would be consequential to an enhancement of the serotonergic and endocannabinoid systems. Thus, paracetamol, is very well-tolerated and also has a good safety profile: In fact, it should be considered the drug of choice in renal failure, keeping however in mind, that in the elderly stroke patient even paracetamol could predispose to new cerebrovascular episodes.

The recommended dose is 1000 mg up to 3–4 times daily [15].

NSAIDs are contraindicated in prolonged administration because of their known effects on the renal system, cardiovascular system, hemo-coagulative system, and their gastro-lesiveness.

At high doses, NSAIDs inhibit endothelial COX-1 (constitutive) and COX-2 (inducible) increasing cardiovascular risk; they are also contraindicated in patients being treated with acetylsalicylic acid or oral anticoagulants for primary or secondary prevention for thrombo-embolic events.

Also to be considered, especially in the orthopedic setting, is the retarding effect on tissue repair and thus ossification that might be associated with overuse of anti-inflammatory drugs.

In any case, NSAIDs do not increase surgical bleeding complications if limited to post-surgery (and avoided before or during surgery) and if given in low doses in short cycles;

Short courses of NSAIDs for postoperative pain management do not expose patients with normal renal function to an appreciable risk of acute kidney damage.

Safety is not as clear in patients with preexisting renal dysfunction.

Gastrointestinal complications from NSAIDs, particularly ibuprofen, are not found to be increased if treatment is limited to less than 7 days.

Thus, their analgesic power remains valid and their use should be contextualized to the type of pain, age, and comorbidities of the patient and clearly limited to short periods of treatment, especially in acute phases [16, 17].

18.5.2 The Opioids

They are indicated in the treatment of moderate-severe pain, and their dosage should be titrated and dosed appropriately according to the patient's age, sex, and comorbidities because of the greater sensitivity older people may have from their use.

Fear of the adverse effects to them associated leads physicians to underdose them.

They are used for their effect on *μ-opioid receptor* (MOR) receptors in the central nervous system and to treat peripheral nociceptive pain due to MOR receptor overexpression triggered by the local inflammatory process. "Weak" opioids (codeine and tramadol) and "strong" opioids have the same common side effects (nausea, vomiting, drowsiness, dizziness, and constipation) and severe side effects (respiratory depression), which can be minimized by using the lowest effective dose of drug, choosing molecules with lower MOR activity, and preferring polypharmacy possibly in combination.

Tramadol at therapeutic dosages, up to 400 mg/day, may have the typical side effects of opioids manifesting, particularly in the elderly, with mental confusion, behavioral alterations, and constipation and could cause a serotonergic syndrome especially when combined with inhibitors to SSRIs and SNRIs.

The winning strategy is to use these drugs at low dosages and to increase the dosage according to pain response.

In the elderly, all drugs belonging to this class can be used starting with low-dose formulations, e.g., tapentadol with a minimum dosage of 25 mg every 12 h; the combination oxycodone/naloxone at the minimum dosage of 5 mg/2.5 mg every 12 h; ending with buprenorphine, which offers the advantage of being used in the patient with renal failure at the minimum starting dose of 5 mcg/h in TTS.

The essential parameter for choosing the appropriate analgesic is *glomerular filtration rate* (eGFR) monitoring.

Once tolerability to a given drug has been tested, the dosage should be titrated and adjusted gradually until the desired degree of analgesia is achieved.

Despite the tendency of opioids to induce drowsiness and cognitive impairment, their effect on improving pain intensity reduces behavioral problems such as aggression and delirium in older population [18].

Again, their use in combination allows for reduced dosage and increased tolerability.

The side effects most responsible for nonadherence to treatment include constipation and urinary retention, which are easily treated by increasing fluid intake, prescribing osmotic laxatives, using peripheral antagonists such as naldemedine and naloxegol, up to the administration of evacuative enemas.

Opioids can also, stimulating midbrain chemoreceptors, cause nausea and vomiting, which can be treated by administering antiemetic or antipsychotic medications, always keeping in mind comorbidities in which use may be inadvisable.

Analgesic tolerance is often insignificant and, in the elderly, pain control can be achieved with stable doses for many years [19].

18.5.3 Adjuvants Drugs

Tissue damage is often associated with neuropathic pain resulting from injury or dysfunction of the central and peripheral nervous system caused by the damage itself. This type of pain is often resistant to conventional therapies with common analgesics. Two categories of drugs can help us control this type of pain and associated cognitive-behavioral disorders: antidepressants and anticonvulsants.

Their use in the management of acute postoperative pain falls under "preemptive analgesia techniques" which are those analgesic techniques administered before the painful stimulus occurs to reduce postoperative pain and the consumption of NSAIDs and analgesics.

Gabapentinoids have been extensively studied for their immediate effect in reducing opioid consumption in the postoperative period and preventing pain chronification.

Their action manifests itself at generous dosages and has to be administered at least 2 h before surgery (*gabapentin up to 1200 mg and pregabalin from 300 and up to 600–900 in a single administration*) to also take advantage of the appreciated sedative effect that can occur at high dosages.

18.5.4 Antidepressants

These medications act by potentiating the descending inhibitory pathways increasing the presence of norepinephrine and serotonin in the spinal cord, locus coeruleus, and potentiating the descending inhibitory noradrenergic system.

Their action on α1 adrenergic, H1 histaminergic, and muscarinic cholinergic receptors is responsible for most of their side effects: sedation, constipation, and weight gain.

Depending on their dosage, antidepressants can be arrhythmogenic and can induce seizures themselves.

The combined use of serotonin reuptake inhibitors with tramadol, MAOI inhibitors, and triptans should be avoided because of the increased risk of serotonergic syndrome carrying increased serotonergic activity.

Serotonin-noradrenaline reuptake inhibitors (SNRIs) are very useful in the treatment of neuropathic pain including persistent postoperative pain. Of these, the most widely used molecule is duloxetine at the initial dosage of 30 mg/day, which can be increased after testing tolerability to 60 mg/day [20].

18.6 Conclusions

Demographic changes say that the "frail persons" are steadily increasing, leading to a correlated increase in conditions that, by causing pain, limit activities and reduce quality of life. Pain therapy can be a lifeline, triggering a virtuous circle that tends to limit disability. However, the multi-problem nature of frail individuals requires a rigorous individualized approach, taking into account, in addition to contraindications related to underlying diseases, medications taken on an ongoing basis and medications prescribed to control pain.

This approach greatly benefits from pain identification which, by identifying the "pain generator" allows rational choice of medications.

A critical area is the treatment of *postoperative pain* (POD), which remains a major problem despite great progress in understanding the physiology of acute pain. The intensity of acute pain may predict the risk of developing a chronic post-surgical pain state [21]. Consequently, it may be important to identify preoperatively patients who might experience severe postoperative pain, because we may provide them with more aggressive analgesic treatment than standardized. Previous studies have focused on preoperative pain level, type of surgery, gender, age, and anxiety level.

The acute pain stimulus results in the activation of sympathetic physiological mechanisms that once again result in tachycardia and hypertension, which increase myocardial oxygen consumption and thus expose patients to the risk of cardiac ischemic events.

Postoperative pain and immobility influence each other by exposing the patient to the risk of deep vein thrombosis and subsequent possible thrombo-embolic events. In thoracic surgery, inadequate postoperative pain control leads to decreased/abolished coughing, limited respiratory driving with very shallow ventilatory excursions, and increasing the risk of atelectasis and pulmonary infectious complications.

The multimodal approach to multidisciplinary perioperative management as outlined in the ERAS (enhanced recovery after surgery) protocols provides for each type of surgery a series of interventions aimed at preservation and maintenance of preoperative organ function in order to reduce the surgical stress response and early discharge of the patient resulting in improved outcome and valuable resource savings.

Thus, pain management begins preoperatively with the administration of pharmacologic analgesics or the application of peripheral analgesia techniques, minimization of the surgical insult, and adequate postoperative analgesia that will allow early mobilization and rapid resumption of oral nutrition [22].

References

1. Bernfort L, Gerdle B. et al. Severity of chronic pain in an elderly population in Sweden. Pain. 2015;156(3):521–527. https://doi.org/10.1097/01.j.pain.0000460336.31600.01.
2. Ferrel B. Pain management in elderly people. J Am Geriatr Soc. 1991;39:64–73.
3. Amidelfan K, Pope JE, Gunn J, Hill MM et al. Clinical Validation of a Multi-Biomarker Assay for the Evaluation of Chronic Pain Patients in a Cross-Sectional, Observational Study. Pain Ther. 2020;9(2):511–529. https://doi.org/10.1007/s40122-020-00175-3. Epub 2020 Jun 3.
4. Raja SN, Carr DB, Cohen M, et al. The revised International Association for the Study of Pain definition of pain: concepts, challenges, and compromises. Pain. 2020;161:1976–82. https://doi.org/10.1097/j.pain.0000000000001939.
5. Cugno S, Forni V, Rovaris D, Cuzziol P, Molinari E, Castelnuovo G. Pain classification systems. In: Clinical psychology of pain. Milano: Springer; 2010.
6. WHO international statistical Classification of diseases and related health problems (ICD-11) (https://wwww.who.int/classifications/icd/en/. Accessed 13 Nov 2020).
7. Chronic pain in general medicine. Agenas 2013. www.salute.gov.it/imgs/C_17_publications_2076_attached.pdf
8. Woolf CJ. Evidence for a central component of post-injury pain hyper-sensitivity. Nature. 1983;306:686–8.
9. Bieri D, Reeve RA, Champion GD, Addicoat L, Ziegler JB. The Faces Pain Scale for the self-assessment of the severity of pain experienced by children: development, initial validation, and preliminary investigation for ratio scale properties. Pain. 1990;41:139–50.
10. McGuire DB. Measuring pain. In: Frank-Stromborg M, Olsen S, editors. Instruments for health-care research. Boston: Jones and Bartlett; 1999. p. 528–61.
11. Pengel LH, Refshauge KM, Maher CG. Responsiveness of pain, disability, and physical impairment outcomes in atients with low back pain. Spine. 2004;29:879–83.
12. Warden V, Hurley AC, Volicer L. Development and psychometric evaluation of the pain assessment in advanced dementia (Painad) scale. J Am Med Dir Assoc. 2003;4(1):9–15.
13. Costardi D, Rozzini L, Costanzi C, et al. The Italian version of the pain assessment in advanced dementia (Painad) scale. Arch Gerontol Geriatr. 2007;44(2):175–80.
14. Mao J, Gold MS, Backonja MM. Combination drug therapy for chronic pain: a call for more clinical studies. J Pain. 2011; "modulation" 12:157–66.
15. Raffa RB, et al. Acetaminophen (paracetamol) oral absorption and clinical influences. Pain Pract. 2014;14(7):668–77. https://doi.org/10.1111/papr.12130. Epub 2013 Oct 28.9
16. Chang RW, Tompkins DM, Cohn SM. Are NSAIDs safe? Assessing the risk-benefit profile of nonsteroidal anti-inflammatory drug use in postoperative pain management. Am Surg. 2021;87(6):872–9. https://doi.org/10.1177/0003134820952834. Epub 2020 Nov 26
17. Murphy PB, et al. Efficacy and safety of non-steroidal anti-inflammatory drugs (NSAIDs) for the treatment of acute pain after orthopedic trauma: a practice management guideline from the eastern Association for the Surgery of trauma and the orthopedic trauma association. Trauma Surg Acute Care Open. 2023; PMID: 368443
18. Grenald SA, Young MA, Wang Y, et al. Synergistic attenuation of chronic pain using mu opioid and cannabinoid receptor 2 agonists. Neuropharmacology. 2017;116:59–70.
19. Kaye AD, Baluch A, Scott JT. Pain management in the elderly population: a review. Ochsner J. 2010;10:179–87.
20. Kehlet H, Wilmore DW. Multimodal strategies to improve surgical outcome. Am J Surg. 2002;183(6):630–41. https://doi.org/10.1016/s0002-9610(02)00866-8.
21. Dolin SJ, Cashman JN, Bland JM. Effectiveness of acute postoperative pain management: I. Evidence from published data. Br J Anaesth. 2002;89(3):409–23.
22. Savoia G, Ambrosio F, et al. SIAARTI recommendations for the treatment of postoperative pain. Minerva Anesthesiol. 2002;68:735–50.

Postoperative Delirium

19

Teodosio Pafundi, Ilaria Martis, and Andrea Fabbo

Abbreviations

POD	Postoperative delirium
POCD	Postoperative cognitive decline
DSM-V	Diagnostic and Statistical Manual of Mental Disorders—fifth edition
IL-6	Interleukin-6
TNF-alpha	Tumor necrosis factor-alpha
GABA	Gamma-aminobutyric acid
CAM	Confusion assessment method
Nu-Desc	Nurse-based delirium assessment tool
PACU	Post-anesthesia care unit
NRS	Numeric Pain Rating scale
VAS	Visual Analog Scale
NOPPAIN	Non-Communicative Patient's Pain Assessment Instrument
NSAIDs	Nonsteroidal anti-inflammatory drugs
COX 2	Cyclooxygenase inhibitors
BIS	Bispectral index (Bis-guided anesthesia)
MNA-SF	Mini-Nutritional Assessment
ERAS	Enhanced recovery after surgery
MCI	Mild cognitive impairment
MMSE	Mini-Mental State Examination
CDT	Clock drawing test
4AT	Delirium assessment tool

T. Pafundi · I. Martis · A. Fabbo (✉)
Territorial Geriatric Unit, Health Authority and Services of Modena, Modena, Italy

V. Boccardi, L. Marano (eds.), *The Frail Surgical Patient*, Practical Issues in Geriatrics, https://doi.org/10.1007/978-3-031-77707-3_19

According to the DSM-5, delirium is a global cognitive disorder with acute onset and transient duration, manifested by alterations in cognitive functions (attention, memory, thinking, perception), associated with an ongoing clinical condition or the use/suspension of medication (diffuse metabolic brain disorder). There are three forms of delirium: hyperkinetic, hypokinetic, and mixed (hypo-hyperkinetic). Hyperkinetic delirium is characterized by symptoms such as psychomotor agitation, state of alertness, increased response to external stimuli (e.g., light, sound), and hallucinations.

Hypokinetic delirium's symptoms are lethargy, a soporific state to the point of coma, reduced psychomotor activity, and reduced response to external stimuli, and are therefore more difficult to diagnose. The mixed form, which is the most frequent, presents characteristics of both with sometimes "unpredictable" alternation of lethargy and agitated state [1].

19.1 Incidence

The incidence of postoperative delirium (POD) is high, and the prevalence increases with the severity of the surgical insult [2]. According to the DSM-5, the incidence of POD in non-cardiac surgery is between 15% and 54% depending on the screening test used. Regarding the patients admitted to intensive care, the incidence of postoperative delirium reaches peaks of 80%. Several studies report that delirium occurs in 12–61% of patients with hip fracture, before and after surgery, respectively [3–5].

19.2 Physiopathology

Surgery causes the release of psychoactive inflammatory markers, including interleukin-6 (IL-6), tumor necrosis factor-alpha (TNF-alpha), and IL-1 beta, which may contribute to the development of delirium via dopamine-, GABA-, or choline-mediated pathways. In addition, general anesthesia exposes the brain to cognitively active drugs that alter the sleep/wake rhythm, so the incidence of delirium is lower in patients exposed to light sedation than in deep sedation [6].

19.3 Risk Factors

The risk of POD occurrence is the product of predisposing and precipitating factors as shown in Table 19.1. Several drugs are associated with the risk of onset of delirium, including:

- Psychotropic Drugs: Phenothiazine, clozapine, lithium, tricyclics, trazodone, and sedative hypnotics
- Anti-convulsant Drugs: Phenobarbital, phenytoin, valproate, and carbamazepine

Table 19.1 Predisposing and precipitating factors of POD

Predisposing factors	Precipitating factors
Advanced age	Prolonged preoperative fasting
Comorbidity	Invasive surgery and/or performed in emergency, site of surgery (abdomen/chest/appendicular), duration of surgery
Diagnosis of dementia and/or depression/ anxiety	Uncontrolled pain
Disability	Infections
Frailty	Preoperative blood glucose value (particularly in the context of cardiac surgery)
Malnutrition	Level of intra-operative bleeding
Dehydration	Intra-operative hypothermia (particularly for forms of hypoactive delirium)
Sensory deficits (vision and hearing)	Postoperative hypoxia (e.g., due to the need for analgesic use)
Multi-organ dysfunction pre-surgery (respiratory, cardiac, renal failure; presence of anemia)	Excessive depth of anesthesia planes
Potentially inappropriate medications (e.g., anticholinergics)	Excessive fluctuations in blood pressure
Hydroelectrolyte alterations (hypo- or hypernatremia in particular)	Inappropriate drug therapies (e.g., excessive use of opioids, neuroleptics, and psychotropic medications)
History of alcohol abuse	Type of care setting (inpatient vs outpatient)

- Substances of Abuse: Alcohol, caffeine, hallucinogens, amphetamines, cocaine, meperidine, and narcotics
- Other Drugs: Steroids, anticholinergics, antihistamines, cimetidine, acyclovir, digoxin, β-blockers, salicylate, ergot alkaloids, and methyldopa

In addition to being perceived as a highly "unique," "traumatic, frightening, and unpleasant" experience in patients who retain the memory of it, delirium is associated with significantly increased mortality, cognitive and noncognitive postoperative complications, and consequent prolonged hospitalization time and healthcare costs.

There is also evidence that delirium is strongly associated with reduced functional recovery (up to 12 months after discharge) after hip fracture [7].

19.4 Delirium and Postoperative Cognitive Dysfunction (POCD)

There is evidence that POD is associated with postoperative cognitive decline (POCD), a decline in cognitive performance both in the short (months) and long term (1 year) after the POD episode. Some studies have also associated POD with an increased risk of developing even severe dementia disease, up to 5 years after the POD episode with consequent need for hospitalization in nursing home and a reduction in quality of life [8].

19.5 Diagnosis

Early screening and prevention is the main strategy for managing delirium and limiting its adverse effects. The diagnosis of delirium is based on two elements [9, 10]:

- Assess alterations in consciousness early.
- Changes must occur either (hours, days, 1–2 weeks) or have fluctuating trends.

The available diagnostic tests are as follows:

- **4AT** (4 'A's test) is often the most preferred for routine use because it is simple and quickly administered (time less than 5 min), does not require specific training for its administration, and incorporates brief elements of cognitive testing. 4AT allows assessment of drowsy or agitated patients who cannot be tested by other tests [11];
- **CAM** (confusion assessment method), which has a reduction in its sensitivity if not used by specially trained personnel [12];
- **Nu-DESC** (Instrument Nursing Delirium Screening Scale) used by nurses [13].

Specifically, the CAM items are as follows:

1. **Acute Onset and Fluctuating Course**: Delirium quickly spreads within a few hours and to have fluctuating course during the 24 h. Changes are often noticed during the night hours. Knowing the patient's previous mental state is crucial, and information should be provided by the family member or caregiver.
2. **Deficit of Attention**: The patient has problems maintaining attention on external stimuli, easy distractibility, and difficulty being engaged in conversation.
3. **Disorganization of Thought**: Usually manifests as incoherence or disorganized speech.
4. **Impaired State of Consciousness**: Change from an alert state to lethargy, to a state of coma.

The 4AT investigates the following four aspects: (1) vigilance state: An alteration of the same is highly suggestive for the presence of delirium in the hospital setting; (2) 4-item Abbreviated Mental State AMT4: Questions are asked of the patient about his/her age, date of birth, location, and current year; (3) level of alertness; (4) acute change or fluctuating course regarding attention, comprehension, or other mental functions (e.g., paranoia and hallucinations). In dementia patients, a fluctuation in cognitive status can occur even in the absence of delirium, but marked fluctuation generally indicates delirium. Screening for POD should begin as early as the postoperative recovery area (PACU) and then be repeated at least every 8 h and continued for the first 5 postoperative days. Patients should not leave the recovery room without being screened for POD.

19.6 Management

Treatment of delirium should begin as soon as objectifiable changes occur via CAM or 4AT. Evidence-based guidelines for appropriate medical treatment are scarce, and wide variability in management patterns has been observed. The key strategy seems to be the adoption, as a first approach, of nonpharmacological preventive measures, which are as follows:

19.6.1 Perform Surgery Early

For example, in the case of hip fracture, perform surgery within 48 h of the injury.

19.6.2 Optimize Analgesic Therapy

The presence of pain should be investigated through validated scales (e.g., NRS or VAS, PAINAD, or NOPPAIN), before and after surgery, and before and after the administration of analgesic therapy [14–18].

Current indications are to use a multimodal approach (use of different analgesic and anesthetic modalities strategically combined to block pain perception). Paracetamol represents the first-line drug treatment. Nonsteroidal anti-inflammatory drugs (NSAIDs) and cyclooxygenase (COX 2) inhibitors should be used with caution and only for short periods, particularly in individuals with impaired renal, hepatic, or cardiac function. Opioids should be administered as a "rescue" strategy in case of failed analgesia with other drugs considering their possible side effects (induction of excessive sedation and postoperative nausea/vomiting) [19].

19.6.3 Identify and Correct Sensory Deficits

Evaluate sensory by paying attention to certain details such as intolerance to background noise, "strained" ears, frequent request to repeat information, presence of embarrassment, insecurity, aggression, anger, and possible presence of earwax plugs or by using specific instruments (Whispered voice test) [20]. Essential is the use of visual and hearing aids (devices always available to the patient, easily accessible, and their use until the moment of entry into the operating room).

The nurse or medical doctor, in the presence of such a deficit, must also facilitate patient comprehension by increasing the time available to provide information and reducing the presence of background noise or distracting elements, possibly including the use of written pages/images.

19.6.4 Avoid Inappropriate Medications

Re-evaluate drug therapy by eliminating inappropriate medications, in accordance with STOP/START criteria and the Beers' List. For example, avoid premedication with benzodiazepines routinely, except for patients with severe anxiety disorder; discontinue therapies with anticholinergic activity if possible (see Table 19.2) [21].

19.6.5 Monitoring the Depth of Anesthesia

Use by the anesthesiologist of assessment tools such as the bispectral index (BIS-guided anesthesia) [22].

19.6.6 Avoid Prolonged Fasting and Dehydration, Re-Feeding Early in the Postoperative Period

Malnutrition is known to lead to an increased risk of complications such as delirium, complex discharge, loss of functional autonomy, and mortality after surgery. Furthermore, regardless of preoperative nutritional status, prolonged intrahospital fasting and dehydration are additional negative prognostic factors.

Much scientific evidence supports the effectiveness of nutritional screening and intervention during hospital stay. The Mini-Nutritional Assessment-Short Form (MNA-SF) represents the preferred screening tool in clinical practice in addition to the use of nutrition-specific serum biomarkers, such as vitamin D and albumin [23].

In general, a proper nutritional approach in the perioperative setting should have the following objectives:

- Avoid insufficient or inadequate food intake.
- Reduce metabolic changes induced by the surgical stress response (altered glucose metabolism, accelerated muscle catabolism, and increased demand for amino acids).
- Minimize the inflammatory response related to surgical stress.

Fasting before performing a general anesthesia procedure is aimed at reducing the volume and acidity of gastric contents in order to reduce the risk of regurgitation and aspiration. However, dehydration and prolonged fasting are associated with increased metabolic complications and mortality.

Anesthesia societies currently recommend the intake of solid foods up to 6 h before anesthesia and clear liquids up to 2 h before.

Administration of carbohydrate beverages (the night before and 2 h before the procedure) does not increase the risk of aspiration, reduces preoperative hunger and anxiety, attenuates the occurrence of insulin resistance, preserves muscle mass, and improves the patient's preoperative well-being. Therefore, the administration of these drinks is currently recommended by the Enhanced Recovery. After Surgery

Table. 19.2 Drugs believed to cause or prolong delirium or confusional states

Analgesics	NSAIDs Opioids (especially meperidine)
Antibiotics and antivirals	Acyclovir Aminoglycosides Amphotericin B Antimalarials Cephalosporins Cycloserine Fluoroquinolones Isoniazid Interferon Linezolid Macrolides Metronidazole Nalidixic acid Penicillins Rifampin Sulfonamides
Anticholinergics	Atropine Benztropine Diphenhydramine Scopolamine Trihexyphenidyl
Antiseizure medications	Carbamazepine Levetiracetam Phenytoin Valproate Vigabatrin
Antidepressants	Mirtazapine Selective serotonin reuptake inhibitors Tricyclic antidepressants
Càrdiovascular and hypertension drugs	Antiarrhythmics Betablockers Clonidine Digoxin Diuretics Methyldopa
Corticosteroids	
Dopamine agonists	Amantadine Bromocriptine Levodopa Pergolide Pramipexole Ropinirole

(continued)

Table. 19.2 (continued)

Gastrointestinal agents	Antiemetics Antispasmodics Histamine 2 receptor blockers Loperamide
Herbal preparations	Atropa belladonna extract Henbane Mandrake Jimson weed St. John's wort Valerian
Hypoglycemics	
Hypnotics and sedatives	Barbiturates Benzodiazepines
Muscle relaxants	Baclofen Cyclobenzaprine
Other CNS-active agents	Disulfiram Cholinesterase inhibitors (e.g., donepezil) Interleukin-2 Lithium Phenothiazines

(ERAS) protocol. The use of high-protein and high-calorie supplements, in addition to limiting the negative effect of perioperative fasting, may be helpful in achieving adequate postoperative nutritional intake, and in reversing the catabolic state induced by surgical stress.

Resumption of hydration and feeding per os as soon as possible after surgery is also recommended [24].

19.6.7 Start Early Postoperative Mobilization

Early mobilization and early physical rehabilitation (i.e., starting the same day or the day after surgery) improves shorter hospital stay times and is associated with lower complication rates, better post-discharge physical performance, and ultimately lower mortality.

Therefore, the rehabilitation plan must be carefully tailored to each patient, and this requires a psychiatric and physiotherapeutic evaluation, aimed at developing an individual rehabilitation plan that takes into account the patient's clinical condition, degree of functional autonomy preacute event, type and timing of surgery, and provides for early referral (within 12–24 h of surgery).

It is also advisable to remove those medical devices (e.g., drains, bladder catheter, and vascular accesses) as soon as possible since they may impair movement.

In the rehabilitation process, in addition to the physiotherapist, other paramedical figures (nurses, social and health workers, and occupational therapists) need to be involved, particularly if subjects with cognitive pathology are involved, as these are at greater risk of worse functional outcomes than cognitively intact subjects. Among currently available rehabilitation models, an interdisciplinary approach is considered the most appropriate for individuals with dementia undergoing surgery (e.g., for hip fracture). This intervention consists of a physical rehabilitation program focused, as much as possible, on intense exercise activities in combination with occupational therapy, and it has been shown to be associated with both reduced length of hospital stay, reduced risk of delirium, and finally improved postoperative functional independence [25, 26].

19.6.8 Limiting the Use of Devices

Bladder catheter use is the major risk factor for urinary infections that are associated with an increased risk of delirium and prolonged hospital stay. Once in place, the bladder catheter should be removed as soon as possible after surgery to prevent urinary tract infections and facilitate mobilization. Early removal, however, has been associated with an increased risk of urinary retention particularly in male subjects with a higher incidence if the catheter is removed within 12 h of spinal anesthesia. In addition, bladder catheter placement is often a trigger for the onset of delirium in the subject with dementia with possible consequent harm related to frequent attempts at self-removal. Based on this evidence, the bladder catheter should not be used routinely but only in selected cases (e.g., patients with sacral decubitus injuries, need for diuresis monitoring in cardiac or nephropathic patients) and should be removed within 12–24 h after surgery.

When acute urinary retention occurs following bladder catheter removal, fast bladder ultrasound can be used to estimate urinary residual; in any case, the use of intermittent catheterization should be preferred to avoid reinsertion of a permanent catheter.

The same applies to the placement of other devices (vascular catheters or nasogastric tube), which should be reserved for strictly necessary cases, proceeding as soon as possible to their removal [27].

19.6.9 Maintain Sleep-Wake Rhythm

Avoid sleep deprivation (e.g., avoid waking the patient for routine blood draws).

19.6.10 Implement Reorientation Strategies

Encourage use of clock and calendar, frequently orient the patient to time, place, and date, suggest bringing personal items to the hospital, effectively communicate information while respecting the patient's schedule.

19.6.11 Reduce Noisy Stimuli

19.6.11.1 Improve Psychological/Social Support for the Frail Patient and Avoid Prolonged Periods of Isolation

Promote perioperative psychological support, e.g., with visit by operating room nurses the day before surgery, accompanying the patient to the operating room by a family member; promoting socialization with other patients and early contact with family members (caregiver involvement).

19.7 Pharmacological Treatment of Delirium

If the nonpharmacological approach proves ineffective, a pharmacological type of treatment can be carried out, which involves avoiding the use of benzodiazepines (except in cases of alcohol withdrawal), preferring instead low doses of haloperidol according to precise schedules (no more than 6 mg/day) aimed at averting adverse effects or atypical neuroleptics such as olanzapine (their routine use for preventive purposes is not currently recommended).

19.8 Conclusions

In conclusion, the management of POD is necessary and is an integrated, structured multidisciplinary approach with the geriatrician at the center of the team. The geriatrician addresses the complexity of the elderly surgical patient, in order to provide a multiprofessional care based on patient's needs, to produce good results in terms of clinical effectiveness (mortality and complications) and cost, with reduction of the average hospital stay and utilization of services in the period successive to hospitalization. The model, managed by a multiprofessional and multidisciplinary team that includes the surgeon, anesthesiologist, geriatric physician, physiatrist, nurse, physical therapist, social worker, and occupational therapist (when present), involves:

- The management of intercurrent medical problems with the goal of stabilizing the patient by avoiding delays in surgery and facilitating early rehabilitation care.
- Performing a comprehensive multidimensional assessment (cognitive, functional, nutritional, and social), secondary prevention of new falls and fractures, organizing the post-discharge pathway, and especially preventing and managing pain and delirium.

In the patient who is to undergo elective surgery, performing a geriatric assessment, in the prehospitalization phase, allows to analyze the elderly person's global situation, establish their degree of frailty, and better predict their surgical outcome, as well as, to implement prehabilitation strategies aimed at increasing resistance to surgical stress and inactivity in the post-surgical period through the enhancement of functional reserves in the perioperative period particularly in individuals with mild cognitive impairment (MCI). In the prehospitalization phase, performing MMSE and CDT would allow the detection of misrecognized mild cognitive deficits, which could, in the course of hospitalization, place patients at higher risk of cognitive complications such as POD and POCD. Early detection of these deficits would allow: (a) plan nonpharmacological delirium prevention strategies: reorientation strategies, involvement of family members, suggestion to bring personal items to the hospital; (b) set up preventive therapies: e.g., taking palmitoylethanolamide/luteolin in MCI patients seems to have demonstrated a reduction in the incidence of delirium; (c) set cognitive training courses [28].

19.9 Conclusive Remarks

Milestone in management of postoperative delirium once it is onset remains the treatment of underlying clinical conditions associating with multiple interventions. Pharmacological control of agitation can be initiated if the consequences of agitation can be dangerous for patient health. The management of delirium starts before the event considering people at risk, promoting early non pharmacological prevention and, when it occurs, consider medical and nursing management, environmental and general measures, and eventually pharmacological treatment of delirium symptoms [29, 30]. It is therefore crucial identify and correct these elements to reduce the occurrence of the delirium and improve patient outcomes.

References

1. American Psychiatric Association. Diagnostic and statistical manual of mental disorders (5th ed.) 2013. https://doi.org/10.1176/appi.books.9780890425596.
2. Bettelli G. Perioperative care of the elderly. Cambridge Medicine Cap. 2018 14 e 38.
3. De Vincentis A, et al. Orthogeriatric comanagement for the care of older subjects with hip fracture: recommendations from an Italian intersociety consensus. Aging Clin Exp Res. 2021;33(9):2405–24.
4. Aceto P, et al. Perioperative Management of Elderly patients (PriME): recommendations from an Italian intersociety consensus. Aging Clin Exp Res. 2020;32(9):1647–73.
5. Alan DK, et al. Enhanced recovery pathways in orthopedic surgery. Anaesthesiol Clin Pharmacol. 2019;35(Suppl 1):S35–9.
6. Maldonado JR. Pathoetiological model of delirium: a comprehensive understanding of the neurobiology of delirium and an evidence-based approach to prevention and treatment. Crit Care Clin. 2008;24(4):789–856.
7. Aldecoa C, Bettelli G, et al. European Society of Anaesthesiology evidence-based and consensus-based guideline on postoperative delirium. Eur J Anaesthesiol. 2017;34(4):192–214.
8. Morandi A, et al. Association between delirium, adverse clinical events and functional outcomes in older patients admitted to rehabilitation settings after a hip fracture: a multi-center retrospective cohort study. Geriatr Gerontol Int. 2019;19:404–8.
9. Attard A, Ranjiith G, et al. Delirium and its treatment. CNS. 2008;22:631–44.
10. Quispel-Aggenbach DWP, et al. Attention, arousal and other rapid bedside screening instruments for delirium in older patients: a systematic review of test accuracy studies. Age Ageing. 2018;47:644–53.

11. Tieges Z, Maclullich AMJ, Anand A, Brookes C, Cassarino M, O'connor M, Ryan D, Saller T, Arora RC, Chang Y, Agarwal K, Taffet G, Quinn T, Shenkin SD, Galvin R. Diagnostic accuracy of the 4AT for delirium detection in older adults: systematic review and meta-analysis. Age Ageing. 2021;50(3):733–43. https://doi.org/10.1093/ageing/afaa224. PMID: 33951145; PMCID: PMC8099016.
12. Inouye SK, van Dyck CH, Alessi CA, Balkin S, Siegal AP, Horwitz RI. Clarifying confusion: the confusion assessment method. A new method for detection of delirium. Ann Intern Med. 1990;113(12):941–8. https://doi.org/10.7326/0003-4819-113-12-941.
13. Lütz A, Radtke FM, Franck M, Seeling M, Gaudreau JD, Kleinwächter R, Kork F, Zieb A, Heymann A, Spies CD. Die Nursing Delirium Screening Scale (Nu-DESC)—Richtlinienkonforme Ubersetzung für den deutschsprachigen Raum [The Nursing Delirium Screening Scale (NU-DESC)]. Anasthesiol Intensivmed Notfallmed Schmerzther. 2008;43(2):98–102. German. https://doi.org/10.1055/s-2008-1060551.
14. Chin RP-H, et al. Scheduled analgesic regimen improves rehabilitation after hip fracture surgery. Clin Orthop Relat Res. 2013;471:2349–60.
15. Hjermstad MJ, Fayers PM, Haugen DF, Caraceni A, Hanks GW, Loge JH, Fainsinger R, Aass N, Kaasa S. European palliative care research collaborative (EPCRC). Studies comparing numerical rating scales, verbal rating scales, and visual analogue scales for assessment of pain intensity in adults: a systematic literature review. J Pain Symptom Manag. 2011;41(6):1073–93. https://doi.org/10.1016/j.jpainsymman.2010.08.016.
16. Heller GZ, Manuguerra M, Chow R. How to analyze the visual analogue scale: myths, truths and clinical relevance. Scand J Pain. 2016;13:67–75. https://doi.org/10.1016/j.sjpain.2016.06.012. Epub 2016 Jul 27.
17. Warden V, Hurley AC, Volicer L. Development and psychometric evaluation of the pain assessment in advanced dementia (PAINAD) scale. J Am Med Dir Assoc. 2003;4(1):9–15. https://doi.org/10.1097/01.JAM.0000043422.31640.F7.
18. Snow AL, Weber JB, O'Malley KJ, Cody M, Beck C, Bruera E, Ashton C, Kunik ME. NOPPAIN: a nursing assistant-administered pain assessment instrument for use in dementia. Dement Geriatr Cogn Disord. 2004;17(3):240–6. https://doi.org/10.1159/000076446. Epub 2004 Jan 27.
19. Morrison RS, et al. Relationship between pain and opioid analgesics on the development of delirium following hip fracture. J Gerontol A Biol Sci Med Sci. 2003;58:76–81.
20. Labanca L, Guimarães FS, Costa-Guarisco LP, Couto EAB, Gonçalves DU. Screening of hearing in elderly people: assessment of accuracy and reproducibility of the whispered voice test. Cien Saude Colet. 2017;22(11):3589–98. Portuguese, English. https://doi.org/10.1590/1413-812320172211.31222016.
21. Clegg A, Young JB. Which medications to avoid in people at risk of delirium: a systematic review. Age Ageing. 2011;40:23.
22. Oliveira CR, Bernardo WM, Nunes VM. Benefit of general anesthesia monitored by bispectral index compared with monitoring guided only by clinical parameters. Systematic review and meta-analysis. Braz J Anesthesiol. 2017;67(1):72–84. https://doi.org/10.1016/j.bjane.2015.09.001. Epub 2016 Apr 14.
23. Weimann A, et al. ESPEN guideline: clinical nutrition in surgery. Clin Nutr. 2017;36(3):623–50.
24. Mazzola P, et al. Association between preoperative malnutrition and postoperative delirium after hip fracture surgery in older adults. J Am Geriatr Soc. 2017;65:1222–8.
25. Su B, et al. Associations between post-operative rehabilitation of hip fracture and outcomes: national database analysis. BMC Musculoskelet Dis. 2018;19:211.
26. Smith TO, et al. Enhanced rehabilitation and care models for adults with dementia following hip fracture surgery. Cochrane Database Syst Rev. 2020;2:CD010569.
27. Kwak DK, et al. Would early removal of indwelling catheter effectively prevent urinary retention after hip fracture surgery in elderly patients? J Orthop Surg Res. 2019;14:315.
28. Lunardelli ML, et al. Co-ultraPEALut: role in preclinical and clinical delirium manifestations. CNS Neurol Disord Drug Targets. 2019;18(7):530–54.

29. Cecília Carboni Tardelli Cerveira1, Cláudia Cristina Pupo2, Sigrid De Sousa dos Santos3, José Eduardo Mourão Santos3 Delirium in the elderly A systematic review of pharmacological and non-pharmacological treatments Dement Neuropsychol 2017 September;11(3):270–275.
30. Siddiqi N, Harrison J, Clegg A, et al. Pharmacologic approaches for prevention delirium has none convincing evidence that are effective. Interventions for preventing delirium in hospitalized non-ICU patients. Cochrane Database Syst Rev. 2016;3:CD005563.

Fluid and Electrolyte Balance 20

Mariagiovanna Cozza

20.1 Introduction

Fluid management has an interesting and widely investigated area of research in the general population and can be particularly challenging in older patients. Depending on cardiac and renal abnormalities, geriatric patients often have poor tolerance for both hypervolemia and dehydration (overload) and hypovolemia or (underload) [1]. Strong experimental evidence shows that hypovolemia results in insufficient oxygen delivery and flow-dependent organ dysfunction whereas hypervolemia leads to interstitial edema with impaired oxygen diffusion and poor collagen regeneration in surgery [2].

Dehydration rates among older adults in hospitals vary significantly, ranging from 4% to 58% according to Volkert et al. [3]. It is important to note that frailty emerges as a significant and independent predictor for postoperative complications, mortality, prolonged hospital stays, and disability development, as established by McIsaac et al. [4]. Conversely, it is worth recognizing that dehydration and fluid/electrolyte imbalances can themselves contribute to the development of frailty in surgical scenarios. A recent observational study involving older patients with hip fractures, which used preoperative dehydration identified by serum-calculated osmolarity as an indicator, revealed a strong association with severe frailty upon discharge and extended hospitalization [5]. Furthermore, in a retrospective observational study encompassing a substantial cohort of older patients who underwent surgery for hip fractures, the postoperative phase witnessed a surge in dehydration prevalence within the high-risk Multi Prognostic Index subgroup, an increase that independently correlated with extended hospital stays and medium- to long-term mortality [6]. The challenge of identifying dehydration in frail surgical patients depends on the observation that, even in the general geriatric population, there is no

M. Cozza (✉)
UOC Intermediate Care, Integration Department, Ausl, Bologna, Italy

V. Boccardi, L. Marano (eds.), *The Frail Surgical Patient*, Practical Issues in Geriatrics, https://doi.org/10.1007/978-3-031-77707-3_20

accurate diagnostic test useful in determining whether older population are dehydrated and some tests should not be used to indicate dehydration (these include dry mouth, feeling thirsty, heart rate, urine color, and urine volume) [7]. The objective of this chapter is to elucidate the unique factors that render frail patients particularly vulnerable to dehydration and acid-base balance disorders during surgical procedures, whether in emergent or elective settings. Additionally, it aims to offer practical guidance, drawing from the Multidimensional Geriatric Assessment, on strategies that can be employed to avert these complications, thus safeguarding the surgical process and yielding positive outcomes in terms of functionality, mortality, hospital stay, and overall well-being. The Perioperative Management of Elderly Patients (PriME) recommendations have put forth a comprehensive model of Comprehensive Geriatric Assessment (CGA), which encompasses physical, functional, psychological, and social considerations. This holistic approach serves as a framework for making decisions that enhance clinical outcomes and functional capacity in older patients [8].

20.2 Age-Related Alterations in Fluid and Electrolyte Homeostasis Control Among Perioperative Frail Patients

20.2.1 Renal Senescence

The glomerular filtration rate (GFR) and renal blood flow (RBF) in healthy 80-year-olds decline due to several factors, including vascular and atherosclerotic sclerosis, immunological damage, advanced glycosylation end products, and inflammatory markers [9]. This decline results in the loss of renal mass and nephrons due to ischemia, reduced tubular function, and a diminished medullary concentration gradient, leading to a reduced kidney concentrating ability. Notably, serum creatinine concentration, commonly used to measure renal function, does not change significantly with aging, primarily due to a decrease in muscle mass. Therefore, an elevated creatinine level in older patients may indicate a lower GFR. These age-related changes make frail patients prone to hypovolemia, electrolyte imbalances (such as dysnatremia and potassium secretion), and acid-base imbalances (hydrogen ion excretion), potentially resulting in iatrogenic fluid overload [10].

During surgery, the GFR is closely tied to cardiac output, and factors like fluid losses or induced hypothermia, especially in urgent surgical cases, can lead to a drop in blood pressure, reducing renal blood flow. Acute renal failure is observed in 30% of older adults undergoing cardiac surgery and 15% undergoing noncardiac surgery, with 70% of survivors requiring dialysis within 2 years postsurgery [11]. Three types of surgery are commonly associated with intrinsic renal failure, often referred to as acute tubular necrosis (ATN): cardiac surgery, aortic aneurysm repair, and biliary tract surgery for obstructive jaundice. In cardiac surgery, higher preoperative glomerular filtration rates in older patients, preoperative correction of anemia, discontinuation of angiotensin-converting enzyme inhibitors, and surgical techniques that reduce cardiopulmonary bypass time have been associated with better outcomes [12].

Renal failure (69%), prolonged mechanical ventilation (65%), respiratory failure (52%), pneumonia (40%), and sepsis (38%) are the most common complications observed in frail patients undergoing surgery, where frailty is defined by the presence of indicators from all three major categories: phenotypic (difficulty walking, falls, weight loss, malnutrition), physiologic (dementia, severe visual impairment, decubitus ulcers, urinary retention or incontinence, fecal incontinence), and psychosocial (lack of housing, inadequate material resources) [13]. In abdominal aortic aneurysm surgery, renal failure may occur in emergency cases due to hypotension and is dependent on the duration of aortic cross-clamping. Another factor contributing to renal failure is material from atheromatous plaques that can obstruct multiple small arteries. The most significant risk factor for perioperative acute tubular necrosis is hypovolemia. Interaction between frailty and high surgical stress has been found to be a significant predictor of adverse outcomes within 1 year after vascular surgery [14].

Perioperative relatively oliguria during surgery and in the immediate postoperative period, which is an expression of the physiological response to trauma, exposure to anesthetic agents, fluid loss, and reduced kidney concentration ability, should not lead the clinician to employ excessive volume resuscitation or diuretics and volume expanders [15]. Instead, it should be guided by dynamic parameters.

However, two clinical scenarios must be considered in frail patients, which include the risk of polyuria following the operation due to tubular injury and electrolyte loss, as well as bladder outlet obstruction [16].

Antibiotics, such as aminoglycosides for infections and nonsteroidal anti-inflammatory drugs used to manage pain, should be avoided. Renal ultrasound should be performed if upper tract obstruction is suspected. High azotemia should be identified and corrected to mitigate prerenal or postrenal factors before, during, and after surgery. To prevent problems related to fluid and electrolyte imbalance, it is essential to regularly monitor urea and electrolytes, weight, blood pressure (both standing and lying), and review drug charts regularly [17].

20.2.2 Water and Body Composition

The percentage of total body water (TBW) is reduced, with one study suggesting it may be as low as 46% in older males and 43% in older females [18], as shown in Fig. 20.1.

Fluid loss primarily occurs through the urinary system, but variable amounts are attributed to insensible losses, which can reach up to 800 mL in 24 h, through the skin, gastrointestinal tract, and lungs. Age-related skin changes, such as reduced water in the stratum corneum and increased transepidermal water loss, make older adults vulnerable to extreme changes in environmental temperature, potentially leading to hypothermia. Normal older subjects often do not perceive thirst in response to water deprivation, possibly due to blunted osmotic and baroreceptor sensitivity in the left atrium and an elevated concentration of atrial natriuretic peptide (ANP), resulting in a persistent hyperosmolar state. Under normal conditions, fluid consumption is also influenced by social determinants and the level of functional autonomy. Therefore,

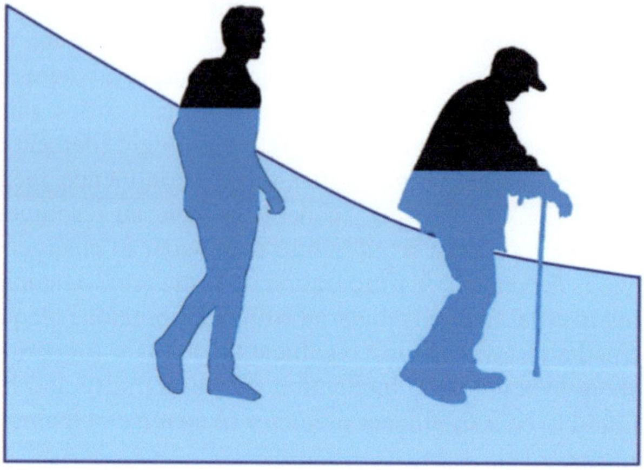

Fig. 20.1 Body water composition. The amount of body water decreases by approximately 15% (about 6 L) between the ages of 20 and 80

frail patients, such as those with dementia or limited mobility, may be at risk of dehydration, particularly in stressful situations [19]. Additionally, many patients take diuretics without proper monitoring, which can result in over- or under-diuresis [20].

Given that many frail patients may already be dehydrated before surgery, it is crucial to schedule surgery as soon as possible and be vigilant for signs of cerebral dehydration symptoms, such as delirium [21]. Some surgical scenarios can exacerbate dehydration in frail patients, such as vomiting with a loss of small bowel fluid, small bowel obstructions, diarrhea, bowel preparations, decreased fluid intake, and insensible losses from respiration, evaporation, or open body cavities. The presence of geriatric syndromes, like delirium, dementia, and incontinence, can hinder timely clinical recognition.

Muscle loss has been estimated at 8% per decade until the age of 70 years, after which the rate of loss increases to 15% per decade [22]. When a sarcopenic patient undergoes major surgery, they face a higher risk of complications and postoperative mortality due to reduced resistance to surgical stress [23].

20.2.3 Hormonal Changes

With aging, atrial natriuretic peptide (ANP), responsible for regulating blood pressure and right atrial filling, increases, leading to a reduction in serum renin and aldosterone concentrations; conversely, antidiuretic hormone, ADH, is not suppressed (no age-related changes in cerebrospinal fluid in older population, except for the absent diurnal variation), but there is a failure of normal renal responsiveness to ADH for decreased medullary solute gradient or a decreased tubular response to ADH at the receptor level [24].

The stress response (pain, incision of the skin, abdominal compression, visceral traction, changes in serum osmolality, hemorrhage, positive pressure breathing, hypoxia, hypercapnia, adrenergic stimulation, vagal stimulation) induced by surgery enhances the secretion of antidiuretic hormone, ADH, from the posterior pituitary and activates sympathetic efferent activity, resulting in increased renin secretion and aldosterone production [25].

These two mechanisms contribute to salt and fluid overload, and the response of aldosterone to hyperkalemia is diminished in the older population. The age-related decrease in renin activity is caused by alterations in kidney glomerulosclerosis, a reduced number of functional nephrons, decreased synthesis of angiotensinogen by the liver, and an increase in ANP levels. The suppressed increase in plasma renin activity (PRA) during anesthesia in older patients is not only a result of elevated plasma ANP levels but is also associated with the diminished response to volume expansion or sodium due to age-related suppression and the inhibition of an increase in renal sympathetic drive, attributed to the downregulation of beta-adrenergic receptors [26]. The immune system also undergoes age-related decline, rendering it less capable of responding during periods of acute inflammation [27].

20.2.4 Cardiovascular Changes

The progressive stiffening of arteries that accompanies the aging process, along with heightened sympathetic nervous system (SNS) activity and reduced β-adrenergic responsiveness, triggers an increase in left ventricular (LV) wall thickness. This alteration in myocardial contractile efficiency shifts the diastolic portion of the pressure/volume loop (compliance curve) to the left and upward, leading to pulmonary congestion [28]. Autonomic dysregulation is a contributing factor to increased perioperative complications among the frail population [29]. Catecholamine hypersecretion forms the basis for cardiovascular complications such as instability, ischemia, vasospasm, and hypercoagulation [30]. Prolonged hypotension can be attributed, in part, to diastolic heart failure with decreased venous compliance, which is commonly observed in the older population [31]. N-terminal-pro-brain-natriuretic peptide (NT-pro-BNP), a hormone secreted by the heart's musculature in response to ventricular stretching to promote natriuresis, traditionally sees elevated levels in congestive heart failure and is used to assess the response to diuretic treatment. NT-pro-BNP increases with age, and the surge in aldosterone due to surgical stress places the patient in a hormonal state resembling congestive heart failure, particularly if already overloaded with crystalloid intravenous fluids [32]. Surgical interventions designed to address heart failure, such as left ventricular assist devices or percutaneous aortic valve placement to alleviate aortic stenosis, may offer treatment strategies that can reverse the frailty associated with congestive heart failure [33].

20.3 The Role of Geriatric Syndromes in Fluid and Electrolyte Homeostasis Control Among Perioperative Frail Patients

Geriatric syndromes are pathological conditions, typical of the older patients, which tend to present recurrently and recognize a genesis multifactorial and occurring when the accumulation of alterations at the level of different systems makes older population vulnerable to stressful situations (change, stimulus) [34]. Geriatric syndromes in themselves affect the older response to changes in body composition and acid-base balance, so dehydration occurs when physiological changes associated with aging interact with a variety of disease processes and syndromes. Problems may arise when the older patient is placed in a state of fluid deprivation or iatrogenic insult [24].

Sarcopenia, frailty, malnutrition, dementia, polypharmacy, and in particular sedatives/psychotropic drugs tend to reduce respiratory drive, both central and peripheral (respiratory muscles, impaired gas exchange, and compromised flow rates), with consequent alveolar hypoventilation and an increase in $paCO_2$, resulting in acidosis respiratory or anemia and acute or chronic cardiopulmonary diseases (hypoxia) resulting in respiratory alkalosis.

In older patients, frailty is linked to breakdown in salt and water homeostasis, similarly sarcopenia and cognitive problems promote the development of hyponatremia [35], euvolemic hyponatremia due to the reduced introduction of water and the attenuation of the thirst mechanism, with the progressive loss of the osmoreceptors, is empowered by geriatric syndromes, such as alterations in cognitive status (delirium), lack of autonomy, and immobilization.

Poor muscle strength with incident functional limitation in older adults is promoted by chronic kidney disease (CKD), and subsequent metabolic acidosis may be as a potential cause of physical function impairment and slow gait speed and falls.

Frail patients are afflicted with chronic illness and morbidity that impair renal potassium handling with secondary hyperkaliemia, such as diabetes mellitus with hyporeninemic hypoaldosteronism, obstructive uropathy, and secondary renal insufficiency from hypertension or long-standing diabetes, or hyperkalemia may be caused by potassium-altering medications and polypharmacy [36]. Volume overload and malnutrition are closely linked. Fluid overload is associated with poor blood pressure control, increase in left ventricular mass, and compromised patient survival [37]. Figure 20.2 summarizes aging changes.

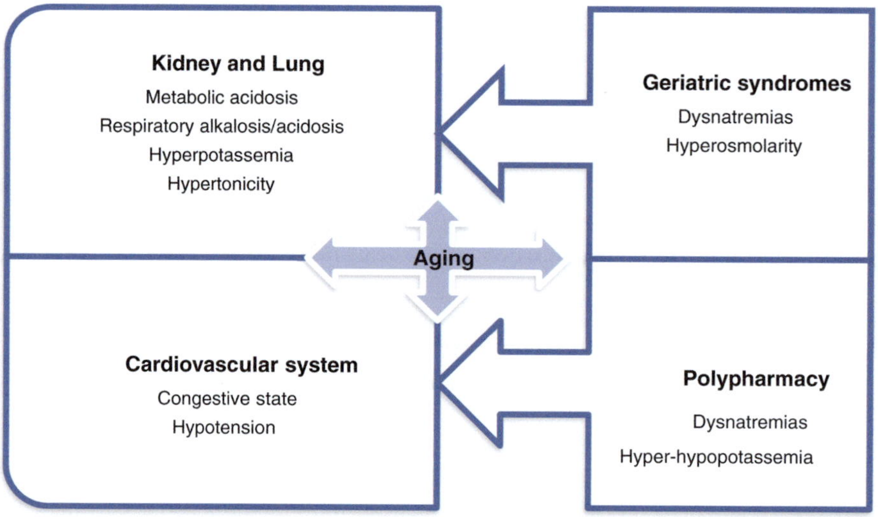

Fig. 20.2 Clinical predisposition of hydration status and acid-base balance in frail patients. Frail patients are more at risk, due to complexity, comorbidity, and presence of geriatric syndromes, of developing electrolyte disorders

20.4 Hydration and Fluid Balance in Surgical Setting

The term dehydration is widely used, but includes each of the following terms:

- Fluid deficit: loss of water with or without electrolytes [38];
- Volume depletion (or extracellular volume depletion): loss of extracellular water especially from the intravascular compartment, accompanied by normal, increased, or reduced serum sodium [38];
- true dehydration (or intracellular volume depletion): deficit of total body water, with loss of fluid from the intracellular (and interstitial) compartments which causes cellular desiccation [39], often associated with high sodium levels and hypernatremia.

Hypovolemia or underload is the loss of the intravascular compartment (10% of body water); it is not the whole volume total blood, but only that small part of the circulating blood volume that fills the vascular bed of the large intrathoracic and abdominal vessels, on which the activation of the so-called receptors depends of the volume that verify the "status of fullness" of the circulatory vessels (the driving force for venous return to the heart) and regulate the preload cardiac and output. The effective blood volume consists of 3 L of plasma and 1 L of transcellular fluid (extracellular fluid). Effective volume restoration, unlike osmolality regulation, is based on the retention of both water and sodium, so volume depletion, leading to loss of extracellular fluid but not intracellular fluid, keeps osmolality normal or low. Hypovolemia, maintaining effective blood volume, is the absolute priority provoking reduced cardiac output and tissue perfusion, and finally shock and multiorgan failure with risk of splanchnic ischemia and anastomotic breakdown. In older frail patients, hypovolemia is likely due to a combination of an inadequate intake, especially in emergency surgery, and excessive fluid loss. Preoperative fasting (with risk of sarcopenia and malnutrition), intraoperative insensible losses, vasomotor depressive effects of anesthesia, hypertonic intestinal preparations, positive pressure ventilation all predispose frail patients to hypovolemia [31]. In consideration of the poor tolerance of losses, in the presence of cardiovascular abnormalities, it is important to establish the duration of this situation, severity of volume deficits, clinical and hemodynamic symptoms, laboratory parameters, taking into consideration that in frail patients, clinical parameters (e.g., thirst, postural dizziness, lethargy, confusion) are unavailable. Some surgery-related factors are particularly dangerous and life threatening in older population to the extent that they favor hypovolemia, above all prolonged duration of surgery, hypothermia that encourage coagulopathy or necessity to use positive pressure mechanic ventilation. Common complaints of fluid loss may be chest pain, abdominal pain, and confusion.

Dehydration is the loss of intracellular water due to movements of water from the intracellular and interstitial spaces that can produce overall hypertonicity. Dehydration refers to a loss of total body water-producing hypertonicity, with a disproportionate fall in water (intracellular volume contraction) relative to sodium and potassium-producing hypernatremia. Many dehydrated patients can also have volume depletion.

Hypervolemia or overload, as an excessive blood volume, causes fluid loss into the interstitial resulting in some edema formation. Overload dehydration can be iatrogenic (IV fluids, steroids, blood transfusions) or caused by several diseases including heart failure, kidney failure, and protein deficiency. It is life threatening and is the promoting factor of heart failure and pulmonary edema; in surgical patients, fluid and salt overload have negative impact on morbidity and mortality [40]. The pathophysiology of volume overload, regardless the main mechanism (traumatic events, myocardial ischemia, hypertensive episodes, changes in medication regimen, worsening renal function, and increased neurohormonal-sympathetic activation), is the persistent volume overload of the intravascular and the interstitial compartments and consequently, through modulating neurohormonal and hemodynamic, increase in venous tone (decreased venous capacitance), with redistribution of fluid from a peripheral venous to the central cardiopulmonary circulation with clinical symptoms of congestion.

Hypervolemia is not synonymous of fluid overload [41], due to composition of intravascular volume expansion, with or without contribution of red blood cell mass excess that is the basis for marked heterogeneity in volume overload profiles and for treatment plan (diuretics should be used for fluid removal, not only for edema) [42].

Typical complications of hypervolemia affect brain with delirium, impaired cognition, altered sleep, intracranial hypertension, lungs with impaired gas exchange, decreased lung volumes, increased work of breathing, kidneys with impaired renal perfusion, salt and water retention, elevated interstitial pressure, intestines with ileus, bacterial translocation, impaired drug absorption, intra-abdominal hypertension, liver with cholestasis, ischemic hepatitis, impaired synthetic function, skin/connective tissue with wound infection, pressure ulcers, poor wound healing, heart with decreased contractility, conduction abnormalities, diastolic dysfunction, and mechanical compression of left ventricle by enlarged right ventricle [43]. Figure 20.3 describes main biochemical differences of these two conditions (hypovolemia and dehydration).

20.4.1 Indication for the Right Fluid Balance

The three current options fluid management are restrictive fluid therapy (RFT), goal-directed fluid therapy (GDT), and liberal fluid therapy (LFT).

Until 20 years ago, the concept of loss of the third space prevailed in surgery, according to the liquid infusion algorithm which started at the rate of 15 mL per kilogram per hour for the first hour, and was reduced to 7 mL per kilogram the next hour of surgery, with patients often developing pulmonary congestion, atrial fibrillation, and pulmonary edema. In the surgical trauma, the concept of the "loss to third space" was abandoned for the risk of edema and pulmonary congestion [21]. Many studies have demonstrated that fluid overload is associated with infection risks, impaired wound healing and cardiorespiratory complications, with significant damage in the same surgical procedures (mesenteric oedema, intestinal failure, and inhibiting anastomotic healing) [10] and impaired gas exchange due to pulmonary

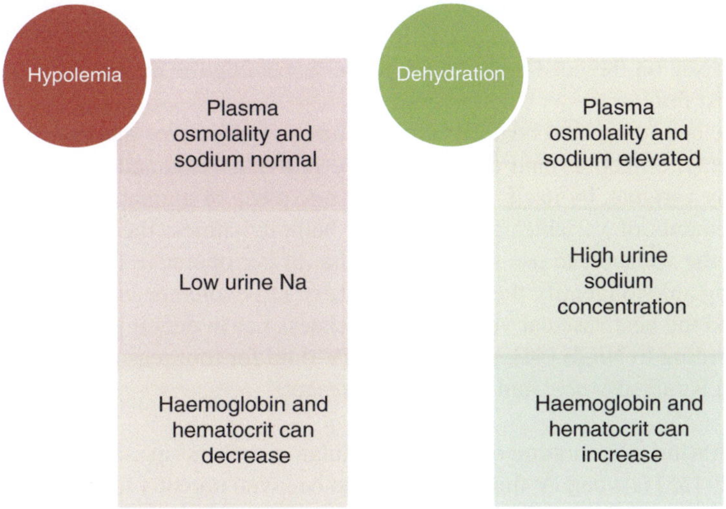

Fig. 20.3 Biochemical differences between hypovolemia and dehydration. Through a simple blood and urine test, we can make a first differential diagnosis of forms of dehydration

interstitial edema, alveolar edema, and/or large collections of pleural or ascitic fluid [44].

The term "zero balance" describes a restrictive regimen aiming to avoid postoperative fluid retention [45]; in a trial [46], the restrictive regimen, despite not demonstrating a difference in 1-year disability-free survival, shows more renal failures. Multicenter RCT involving patients ≥75 years old (the OPTI-AGED study) identified a considerable gap between clinical practice and the relevant guidelines for anesthetic optimization [47].

Goal-directed fluid therapy is based on optimization of preload to achieve a certain goal in stroke volume, cardiac index, or oxygen delivery [48], based on the Frank-Starling physiology, if the stroke volume or cardiac output increases by at least 10%, this is highly predictive of significant cardiac output increase with additional intravascular fluid administration, as the patient is likely hypovolemic and is on the steeper part of the Frank-Starling curve. The step-by-step GDT process is recommended for poorly prepared or high-risk patients or those undergoing more complex surgery. Modern Enhanced Recovery Protocols after Surgery Programs (ERAS programs) are based on these evidences, and current recommendations of fluid therapy in ERAS-programs recommend zero fluid balance and no more than 2–2.5 kg body weight gain [49].

Recent geriatric Intersocietary Italian guidelines recommend perioperative GDT to reduce morbidity and possibly mortality in high-risk patients [8, 50].

In perioperative period, frail patients must be encouraged to clear liquids until 2 h before induction of anesthesia, thereby minimizing the need for intravenous compensation [51, 52]. The patients should be fed orally after surgery, and not by feeding tube (unless special indication).

Therefore, rather than choosing a liberal or restrictive regime, given the reduced ability of frail patients to regulate body fluid, current attention is focused on the type of fluid loss, on the need to replenish while respecting the composition of the loss of the lost fluid.

There are no optimal hemodynamic values and objectives that are applicable to all patients; objectives and alarms must be individualized and re-evaluated regularly; any variable, by itself, provides only one piece of a great puzzle; continuous measurements of variables are preferable hemodynamics; there are little data to support the widespread use of a fixed regime of perioperative fluids; what matters is—being able to identify the onset of a state of hypovolemia and tissue hypoperfusion; find the best vascular volume, nor in excess nor in deficit [53].

According to NICE [54], patients need IV fluid for four reasons, with also a fifth R which is reassessment and continually present.

Resuscitation Restoration of the extracellular space's intravascular volume that is a priority [55] is when IV fluids may need to be given urgently to restore circulation to vital organs following loss of intravascular volume due to bleeding, plasma loss, or excessive external fluid and electrolyte loss, usually from the gastrointestinal (GI) tract, or severe internal losses (e.g., from fluid redistribution in sepsis). The BUN/Cr ratio is relatively proper specificity and positive predictive in cases of bleeding [56].

In this situation it's useful a nonhyponatremic crystalloid solution quickly, or consider human albumin solution 4–5% only for resuscitation in patients with severe sepsis and has been demonstrated to be effective with large-volume paracentesis (>5 L), acute hepatic failure in the pretransplant setting, and in combination with antimicrobials for the management of spontaneous bacterial peritonitis [57].

The hypovolemic hypertonic patient presents an extracellular volume contraction and objectives of the therapy are the correction of the water deficit, the restoration of extracellular volume, and reduction of blood sodium. The contraction of the extracellular volume (hypovolemia), in the first instance, is more dangerous than its hypertonicity; therefore, it is necessary first of all, the correction of blood volume, which is why it must saline solution 0.9% / IV should be used which, despite the patient's hypertonicity characteristics in question, will always be "hypotonic" with respect to the recipient plasma. Once the volume is restored, with raising of blood pressure and resumption of diuresis, it will go correct hyperosmolality by continuing hydration with hypotonic solutions (glucose 5% or saline 0.45%). Best practice guidelines for the perioperative care of the older population from the Association of Anaesthetists recommend that intraoperative hypotension should be avoided in patients aged ≥65y and define intraoperative hypotension as a 20% decrease in systolic blood pressure [58].

Routine Maintenance IV fluids are sometimes needed for patients who simply cannot meet their normal fluid or electrolyte needs by oral or enteral routes but who are otherwise well in terms of fluid and electrolyte balance and handling.

The guidelines suggest giving 25–30 mL/kg of fluid (i.e., 2 L for an average adult, 25 mL/kg/day fluid for patients who are older or frail have renal impairment or cardiac failure) and not more than that with a lot less sodium than normal.

Nice guidelines highlight to consider prescribing less fluid (for example, 20–25 mL/kg/day fluid) for patients who:

- are older or frail,
- have renal impairment or cardiac failure,
- are malnourished and at risk of refeeding syndrome.

The NICE consider besides delivering IV fluids for routine maintenance during daytime hours to promote sleep and well-being.

Replacement In some patients, IV fluids to treat losses from intravascular and/or other fluid compartments are not needed urgently for resuscitation, but are still required to correct existing water and/or electrolyte deficits or ongoing external losses. These losses are usually from the GI or urinary tract, although high insensible losses occur with fever, and burns patients can lose high volumes of what is effectively plasma. Sometimes, these deficits have developed slowly with associated compensatory adaptations of tissue electrolyte and fluid distribution that must be considered in subsequent replacement regimens.

Redistribution In addition to external fluid and electrolyte losses, patients who are septic, critically ill, post-major surgery or those with major cardiac, liver, or renal comorbidity can have fluid distribution changes or abnormal fluid handling.

Frail patients, undergoing high-risk surgeries, could benefit of invasive monitoring such as transesophageal Doppler may be considered to accurately monitor patient's fluid status and to predict the most effective intervention should the patient develops hypotension or hypoperfusion [31], because waiting for hypotension to diagnose the shock, one may have already occurred tissue hypoperfusion and hypotension cannot be considered as an automatic trigger for administration of liquids, because not all hypotensive events are due to hypovolemia.

The most commonly used resuscitation crystalloids are 0.9% normal saline and lactated ringer (LR). It is necessary to infuse large volume to expand the intravascular compartment, with the risk to higher amount of chloride in comparison with plasma resulting in hyperchloremic acidosis [59].

The physiological solution, therefore, presents, per itself, a pH tending towards acidity, but the infusion of 1–2 L per day does not change the acidity of the recipient substantial manner, while the infusion of generous doses of physiological saline solution (as can happen in cardiac surgery, during dialysis or therapy intensive, etc.) is influential on the state of the acid-base balance and can facilitate induction of an acidosis, even to a condition of academia [when the H+ concentration becomes equal to or greater than 45 nEq/L (corresponding to a pH equal to or less than 7.35)] [53].

Table 20.1 Types of intravenous solution. The choice of solutions in the clinical management of dehydration varies depending on the solute composition and osmolality.

Types of solution	Composition	mOsm/L
5% glucosate	50 g glucose	278
20% glucosate	200 g glucose	1112
3% NaCl	Na and Cl 513 mEq	1026
0.9% NaCl	Na and Cl 154 mEq/L	308
Lactated Ringers (Lac 28)	Na 130 Cl 109 mEq/L	274–5
Hartmann solution (Lac 29)	Na 131 Cl 111 mEq/L	278
Plasma Lyte	Na 140 Cl 98 mEq/L	295
0.45% Normal Saline	Na and Cl 77 mEq/L	155

When hyperchloremia is present in the afferent renal arteriole, chloride is filtered through the glomerulus and not reabsorbed in the proximal tubule; in front of the distal tubule the chloride causes releasing of adenosine with vasoconstriction, increased arterial resistance, and a decrease in renal blood flow and perfusion. In addition to the effects on the kidney, saline excess and the resultant hyperchloremic acidosis have adverse effects on various metabolic processes and organ functions [60]: gastric blood flow, renal blood flow and perfusion, blood loss and need for blood product transfusion, cardiac contractility, damage of glycocalyx, with prolonged postoperative recovery. Excess crystalloid fluid compromises anastomotic stability by decreasing collagen formation and increasing inflammation, at least in experimental studies [61]. Alternative crystalloids such as plasma lyte or lactated ringer's, with lower sodium and chloride concentrations, or colloids may be considered. (Table 20.1 describes types of IV solution.) A special problem occurs in the patient with intestinal obstruction, who has from 4 to 5 L of fluid trapped in loops of bowel, not only water but also electrolytes; in this patient administration of sodium chloride is continued monitoring urinary chloride level [62].

In addition to the indispensable attention to tonicity, the acid-base state must never be neglected; it becomes essential to ask if fluid losses (vomiting, either from diarrhea or from excessive discharge through drainage) were rich in acidic substances or basic substances, because, in case of acid losses (e.g., gastric vomiting) the patient loses hydrogen and chloride (HCl) and becomes "alkalemic," due to an increase in bicarbonates that go to compensate for the chlorine deficiency in the right column of the Gamble ionogram, so normal saline is useful to change bicarbonates with chloride; instead, vomiting of bile liquid, notoriously rich in alkaline substances, can lead to acidemia and should be not corrected with saline solution [63] (Table 20.2).

20.4.2 Hyponatremia and Hypernatremia

Serum Na+ clinically is a surrogate marker of tonicity. Osmolarity is a measure of the concentration of all solutes per unit of solution volume; tonicity referring to the concentration (per unit of solution volume) [64].

Table 20.2 Changes in electrolytes according to losses. In basis of type of surgery, we can observe different electrolyte losses.

	Gastric losses	Pancreatic fistula	Small intestine fistula	Biliary fistula	Diarrhea
Na	–	–	–	–	++
K	–	–	–	–	–
HCO_3	++	–	–	=	–
Cl	–	=	–	–	++

The gold standard to both screen for and diagnose low-intake dehydration is direct measurement of serum/plasma osmolality (pOsm), using a threshold of >300 mOsm/kg. When direct measurement of osmolality is not available, the osmolarity equation (pOsm = 1.86 × (Na+ + K+) + 1.15 × glucose + urea +14, all measured in mmol/L) should be used for diagnosis, using a threshold of >295 mmol/L, across healthy and frail older people, those in and out of hospital, with and without diabetes, with and without poor renal function, at all levels of directly measured serum osmolality (or dehydration) and in men and women [7].

Dysnatremia is highly prevalent during hospitalization of older surgical patients, significantly higher in the cognitively and functionally impaired patients, with 2.3 times higher mortality, compared to patients without such abnormalities [65], and patients taking selective serotonin reuptake inhibitors, proton pump inhibitors, opioids or chlorpropamide potentially at increased risk of postoperative hyponatremia [66]. The digestive tract surgery in frail older individuals, with the increased nonosmotic vasopressin (AVP) secretion stimulated by volume depletion (due to gastrointestinal fluid losses or the third spacing of fluids) and the reduced oral sodium intake may contribute to the development of hyponatremia in this patient population [67]. Postoperative electrolyte disorders (hyponatremia and hypocalcemia) are risk factors for postoperative delirium in patients undergoing orthopedic surgeries [68].

It is necessary to find confounders such as hyperglycemia, in diabetic ketoacidosis and in hyperglycemic, hyperosmolar nonketotic states.

The plasma Na must be corrected for the glucose using the following formula:

$$\begin{aligned}&\text{Na corrected} = \text{Na measured} + 0.016 \times (\text{Glucose} - 100)\\&\text{if the glucose is} < 400\,\text{mg\%}\end{aligned}$$

For glucoses greater than 400 mg/dL, the relationship is nonlinear and the following formula should instead be used:

$$\text{Na corrected} = \text{Na measured} + 0.024 \times (\text{Glucose} - 100)$$

The mean decreases in serum sodium concentration averaged 2.4 meq/L for every 100 mg/dL increase in glucose concentration [69].

The classic 5% glucose solution is "isotonic at origin" (pOsm = 278) but it is sugar, as soon as it penetrates the plasma, it immediately enters the cells and is immediately used by cellular metabolism. This is why solution infusions of excess glucose help dilute electrolytes existing in the plasma, with serious general harm and, in particular, they can become responsible of serious clinical conditions of hyponatremia. The use of these "drips" is very dangerous (even *quoad vitam*) in those patients with hypo-osmolar syndromes, such as in symptomatic hyponatremia or even initially asymptomatic, and even more so in the perioperative phases.

The syndrome of inappropriate ADH secretion is characterized by isovolemic hyponatremia and elevated ADH levels despite subnormal plasma osmolality levels, such as in central nervous system disorders, infection, pharmacologic agents, and malignancies. Figure 20.4 describes diagnostic algorithm of hyponatremia.

Serious manifestations of hyponatremia are generally associated with plasma sodium concentrations less than 120 mEq/L.

The following formula may be used to estimate the anticipated change in serum Na when correcting hyponatremia using intravenous fluids.

- Change in serum Na = (infusate Na—serum Na)/(total body water +1).
- Total body water = weight (kg) × 0.6 [or ×0.5 in women, or 0.4 in frail elderly].

For acute form (<48 h), and symptomatic form, with [Na+] < 120 mEq/L, the risk of hyponatremia exceeds the risk of treatment, so it is necessary a rapid correction, 1–2 mEq/L/every hour, with hypertonic saline solution (Fig. 20.5 illustrates how to prepare hypertonic saline starting from saline 0.9%); while in chronic form (>48 h), the risk of treatment usually outweighs the risk of hyponatremia, so it occurs a slow correction, 0.4 mEq/L/every hour, no more than 10 mEq/L in the first 24 h and no more than 18 mEq/L in the first 48 h. The correction must take place without exceeding the variation of 1–2 mEq/L/h, until the acute symptoms regress. Once this goal is achieved, do not exceed an increase of 0.4 mEq/L/h [70].

Excessively rapid correction of hyponatremia has been associated with demyelinating lesions in the pons (central pontine myelinolysis), and more generally in both pontine and extrapontine central nervous system structures (osmotic demyelination syndrome), resulting in both temporary and permanent neurological sequelae [71].

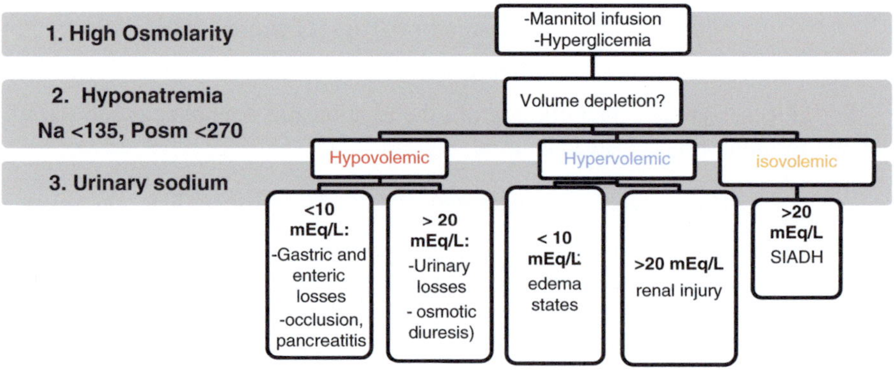

Fig. 20.4 Management of hyponatremia. The main steps of investigating the etiopathogenesis of hyponatremia are to recognize true hyponatremia by the presence of others solutes, identify the presence of volume depletion and subsequently urinary sodium

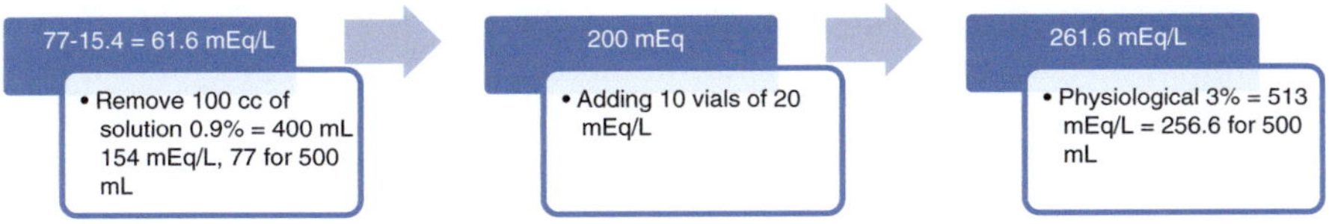

Fig. 20.5 Hypertonic saline composition. It's possible obtain hypertonic saline starting from saline 0.9%

Hypernatremia is often for aging changes at the beginning of the hospitalization [72] and is usually iatrogenic. The first question to ask, therefore, is the following: Has total sodium really increased or has water decreased?

In frail patients, hypernatremia euvolemic may be a marker for severe associated systemic illness and represents the most common form, due to the reduced introduction of water caused by the attenuation of the thirst mechanism, alterations in cognitive status, lack of autonomy, immobilization, absence of caregiver [73]. If there are clinically evident edemas (associated with hypernatremia), it is an increase in total sodium and, in first of all, we must think of an iatrogenic hypothesis, due to excessive administration of saline solutions (hypertonic sodium). If hypernatremic patient is dehydrated, the second crucial question must be asked: Is he urinating little or is he urinating a lot? If the patient is urinating little (diuresis <500 cc/24 hours), your urine will be very concentrated and will have a specific gravity >1.020 and/or a high osmolality (>700 mOsm/kg). If urine output is little, despite having introduced liquids in quantity adequate, and patient is dehydrated, it is intuitive that the patient will have lost a lot of fluids extrarenal or renal. If the excretion of solutes (sugars, urea, sodium, etc.) exceeds 750 mOsm per day, a more abundant osmotic diuresis occurs which is also called "solute polyuria" and excludes the involvement of ADH.

The hypovolemic form of hypernatremia is essentially due to the loss of free water associated with dehydration. Diarrhea represents the most common form of gastrointestinal hypernatremia; osmotic diarrhea (induced by lactulose, sorbitol or carbohydrate malabsorption) and gastroenteritis cause losses of water in excess of the secretion of sodium and potassium. Kidney leaks are even more common and are linked to osmotic diuresis, medications, and diabetes insipidus. The presence of nonreabsorbable solutes in the renal tubule causes a forced elimination of free water and is found above all in glycosuria due to glycometabolic decompensation, mannitol therapy, and diets with a high protein content. Diabetes insipidus represents a pathological condition characterized by deficiency in the action of antidiuretic hormone due to impaired secretion of antidiuretic hormone (central diabetes insipidus) or due to the insensitivity of the renal tubule to hormonal action (neurogenic diabetes insipidus) [74].

To calculate what is the free water deficit that must be infused to treat hypernatremia, the formula used is:

$$\text{Water deficit} = \text{current TBW}\left(= \text{approx } 50\%\text{lean body weight}\right) \\ \times\left(\left[\text{Serum Na} / 140\right] - 1\right).$$

This formula presents limitation, because it does not include estimated losses from sweat, isosmotic loss in diarrhea, or osmotic diuresis.

If patients are symptomatic, deficit must replace in 24 h, with hourly infusion rate (mL/h) > water deficit in mL ÷ 24 h, measuring serum Na every 1–2 h until 145 meq.

For chronic correction, goal is approximately 10 eq/L/24 h; measuring serum Na every 6 h.

In hypertonic states with hypovolemia, attention must prevail towards blood volume which must be corrected first of all, and saline solution must be administered even in the presence of possible hypernatremia. Only when the most serious symptoms and signs of hypovolemia have subsided is it possible also think about correcting hypertonicity [74].

20.4.3 Hypokalemia/Hyperkalemia

Elevated plasma levels of potassium in older patients undergoing open abdominal surgery were predictive of increased 30-day mortality [75]. Some patients with high normal serum potassium concentration at the admission remain asymptomatic, but rhabdomyolysis, vascular procedures with tissue ischemia, polypharmacy (potassium-sparing, nonsteroidal anti-inflammatory drugs, angiotensin-converting enzyme inhibitors, blockers, heparin, digoxin, and trimethoprim sulfate), blood product resuscitation, parenteral nutrition formulations and intravenous amino acids, medication-induced hyperosmolarity (with tonicity-induced changes in intracellular metabolism that impair transcellular potassium gradients) make hyperkalemia resulting with acute renal failure, especially in frail patients with certain acute conditions and chronic comorbidities, such as the same chronic kidney disease, diabetes mellitus and insulin resistance, metabolic acidosis, and hypoventilation-induced respiratory acidosis during anesthesia especially in chronic obstructive pulmonary disease (COPD), sarcopenia, restrictive pathologies, immobilization [76]. Figure 20.6 illustrates the main pathogenesis of hyperkaliemia.

Patients with preoperative serum potassium level > 6 mEq/L should not be recommended for elective surgery [77].

The incidence of preoperative hypokalemia in gastrointestinal surgery is significantly higher than that of general inpatients, with risk factors included the use of potassium-removing diuretics before surgery, inability to eat for more than 3 days or intestinal obstruction, diarrhea for more than 48 h and hypokalemia on admission, the use of two or more bowel preparation (polyethylene glycol) medications and laxative (lactulose and mannitol prior to hospitalization for constipation) especially for laparoscopic radical gastrectomy, insufficient intake [78]. ERAS also recommends prophylactic potassium supplementation [79] (Fig. 20.7).

20.4.4 Hypomagnesemia

Isolated hypomagnesemia should be corrected prior to elective procedures because of its potential for causing cardiac arrhythmias and could be a good predictor of incident delirium [80]. Mg replacement therapy is recommended for those patients

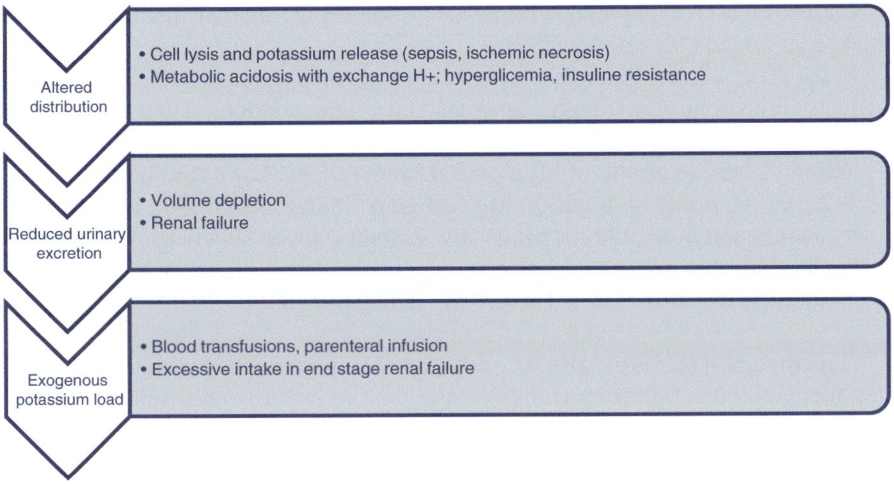

Fig. 20.6 Causes of hyperpotassemia in frail surgical patients. In the perioperative period, frail patients may face the risk of hyperkaliemia, as well as by for iatrogenesis, also due to difficulties in redistribution or excretion

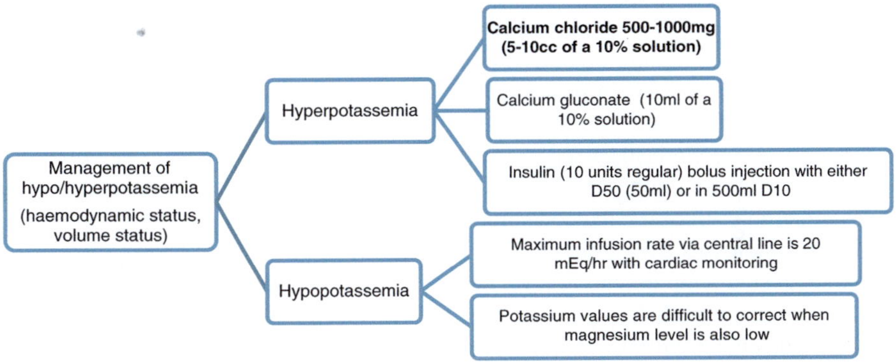

Fig. 20.7 Treatment of hypo/hyperpotassemia. Frail patients are unable to tolerate hypo/hyperpotassemia for a long time, so interventions to promptly correct these electrolytes disorders should be implemented. D = glucosate infusion

with serum Mg values of 1 mEq/dL or less [81]. Several conditions commonly seen in the ICU patients can cause gastrointestinal loss of Mg leading to significant Mg depletion, such as vomiting and nasogastric suction, diarrhea, enteritis, inflammatory bowel disease, intestinal and biliary fistulas, use of diuretics, intestinal surgery resections, and pancreatitis, common after cardiac surgery with decreased value for about 24 h postoperatively. Extracellular magnesium is protein bound; poor protein values may be a contributor. Hypomagnesemia may lead to hypokalemia; thus, treating magnesium levels is important while supplementing potassium and also calcium levels should be checked and addressed when evaluating magnesium values.

Cardiac effects of hypomagnesemia are prolonged QT interval and tachyarrhythmias (e.g., torsades de pointes) [82].

In the acute clinical settings with hemodynamically unstable patients, including patients with severe arrhythmias, established recommendations suggest:

- giving 16 mEq (8 mmol) of Mg over 2–15 min followed by a continuous infusion 1–2 g [8–16 mEq] (4–8 mmol) MgSO4 given initially over 5–60 min followed by an infusion 4–8 g [32–64 mEq] (16–32 mmol) given slowly over 12–24 h;
- magnesium therapy should be considered in patients with moderately reduced glomerular filtration rate and severe Mg deficiency [83].

Hypermagnesemia is usually iatrogenic and is reported along with impaired kidney function, bowel disorders, and old age. Severe hypermagnesemia can lead to respiratory and cardiac arrest.

20.4.5 Hypophosphatemia

Many older frail people are undernourished; postoperative hypophosphatemia, from the intracellular movement of phosphate for the formation of ATP and other anabolic demands, can be a result of hemodilution caused by bleeding or fluid administration during surgery, diabetic ketoacidosis, refeeding syndrome, and severe respiratory alkalosis [84]. A postoperative complication may be mechanical ventilation because of muscle weakness; therefore, supplementation with phosphate-containing compounds has been shown to improve respiratory muscle function [85] and myocardial function [86]. The choice of replacement fluid is thereby especially relevant, with preferred balanced solutions as option, except when replacing gastric and/or fistula losses over stoma [87].

A suggested supplementation regimen for mild deficiency is 0.61–0.8 mmol/L oral replacement with 0.3 mmol/kg/day PO4 (divided doses to minimize diarrhea) or i.v. replacement with 0.3 mmol/kg/day PO4 (as K3PO4 or Na3PO4) over 8–12 h, for value below 0.32 mmol, i.v. replacement with 0.6 mmol/kg/day PO4 (as K3PO4 or Na3PO4) over 8–12 h.

20.5 Conclusion

Dehydration is a marker of frailty; the interplay between age, polypharmacy and geriatric syndromes, and reduced homeostasis predispose older adults to significant fluid and electrolyte abnormalities in the course of surgical stress. In addition to expected surgery complications, inadequate fluid management can worse, rather than improve, volume and sodium intake, with risk of overhydration and underhydration.

It is difficult to right balance between hypovolemia and consequent tissue perfusion and meanwhile not worsening interstitial and pulmonary oedema [88]. ERAS programs establish a physiological treatment regimen on the surgical ward, including Comprehensive Geriatric Assessment (CGA), in order to consider patient-goal centered and not only the surgical procedure; in this point of view, fluid lost should be replaced with fluid resembling the loss in volume and electrolyte composition [21], due to older difficulty to restore alterations.

The decision of high-risk surgery, if a patient is critically ill, should be evaluated in a multidisciplinary approach and considering above all patients and their families [89].

References

1. Staheli B, Rondeau B. Anesthetic considerations in the geriatric population. In: StatPearls [internet]. Treasure Island (FL): StatPearls Publishing; 2023.
2. Licker M, Triponez F, Ellenberger C, et al. Fluid therapy in thoracic surgery: a zero-balance target is always best! Turk J Anaesthesiol Reanim. 2016;44(5):227–9. https://doi.org/10.5152/TJAR.2016.006.
3. Volkert D, Beck AM, Cederholm T, et al. ESPEN guideline on clinical nutrition and hydration in geriatrics. Clin Nutr. 2019;38(1):10–47. https://doi.org/10.1016/j.clnu.2018.05.024.
4. McIsaac DI, Taljaard M, Bryson GL, et al. Frailty as a predictor of death or new disability after surgery: a prospective cohort study. Ann Surg. 2020;271:283–9. https://doi.org/10.1097/sla.0000000000002967.
5. Sabanovic K, Skjøde Damsgaard EM, et al. Preoperative dehydration identified by serum calculated osmolarity is associated with severe frailty in patients with hip fracture. Clin Nutr ESPEN. 2022;52:94–9. https://doi.org/10.1016/j.clnesp.2022.10.006.
6. Zanetti M, De Colle P, Omiciuolo C, et al. Postoperative dehydration is associated with frailty and decreased survival in older patients with hip fracture. Nutrients. 2022;14(4):820. https://doi.org/10.3390/nu14040820.
7. Hooper L, Abdelhamid A, Attreed NJ, et al. Clinical symptoms, signs and tests for identification of impending and current water-loss dehydration in older people. Cochrane Database Syst Rev. 2015;2015(4):CD009647. https://doi.org/10.1002/14651858.CD009647.pub2.
8. Aceto P, Antonelli Incalzi R, Bettelli G, Società Italiana di Anestesia Analgesia Rianimazione e Terapia Intensiva (SIAARTI), Società Italiana di Gerontologia e Geriatria (SIGG), Società Italiana di Chirurgia (SIC), Società Italiana di Chirurgia Geriatrica (SICG) and Associazione Italiana di Psicogeriatria (AIP), et al. Perioperative Management of Elderly patients (PriME): recommendations from an Italian intersociety consensus. Aging Clin Exp Res. 2020;32(9):1647–73. https://doi.org/10.1007/s40520-020-01624-x. Erratum in: Aging Clin Exp Res. 2020 Sep 10.
9. Weinstein JR, Anderson S. The aging kidney: physiological changes. Adv Chronic Kidney Dis. 2010;17(4):302–7. https://doi.org/10.1053/j.ackd.2010.05.002.
10. El-Sharkawy AM, Sahota O, Maughan RJ, et al. The pathophysiology of fluid and electrolyte balance in the older adult surgical patient. Clin Nutr. 2014;33(1):6–13. https://doi.org/10.1016/j.clnu.2013.11.010.
11. Bettelli G. Perioperative care of the elderly: clinical and organizational aspects. 1st ed. Cambridge University Press; 2017.
12. Carrascal Y, Laguna G, Blanco M, et al. Acute kidney injury after heart valve surgery in elderly patients: any risk factors to modify? Braz J Cardiovasc Surg. 2021;36(1):1–9. https://doi.org/10.21470/1678-9741-2019-0483.
13. Dewan KC, Navale SM, Hirji SA, et al. The role of frailty in failure to rescue after cardiovascular surgery. Ann Thorac Surg. 2021;111(2):472–8. https://doi.org/10.1016/j.athoracsur.2020.06.065.

14. Gilbertson EA, Bailey TR, Kraiss LW, et al. Long-term impact of vascular surgery stress on frail older patients. Ann Vasc Surg. 2021;70:9–19. https://doi.org/10.1016/j.avsg.2020.06.048.
15. Mendes RS, Suassuna J. Perioperative oliguria: adequate physiological response or risk for acute kidney injury? J Bras Nefrol. 2021;43(1):1–2. https://doi.org/10.1590/2175-8239-JBN-2020-E001.
16. Beck LH. Perioperative renal, fluid, and electrolyte management. Clin Geriatr Med. 1990;16(3):557–69.
17. Oliver D. Medical input, rehabilitation and discharge planning for patients with hip fracture: why traditional models are not fit for purpose and how things are changing. Curr Anaesth Crit Care. 2005;16(1):11–22.
18. Virgili F, D'Amicis A, Ferro-Luzzi A. Body composition and body hydration in old age estimated by means of skinfold thickness and deuterium dilution. Ann Hum Biol. 1992;19:57–66.
19. Edmonds CJ, Foglia E, Booth P, et al. Dehydration in older people: a systematic review of the effects of dehydration on health outcomes, healthcare costs and cognitive performance. Arch Gerontol Geriatr. 2021;95:104380. https://doi.org/10.1016/j.archger.2021.104380.
20. Thomsen LA, Winterstein AG, Sondergaard B, et al. Systematic review of the incidence and characteristics of preventable adverse drug events in ambulatory care. Ann Pharmacother. 2007;41:1411e26. https://doi.org/10.1345/aph.1H658.
21. Brandstrup B, Møller AM. The challenge of perioperative fluid Management in Elderly Patients. Curr Anesthesiol Rep. 2019;9(4):406.
22. Kim TN, Choi KM. Sarcopenia: definition, epidemiology, and pathophysiology [internet]. J Bone Metab. 2013;1 https://doi.org/10.11005/jbm.2013.20.1.1.
23. Pinotti E, Montuori M, Borrelli V, et al. Sarcopenia: what a surgeon should know. Obes Surg. 2020;30(5):2015–20. https://doi.org/10.1007/s11695-020-04516-1.
24. Luckey AE, Parsa CJ. Fluid and electrolytes in the aged. Arch Surg. 2003;138(10):1055–60. https://doi.org/10.1001/archsurg.138.10.1055.
25. Hiner HH, Suki WN. Fluid and electrolyte disorders in the surgical patient. In: Suki WN, Massry SG, editors. Therapy of renal diseases and related disorders. Boston, MA: Springer; 1991. https://doi.org/10.1007/978-1-4613-0689-4_16.
26. Tsunoda K, Abe K, Goto T, et al. Effect of age on the renin-angiotensin- aldosterone system in normal subjects: simultaneous measurement of active and inactive renin, renin substrate and aldosterone in plasma. J Clin Endocrinol Metab. 1986;62:384–9.
27. Clegg A, Young J, Iliffe S, et al. Frailty in elderly people. Lancet. 2013;381(9868):752–62. https://doi.org/10.1016/S0140-6736(12)62167-9.
28. Strait JB, Lakatta EG. Aging-associated cardiovascular changes and their relationship to heart failure. Heart Fail Clin. 2012;8(1):143–64. https://doi.org/10.1016/j.hfc.2011.08.011.
29. James L, Levin M, Lin H, et al. Association of preoperative frailty with intraoperative hemodynamic instability and postoperative mortality. Anesth Analg. 2019;128:1279–85. https://doi.org/10.1213/ANE.0000000000004085.
30. Crucitti A. Surgical management of elderly patient. 1st ed. Cham: Springer; 2018.
31. Jin Z, Rismany J, Gidicsin C, et al. Frailty: the perioperative and anesthesia challenges of an emerging pandemic. J Anesth. 2023;37(4):624–40. https://doi.org/10.1007/s00540-023-03206-3.
32. Kudoh A, Ishihara H, Matsuki A. Renin-aldosterone system and atrial natriuretic peptide during anesthesia in orthopedic patients over 80 years of age. J Clin Anesth. 1999;11:101–7. https://doi.org/10.1016/S0952-8180(99)00012-4.
33. Robinson TN, Walston JD, Brummel NE, et al. Frailty for surgeons: review of a National Institute on aging conference on frailty for specialists. J Am Coll Surg. 2015;221(6):1083–92. https://doi.org/10.1016/j.jamcollsurg.2015.08.428.
34. Inouye SK, Studenski S, Tinetti ME, et al. Geriatric syndromes: clinical, research, and policy implications of a core geriatric concept. J Am Geriatr Soc. 2007;55:780–91. https://doi.org/10.1111/j.1532-5415.2007.01156.x.

35. Karakousis ND, Kostakopoulos NA. Hyponatremia in the frail. J Frailty Sarcopenia Falls. 2021;6(4):241–5. https://doi.org/10.22540/JFSF-06-241.
36. Perazella MA, Mahnensmith RL. Hyperkalemia in the elderly: drugs exacerbate impaired potassium homeostasis. J Gen Intern Med. 1997;12(10):646–56. https://doi.org/10.1046/j.1525-1497.1997.07128.x.
37. Chan GC, Fung WW, Szeto CC, et al. From MIA to FIFA: the vicious matrix of frailty, inflammation, fluid overload and atherosclerosis in peritoneal dialysis. Nephrology (Carlton). 2023;28(4):215–26. https://doi.org/10.1111/nep.14150.
38. Sarhill N, Walsh D, Nelson K, Davis M. Evaluation and treatment of cancer-related fluid deficits: volume depletion and dehydration. Support Care Cancer. 2001;9(6):408–19. https://doi.org/10.1007/s005200100251.
39. Thomas DR, Tariq SH, Makhdomm S, et al. Physician misdiagnosis of dehydration in older adults. J Am Med Dir Assoc. 2004;5(2 Suppl):S30–S4. https://doi.org/10.1097/01.JAM.0000083444.46985.16.
40. Raghunathan K, McGee WT, Higgins T. Importance of intravenous fluid dose and composition in surgical ICU patients. Curr Opin Crit Care. 2012;18:350–7. https://doi.org/10.1097/MCC.0b013e328355598c.
41. Vincent JL, Pinsky MR. We should avoid the term "fluid overload". Crit Care. 2018;22:214. https://doi.org/10.1186/s13054-018-2141-7.
42. Miller WL. Fluid volume overload and congestion in heart failure: time to reconsider pathophysiology and how volume is assessed. Circ Heart Fail. 2016;9(8):e002922. https://doi.org/10.1161/CIRCHEARTFAILURE.115.002922.
43. Koratala A, Ronco C, Kazory A. Diagnosis of fluid overload: from conventional to contemporary concepts. Cardiorenal Med. 2022;12(4):141–54. https://doi.org/10.1159/000526902.
44. Butterworth IV JF, Mackey DC, Wasnick JD(Eds.). Management of patients with fluid & electrolyte disturbances. Morgan & Mikhail's Clinical Anesthesiology, 6e. McGraw Hill. 2018. https://accessmedicine.mhmedical.com/content.aspx?bookid=2444&sectionid=193556802.
45. Gupta R, Gan TJ. Peri-operative fluid management to enhance recovery. Anaesthesia. 2016;71(Suppl 1):40–5. https://doi.org/10.1111/anae.13309.
46. Myles PS, Bellomo R, Corcoran T, et al. Australian and New Zealand College of Anaesthetists Clinical Trials Network and the Australian and New Zealand Intensive Care Society Clinical Trials Group. Restrictive versus liberal fluid therapy for major abdominal surgery. N Engl J Med. 2018;378:2263–74. https://doi.org/10.1056/NEJMoa1801601.
47. Molliex S, Passot S, Futier E, et al. Stepped wedge cluster randomised controlled trial to assess the effectiveness of an optimisation strategy for general anaesthesia on postoperative morbidity and mortality in elderly patients (the OPTI-AGED study): a study protocol. BMJ Open. 2018;8(6):e021053. https://doi.org/10.1136/bmjopen-2017-021053.
48. Shoemaker WC, Appel PL, Kram HB, et al. Prospective trial of supranormal values of survivors as therapeutic goals in high-risk surgical patients. Chest. 1988;94(06):1176–86. https://doi.org/10.1378/chest.94.6.1176.
49. Feldheiser A, Aziz O, Baldini G, et al. Enhanged recovery after surgery (ERAS) in gastrointestinal surgery, part 2: consensus statement for anaesthesia practice. Acta Anesthesiol Scand. 2016;60(3):289–334. https://doi.org/10.1111/aas.12651. Epub 2015 Oct 30.
50. Giglio M, Manca F, Dalfino L, et al. Perioperative hemodynamic goal-directed therapy and mortality: a systematic review and meta-analysis with meta-regression. Minerva Anestesiol. 2016;82:1199–213.
51. Miller TE, Myles PS. Perioperative fluid therapy for major surgery. Anesthesiology. 2019;130:825–32. https://doi.org/10.1097/ALN.0000000000002603. Erratum in: Anesthesiology. 2020 Feb;132(2):405. https://doi.org/10.1097/ALN.0000000000003066.
52. Voldby AW, Brandstrup B. Fluid therapy in the perioperative setting—a clinical review. J Intensive Care. 2016;4:27. https://doi.org/10.1186/s40560-016-0154-3.
53. Sgambato F, Pinna G, Prozzo P, et al. Pre-intra-post-operative infusion therapy: just a problem for the anesthetist? Notebooks Ital J Med. 2017;5(2):e15.

54. National Institute for Health and Care Excellence. Intravenous fluid therapy in adults in hospital [CG174]. 2013., https://www.nice.org.uk/guidance/cg174.
55. Bhave G, Neilson EG. Volume depletion versus dehydration: how understanding the difference can guide therapy. Am J Kidney Dis. 2011;58(2):302–9. https://doi.org/10.1053/j.ajkd.2011.02.395.
56. Tomizawa M, Shinozaki F, Hasegawa R, et al. Patient characteristics with high or low blood urea nitrogen in upper gastrointestinal bleeding. World J Gastroenterol: WJG. 2015;21(24):7500–5. https://doi.org/10.3748/wjg.v21.i24.7500.
57. Narula N, Tsoi K, Marshall JK. Should albumin be used in all patients with spontaneous bacterial peritonitis? Can J Gastroenterol. 2011;25(7):373–6. https://doi.org/10.1155/2011/586702.
58. Luca E, Schipa C, Cambise C, et al. Implication of age-related changes on anesthesia management. Saudi J Anaesth. 2023;17(4):474–81. https://doi.org/10.4103/sja.sja_579_23.
59. Piper GL, Kaplan LJ. Fluid and electrolyte management for the surgical patient. Surg Clin North Am. 2012;92(2):189–205. https://doi.org/10.1016/j.suc.2012.01.004.
60. Lobo DN. The 2023 Sir David Cuthbertson Lecture. A fluid journey: experiments that influenced clinical practice. Clin Nutr. 2023;42(11):2270–81. https://doi.org/10.1016/j.clnu.2023.09.029. Epub 2023 Oct 3.
61. Kulemann B, Timme S, Sifert G, et al. Intraoperative crystalloid overload leads to substantial inflammatory infiltration of intestinal anastomosis—a histomorphological analysis. Surgery. 2013;154(3):596–603. https://doi.org/10.1016/j.surg.2013.04.010.
62. Thomas EG, Ledwich TW, Hunnicutt AJ. The fluid, electrolyte and nutritional management of the elderly surgical patient. J Am Geriatr Soc. 1955;3(5):311–5. https://doi.org/10.1111/j.1532-5415.1955.tb00401.x.
63. Sgambato F, Prozzo S, Sgambato E. The existing (and unavoidable) interrelationships between hydro-electrolyte, acid-base, osmolar and volume balances. Chapter 40 in The ABC of "humanized" acid-base balance without logarithms. Incontri al Casale, Maddaloni, 2016, 229–234.
64. Lacey J, Corbett J, Forni L, et al. A multidisciplinary consensus on dehydration: definitions, diagnostic methods and clinical implications. Ann Med. 2019;51(3–4):232–51. https://doi.org/10.1080/07853890.2019.1628352.
65. Antonelli Incalzi R, Gemma O, Capperella I, et al. Post-operative electrolyte imbalance: its incidence and prognosis implications for elderly orthopaedic patients. Age Ageing. 1993;22:325–31. https://doi.org/10.1093/ageing/22.5.325.
66. Rudge JE, Kim D. New-onset hyponatremia after surgery for traumatic hip fracture. Age Ageing. 2014;43(6):821–6. https://doi.org/10.1093/ageing/afu069.
67. Verbalis JG, Goldsmith SR, Greenberg A, et al. Diagnosis, evaluation, and treatment of hyponatremia: expert panel recommendations. Am J Med. 2013;126(10 Suppl 1):S1–42. https://doi.org/10.1016/j.amjmed.2013.07.006.
68. Wang LH, Xu DJ, Wei XJ, et al. Electrolyte disorders and aging: risk factors for delirium in patients undergoing orthopedic surgeries. BMC Psychiatry. 2016;16:418. https://doi.org/10.1186/s12888-016-1130-0.
69. Hillier TA, Abbott RD, Barrett EJ. Hyponatremia: evaluating the correction factor for hyperglycemia. Am J Med. 1999;106(4):399–403. https://doi.org/10.1016/s0002-9343(99)00055-8.
70. Adrogué HJ, Madias NE. Hyponatremia. N Engl J Med. 2000;342(21):1581–9. https://doi.org/10.1056/NEJM200005253422107.
71. Danyalian A, Heller D. Central pontine Myelinolysis. 8. In: StatPearls [internet]. Treasure Island (FL): StatPearls Publishing; 2023.
72. Bagshaw SM, Townsend DR, McDermid RC. Disorders of sodium and water balance in hospitalized patients. Can J Anaesth. 2009;56(2):151–67. https://doi.org/10.1007/s12630-008-9017-2.
73. Barbagallo M et al. Acid base balance and electrolyte imbalances. Short manual of Geriatrics. Ed. Universo 2012.
74. Sgambato F, Prozzo S, Caporaso C, et al. Clinical physiopathology of hypernatremia. Relazione all'XI Congresso Nazionale FADOI, Workshop "Approccio clinico al paziente con ipersodiemia" (Torino, 19 maggio 2006) 2006.

75. Ebrahim M, Larsen PB, Hannani D, et al. Preoperative risk factors including serum levels of potassium, sodium, and creatinine for early mortality after open abdominal surgery: a retrospective cohort study. BMC Surg. 2021;21:62. https://doi.org/10.1186/s12893-021-01070-0.
76. Ayach T, Nappo RW, Paugh-Miller JL, et al. Postoperative hyperkalemia. Eur J Intern Med. 2015;26(2):106–11. https://doi.org/10.1016/j.ejim.2015.01.010.
77. Lema GF, Tesema HG, Fentie DY, et al. Evidence-based perioperative management of patients with high serum potassium level in resource-limited areas: A systematic review. Int J Surg. 2019. 21:21-29.
78. Yang M, Li Q, Zhou Y, et al. Risk factors for hypokalemia and its association with postoperative recovery in patients scheduled for radical gastrectomy: a retrospective study. BMC Anesthesiol. 2023;23:285. https://doi.org/10.1186/s12871-023-02246-2.
79. Boersema GS, van der Laan L, Wijsman JH. A close look at postoperative fluid management and electrolyte disorders after gastrointestinal surgery in a teaching hospital where patients are treated according to the ERAS protocol. Surg Today. 2014;44:2052–7. https://doi.org/10.1007/s00595-013-0794-z.
80. Boccardi V, Ercolani S, Serra R. Hypomagnesemia and incident delirium in hospitalized older persons. Aging Clin Exp Res. 2023;35(4):847–53. https://doi.org/10.1007/s40520-023-02357-3.
81. Chernow B, Bamberger S, Stoiko M, et al. Hypomagnesemia in patients in postoperative intensive care. Chest. 1989;95(2):391–7. https://doi.org/10.1378/chest.95.2.391. Erratum in: Chest 95(6):1362.
82. Negru AG, Pastorcici A, Crisan S, et al. The role of hypomagnesemia in cardiac arrhythmias: a clinical perspective. Biomedicines. 2022;10(10):2356. https://doi.org/10.3390/biomedicines10102356.
83. Hansen BA, Bruserud Ø. Hypomagnesemia in critically ill patients. J Intensive Care. 2018;6:21. https://doi.org/10.1186/s40560-018-0291-y.
84. Dwyer K, Barone JE, Rogers JF. Severe hypophosphatemia in postoperative patients. Nutr Clin Pract. 1992;7:279–83. https://doi.org/10.1177/0115426592007006279.
85. Nava S, Fuccella LM, Viglianti B. Physiological effects of intravenous fructose 1,6-diphosphate on diaphragmatic function in malnourished patients with COPD. Monaldi Arch Chest Dis. 2004;61(4):203–8. https://doi.org/10.4081/monaldi.2004.682.
86. Dhingra R, Sullivan LM, Fox CSJM, et al. Relations of serum phosphorus and calcium levels to the incidence of cardiovascular disease in the community. Arch Intern Med. 2007;167:879–5. https://doi.org/10.1001/archinte.167.9.879.
87. Kagansky N, Levy S, Koren-Morag N, et al. Hypophosphataemia in old patients is associated with the refeeding syndrome and reduced survival. J Intern Med. 2005;257:461–8. https://doi.org/10.1111/j.1365-2796.2005.01457.x.
88. Boulain T, Cecconi M. Can one size fit all? The fine line between fluid overload and hypovolemia. Intensive Care Med. 2015;41:544–6. https://doi.org/10.1007/s00134-015-3683-7.
89. Chan SP, Ip KY, Irwin MG. Peri-operative optimisation of elderly and frail patients: a narrative review. Anaesthesia. 2019;74(Suppl 1):80–9. https://doi.org/10.1111/anae.14512.

Postoperative Stress, Metabolism, and Catabolism

21

Riccardo Calvani, Anna Picca, Hélio José Coelho-Júnior, Matteo Tosato, and Emanuele Marzetti

21.1 Introduction

The number of older adults undergoing major surgery has steadily increased in recent decades [1, 2]. Recent data show that in the United States the incidence and 5-year cumulative risk of major surgery in community-dwelling older adults are 8.8 per 100 person-years and 13.8%, respectively, with the highest figures found in highly vulnerable groups (e.g., individuals living with frailty or dementia) [1].

Advancing age, frailty, dementia, and other age-related conditions or risk factors (e.g., multimorbidity, polypharmacy) are associated with postsurgery complications and negative outcomes, including delirium, infections, functional decline, and mortality [3–8].

In a recent systematic review and meta-analysis of 54 studies involving nearly 21,000 older non-cardiac surgical patients, the overall incidence of postoperative delirium was 19% after elective surgery and 32% after emergency surgery [8]. Postsurgical delirium was associated with higher odds of intensive care unit

R. Calvani (✉) · E. Marzetti
Department of Geriatrics, Orthopedics and Rheumatology, Università Cattolica del Sacro Cuore, Rome, Italy

Fondazione Policlinico Universitario "Agostino Gemelli" IRCCS, Rome, Italy
e-mail: riccardo.calvani@unicatt.it; emanuele.marzetti@unicatt.it

A. Picca
Fondazione Policlinico Universitario "Agostino Gemelli" IRCCS, Rome, Italy

Department of Medicine and Surgery, LUM University, Casamassima, Italy
e-mail: picca@lum.it

H. J. Coelho-Júnior · M. Tosato
Fondazione Policlinico Universitario "Agostino Gemelli" IRCCS, Rome, Italy
e-mail: matteo.tosato@policlinicogemelli.it

V. Boccardi, L. Marano (eds.), *The Frail Surgical Patient*, Practical Issues in Geriatrics, https://doi.org/10.1007/978-3-031-77707-3_21

admissions, longer hospital stays, non-home discharge, and mortality [8]. In older adults, the rate of surgical site infections, the second most common type of healthcare-associated infections, was estimated to be around 1.2–3.7% [9]. In a cohort of 2013 adults aged 80 years and older who underwent non-orthopedic surgical procedures, around 20% experienced postoperative functional decline at 30 days [10]. Age-related factors independently associated with reduced functional abilities included both preoperative conditions (i.e., mobility aid use and malnutrition) and postoperative factors (i.e., delirium, pressure ulcers, and the need for mobility aid at discharge) [10]. A recent study on nearly 5600 American community-dwelling older adults who underwent major surgery showed that 13.4% of all patients died within one year [5]. Mortality rates were higher among those with probable dementia (32.7%) and frailty (27.8%). Patients aged 85–89 years or 90 years and older were three to six times more likely to die than those aged 65–69 years, respectively [5].

Postoperative stress or surgical stress refers to the organismal response to direct and indirect injuries following surgery [11]. Direct injuries stem from surgical procedures (e.g., site access, tissue manipulation and/or dissection), while indirect injuries are mainly secondary to changes in local or global perfusion and immune system response [11].

Surgical stress response is an evolutionarily conserved process that limit surgical-induced injury, preserve fluid, and mobilize substrates to facilitate the restoration of tissue homeostasis [11]. This multi system phenomenon involves a complex interplay among between endocrine, immune, and metabolic systems [12].

In older adults, surgical procedures induce a perturbed stress response, which is characterized by altered glucose metabolism, protein catabolism, and immune and hormonal dysregulation [13]. This, in turn, may aggravate preexisting age-related conditions, including sarcopenia [14], and induce an accelerated aging phenotype [15].

In the present chapter, the impact of aging on stress response to surgery will be summarized, with a specific focus on muscle anabolism/catabolism. Finally, novel therapeutic options, including the use of geroprotectors (i.e., molecules targeting biological pillars of aging), will be briefly introduced.

21.2 Stress Response to Surgery: Moving Beyond the "Ebb and Flow" Paradigm

The stress response to surgery is a set of interconnected physiological adaptations that hosts put in place in response to surgical insults. It involves a mixture of overlapping immune, neuroendocrine, metabolic, hemodynamic, and coagulation processes that promote the restoration of tissue and systemic homeostasis [16].

The systemic response to surgery is influenced by both exogenous and endogenous factors [11]. Exogenous factors are those associated with surgical procedures and include type and invasiveness (e.g., laparoscopic vs open surgery), duration, anesthetic technique, and fluid administration. Endogenous (host) factors include demographic factors (such as age and sex) and clinical parameters (e.g., comorbidities, concomitant therapies, cognitive and mood status).

Interactions between endogenous and exogenous factors are major contributors to the wide variety of postoperative outcomes and recovery trajectories observed after surgery [13, 17].

The concept of stress response to surgery derives from the theoretical framework conceived by Cuthbertson in the late 1930s [18, 19]. In his seminal observations in patients with lower limb fractures, Cuthbertson described the host response to traumatic injury as the sequential occurrence of two different stages, termed "ebb" and "flow" [20]. According to this model, immediately after the injury, a short (1–2 days) *ebb* phase occurs, which is characterized by a systemic reduction in metabolic activity, low oxygen consumption, and fluid retention to support vital organs. Then, a longer (7–10 days) *flow* phase starts, which develops as a hypermetabolic state characterized by accelerated catabolism, increase in cardiac output and ventilation, and high oxygen consumption, with the aim of providing substrates and energy for recovery pathways.

A late response phase then ensues, which suppresses previously activated processes to allow return of the organism to its preinjury state.

The ebb-flow model was subsequently applied to surgery and perioperative setting [19, 21, 22]. Evidence acquired over time led to the definition of the physiological mechanisms involved in the surgical stress response and the traditional model was revisited [21–23].

It is now widely acknowledged that following surgical insult at site of access, a multilevel cascade of events occurs, which involves local inflammatory processes, and afferent stimuli from both somatic and autonomic nervous system. This, in turn, activates systemic immune and neuroendocrine responses [21, 23].

Surgical injury at the site of access activates both innate and adaptive immune response. Damaged cells and tissue may release a vast array of mediators, including heat-shock proteins (HSPs), high-mobility group protein Box 1 (HMGB1), adenosine triphosphate (ATP), uric acid crystals, fatty acids, fibronectin, extracellular vesicles, and nuclear and mitochondrial DNA (mtDNA), also termed damage-associated molecular patterns (DAMPS) [24, 25]. DAMPS are detected by pattern recognition receptors (PRRs) on multiple immune cell types (i.e., monocytes/macrophages, dendritic cells, neutrophils, mast cells, natural killer cells, and eosinophils), but also on non-immune cells, such as epithelial cells, endothelial cells, and fibroblasts, and lead to the release of interferons, cytokines and chemokines, the recruitment of inflammatory cells, the activation of complement, and the promotion of defensive immunothrombosis [26–28].

This "sterile" (i.e., not pathogen-associated) inflammatory response limits the possibility of opportunistic infections and plays a crucial role in tissue repair and regeneration.

Local injury (e.g., activation of nociceptors, peripheral nerve injury, inflammatory mediators) stimulates sympathoadrenal response and activates the hypothalamic-pituitary-adrenal (HPA) axis. Activation of sympathetic autonomous nervous system leads to the release of noradrenaline and adrenaline, which increase blood pressure and heart rate [29]. Hepatic, pancreatic, and renal function are also affected, with a net increase in glucagon levels, a reduction in insulin secretion, and activation of the renin-angiotensin-aldosterone axis.

HPA axis stimulation determines a rapid increase in circulating levels of cortisol, growth hormone, vasopressin, and prolactin. In particular, cortisol levels are amplified by the synergistic action of multiple processes that regulate its synthesis, transport, and clearance [30, 31]. Following a surgical insult, the hypothalamic paraventricular nucleus (PVN) receives afferent information from various brain areas (e.g., limbic areas and brainstem structures) conveying cognitive and emotional stressors, pain, and inflammatory stimuli [30, 31]. Parvocellular neurons, a specific type of neuroendocrine cells in the PVN, secrete corticotrophin-releasing hormone (CRH), which stimulates the release of adrenocorticotrophic hormone (ACTH) by anterior pituitary into the systemic circulation. ACTH in turn induces the synthesis and release of cortisol by the adrenal cortex. High levels of inflammatory cytokines (e.g., tumor necrosis factor-α, TNF-α, interleukin (IL)-1 and -6) cause a direct stimulation of both CRH and ACTH. In the first day postsurgery, physiological ultradian pulses in ACTH and cortisol are amplified. While circulating ACTH returns to normal within the first 48 h, cortisol persists at elevated levels [32], which suggests that adrenal release of cortisol may be uncoupled from HPA axis stimuli following systemic inflammation [33, 34]. Moreover, fever, elastase released by activated neutrophil, and local changes in pH induced by inflammation may reduce the availability and/or the affinity for cortisol of its main plasma transport protein, i.e., cortisol-binding globulin (CBG) and albumin [35]. Cortisol clearance is also reduced (up to 50%) following surgery, due to the suppression of the expression/activity of cortisol-metabolizing enzymes in liver and adipose tissue [36].

Collectively, perioperative neuroendocrine response leads to a rapid mobilization of energy substrates (i.e., protein, fat, and carbohydrates) from their body stores to increase blood glucose levels and the renal reabsorption of sodium to promote fluid retention.

The surgical stress response is often a self-limiting process that resolves over time. The resolution of surgical stress response is a multistep process which involves specific neuroimmune processes, such as the "cholinergic anti-inflammatory pathway" or "vagal inflammatory reflex," through which efferent activity in the vagus nerve halts the release of inflammatory mediators by macrophages, monocytes, dendritic and T cells, and endothelial cells that express nicotinic acetylcholine receptors [37]. Somatosensory and autonomic regulation of the immune response prevents overactivity of the immune system and promotes the resolution of inflammation [38, 39]. Inhibition of the HPA axis is mainly mediated by negative feedback processes at the PVN [31]. Both "fast" (gene transcription-independent) and "slow" (genomic "delayed feedback") mechanisms have been described, which involve glucocorticoid receptors (GRs), endocannabinoids, and GABAergic inhibitory signals on CRH-releasing neurons [31].

However, when the magnitude of the insult is particularly relevant (e.g., cardiac surgery) and/or due to specific patient-related factors, including (biological) age and frailty status, the stress response may be exaggerated or suppressed and cause further organ damage [21, 40, 41]. For instance, unresolved chronic sterile inflammation can lead to metabolic disorders as well as neurodegenerative and autoimmune diseases [42].

In the next section, the characteristics of stress response in older adults will be summarized, with a particular focus on the interactions between postoperative inflammatory and neuroendocrine response and the biological processes underlying aging.

21.2.1 Postsurgical Response in Older Adults: "Stressing Out" the Hallmarks of Aging

Aging process is characterized by a constellation of interconnected phenomena at the cellular and molecular level, collectively termed as "hallmarks of aging" [43]. Twelve biological pillars of aging have been proposed, i.e., genomic instability, telomere attrition, epigenetic alterations, loss of proteostasis, disabled macroautophagy, deregulated nutrient-sensing, mitochondrial dysfunction, cellular senescence, stem cell exhaustion, altered intercellular communication, chronic inflammation, and dysbiosis [44]. According to the "geroscience" hypothesis, the hallmarks of aging are functionally related to each other and determine the erosion of the so-called "hallmarks of health," including the maintenance of spatial compartmentalization and organismal homeostasis over time, and an adequate response to stress stimuli [44].

Aging-related processes modify the response to surgical injury, mainly acting on immune and neuroendocrine-metabolic systems [13].

Aging is associated with profound changes in immune system, which affect both innate and adaptive response, due to a phenomenon called immunosenescence [45]. A progressive decline in T-cell repertoire secondary to thymic involution, abnormal lymphocyte metabolism, and increased secretion of senescence-associated mediators (including pro-inflammatory and pro-thrombotic molecules) are distinctive features of the immunosenescence process, which is associated with impaired immune response, increased infection susceptibility, poor vaccine response, and higher risk of chronic (age-related) diseases [45]. Older adults show perturbed acute-phase response following endotoxin challenge, which is characterized by hyperreactivity, prolonged secretion of inflammatory mediators, enhanced febrile response, and hypotension [46, 47]. Immunosenescence is also characterized by the presence of a chronic sterile low-grade inflammatory status, termed "inflammaging" [48]. A main feature of inflammaging is the prolonged activation of the innate immune system [48], which is primarily driven by endogenous stimuli, such as DAMPs [49]. This in turn determines the activation of multiple PRRs and intracellular multiprotein complexes, such as the inflammasome, which leads to the synthesis and release of pro-inflammatory cytokines (e.g., IL-1 and IL-6 and TNF-α) [26]. Notably, several hallmarks of aging, including cellular senescence, mitochondrial dysfunction, defective cellular quality control (e.g., disrupted autophagy and mitophagy), and gut dysbiosis, may synergistically interact with inflammaging and increase its negative effects on health [48].

Collectively, immunosenescence and inflammaging may contribute to exacerbating the immune component of surgical stress response. For instance, age-related increase in circulating DAMPs may combine to those associated with surgery, leading to hyperactivation of postoperative inflammatory response and increased risk of complications [24]. In older adults undergoing cardiac bypass surgery, higher plasma levels of mtDNA (>650 copies/μL) at the beginning of surgery were associated with a fivefold greater risk for postoperative atrial fibrillation independent of the type of intervention [50]. Circulating mtDNA was also found to be associated with the severity of multiorgan failure in patients with valvular heart disease undergoing cardiac surgery [51].

High circulating mtDNA levels following pancreaticoduodenectomy were associated with increased postoperative inflammation and fever in older adults with borderline resectable pancreatic adenocarcinoma [52]. In a group of patients with peritoneal metastasis undergoing cytoreductive surgery combined with hyperthermic intraperitoneal chemotherapy, massive release of DAMPs (including HSP70 and HMGB1) was found after surgery, which was associated with immune suppression [53]. Notably, higher plasma HMGB1 levels were observed in those who developed postoperative infections.

Major perturbations in neuroendocrine systems occur with aging that may alter postoperative response to surgery. An imbalance between sympathetic and parasympathetic components of the autonomic nervous system is frequently observed with advancing age [54, 55]. The most distinctive feature of age-related autonomic alterations is sympathetic overdrive, which is mainly driven by increased activity of noradrenergic neurons in specific subcortical areas [56]. Sympathetic activity appears to increase across several organs, including heart, skeletal muscle, and gut, due to the combination of increased frequency of bursts of muscle sympathetic nervous activity (MSNA) [57], reduced clearance of adrenaline, and reduced neuronal reuptake of noradrenaline [56]. Paradoxically, sympathoadrenal response to acute stress may be attenuated in older adults [56, 58]. However, this is not reflected by lower levels of circulating adrenaline because of its reduced clearance. Sympathetic overdrive is paralleled by diminished parasympathetic activity [55]. Reduced vagal tone is associated with dampened inflammatory reflex, which fuels pro-inflammatory pathways and inflammaging [54, 55]. Surgical procedures may further weaken vagal activity [59]. Remarkably, the concomitant overactivation of sympathetic system and parasympathetic downflow are considered risk factors for the development of chronic conditions, such as cardiovascular diseases, obesity, and metabolic disorders [60–62].

Aging is also associated with alterations in HPA axis [63]. Older adults have higher basal cortisol levels due to several mechanisms that involve the biological hallmarks of aging [63].

Genomic instability, epigenetic changes [64], inflammaging [65], mitochondrial dysfunction [66], cell senescence [67], and gut dysbiosis [68] have been involved in the age-related dysregulation of HPA response, which is characterized by blunted negative feedback due to the loss of GRs in the CNS, reduced inhibitory signaling at the PVN, increased expression of CRH (and vasopressin), and altered diurnal variation of cortisol [31, 63]. Moreover, age-related decline in CBG and cortisol-metabolizing enzymes (i.e., 11b-hydroxysteroid dehydrogenases) further contributes to higher free cortisol levels [63]. Not surprisingly, older adults have higher perioperative cortisol levels compared with younger patients [69], which is associated with greater risk of complications, including cognitive decline, delirium, longer length of stay, and mortality [70–72].

Postoperative stress response may also be associated with an accelerated aging phenotype in older adults [15]. In a cohort of older adults undergoing surgery repair for traumatic hip fracture, a transient increase in biological age markers (i.e., second-generation DNA methylation clocks) occurred in the first 24 h, which was followed by a return to baseline at 4–7 days postsurgery [15].

In conclusion, older adults show perturbed postoperative stress response due to a self-reinforcing cycle between local and systemic response to surgical injury and the biological hallmarks of aging. This leads to a cascade of events at the immunological and neuroendocrine level, such as the increase in pro-inflammatory and pro-thrombotic mediators, and the enhanced release of stress hormones (especially cortisol and adrenaline), which hinders recovery, induces impaired wound healing, promotes catabolism, and increases overall risk of adverse events and death. Postoperative stress response may also accelerate biological aging and aggravate preexisting conditions, including frailty and sarcopenia [16, 73]. In the following sections, the mechanisms associated with surgery-related loss of muscle mass and strength/function will be discussed, with a glance on potential treatment options based on novel geroscience-based approaches.

21.3 Postoperative Muscle Wasting in Older Adults: The Elephant in the Room

Loss of muscle mass is a common (and often overlooked) consequence of major surgery, especially in older patients [14, 74]. Numerous studies have assessed both acute and long-term changes in muscle mass after surgery. In older patients undergoing elective total hip arthroplasty, a substantial decline in quadriceps (–3.4%) and thigh muscle cross-sectional area (−4.2%) was reported in the non-operated leg after 5–6 days of hospitalization [75]. Muscle decline was also observed in non-orthopedic settings. Whole-body fat-free mass decreased significantly (−1.9 kg) at 3 weeks after coronary artery bypass graft surgery, especially in those with elevated postoperative blood cortisol-to-testosterone ratio [76]. A significant reduction in psoas muscle area (−21%) was observed in older adults after endovascular aortic repair over a 3-year follow-up, which was steeper during the first postoperative year [77]. Among older patients undergoing surgery for non-metastatic colorectal cancer, around 14% developed muscle wasting (operationalized as a reduction of at least 5.7% in muscle mass) over a 12-month follow-up [78]. Approximately 20% of patients with stage I–III colorectal cancer who underwent resection for colorectal cancer experienced large reduction in muscle mass at 14 months after surgery [79].

Surgery-related muscle loss is associated with a reduction in muscle strength/function, which increases the risk of developing sarcopenia [14, 74]. In turn, sarcopenia increases the risk of perioperative and postoperative complications in surgical patients [80, 81]. Recent systematic reviews and meta-analysis assessed the prevalence of sarcopenia and its impact on postoperative outcomes across all surgical specialties [81, 82]. In people undergoing gastrointestinal surgery, the prevalence of sarcopenia ranged from 6.8% to 35.9% [82]. The presence of sarcopenia was associated with increased risk of complications (odds ratio [OR] = 3.0, 95% confidence interval [CI] 2.6–3.6) and hospital readmission at 30 days (OR = 2.2, 95% CI 1.4–3.4) after surgery. A recent systematic review and meta-analysis examined data from 97,643 patients (of which 33,070 had sarcopenia) with oncological, gastrointestinal, cardiovascular, transplant, and emergency surgery [81]. The pooled analysis showed that older adults with sarcopenia had poorer postoperative outcomes, including longer hospital stay (mean difference [MD] = +1.7 days; 95% CI: 1.2–2.2), higher complication incidence (OR 1.7; 95% CI: 1.5–1.9), reduced rate of home discharge (78.2 vs. 90.0%; OR 0.5; 95% CI: 0.4–0.6), and higher mortality compared with those without sarcopenia [81]. Lower survival rate was observed in patients with sarcopenia at one (78.2 vs. 90.0%; OR 0.5; 95% CI: 0.4–0.5), three (57.9 vs. 70.2%; OR 0.4; 95% CI: 0.3–0.6), and five (63.5 vs. 75.9%; OR 0.6; 95% CI: 0.5–0.7) years postsurgery compared with non-sarcopenic peers. Subgroup and sensitivity analyses confirmed a higher incidence of complications and mortality in older adults with sarcopenia irrespective of the type of surgery [81].

From a pathophysiological point of view, surgery-related muscle atrophy is characterized by the interaction of multiple pathways that shift anabolic/catabolic balance toward net muscle loss. This phenomenon may derive either by a reduction in muscle protein synthesis (MPS) or an increase in muscle protein breakdown (MPB) [14]. Substantial muscle loss mainly occurs in the first postoperative week(s) due to several factors, including prolonged bed rest, processes associated with postoperative stress response, inadequate protein/energy nutrition [83–86].

Prolonged bed rest leads to deconditioning of multiple physiological systems and is a major independent contributor of many chronic conditions, including cardiovascular disease and metabolic disorders [87]. Loss of muscle mass has been extensively reported in otherwise healthy subjects following periods of bed rest [88–90]. In middle-aged adults, fourteen days of bed rest induced a reduction of muscle cross-sectional area, satellite cell, myonuclear content, and capillary density [89]. In healthy older adults, 10-day bed rest was associated with a significant decrease in MPS (-30%), whole body and lower extremity lean mass (−1.50 kg and −0.95 kg, respectively), and knee extension strength (−15.6%) [88]. A five-day bed rest challenge showed that older adults were more susceptible than younger adults to muscle loss after short-term bed rest [90]. Muscle biopsies collected before and after bed rest showed that this phenomenon may be partially explained by the suppression of MPS (i.e., inhibition of mammalian target of rapamycin complex 1 (mTORC1)-dependent pathway) and increased MPB, as witnessed by the expression of markers related to muscle proteolysis (e.g., muscle atrophy F-box (MAFbx)/atrogin-1). A recent study elegantly described the effects of short- (6 days) and long-term (55 days) bed rest in a cohort of healthy adults [91]. In the first days of bed rest, physical inactivity determines the reduction in muscle energy consumption, which is associated with the accumulation of intracellular glycogen and lipids droplets. This leads to a reduction in insulin sensitivity and a decrease in the translocation of glucose transporter type 4 at the cell membrane. Bed rest is associated with loss of lean muscle mass, which is accompanied by the intramuscular generation of pro-inflammatory lipotoxic lipid species, including ceramide and sphingomyelin, that accumulate close to mitochondria. A parallel increase in circulating levels of IL-6 and TNF-α is also observed. Long-term bed rest is characterized by a metabolic shift toward glucose oxidation, decreased mitochondrial size and density, and reduced supercomplex formation, which ultimately results in blunted oxidative phosphorylation (OXPHOS) capacity [91].

Notably, lipotoxicity, mitochondrial dysfunction, reduced OXPHOS capacity, and systemic inflammation have also been recognized as cardinal pathophysiological features of sarcopenia [92–95], which highlights the prominent role of bed rest for the development and/or progression of the condition [96].

Several processes that characterize postsurgery stress response may exacerbate the detrimental effects of bed rest on muscle and/or promote muscle wasting. For instance, hypercortisolemia stimulates muscle catabolism and can be associated with reduced muscle strength and function [97]. High cortisol levels may co-occur with age-related decline in dehydroepiandrosterone sulfate (DHEAS). DHEAS is a precursor of sex steroid hormones that enhances MPS and anabolic processes [98]. Circulating levels of DHEAS are independently associated with muscle strength and mass in older adults [99]. A high cortisol/DHEAS ratio is considered a risk factor for the development of sarcopenia [100]. Increase in cortisol: DHEAS ratio has been found in older adults with hip fracture and was associated with reduced neutrophil superoxide generation and perturbed immune function [101]. Unbalanced sympatho-vagal activity (i.e., high MRSA and/or low heart rate variability) is associated with reduced muscle mass and strength/function in older adults [102, 103]. Both local and systemic inflammation may negatively influence MPS/MPB balance through several pathways, including inhibition of mTORC1 signaling [104] and upregulation of ubiquitin-proteasome pathway [105].

It is widely acknowledged that sarcopenia recapitulates all the hallmarks of aging [106, 107]. Altered epigenetic landscape (i.e., hypermethylation on genes involved in musculoskeletal growth, including phosphatidylinositol 3-AKT-protein kinase B-mammalian target of rapamycin [PI3K-AKT-mTOR], Hippo-signaling pathway and HOX genes) was found in muscle of older adults [107, 108]. Perturbed muscle methylome was also associated with sarcopenia and individual measures of muscle mass, strength, and function in older individuals from the Hertfordshire Sarcopenia Study [109]. Decline in mitochondrial function is a major driver of sarcopenia [110, 111]. Older adults with sarcopenia show transcriptional signature of mitochondrial bioenergetic dysfunction (e.g., downregulation of OXPHOS and mitochondrial proteostasis genes), which was associated with reduced number of mitochondria, decline in mitochondrial respiratory complex activity, and perturbed nicotinamide adenine dinucleotide [NAD+] homeostasis [94].

Lower muscle oxidative capacity was found to predict mobility decline in older adults from the Baltimore Longitudinal Study of Aging (BLSA) [111]. In BLSA participants, low mitochondrial function was also associated with chronic inflammation and excess production of reactive oxygen species (ROS) [112]. Moreover, circulating levels of mtDNA were found to be an independent risk factor for sarcopenia [113]. Mitochondrial quality control processes, such as clearance of damaged/dysfunctional mitochondria via autophagy/mitophagy, may be impaired in skeletal muscles of older adults due to perturbations in anabolic/catabolic stimuli (e.g., hyperactivation of mTORC1 signaling) [114, 115]. Higher circulating levels of components of the senescence-associated secretory phenotype (SASP), including Activin A, intercellular adhesion molecule 1, matrix metallopeptidase 7, vascular endothelial growth factor A, were associated with lower grip strength, and reduced physical performance (i.e., lower total score at the Short Physical Performance Battery [SPPB], higher 400 m walk test time) in over 1300 older adults form the LIFE study [116]. In the same cohort, SASP mediators predicted the onset of mobility disability and the decline in SPPB total score at 12 and 24 months [117]. In this scenario, postsurgery response may exacerbate hallmarks of aging and aggravate muscle loss in older adults with sarcopenia [107].

Finally, inadequate ingestion of energy and protein with diet is a critical factor for the development of sarcopenia [118]. Low energy/protein intake in the immediate postoperative period is associated with loss of muscle mass in older adults [86]. After colorectal surgery, older patients who consumed a significantly lower amount of energy (25%) and protein (12%) than recommended by the European Society for Clinical Nutrition and Metabolism (ESPEN) [119] lost approximately 10% of vastus lateralis muscle mass in the first 5 postoperative days [86].

In conclusion, older adults undergoing major surgery are at high risk of losing muscle mass, strength/function, and developing sarcopenia due to a combination of prolonged bed rest, neuroimmune pathways associated with postoperative stress response, and malnutrition. These processes overstimulate the biological hallmarks of aging and promote accelerated muscle aging.

In the next section, interventions to reduce detrimental consequences of surgery in older patients will be discussed, with a focus on current guidelines and potential novel treatments targeting the hallmarks of aging.

21.4 Strategies to Manage Postoperative Stress Response and Preserve Muscle Mass in Older Adults

Current strategies to manage postoperative stress response are based on the guidelines by the Enhanced Recovery After Surgery (ERAS) Society [120]. ERAS recommendations are built on a multimodal approach that was originally theorized and implemented by Henrik Kehlet in colorectal surgery in Denmark in the late 1990s

[121, 122]. ERAS multimodal care pathway aims to reduce surgery-associated stress and achieve early recovery through the adoption of pre-, intra-, and postoperative measures, which include comprehensive preoperative counseling, prehabilitation, minimally invasive surgery, use of short-acting anesthetic agents, shorter fasting interval, early re-establishment of oral nutrition, and mobilization [11, 123]. Specific guidelines have been published for most surgical specialties and can be found on the ERAS Society website (https://erassociety.org/guidelines/). Higher adherence/compliance to ERAS protocols is associated with shorter length of hospital stay [124, 125], reduced risk of complications and readmissions [126, 127], decreased costs [128], and improved patient experience [129].

Prehabilitation aims at improving physical, nutritional, and psychological health of patients between the time of diagnosis and the surgery and is based on the design of an individualized multicomponent intervention including diet, physical exercise, and stress-reducing psychological component [130]. In older high-risk patients undergoing major abdominal surgery, a multimodal intervention comprising motivational interview, supervised high-intensity endurance training, and personalized promotion of physical activity administered prior to the intervention was able to improve aerobic capacity and reduce postoperative complications compared to the standard of care [131]. Systematic reviews and meta-analyses have shown that prehabilitation has a significant impact in shortening LOS and reducing postoperative complications in frail and high-risk patients undergoing major abdominal surgery [132, 133]. Pre- and postoperative nutrition care pathway is critical to preserve muscle mass, strength/function, and reduce surgical complications [119]. ESPEN practical guidelines for clinical nutrition in surgery recommend to limiting preoperative fasting and fluid intake restrictions to 2 h for fluids and 6 h for solids, respectively [119]. Early oral nutrition is a key component of both ESPEN and ERAS recommendations [119, 123]. In most cases, oral nutrition (e.g., standard hospital diet and/or nutritional supplements) can be re-established immediately after surgery. Retrospective studies and randomized clinical trials that assessed the clinical impact of specific ERAS components have indicated early oral nutrition as a strong predictor for shortened LOS [134–137]. Early postoperative mobilization (possibly within the first 24 h) is crucial to preserve muscle mass and to accelerate functional recovery. An early mobilization postoperative program based on supervised aerobic exercise, resistance, and flexibility training led to greater improvement in physical function (i.e., reduced risk of inability to walk independently at discharge) compared to standard of care in older adults after major abdominal cancer surgery [138]. In older adults hospitalized for acute decompensated heart failure, a rehabilitation intervention started during or immediately after admission and that included four domains of physical function (strength, balance, mobility, and endurance) led to higher scores on the SPPB than usual care at 3 months [139].

Accumulating evidence showed that the adoption of ERAS protocols may positively influence several components of the postoperative stress response, including inflammation, neuroimmune pathways, and anabolic/catabolic balance in older adults. In patients with colorectal cancer, those who were followed using ERAS protocols showed lower levels of inflammatory markers, including TNF-α, IL-6,

CRP, and white blood cell counts, which were also associated with reduced LOS and less complications than non-ERAS group [127, 140]. Early mobilization/rehabilitation was associated with improved vagal activity and reduced inflammation through the restoration of inflammatory reflex [59]. Greater adherence to ESPEN nutritional recommendations (i.e., ingestion of at least 25 kcal/kg/day of energy and 1.5 g protein/kg/day) in the immediate postoperative period was associated with reduced loss of muscle mass in older adults after surgical resection of colorectal cancer [86].

Notably, multicomponent interventions involving physical activity (in particular, resistance training) and nutrition are the standard of care for the prevention and management of sarcopenia and physical frailty in older adults [118, 141].

According to the geroscience hypothesis, interventions that target biological mechanisms of aging may prevent, treat, or mitigate multiple age-related conditions simultaneously [142]. This concept may also be applied to the management of post-surgical stress response in older adults.

Exercise can attenuate major hallmarks of aging, including chronic inflammation, mitochondrial dysfunction, and cellular senescence [143]. Recent meta-analysis showed that exercise was able to improve mitochondrial quality, density, dynamics, oxidative, and antioxidant capacity in older adults [144]. A 12-week structured physical activity intervention encompassing progressive strength and endurance training (for 2 days/week) reduced circulating levels of SASP mediators in older adults, which was paralleled by improvement in body composition and physical function (i.e., higher handgrip strength, better performance at chair stand, and timed up and go tests) [145].

Interestingly, some FDA-approved medications and nutraceuticals are being evaluated for their geroscience potential [146, 147]. Metformin, a biguanide that is commonly used to treat type 2 diabetes, can stimulate mitochondrial biogenesis and autophagy, reduce the release of ROS and advanced glycation end products, limit macromolecular damage, and exert anti-inflammatory and senolytic effects through the downregulation on pro-inflammatory NF-kB signaling [148]. Observational studies have shown that metformin has beneficial effects on several age-related diseases, including cardiovascular disease, cancer, and neurodegenerative diseases [149, 150]. Recent evidence showed that perioperative use of metformin was associated with lower risk of postoperative complications and mortality in patients with type 2 diabetes undergoing major surgery [151, 152].

Food-derived bioactive substances may target main hallmarks of aging and "mimic" some of the health-promoting effects of physical activity [118, 153]. Several nutraceuticals, including apigenin (a trihydroxyflavone found in edible plants, such as parsley, celery, and grapefruit) [154], fisetin (a flavonol found in strawberries) [155], hesperidin (a flavanone glycoside abundant in the peel of citrus fruits) [156], nicotinamide riboside (a trace element in milk and precursor of NAD+) [157], quercetin (a flavonoid from onions and red fruits) [158], resveratrol (a polyphenol found in grape skin) [159, 160], urolithins (compounds produced by the gut bacteria from ingested ellagitannins and ellagic acid from pomegranate) [161, 162], and ursolic acid (a lipophilic pentacyclic triterpene from apple peel, berries and herbs) [163], are increasingly studied for their promising effects on multiple conditions associated with muscle wasting. Although preclinical studies have shown positive results, evidence in human muscle aging is still scarce.

More research is needed to assess the potential use of substances with geroprotective activities to support multimodal intervention in the management of postoperative stress response.

21.5 Conclusions

In recent decades, there has been a significant increase in the number of older people undergoing major surgery. Older adults are at higher risk for perioperative complications and negative outcomes due to the combination of multimorbidity, frailty, and a perturbed port surgery response. The latter may combine with the hallmarks of aging to hamper recovery, aggravate preexisting conditions, and accelerate biological aging. Muscle is particularly vulnerable to factors associated with surgery, such as prolonged bed rest and hypercatabolism. In older adults, surgery-associated loss of muscle mass, strength, and function negatively affects postoperative outcomes. Strategies to manage postoperative stress and promote recovery of older adults undergoing major surgery are based on the combination of multiple interventions that timely target all possible sources of perioperative stress to reduce inflammation, limit catabolism, and promote muscle anabolism. A multidisciplinary team composed by surgeons, anesthesiologists, geriatricians, nurses, and other health professionals (nutritionists, physiotherapists, etc.) is needed to design individualized pathways of care that match older patients' needs. Multimodal interventions may also exert positive effects on the biological pillars of aging. In this scenario, novel substances targeting the hallmarks of aging are being investigated to support recovery from surgery.

References

1. Becher RD, Vander Wyk B, Leo-Summers L, Desai MM, Gill TM. The incidence and cumulative risk of major surgery in older persons in the United States. Ann Surg. 2023;277:87–92. https://doi.org/10.1097/SLA.0000000000005077.
2. Fowler AJ, Abbott TEF, Prowle J, Pearse RM. Age of patients undergoing surgery. Br J Surg. 2019;106:1012–8. https://doi.org/10.1002/BJS.11148.
3. Gajdos C, Kile D, Hawn MT, Finlayson E, Henderson WG, Robinson TN. Advancing age and 30-day adverse outcomes after nonemergent general surgeries. J Am Geriatr Soc. 2013;61:1608–14. https://doi.org/10.1111/JGS.12401.
4. McIsaac DI, Taljaard M, Bryson GL, Beaulé PE, Gagné S, Hamilton G, et al. Frailty as a predictor of death or new disability after surgery: a prospective cohort study. Ann Surg. 2020;271:283–9. https://doi.org/10.1097/SLA.0000000000002967.
5. Gill TM, Vander Wyk B, Leo-Summers L, Murphy TE, Becher RD. Population-based estimates of 1-year mortality after major surgery among community-living older US adults. JAMA Surg. 2022;157:E225155. https://doi.org/10.1001/JAMASURG.2022.5155.

6. Ho VP, Bensken WP, Warner DF, Claridge JA, Santry HP, Robenstine JC, et al. Association of complex multimorbidity and long-term survival after emergency general surgery in older patients with medicare. JAMA Surg. 2022;157:499–506. https://doi.org/10.1001/JAMASURG.2022.0811.
7. Lertkovit S, Siriussawakul A, Suraarunsumrit P, Lertpipopmetha W, Manomaiwong N, Wivatdechakul W, et al. Polypharmacy in older adults undergoing major surgery: prevalence, association with postoperative cognitive dysfunction and potential associated anesthetic agents. Front Med (Lausanne). 2022:9. https://doi.org/10.3389/FMED.2022.811954.
8. Yan E, Veitch M, Saripella A, Alhamdah Y, Butris N, Tang-Wai DF, et al. Association between postoperative delirium and adverse outcomes in older surgical patients: a systematic review and meta-analysis. J Clin Anesth. 2023:90. https://doi.org/10.1016/J.JCLINANE.2023.111221.
9. Calderwood MS, Kleinman K, Bratzler DW, Ma A, Bruce CB, Kaganov RE, et al. Use of Medicare claims to identify US hospitals with a high rate of surgical site infection after hip arthroplasty. Infect Control Hosp Epidemiol. 2013;34:31–9. https://doi.org/10.1086/668785.
10. Zhang LM, Zhang LM, Hornor MA, Robinson T, Rosenthal RA, Ko CY, et al. Evaluation of postoperative functional health status decline among older adults. JAMA Surg. 2020;155:950–8. https://doi.org/10.1001/JAMASURG.2020.2853.
11. Scott MJ, Miller TE. Pathophysiology of major surgery and the role of enhanced recovery pathways and the anesthesiologist to improve outcomes. Anesthesiol Clin. 2015;33:79–91. https://doi.org/10.1016/J.ANCLIN.2014.11.006.
12. Moor D, Aggarwal G, Quiney N. Systemic response to surgery. Surgery (United Kingdom). 2017;35:220–3. https://doi.org/10.1016/j.mpsur.2017.01.013.
13. Hashmi NK, Podgoreanu MV. Stress response to surgery in the elderly. Principles of geriatric critical care 2018:168–86. https://doi.org/10.1017/9781316676325.013.
14. Shrestha A, Dani M, Kemp P, Fertleman M. Acute sarcopenia after elective and emergency surgery. Aging Dis. 2022;13:1759–69. https://doi.org/10.14336/AD.2022.0404.
15. Poganik JR, Zhang B, Baht GS, Tyshkovskiy A, Deik A, Kerepesi C, et al. Biological age is increased by stress and restored upon recovery. Cell Metab. 2023;35:807–20 .e5. https://doi.org/10.1016/J.CMET.2023.03.015.
16. Finnerty CC, Mabvuure NT, Kozar RA, Herndon DN. The surgically induced stress response. JPEN J Parenter Enteral Nutr. 2013;37:21S–9S. https://doi.org/10.1177/0148607113496117.
17. Podgoreanu MV, Schwinn DA. New paradigms in cardiovascular medicine: emerging technologies and practices: perioperative genomics. J Am Coll Cardiol. 2005;46:1965–77. https://doi.org/10.1016/J.JACC.2005.08.040.
18. Cuthbertson DP, Angeles Valero Zanuy MA, León Sanz ML. Post-shock metabolic response. 1942. Nutricion Hospitalaria. 2001;16(5):176.
19. Wilmore DW. From Cuthbertson to fast-track surgery: 70 years of progress in reducing stress in surgical patients. Ann Surg. 2002;236:643–8. https://doi.org/10.1097/00000658-200211000-00015.
20. Cuthbertson DP. Observations on the disturbance of metabolism produced by injury to the limbs. QJM. 1932;1:233–46. https://doi.org/10.1093/OXFORDJOURNALS.QJMED.A066583/2/1-2-233.PDF.GIF.
21. Kohl BA, Deutschman CS. The inflammatory response to surgery and trauma. Curr Opin Crit Care. 2006;12:325–32. https://doi.org/10.1097/01.CCX.0000235210.85073.FC.
22. Desborough JP. The stress response to trauma and surgery. Br J Anaesth. 2000;85:109–17. https://doi.org/10.1093/BJA/85.1.109.
23. Manou-Stathopoulou V, Korbonits M, Ackland GL. Redefining the perioperative stress response: a narrative review. Br J Anaesth. 2019;123:570–83. https://doi.org/10.1016/J.BJA.2019.08.011.
24. Caballero-Herrero MJ, Jumilla E, Buitrago-Ruiz M, Valero-Navarro G, Cuevas S. Role of damage-associated molecular patterns (DAMPS) in the postoperative period after colorectal surgery. Int J Mol Sci. 2023:24. https://doi.org/10.3390/IJMS24043862.

25. Picca A, Guerra F, Calvani R, Coelho-Júnior HJ, Landi F, Bernabei R, et al. Extracellular vesicles and damage-associated molecular patterns: a Pandora's box in health and disease. Front Immunol. 2020:11. https://doi.org/10.3389/FIMMU.2020.601740.
26. Gong T, Liu L, Jiang W, Zhou R. DAMP-sensing receptors in sterile inflammation and inflammatory diseases. Nat Rev Immunol. 2020;20:95–112. https://doi.org/10.1038/S41577-019-0215-7.
27. Ito T. PAMPs and DAMPs as triggers for DIC. J Intensive Care. 2014:2. https://doi.org/10.1186/S40560-014-0065-0.
28. Engelmann B, Massberg S. Thrombosis as an intravascular effector of innate immunity. Nat Rev Immunol. 2013;13:34–45. https://doi.org/10.1038/NRI3345.
29. Burton D, Nicholson G, Hall G. Endocrine and metabolic response to surgery. Cont Educ Anaesth Crit Care Pain. 2004;4:144–7. https://doi.org/10.1093/BJACEACCP/MKH040.
30. Miller T, Gibbison B, Russell GM. Hypothalamic–pituitary–adrenal function during health, major surgery, and critical illness. BJA Educ. 2017;17:16–21. https://doi.org/10.1093/bjaed/mkw042.
31. Herman JP, McKlveen JM, Ghosal S, Kopp B, Wulsin A, Makinson R, et al. Regulation of the hypothalamic-pituitary-adrenocortical stress response. Compr Physiol. 2016;6:603–21. https://doi.org/10.1002/CPHY.C150015.
32. Gibbison B, Spiga F, Walker JJ, Russell GM, Stevenson K, Kershaw Y, et al. Dynamic pituitary-adrenal interactions in response to cardiac surgery. Crit Care Med. 2015;43:791–800. https://doi.org/10.1097/CCM.0000000000000773.
33. Peeters B, Boonen E, Langouche L, Van den Berghe G. The HPA axis response to critical illness: new study results with diagnostic and therapeutic implications. Mol Cell Endocrinol. 2015;408:235–40. https://doi.org/10.1016/J.MCE.2014.11.012.
34. Bornstein SR, Engeland WC, Ehrhart-Bornstein M, Herman JP. Dissociation of ACTH and glucocorticoids. Trends Endocrinol Metab. 2008;19:175–80. https://doi.org/10.1016/J.TEM.2008.01.009.
35. Henley DE, Lightman SL. New insights into corticosteroid-binding globulin and glucocorticoid delivery. Neuroscience. 2011;180:1–8. https://doi.org/10.1016/J.NEUROSCIENCE.2011.02.053.
36. Boonen E, Vervenne H, Meersseman P, Andrew R, Mortier L, Declercq PE, et al. Reduced cortisol metabolism during critical illness. N Engl J Med. 2013;368:1477–88. https://doi.org/10.1056/NEJMOA1214969.
37. Tracey KJ. The inflammatory reflex. Nature. 2002;420:853–9. https://doi.org/10.1038/NATURE01321.
38. Udit S, Blake K, Chiu IM. Somatosensory and autonomic neuronal regulation of the immune response. Nat Rev Neurosci. 2022;23:157–71. https://doi.org/10.1038/S41583-021-00555-4.
39. Rolls A. Immunoception: the insular cortex perspective. Cell Mol Immunol. 2023;20:1270–6. https://doi.org/10.1038/S41423-023-01051-8.
40. Bartels K, Karhausen J, Clambey ET, Grenz A, Eltzschig HK. Perioperative organ injury. Anesthesiology. 2013;119:1474–89. https://doi.org/10.1097/ALN.0000000000000022.
41. Dobson GP. Addressing the global burden of trauma in major surgery. Front Surg. 2015:2. https://doi.org/10.3389/FSURG.2015.00043/FULL.
42. Furman D, Campisi J, Verdin E, Carrera-Bastos P, Targ S, Franceschi C, et al. Chronic inflammation in the etiology of disease across the life span. Nat Med. 2019;25:1822–32. https://doi.org/10.1038/S41591-019-0675-0.
43. López-Otín C, Blasco MA, Partridge L, Serrano M, Kroemer G. The hallmarks of aging. Cell. 2013;153:1194. https://doi.org/10.1016/J.CELL.2013.05.039.
44. López-Otín C, Blasco MA, Partridge L, Serrano M, Kroemer G. Hallmarks of aging: an expanding universe. Cell. 2023;186:243–78. https://doi.org/10.1016/J.CELL.2022.11.001.
45. Liu Z, Liang Q, Ren Y, Guo C, Ge X, Wang L, et al. Immunosenescence: molecular mechanisms and diseases. Signal Transduct Target Ther. 2023:8. https://doi.org/10.1038/S41392-023-01451-2.

46. Krabbe KS, Bruunsgaard H, Hansen CM, Møller K, Fonsmark L, Qvist J, et al. Ageing is associated with a prolonged fever response in human endotoxemia. Clin Diagn Lab Immunol. 2001;8:333–8. https://doi.org/10.1128/CDLI.8.2.333-338.2001.
47. Krabbe KS, Bruunsgaard H, Qvist J, Hansen CM, Møller K, Fonsmark L, et al. Hypotension during endotoxemia in aged humans. Eur J Anaesthesiol. 2001;18:572–5. https://doi.org/10.1046/J.1365-2346.2001.00958.X.
48. Franceschi C, Garagnani P, Parini P, Giuliani C, Santoro A. Inflammaging: a new immune-metabolic viewpoint for age-related diseases. Nat Rev Endocrinol. 2018;14:576–90. https://doi.org/10.1038/S41574-018-0059-4.
49. Picca A, Lezza AMS, Leeuwenburgh C, Pesce V, Calvani R, Landi F, et al. Fueling inflamm-aging through mitochondrial dysfunction: mechanisms and molecular targets. Int J Mol Sci. 2017:18. https://doi.org/10.3390/IJMS18050933.
50. Zajonz T, Koch C, Schwiddessen J, Markmann M, Hecker M, Edinger F, et al. Minimized extracorporeal circulation is associated with reduced plasma levels of free-circulating mitochondrial DNA compared to conventional cardiopulmonary bypass: a secondary analysis of an exploratory, prospective, interventional study. J Clin Med. 2022:11. https://doi.org/10.3390/JCM11112994.
51. Grigoriev E, Ponasenko AV, Sinitskaya AV, Ivkin AA, Kornelyuk RA. Mitochondrial DNA as a candidate marker of multiple organ failure after cardiac surgery. Int J Mol Sci. 2022:23. https://doi.org/10.3390/IJMS232314748.
52. Pencovich N, Nevo N, Weiser R, Bonder E, Bogoch Y, Nachmany I. Postoperative rise of circulating mitochondrial DNA is associated with inflammatory response in patients following pancreaticoduodenectomy. Eur Surg Res. 2021;62:18–24. https://doi.org/10.1159/000514661.
53. Leijte GP, Custers H, Gerretsen J, Heijne A, Roth J, Vogl T, et al. Increased plasma levels of danger-associated molecular patterns are associated with immune suppression and postoperative infections in patients undergoing cytoreductive surgery and hyperthermic intraperitoneal chemotherapy. Front Immunol. 2018:9. https://doi.org/10.3389/FIMMU.2018.00663.
54. Jiang Y, Yabluchanskiy A, Deng J, Amil FA, Po SS, Dasari TW. The role of age-associated autonomic dysfunction in inflammation and endothelial dysfunction. Geroscience. 2022;44:2655–70. https://doi.org/10.1007/S11357-022-00616-1.
55. Giunta S, Xia S, Pelliccioni G, Olivieri F. Autonomic nervous system imbalance during aging contributes to impair endogenous anti-inflammaging strategies. Geroscience. 2024;46:113–27. https://doi.org/10.1007/S11357-023-00947-7.
56. Seals DR, Esler MD. Human ageing and the sympathoadrenal system. J Physiol. 2000;528:407–17. https://doi.org/10.1111/J.1469-7793.2000.00407.X.
57. Keir DA, Badrov MB, Tomlinson G, Notarius CF, Kimmerly DS, Millar PJ, et al. Influence of sex and age on muscle sympathetic nerve activity of healthy normotensive adults. Hypertension. 2020;76:997–1005. https://doi.org/10.1161/HYPERTENSIONAHA.120.15208.
58. Esler M, Kaye D, Thompson J, Jennings G, Cox H, Turner A, Lambert G, Seals D. Effects of aging on epinephrine secretion and regional release of epinephrine from the human heart. J Clin Endocrinol Metab. 1995;80:435–42. https://doi.org/10.1210/JCEM.80.2.7852502.
59. Grote V, Levnajić Z, Puff H, Ohland T, Goswami N, Frühwirth M, et al. Dynamics of vagal activity due to surgery and subsequent rehabilitation. Front Neurosci. 2019:13. https://doi.org/10.3389/FNINS.2019.01116.
60. Dekker JM, Crow RS, Folsom AR, Hannan PJ, Liao D, Swenne CA, et al. Low heart rate variability in a 2-minute rhythm strip predicts risk of coronary heart disease and mortality from several causes: the ARIC study. Atherosclerosis risk in communities. Circulation. 2000;102:1239–44. https://doi.org/10.1161/01.CIR.102.11.1239.
61. Laederach-Hofmann K, Mussgay L, Rúddel H. Autonomic cardiovascular regulation in obesity. J Endocrinol. 2000;164:59–66. https://doi.org/10.1677/JOE.0.1640059.
62. Yu TY, Lee MK. Autonomic dysfunction, diabetes and metabolic syndrome. J Diabetes Investig. 2021;12:2108–11. https://doi.org/10.1111/JDI.13691.

63. van den Beld AW, Kaufman JM, Zillikens MC, Lamberts SWJ, Egan JM, van der Lely AJ. The physiology of endocrine systems with ageing. Lancet Diabetes Endocrinol. 2018;6:647–58. https://doi.org/10.1016/S2213-8587(18)30026-3.
64. Gassen NC, Chrousos GP, Binder EB, Zannas AS. Life stress, glucocorticoid signaling, and the aging epigenome: implications for aging-related diseases. Neurosci Biobehav Rev. 2017;74:356–65. https://doi.org/10.1016/J.NEUBIOREV.2016.06.003.
65. Sergio G. Exploring the complex relations between inflammation and aging (inflammaging): anti-inflammaging remodelling of inflammaging, from robustness to frailty. Inflamm Res. 2008;57:558–63. https://doi.org/10.1007/S00011-008-7243-2.
66. Picard M, McManus MJ, Gray JD, Nasca C, Moffat C, Kopinski PK, et al. Mitochondrial functions modulate neuroendocrine, metabolic, inflammatory, and transcriptional responses to acute psychological stress. Proc Natl Acad Sci USA. 2015;112:E6614–23. https://doi.org/10.1073/PNAS.1515733112.
67. Lunin SM, Novoselova EG, Glushkova OV, Parfenyuk SB, Novoselova TV, Khrenov MO. Cell senescence and central regulators of immune response. Int J Mol Sci. 2022:23. https://doi.org/10.3390/IJMS23084109.
68. Rusch JA, Layden BT, Dugas LR. Signalling cognition: the gut microbiota and hypothalamic-pituitary-adrenal axis. Front Endocrinol (Lausanne). 2023:14. https://doi.org/10.3389/FENDO.2023.1130689.
69. Prete A, Yan Q, Al-Tarrah K, Akturk HK, Prokop LJ, Alahdab F, et al. The cortisol stress response induced by surgery: a systematic review and meta-analysis. Clin Endocrinol. 2018;89:554–67. https://doi.org/10.1111/CEN.13820.
70. Kudoh A, Takase H, Katagai H, Takazawa T. Postoperative interleukin-6 and cortisol concentrations in elderly patients with postoperative confusion. Neuroimmunomodulation. 2005;12:60–6. https://doi.org/10.1159/000082365.
71. Mu DL, Li LH, Wang DX, Li N, Shan GJ, Li J, et al. High postoperative serum cortisol level is associated with increased risk of cognitive dysfunction early after coronary artery bypass graft surgery: a prospective cohort study. PLoS One. 2013:8. https://doi.org/10.1371/JOURNAL.PONE.0077637.
72. Kazmierski J, Banys A, Latek J, Bourke J, Jaszewski R. Cortisol levels and neuropsychiatric diagnosis as markers of postoperative delirium: a prospective cohort study. Crit Care. 2013:17. https://doi.org/10.1186/CC12548.
73. Schricker T, Lattermann R. Perioperative catabolism. Can J Anaesth. 2015;62:182–93. https://doi.org/10.1007/S12630-014-0274-Y.
74. Welch C, Hassan-Smith ZK, Greig CA, Lord JM, Jackson TA. Acute sarcopenia secondary to hospitalisation—an emerging condition affecting older adults. Aging Dis. 2018;9:151–64. https://doi.org/10.14336/AD.2017.0315.
75. Kouw IWK, Groen BBL, Smeets JSJ, Kramer IF, van Kranenburg JMX, Nilwik R, et al. One week of hospitalization following elective hip surgery induces substantial muscle atrophy in older patients. J Am Med Dir Assoc. 2019;20:35–42. https://doi.org/10.1016/J.JAMDA.2018.06.018.
76. Hansen D, Linsen L, Verboven K, Hendrikx M, Rummens JL, van Erum M, et al. Magnitude of muscle wasting early after on-pump coronary artery bypass graft surgery and exploration of aetiology. Exp Physiol. 2015;100:818–28. https://doi.org/10.1113/EP085053.
77. Lindström I, Protto S, Khan N, Sillanpää N, Hernesniemi J, Oksala N. Developing sarcopenia predicts long-term mortality after elective endovascular aortic aneurysm repair. J Vasc Surg. 2020;71:1169–78.e5. https://doi.org/10.1016/J.JVS.2019.05.060.
78. Argillander TE, Spek D, van der Zaag-Loonen HJ, van Raamt AF, van Duijvendijk P, van Munster BC. Association between postoperative muscle wasting and survival in older patients undergoing surgery for non-metastatic colorectal cancer. J Geriatr Oncol. 2021;12:1052–8. https://doi.org/10.1016/J.JGO.2021.04.004.
79. Brown JC, Caan BJ, Meyerhardt JA, Weltzien E, Xiao J, Cespedes Feliciano EM, et al. The deterioration of muscle mass and radiodensity is prognostic of poor survival in stage I-III

colorectal cancer: a population-based cohort study (C-SCANS). J Cachexia Sarcopenia Muscle. 2018;9:664–72. https://doi.org/10.1002/JCSM.12305.
80. Pinotti E, Montuori M, Borrelli V, Giuffrè M, Angrisani L. Sarcopenia: what a surgeon should know. Obes Surg. 2020;30:2015–20. https://doi.org/10.1007/S11695-020-04516-1.
81. Knoedler S, Schliermann R, Knoedler L, Wu M, Hansen FJ, Matar DY, et al. Impact of sarcopenia on outcomes in surgical patients: a systematic review and meta-analysis. Int J Surg. 2023;109:4238–62. https://doi.org/10.1097/JS9.0000000000000688.
82. Pipek LZ, Baptista CG, Nascimento RFV, Taba JV, Suzuki MO, do Nascimento FS, et al. The impact of properly diagnosed sarcopenia on postoperative outcomes after gastrointestinal surgery: a systematic review and meta-analysis. PLoS One. 2020:15. https://doi.org/10.1371/JOURNAL.PONE.0237740.
83. Osaki T, Matsunaga T, Makinoya M, Shishido Y, Miyatani K, Uchinaka E, et al. Impact of gastrectomy on body composition within 1 month in patients with gastric cancer. Surg Today. 2023;53:834–44. https://doi.org/10.1007/S00595-022-02633-1.
84. van Wijk L, van Duinhoven S, Liem MSL, Bouman DE, Viddeleer AR, Klaase JM. Risk factors for surgery-related muscle quantity and muscle quality loss and their impact on outcome. Eur J Med Res. 2021:26. https://doi.org/10.1186/S40001-021-00507-9.
85. Marusic U, Narici M, Simunic B, Pisot R, Ritzmann R. Nonuniform loss of muscle strength and atrophy during bed rest: a systematic review. J Appl Physiol. 1985;2021(131):194–206. https://doi.org/10.1152/JAPPLPHYSIOL.00363.2020.
86. Hardy EJ, Deane CS, Lund JN, Phillips BE. Loss of muscle mass in the immediate postoperative period is associated with inadequate dietary protein and energy intake. Eur J Clin Nutr. 2023;77:503–5. https://doi.org/10.1038/S41430-023-01264-0.
87. Krasnoff J, Painter P. The physiological consequences of bed rest and inactivity. Adv Ren Replace Ther. 1999;6:124–32. https://doi.org/10.1016/S1073-4449(99)70030-0.
88. Kortebein P, Ferrando A, Lombeida J, Wolfe R, Evans WJ. Effect of 10 days of bed rest on skeletal muscle in healthy older adults. JAMA. 2007;297:1772–4. https://doi.org/10.1001/JAMA.297.16.1772-B.
89. Arentson-Lantz EJ, English KL, Paddon-Jones D, Fry CS. Fourteen days of bed rest induces a decline in satellite cell content and robust atrophy of skeletal muscle fibers in middle-aged adults. J Appl Physiol. 1985;2016(120):965–75. https://doi.org/10.1152/JAPPLPHYSIOL.00799.2015.
90. Tanner RE, Brunker LB, Agergaard J, Barrows KM, Briggs RA, Kwon OS, et al. Age-related differences in lean mass, protein synthesis and skeletal muscle markers of proteolysis after bed rest and exercise rehabilitation. J Physiol. 2015;593:4259–73. https://doi.org/10.1113/JP270699.
91. Eggelbusch M, Charlton BT, Bosutti A, Ganse B, Giakoumaki I, Grootemaat AE, et al. The impact of bed rest on human skeletal muscle metabolism. Cell Rep Med. 2024:5. https://doi.org/10.1016/J.XCRM.2023.101372.
92. Carter CS, Justice JN, Thompson LD. Lipotoxicity, aging, and muscle contractility: does fiber type matter? Geroscience. 2019;41:297–308. https://doi.org/10.1007/S11357-019-00077-Z.
93. Picca A, Calvani R, Bossola M, Allocca E, Menghi A, Pesce V, et al. Update on mitochondria and muscle aging: all wrong roads lead to sarcopenia. Biol Chem. 2018;399:421–36. https://doi.org/10.1515/HSZ-2017-0331.
94. Migliavacca E, Tay SKH, Patel HP, Sonntag T, Civiletto G, McFarlane C, et al. Mitochondrial oxidative capacity and NAD+ biosynthesis are reduced in human sarcopenia across ethnicities. Nat Commun. 2019:10. https://doi.org/10.1038/S41467-019-13694-1.
95. Dalle S, Rossmeislova L, Koppo K. The role of inflammation in age-related sarcopenia. Front Physiol. 2017:8. https://doi.org/10.3389/FPHYS.2017.01045.
96. Di Girolamo FG, Fiotti N, Milanović Z, Situlin R, Mearelli F, Vinci P, et al. The aging muscle in experimental bed rest: a systematic review and meta-analysis. Front Nutr. 2021:8. https://doi.org/10.3389/FNUT.2021.633987.
97. Katsuhara S, Yokomoto-Umakoshi M, Umakoshi H, Matsuda Y, Iwahashi N, Kaneko H, et al. Impact of cortisol on reduction in muscle strength and mass: a Mendelian randomization

study. J Clin Endocrinol Metab. 2022;107:E1477–87. https://doi.org/10.1210/CLINEM/DGAB862.
98. Sato K, Iemitsu M. The role of dehydroepiandrosterone (DHEA) in skeletal muscle. Vitam Horm. 2018;108:205–21. https://doi.org/10.1016/BS.VH.2018.03.002.
99. Valenti G, Denti L, Maggio M, Ceda GP, Volpato S, Bandinelli S, et al. Effect of DHEAS on skeletal muscle over the life span: the InCHIANTI study. J Gerontol A Biol Sci Med Sci. 2004;59:466–72. https://doi.org/10.1093/GERONA/59.5.M466.
100. Yanagita I, Fujihara Y, Kitajima Y, Tajima M, Honda M, Kawajiri T, et al. A high serum cortisol/DHEA-S ratio is a risk factor for sarcopenia in elderly diabetic patients. J Endocr Soc. 2019;3:801–13. https://doi.org/10.1210/JS.2018-00271.
101. Butcher SK, Killampalli V, Lascelles D, Wang K, Alpar KE, Lord JM. Raised cortisol:DHEAS ratios in the elderly after injury: potential impact upon neutrophil function and immunity. Aging Cell. 2005;4:319–24. https://doi.org/10.1111/J.1474-9726.2005.00178.X.
102. da Fonseca GWP, Dos Santos MR, de Souza FR, da Costa MJA, von Haehling S, Takayama L, et al. Sympatho-vagal imbalance is associated with sarcopenia in male patients with heart failure. Arq Bras Cardiol. 2019;112:739–46. https://doi.org/10.5935/ABC.20190061.
103. Zheng K, Wang Z, Han P, Chen C, Huang C, Wu Y, et al. Lower heart rate variability is associated with loss of muscle mass and sarcopenia in community-dwelling older Chinese adults. J Formos Med Assoc. 2023; https://doi.org/10.1016/J.JFMA.2023.10.010.
104. Frost RA, Lang CH. mTor signaling in skeletal muscle during sepsis and inflammation: where does it all go wrong? Physiology (Bethesda). 2011;26:83–96. https://doi.org/10.1152/PHYSIOL.00044.2010.
105. Haberecht-Müller S, Krüger E, Fielitz J. Out of control: the role of the ubiquitin proteasome system in skeletal muscle during inflammation. Biomol Ther. 2021:11. https://doi.org/10.3390/BIOM11091327.
106. Picca A, Calvani R, Cesari M, Landi F, Bernabei R, Coelho-Júnior HJ, et al. Biomarkers of physical frailty and sarcopenia: coming up to the place? Int J Mol Sci. 2020;21:1–16. https://doi.org/10.3390/IJMS21165635.
107. Granic A, Suetterlin K, Shavlakadze T, Grounds MD, Sayer AA. Hallmarks of ageing in human skeletal muscle and implications for understanding the pathophysiology of sarcopenia in women and men. Clin Sci (Lond). 2023;137:1721–51. https://doi.org/10.1042/CS20230319.
108. Zykovich A, Hubbard A, Flynn JM, Tarnopolsky M, Fraga MF, Kerksick C, et al. Genome-wide DNA methylation changes with age in disease-free human skeletal muscle. Aging Cell. 2014;13:360–6. https://doi.org/10.1111/ACEL.12180.
109. Antoun E, Garratt ES, Taddei A, Burton MA, Barton SJ, Titcombe P, et al. Epigenome-wide association study of sarcopenia: findings from the Hertfordshire sarcopenia study (HSS). J Cachexia Sarcopenia Muscle. 2022;13:240–53. https://doi.org/10.1002/JCSM.12876.
110. Grevendonk L, Connell NJ, McCrum C, Fealy CE, Bilet L, Bruls YMH, et al. Impact of aging and exercise on skeletal muscle mitochondrial capacity, energy metabolism, and physical function. Nat Commun. 2021:12. https://doi.org/10.1038/S41467-021-24956-2.
111. Tian Q, Mitchell BA, Zampino M, Fishbein KW, Spencer RG, Ferrucci L. Muscle mitochondrial energetics predicts mobility decline in well-functioning older adults: the Baltimore longitudinal study of aging. Aging Cell. 2022:21. https://doi.org/10.1111/ACEL.13552.
112. Zampino M, Brennan NA, Kuo PL, Spencer RG, Fishbein KW, Simonsick EM, et al. Poor mitochondrial health and systemic inflammation? Test of a classic hypothesis in the Baltimore longitudinal study of aging. Geroscience. 2020;42:1175–82. https://doi.org/10.1007/S11357-020-00208-X.
113. Fan Z, Yang JY, Guo Y, Liu YX, Zhong XY. Altered levels of circulating mitochondrial DNA in elderly people with sarcopenia: association with mitochondrial impairment. Exp Gerontol. 2022:163. https://doi.org/10.1016/J.EXGER.2022.111802.
114. Bonifacio A, Mariggiò MA, Marzetti E, Calvani R, Coelho-Júnior HJ, Landi F, et al. Mitochondrial quantity and quality in age-related sarcopenia. Int J Mol Sci. 2024;25:2052. https://doi.org/10.3390/IJMS25042052.

115. Sirago G, Picca A, Calvani R, Coelho-Júnior HJ, Marzetti E. Mammalian target of rapamycin (mTOR) signaling at the crossroad of muscle fiber fate in sarcopenia. Int J Mol Sci. 2022:23. https://doi.org/10.3390/IJMS232213823.
116. Fielding RA, Atkinson EJ, Aversa Z, White TA, Heeren AA, Achenbach SJ, et al. Associations between biomarkers of cellular senescence and physical function in humans: observations from the lifestyle interventions for elders (LIFE) study. Geroscience. 2022;44:2757–70. https://doi.org/10.1007/S11357-022-00685-2.
117. Fielding RA, Atkinson EJ, Aversa Z, White TA, Heeren AA, Mielke MM, et al. Biomarkers of cellular senescence predict the onset of mobility disability and are reduced by physical activity in older adults. J Gerontol A Biol Sci Med Sci. 2024:79. https://doi.org/10.1093/GERONA/GLAD257.
118. Calvani R, Picca A, Coelho-Júnior HJ, Tosato M, Marzetti E, Landi F. Diet for the prevention and management of sarcopenia. Metabolism. 2023:146. https://doi.org/10.1016/J.METABOL.2023.155637.
119. Weimann A, Braga M, Carli F, Higashiguchi T, Hübner M, Klek S, et al. ESPEN guideline: clinical nutrition in surgery. Clin Nutr. 2017;36:623–50. https://doi.org/10.1016/J.CLNU.2017.02.013.
120. Fearon KCH, Ljungqvist O, Von Meyenfeldt M, Revhaug A, Dejong CHC, Lassen K, et al. Enhanced recovery after surgery: a consensus review of clinical care for patients undergoing colonic resection. Clin Nutr. 2005;24:466–77. https://doi.org/10.1016/J.CLNU.2005.02.002.
121. Bardram L, Funch-Jensen P, Jensen P, Kehlet H, Crawford ME. Recovery after laparoscopic colonic surgery with epidural analgesia, and early oral nutrition and mobilisation. Lancet. 1995;345:763–4. https://doi.org/10.1016/S0140-6736(95)90643-6.
122. Kehlet H. Multimodal approach to control postoperative pathophysiology and rehabilitation. Br J Anaesth. 1997;78:606–17. https://doi.org/10.1093/BJA/78.5.606.
123. Gustafsson UO, Scott MJ, Hubner M, Nygren J, Demartines N, Francis N, et al. Guidelines for perioperative care in elective colorectal surgery: enhanced recovery after surgery (ERAS®) society recommendations: 2018. World J Surg. 2019;43:659–95. https://doi.org/10.1007/S00268-018-4844-Y.
124. Liu JY, Perez SD, Balch GG, Sullivan PS, Srinivasan JK, Staley CA, et al. Elderly patients benefit from enhanced recovery protocols after colorectal surgery. J Surg Res. 2021;266:54–61. https://doi.org/10.1016/J.JSS.2021.01.050.
125. Li J, Zhao F, Gao J, Dong W, Yu X, Zhu C, et al. Enhanced recovery after surgery (ERAS) protocol in geriatric patients underwent unicompartmental knee arthroplasty: a retrospective cohort study. Medicine. 2023:102. https://doi.org/10.1097/MD.0000000000032941.
126. Bagnall NM, Malietzis G, Kennedy RH, Athanasiou T, Faiz O, Darzi A. A systematic review of enhanced recovery care after colorectal surgery in elderly patients. Color Dis. 2014;16:947–56. https://doi.org/10.1111/CODI.12718.
127. Han H, Wan R, Chen J, Fan X, Zhang LW. Effects of the enhanced recovery after surgery (ERAS) protocol on the postoperative stress state and short-term complications in elderly patients with colorectal cancer. Cancer Rep (Hoboken). 2024;7 https://doi.org/10.1002/CNR2.1979.
128. Geltzeiler CB, Rotramel A, Wilson C, Deng L, Whiteford MH, Frankhouse J. Prospective study of colorectal enhanced recovery after surgery in a community hospital. JAMA Surg. 2014;149:955–61. https://doi.org/10.1001/JAMASURG.2014.675.
129. Liu JY, Wick EC. Enhanced recovery after surgery and effects on quality metrics. Surg Clin North Am. 2018;98:1119–27. https://doi.org/10.1016/J.SUC.2018.07.001.
130. Singh SJ, Danjoux G, Durrand J. Prehabilitation. Clin Med (Lond). 2019;19:458–64. https://doi.org/10.7861/CLINMED.2019-0257.
131. Barberan-Garcia A, Ubré M, Roca J, Lacy AM, Burgos F, Risco R, et al. Personalised prehabilitation in high-risk patients undergoing elective major abdominal surgery: a randomized blinded controlled trial. Ann Surg. 2018;267:50–6. https://doi.org/10.1097/SLA.0000000000002293.

132. Hughes MJ, Hackney RJ, Lamb PJ, Wigmore SJ, Christopher Deans DA, Skipworth RJE. Prehabilitation before major abdominal surgery: a systematic review and meta-analysis. World J Surg. 2019;43:1661–8. https://doi.org/10.1007/S00268-019-04950-Y.
133. Skořepa P, Ford KL, Alsuwaylihi A, O'Connor D, Prado CM, Gomez D, et al. The impact of prehabilitation on outcomes in frail and high-risk patients undergoing major abdominal surgery: a systematic review and meta-analysis. Clin Nutr. 2024;43:629–48. https://doi.org/10.1016/J.CLNU.2024.01.020.
134. Noorian S, Kwaan MR, Jaffe N, Yaceczko SD, Chau LW. Perioperative nutrition for gastrointestinal surgery: on the cutting edge. Nutr Clin Pract. 2023;38:539–56. https://doi.org/10.1002/NCP.10970.
135. Dag A, Colak T, Turkmenoglu O, Gundogdu R, Aydin S. A randomized controlled trial evaluating early versus traditional oral feeding after colorectal surgery. Clinics (Sao Paulo). 2011;66:2001–5. https://doi.org/10.1590/S1807-59322011001200001.
136. Le ZC, Ye XZ, Zhang CJ, Dong QT, Chen BC, Yu Z. Early versus traditional postoperative oral feeding in patients undergoing elective colorectal surgery: a meta-analysis of randomized clinical trials. Dig Surg. 2013;30:225–32. https://doi.org/10.1159/000353136.
137. Willcutts KF, Chung MC, Erenberg CL, Finn KL, Schirmer BD, Byham-Gray LD. Early oral feeding as compared with traditional timing of Oral feeding after upper gastrointestinal surgery: a systematic review and meta-analysis. Ann Surg. 2016;264:54–63. https://doi.org/10.1097/SLA.0000000000001644.
138. De Almeida EPM, De Almeida JP, Landoni G, Galas FRBG, Fukushima JT, Fominskiy E, et al. Early mobilization programme improves functional capacity after major abdominal cancer surgery: a randomized controlled trial. Br J Anaesth. 2017;119:900–7. https://doi.org/10.1093/BJA/AEX250.
139. Kitzman DW, Whellan DJ, Duncan P, Pastva AM, Mentz RJ, Reeves GR, et al. Physical rehabilitation for older patients hospitalized for heart failure. N Engl J Med. 2021;385:203–16. https://doi.org/10.1056/NEJMOA2026141.
140. Jalloun HE, Lee IK, Kim MK, Sung NY, Al Turkistani SA, Park SM, et al. Influence of the enhanced recovery after surgery protocol on postoperative inflammation and short-term postoperative surgical outcomes after colorectal cancer surgery. Ann Coloproctol. 2020;36:264–72. https://doi.org/10.3393/AC.2020.03.25.
141. Bernabei R, Landi F, Calvani R, Cesari M, Del Signore S, Anker SD, et al. Multicomponent intervention to prevent mobility disability in frail older adults: randomised controlled trial (SPRINTT project). BMJ. 2022:377. https://doi.org/10.1136/BMJ-2021-068788.
142. Rolland Y, Sierra F, Ferrucci L, Barzilai N, De Cabo R, Mannick J, et al. Challenges in developing Geroscience trials. Nat Commun. 2023:14. https://doi.org/10.1038/S41467-023-39786-7.
143. Garatachea N, Pareja-Galeano H, Sanchis-Gomar F, Santos-Lozano A, Fiuza-Luces C, Morán M, et al. Exercise attenuates the major hallmarks of aging. Rejuvenation Res. 2015;18:57–89. https://doi.org/10.1089/REJ.2014.1623.
144. Lippi L, de Sire A, Mezian K, Curci C, Perrero L, Turco A, et al. Impact of exercise training on muscle mitochondria modifications in older adults: a systematic review of randomized controlled trials. Aging Clin Exp Res. 2022;34:1495–510. https://doi.org/10.1007/S40520-021-02073-W.
145. Englund DA, Sakamoto AE, Fritsche CM, Heeren AA, Zhang X, Kotajarvi BR, et al. Exercise reduces circulating biomarkers of cellular senescence in humans. Aging Cell. 2021:20. https://doi.org/10.1111/ACEL.13415.
146. Kulkarni AS, Aleksic S, Berger DM, Sierra F, Kuchel GA, Barzilai N. Geroscience-guided repurposing of FDA-approved drugs to target aging: a proposed process and prioritization. Aging Cell. 2022:21. https://doi.org/10.1111/ACEL.13596.
147. Liu JK. Antiaging agents: safe interventions to slow aging and healthy life span extension. Nat Prod Bioprospect. 2022:12. https://doi.org/10.1007/S13659-022-00339-Y.
148. Kulkarni AS, Gubbi S, Barzilai N. Benefits of metformin in attenuating the hallmarks of aging. Cell Metab. 2020;32:15–30. https://doi.org/10.1016/J.CMET.2020.04.001.

149. Campbell JM, Bellman SM, Stephenson MD, Lisy K. Metformin reduces all-cause mortality and diseases of ageing independent of its effect on diabetes control: a systematic review and meta-analysis. Ageing Res Rev. 2017;40:31–44. https://doi.org/10.1016/J.ARR.2017.08.003.
150. Campbell JM, Stephenson MD, De Courten B, Chapman I, Bellman SM, Aromataris E. Metformin use associated with reduced risk of dementia in patients with diabetes: a systematic review and meta-analysis. J Alzheimers Dis. 2018;65:1225–36. https://doi.org/10.3233/JAD-180263.
151. Reitz KM, Marroquin OC, Zenati MS, Kennedy J, Korytkowski M, Tzeng E, et al. Association between preoperative metformin exposure and postoperative outcomes in adults with type 2 diabetes. JAMA Surg. 2020:155. https://doi.org/10.1001/JAMASURG.2020.0416.
152. Lin CS, Chang CC, Yeh CC, Chang YC, Chen TL, Liao CC. Outcomes after surgery in patients with diabetes who used metformin: a retrospective cohort study based on a real-world database. BMJ Open Diabetes Res Care. 2020:8. https://doi.org/10.1136/BMJDRC-2020-001351.
153. Kim C, Hwang JK. Flavonoids: nutraceutical potential for counteracting muscle atrophy. Food Sci Biotechnol. 2020;29:1619–40. https://doi.org/10.1007/S10068-020-00816-5.
154. Wang D, Yang Y, Zou X, Zhang J, Zheng Z, Wang Z. Antioxidant apigenin relieves age-related muscle atrophy by inhibiting oxidative stress and hyperactive mitophagy and apoptosis in skeletal muscle of mice. J Gerontol A Biol Sci Med Sci. 2020;75:2081–8. https://doi.org/10.1093/GERONA/GLAA214.
155. Liu L, Yue X, Sun Z, Hambright WS, Wei J, Li Y, et al. Reduction of senescent fibro-adipogenic progenitors in progeria-aged muscle by senolytics rescues the function of muscle stem cells. J Cachexia Sarcopenia Muscle. 2022;13:3137–48. https://doi.org/10.1002/JCSM.13101.
156. Oh HJ, Jin H, Lee BY. Hesperidin ameliorates sarcopenia through the regulation of inflammaging and the AKT/mTOR/FoxO3a signaling pathway in 22-26-month-old mice. Cells. 2023:12. https://doi.org/10.3390/CELLS12152015.
157. Lapatto HAK, Kuusela M, Heikkinen A, Muniandy M, van der Kolk BW, Gopalakrishnan S, et al. Nicotinamide riboside improves muscle mitochondrial biogenesis, satellite cell differentiation, and gut microbiota in a twin study. Sci Adv. 2023:9. https://doi.org/10.1126/SCIADV.ADD5163.
158. VanderVeen BN, Cardaci TD, Cunningham P, McDonald SJ, Bullard BM, Fan D, et al. Quercetin improved muscle mass and mitochondrial content in a murine model of cancer and chemotherapy-induced cachexia. Nutrients. 2022:15. https://doi.org/10.3390/NU15010102.
159. Momken I, Stevens L, Bergouignan A, Desplanches D, Rudwill F, Chery I, et al. Resveratrol prevents the wasting disorders of mechanical unloading by acting as a physical exercise mimetic in the rat. FASEB J. 2011;25:3646–60. https://doi.org/10.1096/FJ.10-177295.
160. Hosoda R, Nakashima R, Yano M, Iwahara N, Asakura S, Nojima I, et al. Resveratrol, a SIRT1 activator, attenuates aging-associated alterations in skeletal muscle and heart in mice. J Pharmacol Sci. 2023;152:112–22. https://doi.org/10.1016/J.JPHS.2023.04.001.
161. Ryu D, Mouchiroud L, Andreux PA, Katsyuba E, Moullan N, Nicolet-Dit-Félix AA, et al. Urolithin A induces mitophagy and prolongs lifespan in C. elegans and increases muscle function in rodents. Nat Med. 2016;22:879–88. https://doi.org/10.1038/NM.4132.
162. Rodriguez J, Pierre N, Naslain D, Bontemps F, Ferreira D, Priem F, et al. Urolithin B, a newly identified regulator of skeletal muscle mass. J Cachexia Sarcopenia Muscle. 2017;8:583–97. https://doi.org/10.1002/JCSM.12190.
163. Tao W, Ouyang Z, Liao Z, Li L, Zhang Y, Gao J, et al. Ursolic acid alleviates cancer cachexia and prevents muscle wasting via activating SIRT1. Cancers (Basel). 2023:15. https://doi.org/10.3390/CANCERS15082378.

Nutritional Support and Recovery: Lesson Learned from ERAS

22

Carolina Francesca Bolli

22.1 Introduction

Enhanced Recovery After Surgery (ERAS) protocols are evidence-based protocols developed to standardize and optimize perioperative care to reduce trauma, physiological stress, and organ dysfunctions (metabolic, endocrine, and inflammatory response) as well as reduce protein catabolism induced by surgery [1] (Fig. 22.1).

The concept of mitigating postoperative stress and enhancing the patient's response to surgical trauma dates back to 1990, when first Danish surgeon Henrik Kehlet critically analyzed traditional perioperative management and questioned the related practices that consisted in preoperative fasting, mobility restrictions, bowel preparation, and slow resumption of feeding after surgery [2]. Kehlet therefore devised a protocol he called Fast Track Surgery that was based on abolishing the preoperative procedures used until then and replacing them with new criteria. This protocol resulted in a significantly improved postoperative course, thus reducing the length of hospitalization, metabolic stress, fluid overload, and insulin resistance.

The idea of founding a European group of surgeons to take up, develop, and disseminate the new Fast Track Surgery philosophy came from Kenneth Fearon of the University of Edinburgh and Olle Ljungqvist of Karolinska Institutet, during a congress on perioperative nutrition held in 2001 in London; the ERAS Study Group was born, consisting of surgeons and anesthesiologists who carried out a review of the literature and the current evidence related to optimal perioperative care [3].

By this assumption, they developed a 20-item protocol and published the first ERAS guidelines in 2005 [4]. In 2010, the ERAS Society, a non-profit medical society based in Stockholm, was officially founded.

C. F. Bolli (✉)
UOC Diabetes and Dietetics, Hospital San Filippo Neri, Rome, Italy
e-mail: carolinafrancesca.bolli@aslroma1.it

V. Boccardi, L. Marano (eds.), *The Frail Surgical Patient*, Practical Issues in Geriatrics, https://doi.org/10.1007/978-3-031-77707-3_22

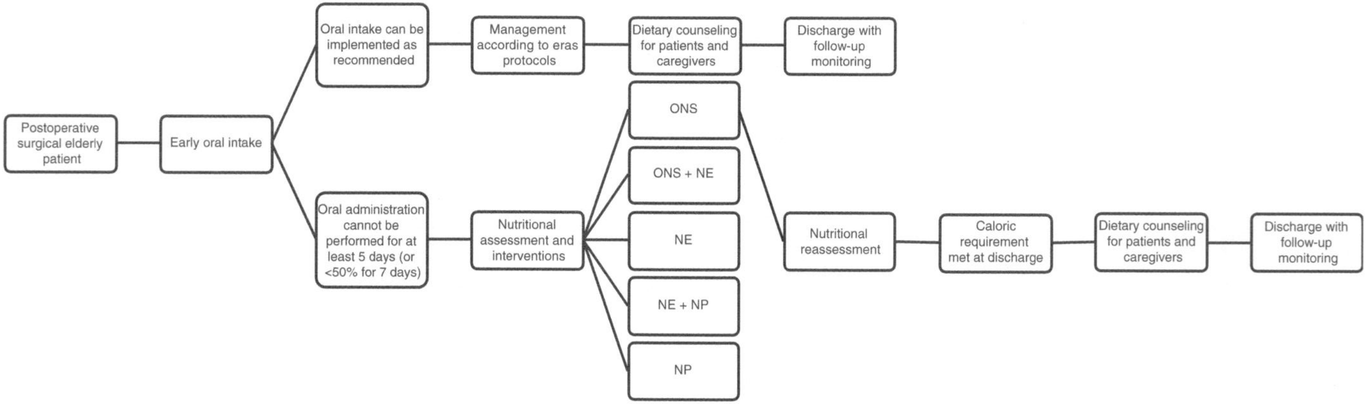

Fig. 22.1 Postoperative nutritional care process for older persons

22.2 The Items of ERAS

The ERAS protocol is an integrated, multidisciplinary approach that first involves the patient, who is properly informed and prepared, and then the hospital team that includes surgeons, anesthesiologists, nursing staff, nutritionists, dietitians, and physical and occupational therapists [5].

The pivotal concept guiding the ERAS protocol is to reduce the stressful impact that elective major surgery has on the patient. The goals are early recovery after surgery and reduced complication rates, which also translates into reduced length of postoperative stay and reduced material and social costs.

The protocol divides the perioperative period into 3 phases: pre-, intra-, and post-operative. Both the 2018 ERAS Society guidelines [6] and the 2019 POIS-Associazione Chirurghi Ospedalieri Italiani joint guidelines [7] point out the 25 items, divided into 4 phases: the preadmission phase, the preoperative phase, the intraoperative phase, and the postoperative phase (Table 22.1).

From a metabolic nutritional perspective, ERAS programs involve a trimodal approach that includes nutrition, exercise, and the psychological component of stress reduction. This approach has demonstrated a significant reduction in the

Table 22.1 ERAS Protocol Items

Preadmission items
1. Information
2. Optimization
3. Prehabilitation
4. Nutrition
5. Anemia screening
Preoperative items
6. Prevention of nausea and vomiting (PONV)
7. Selective premedication
8. Prophylactic antibiotics
9. No bowel preparation
10. Maintaining Euvolemia
11. No fasting and carbohydrate drink
Intraoperative items
12. Standard anesthetic protocol
13. Fluid Normovolemia
14. Normothermia
15. Minimally invasive surgery
16. No drainage
Postoperative items
17. Nasogastric intubation
18. Multimodal analgesia
19. Thromboprophylaxis
20. Fluid Normovolemia
21. Urinary Cath 1–3 D
22. Prevention of postoperative ileus
23. Prevent hyperglycemia
24. Postoperative nutrition
25. Early mobilization

number of complications and reduced length of stay (LOS) in high-risk elderly patients in grades III and IV according to the American Society of Anesthesiologists (ASA) classification [8]. The first key element of the ERAS protocol is patient information: In fact, comprehensive preoperative counseling in which adequate and detailed explanations and information are provided to the patient can reduce anxiety related to the surgical event and the postoperative phase. This requires the involvement of the entire multidisciplinary team whose role is to guide, assist, and inform the patient and relatives in the surgical course before and during hospitalization [6].

A preoperative nutritional assessment of the patient candidate for surgery is essential to detect the possible presence of ongoing malnutrition or risk of malnutrition, this becomes even more important in the geriatric population. This gives us the opportunity to intervene early, improve nutritional status, and correct specific deficits. We have several validated tools available for malnutrition screening (MUST, NRS, Subjective Global Assessment), but the Mini Nutritional Assessment (MNA) is specific for the geriatric population [9].

In patients who had unintentional weight loss of 5–10% and in patients at risk of malnutrition, the risk of postoperative complications is increased so preoperative nutritional treatment is necessary in these cases. Nutritional intervention using oral nutritional supplements (ONS) or enteral nutrition (EN) or parenteral nutrition (PN) has better results if started as early as 7–10 days before surgery and has been associated with a reduction in the prevalence of infectious complications and anastomotic leakage [6]. Therefore, perioperative nutritional therapy should be started even if it is expected that the patient will not be able to feed for more than 5 days in the perioperative period. It is also indicated in patients in whom reduced oral intake is expected and who cannot maintain more than 50% of the recommended intake for more than 7 days. If oral nutrition and the use of ONS are not sufficient to maintain adequate nutritional status, the enteral route should always be preferred over parenteral nutrition. Parenteral nutrition should be administered as soon as possible if there is contraindication to enteral nutrition.

When patients do not cover their energy needs with spontaneous oral feeding, it is recommended to encourage ONS intake during the preoperative period regardless of nutritional status. In the preoperative period, ONS should be given to all malnourished cancer patients and high-risk patients (among whom sarcopenic elderly constitute a special group) who are to undergo major abdominal surgery. Immunomodulatory ONS (which include arginine, omega-3 fatty acids, and nucleotides) may be preferred and administered for 5–7 days in the preoperative period. Patients with severe nutritional risk should receive nutritional therapy before major surgery even if it has been delayed. A period of 7–14 days may be appropriate. Preoperative PN should be given only to patients with malnutrition or severe nutritional risk in whom energy requirements cannot be adequately met by EN. A period of 7–14 days is recommended [8].

Avoiding fasting is a key component of the ERAS protocol. Preoperative fasting from midnight is not necessary in most patients, and patients undergoing surgery who are considered not at specific risk of aspiration can drink clear liquids up to 2 h before anesthesia and solids up to 6 h before anesthesia.

Preoperative intake of a carbohydrate beverage (12.5% maltodextrin) volume of 800 mL the night before and 400 mL 2–4 h before surgery reduces perioperative discomfort—including anxiety—as well as postoperative insulin resistance, length of hospital stays, and improves postoperative well-being [8].

Insulin resistance is a hallmark of the body's physiological response to surgery-induced trauma and can persist several weeks after surgery, as well as it is the cause of postoperative hyperglycemia. Increased insulin resistance and blood glucose levels have been seen to be associated with increased risk of complications and mortality after major abdominal surgery. Insulin resistance and hyperglycemia lead to osmotic fluid passage in the vascular space and increased glucose availability to glucose-dependent tissues, such as white blood cells and the brain.

A large RCT showed that oral carbohydrate loading in the preoperative phase moderated glucose concentrations in the postoperative phase and reduced the need for insulin [10]. Further studies have shown that the application of ERAS protocols in surgery is associated with partial or complete attenuation of postoperative stress. In particular, they found unchanged postoperative nitrogen losses, neutral nitrogen balance, minimal insulin resistance, and preserved normoglycemia during feeding after major colorectal surgery [11].

22.3 Early Mobilization

To date, we can say that early mobilization after surgery is a key component of perioperative care, a key element in the application of the ERAS protocol, and one of the cornerstones in avoiding postoperative complications. Patients derive several benefits from early mobilization: avoidance of muscular and cardiovascular decay, improved mood, decreased risk of developing pulmonary complications, and low incidence of thromboembolic and insulin resistance disorders.

However, although there is plenty of evidence regarding the detrimental effects of immobilization, there is limited evidence regarding the benefit of dedicated interventions specifically designed to increase early mobilization after surgery [6].

Active patient participation is critical in order to reduce overall hospital length of stay, reduce complication rates, and have better tolerance to per os diet as early as the first few hours after surgery, so it may be helpful to find tools that encourage the patient to move. However, patient mobilization is still a critical component of the program, since age, comorbidities, and surgical procedures risk compromising overall performance.

Early mobilization can occur as early as postoperative days 0–3. In fact, it is believed to be safe and effective to achieve mobilization even within a few hours of the end of surgery by stimulating the patient to perform simple initial exercises while remaining in bed, and then later get up and take small steps within the room or ward whenever possible.

An important consideration to make is that failure of early mobilization is caused by a variety of factors including patient motivation and performance that should be improved during prehabilitation and preoperative counseling, preexisting comorbidities, or postoperative factors such as inadequate pain control, continuous intravenous (IV) fluid intake, prolonged indwelling urinary catheter, and inadequate PONV control.

On the other hand, a standard definition of appropriate early mobilization is still lacking, as the goals differ in different local protocols, and there is not yet enough evidence to support the importance of allocating additional resources that can take care of this aspect.

In conclusion, early mobilization through patient education and encouragement is a key component of the ERAS protocol, and prolonged immobilization is associated with a variety of adverse effects [7].

22.4 Postoperative Nutritional Care

In most cases, oral nutrition can begin within a few hours of surgery. This component of the ERAS protocol has demonstrated a significantly reduced rate of complications and LOS [8]. Even after colorectal surgery, early oral nutrition within 24 h can lead to a shorter length of hospital stay and reduce the risk of postoperative complications. Notably, early resumption of oral feeding does not appear to have a detrimental effect on the anastomotic healing process, nor does it increase the rate of colorectal anastomosis leakage [7].

However, it is recommended that oral intake be adjusted according to individual tolerance and the type of intervention performed with particular caution in elderly patients. Notably, the quantity of ingesta should be adapted to the state of gastrointestinal function and individual tolerance [8].

Surgery results in a number of responses to the body including the release of stress hormones and mediators of inflammation (cytokines). The cytokine response to infection and injury has a major impact on metabolism, i.e., it causes catabolism of glycogen, fat, and protein with release into the circulation of glucose, free fatty acids, and amino acids, so that substrates are diverted from their normal purpose of maintaining peripheral protein mass (especially muscle) to the tasks of healing and immune response.

Nutritional therapy can provide the energy for optimal healing and recovery, but in the immediate postoperative phase it can only minimally counteract muscle catabolism. To restore protein masses, the body must adequately deal with the surgical trauma and possible infections, so that there must be adequate nutritional status or support and exercise.

The importance of resuming a normal diet early after surgery is even more stressed by the association between decreased food intake and in-hospital mortality, and between increased morbidity and decreased food intake. Avoiding any additional nutritional therapy also carries the risk of undernutrition during the postoperative course after major surgery, since it is necessary to achieve energy and protein requirements [7].

Further assessment of nutritional status after surgery is recommended, as well as its regular monitoring and follow-up during hospital stay, and, if necessary, continuation of nutritional support therapy and skilled dietary counseling after discharge. If oral intake cannot be implemented for 5 days or if ingestions are less than 50% of requirements for more than 7 days, it is necessary to intervene with nutritional support therapy. Supportive therapy may involve the administration of ONS or consider artificial nutrition.

Early EN within 24 h after surgery should be implemented in patients in whom early oral nutrition cannot be started and in whom oral intake will be inadequate (<50%) for more than 7 days. It is recommended to start EN at a low rate (10–20 mL/h) and increase the rate gradually according to individual tolerance, due to limited intestinal tolerance, while the target may be reached by 5–7 days. Postoperative administration of a specific formula enriched with arginine, omega-3 fatty acids, and ribonucleotides is recommended for malnourished patients undergoing major cancer surgery. If energy and nutrient requirements cannot be met by oral and enteral intake alone for more than 7 days, a combination of EN and NP is recommended. Exclusive NP should be administered if there is contraindication to EN, such as in intestinal obstruction [8].

Thus, there is wide evidence that minimal preoperative fasting, carbohydrate loading, early resumption of normal solid diet, and early mobilization are associated with reduced surgical stress response, as well as reduced morbidity, length of stay, and hospitalization costs.

22.5 Oral Nutritional Supplements (ONS)

Several studies have highlighted the fact that in the immediate postoperative period spontaneous food intake rarely reaches the expected target, and therefore, patients tend to lose weight and especially muscle mass. Therefore, it may be important to try to increase the routine use of oral nutritional supplements (ONS) in ERAS protocols to supplement total food intake. Some randomized controlled trials evaluated the effects of ONS use in postoperative care on nutritional and functional parameters as well as clinical outcomes and healthcare costs. There is some evidence to suggest that ONS improves weight reduction, nutritional intake, lower incidence of complications, and reduced hospital stay [7].

22.6 Immunonutrition

Surgical stress can result in acute arginine deficiency, impair immune function, particularly T cells, compromise wound healing capacity, and increase the risk of postoperative infectious complications. Immunonutrition was developed to improve the perioperative immune-metabolic and inflammatory response. Specifically, it involves the administration of biologically active nutrients with immunomodulatory and anti-inflammatory properties usually administered orally or enterally. Immunonutrient mixtures containing omega-3 fatty acids, arginine, and ribonucleotides are believed to reduce postoperative infectious complications, and favorably modify immune and inflammatory responses. Based on an extensive review of multiple RCTs and meta-analyses, the ESPEN guidelines on perioperative nutrition recommend that peri-or at least postoperative administration of immunonutrients (arginine, n-3 FA, and ribonucleotides) for malnourished patients undergoing major cancer surgery. Therefore, immunonutrition should be encouraged in clinical practice and within ERAS protocols [6, 7].

22.7 Nutritional Management of the Older Patient

The older patient is at increased risk of malnutrition for several causes, such as aging-induced anorexia and the presence of acute and/or chronic diseases that often induce catabolism.

As we have already discussed extensively, malnutrition is related to increased risk of infectious complications, length of hospital stay, morbidity and mortality, as well as the occurrence of dehydration, sarcopenia, and frailty [12]. Therefore, proper nutrition is necessary in this category of patients, especially in those individuals who have undergone surgery.

22.8 Nutritional Needs

In the elderly, an intake of 30 kcal/kg body weight per day is recommended; this value should be adjusted individually according to nutritional status, level of physical activity, and presence of disease [9].

As for protein intake, 1–1.2 g/kg body weight is recommended in order to preserve lean body mass and prevent sarcopenia. In cases of disease, protein requirements appear to be increased due to inflammation and possible ongoing infections, although there is insufficient evidence to suggest increasing protein intakes above those recommended. However, it is important to note that insufficient energy intake increases protein requirements, so it is important to ensure not only adequate protein intake but also adequate energy intake [13].

Elderly patients, also due to the polypharmacotherapy they are subjected to, often suffer from gastrointestinal problems including constipation and diarrhea. Therefore, a daily intake of 25 g of dietary fiber is recommended to help normalize bowel function [9].

Provided there are no specific deficiencies, micronutrients should be provided according to the recommendation of the European Food Safety Authority (EFSA) or corresponding national nutritional societies for healthy elderly people [14].

It is recommended a daily intake of 1.6 L/2 L of water, respectively for women and man, unless there is a clinical condition that requires a different approach (such as in heart and kidney failure that requires restriction of fluid intake; conversely, additional intake is required in the presence of high temperatures, increased physical activity, fever, diarrhea, or vomiting) [9].

22.9 Home and Institutional Nutritional Management

Any healthcare facility specifically for elderly patients should possess a multidisciplinary team that collaborates and communicates synergistically. The expertise of multiple professions allows us to achieve adequate dietary intake, maintain and/or increase body weight, and improve functional and clinical outcomes. In institutional settings, standard operating procedures for nutrition and hydration care should be established and responsibilities should be well regulated. Particular attention should be paid to interface management, as important information regarding nutritional status is often lost as patients transition to another healthcare setting.

The implementation of a screening protocol and the implementation of a nutrition care plan within these facilities have been shown to improve energy and protein intake and, consequently, maintenance of adequate body weight, while at the same time reducing the rate of hospital infections and improving the nutritional status, quality of life, and health of patients.

In addition, it would be important for healthcare providers and caregivers to be offered nutrition education, by dieticians and dietitians, in order to ensure awareness and basic knowledge about nutritional problems, thus promoting appropriate dietary intake of elderly people with malnutrition or at risk of malnutrition so to ensure better care processes [9].

22.10 Screening, Assessment, Intervention, and Monitoring

It is important to screen for nutritional status even in the postoperative phase using validated tests such as the MNA, which is specific to the geriatric population, in order to identify subjects who are malnourished or at risk of malnutrition and intervene to prevent or treat it [15].

Diagnosed subjects should undergo a comprehensive assessment of nutritional status. Then, an individualized nutrition care plan can be developed and implemented from the perspective of a multidisciplinary team approach. All aspects of the patient, both physical and mental/psychological, social, clinical, and ethical, and all options used to ensure adequate dietary intake, should be considered.

The intervention process should be monitored, and re-evaluations should be carried out at regular intervals in order to check whether the goals have been achieved. If not, goals and interventions should be adjusted according to the problems that have arisen. It is important to initiate appropriate nutritional care after discharge so to ensure the continuation of nutritional interventions initiated in the hospital.

In particular, many elderly people present difficulties in independent meal management due to functional and cognitive limitations, therefore, support ranging from positioning patients at the table, encouragement of food intake to direct physical assistance at meals may be needed, which should be provided both in inpatient facilities and at home. Equally important would be encouraging eating in company and creating a family and serene atmosphere during meals: in fact, eating is a social act that is known to stimulate dietary intake, even in the elderly.

Another important element is the nutritional information and education that professionals such as dietitians or dieticians must provide to elderly individuals in order to improve awareness and knowledge of nutritional problems and thus promote adequate nutrition. Finally, older persons with malnutrition or at risk of malnutrition should be encouraged to be physically active and exercise to maintain or improve muscle mass and function. In fact, in such individuals, weight loss occurs at the expense of muscle mass resulting in impaired physical performance. Reduced muscle training and periods of allurement can further exacerbate this condition. Again, it is necessary for a professional to identify the type of training, intensity, and starting level appropriate to the elderly individual's physical condition.

References

1. Paduraru M, et al. Enhanced recovery after surgery (ERAS)—the evidence in geriatric emergency surgery: a systematic review. Chirurgia (Bucur). 2017;112:546. https://doi.org/10.21614/chirurgia.112.5.546.
2. Pędziwiatr M, et al. Current status of enhanced recovery after surgery (ERAS) protocol in gastrointestinal surgery. Med Oncol. 2018;35:95. https://doi.org/10.1007/s12032-018-1153-0.
3. Ljungqvist O, et al. Enhanced recovery after surgery: a review. JAMA Surg. 2017;152(3):292–8. https://doi.org/10.1001/jamasurg.2016.4952.
4. Fearon KCH, et al. Enhanced recovery after surgery: a consensus review of clinical care for patients undergoing colonic resection. Clin Nutr. 2005;24(3):466–77. https://doi.org/10.1016/j.clnu.2005.02.002.
5. Kehlet H, et al. Evidence-based surgical care and the evolution of fast-track surgery. Ann Surg. 2008;248(2):189–98. https://doi.org/10.1097/SLA.0b013e31817f2c1a.
6. Gustafsson UO, et al. Guidelines for perioperative Care in Elective Colorectal Surgery: enhanced recovery after surgery (ERAS) society recommendations: 2018. World J Surg. 2019;43:659–95. https://doi.org/10.1007/s00268-018-4844-y.
7. Ficari F, et al. Enhanced recovery pathways in colorectal surgery: a consensus paper by the Associazione Chirurghi Ospedalieri Italiani (ACOI) and the PeriOperative Italian society (POIS). G Chir. 2019;40(1):1–40.
8. Weimann A, et al. ESPEN guideline: clinical nutrition in surgery. Clin Nutr. 2017;36:623–50. https://doi.org/10.1016/j.clnu.2017.02.013.
9. Volkert D, Beck AM, Cederholm T, Cruz-Jentoft A, Goisser S, Hooper L, Kiesswetter E, Maggio M, Raynaud-Simon A, Sieber CC, Sobotka L, van Asselt D, Wirth R, Bischoff SC. ESPEN guideline on clinical nutrition and hydration in geriatrics. Clin Nutr. 2019;38(1):10–47. https://doi.org/10.1016/j.clnu.2018.05.024. Epub 2018 Jun 18.
10. Gianotti L, Biffi R, Sandini M, et al. Preoperative oral carbohydrate load versus placebo in major elective abdominal surgery (PROCY): a randomized, placebo-controlled, multi-center, phase III trial. Ann Surg. 2018;267:623–30. https://doi.org/10.1097/SLA.0000000000002325.
11. Soop M, Nygren J, Thorell A, et al. Preoperative oral carbohydrate treatment attenuates endogenous glucose release 3 days after surgery. Clin Nutr. 2004;23:733–41. https://doi.org/10.1016/j.clnu.2003.12.007.
12. Agarwal E, Miller M, Yaxley A, Isenring E. Malnutrition in the elderly: a narrative review. Maturitas. 2013;76(4):296–e302.
13. Deutz NE, Bauer JM, Barazzoni R, Biolo G, Boirie Y, Bosy-Westphal A, et al. Protein intake and exercise for optimal muscle function with aging: recommendations from the ESPEN expert group. Clin Nutr. 2014;33:929–e36.

14. EFSA. Dietary reference values for nutrients: summary report. EFSA Support Rep. 2017;2017:e15121.
15. Vellas B, Villars H, Abellan G, et al. Overview of MNA®—its history and challenges. J Nutr Health Aging. 2006;10:466–87.

The Physiotherapist: The Importance of Early Functional Recovery

23

Felice Picariello, Maria Marella Carbone, Luca Barni, Manuel González Sánchez, Alejandro Galán-Mercant, and Patricia Froes Meyer

23.1 Introduction

23.1.1 The Importance of Physical Therapy in the Geriatric Patient

The World Health Organisation, in its World Report on Ageing and Health, emphasized how life expectancy worldwide has increased, estimating that by 2030 one in six people will be 60 years or older. This extension of life expectancy is an incredibly valuable resource, because it offers the opportunity to reconsider not only what old age looks like, but also how our entire lives might unfold. However, the extent of the opportunities arising from these extra years of life depends heavily on one key factor: *health* [1, 2].

F. Picariello (✉)
Health education and sustainable development – UNESCO, Federico II University, Naples, Italy
e-mail: felice.picariello@unina.it

M. M. Carbone
Physiotherapy and Rehabilitation, Rehabil Clinic, Somma Vesuviana, Italy

L. Barni
Physiotherapy, Montecatini Terme, Montecatini Terme, Toscana, Italy

M. G. Sánchez
Physiotherapy, University of Malaga, Malaga, Spain
e-mail: mgsa23@uma.es

A. Galán-Mercant
Nursing and Physiotherapy Department, University of Cadiz, Cadiz, Spain
e-mail: alejandro.galan@uca.es

P. F. Meyer
Physiotherapy, IRG – International Research Group, Natal, Brasil

V. Boccardi, L. Marano (eds.), *The Frail Surgical Patient*, Practical Issues in Geriatrics, https://doi.org/10.1007/978-3-031-77707-3_23

Interventions aimed at achieving optimal health range from preventive medicine to surgery, and, a particularly prominent role has historically been played by physiotherapy. Indeed, starting from prevention to specific therapies in cases of overt disability, it provides interventions aimed at assessing, treating and, more generally, taking care of the patient, guiding them to achieve an improvement in their quality of life. This is particularly important when dealing with a geriatric patient, a term that indicates a condition that is not simply age-related, but one of objective *frailty*.

In fact, the rehabilitation of the sick older person implies, by definition, a complex intervention in which it is necessary to combine technical skills that take into account not only the impairment itself, but also other concomitant pathologies and impairments, past experiences, and the expectations of the patient and family.

But over the years it has been amply demonstrated how physiotherapy intervention, whether it is directed at musculoskeletal, cardiological, respiratory, or neurological aspects, can guarantee to the patient an improvement in quality of life as well as greater autonomy in activities of daily living (ADL) [3–7].

Another area in which physiotherapy plays a key role in preserving the health condition of the geriatric patient is related to hospitalization, particularly before and after surgery. Over the years, it has been shown that hospitalization of the geriatric patient results in several negative consequences, such as cognitive decline, reduced muscle strength and mobility, and worsening respiratory conditions, but there is ample evidence that early physiotherapy intervention can positively interfere with all these aspects.

23.1.2 Hospitalization-Related Risks in the Geriatric Patient

The increase in life expectancy and the consequent increase in the elderly population leads to several consequences, one of which is an increased risk of hospitalization [8].

In line with this, approximately 30–60% of patients aged 65 and over were found to experience functional decline during hospitalization, resulting in decreased autonomy, increased dependence, rise in medical cost and family burden, prolonged hospitalization, growth in readmission rate, and long-term institutionalization in a care facility [9].

This is because frail patients admitted to acute care hospitals, including those who are able to walk independently, spend most of their time in the hospital in bed. However, an individualized, multicomponent exercise program has been shown to be safe and effective in reversing the functional decline associated with hospitalization [10].

The intervention of a physical therapist during hospitalization is necessary to prevent further serious consequences related to bed rest, including the risk of falls. Falls can result in consequences of varying degrees, including minor injuries (such as lacerations, contusions, sprains, and strains) but also more serious injuries such as head trauma, fractures, and death [11]; in addition, anxiety and fear of falling can arise following a fall [12]. Fall prevention programs in the hospital include various strategies such as patient education, adaptation of the environment, use of assistive devices, management of cognitive impairment, and a key intervention is represented by rehabilitation and exercise therapies [13].

An additional critical aspect related to the hospitalization of the geriatric patient is the onset of delirium, which is a medical emergency characterized by a disturbance of attention, awareness, and cognitive function developed over a short period of time. Several studies have reported that up to one third of patients over 70 years of age admitted to any medical unit develop delirium, a percentage that increases up to 50% in surgical units and up to 85% in palliative care units [14]. Since delirium has a multifactorial etiology, a single component approach is not recommended; for this reason, interventions that have proven effective in preventing or treating delirium are multimodal strategies that act on different risk factors of delirium, such as cognitive impairment, sleep deprivation, immobility, dehydration, and vision or hearing impairment.

But considering that it has been widely shown that delirium and physical function are closely related, one of the most widely used prevention strategies is exercise at each of the critical moments, from primary care, during hospital stay and after discharge [14].

Therefore frailty, which represents a new medical concept defined as *"a clinically recognizable state of increased vulnerability that is the result of an aging-related decline in function in multiple physiological organ systems, such that the ability to cope with daily or acute stressors is compromised"* [15] is to date a major challenge for all healthcare professionals. But a meticulous approach based on comprehensive geriatric assessment can ensure countless benefits for older patients and prevent serious consequences related to hospitalization [16].

23.2 Prehabilitation: Role in Geriatric Surgery

Prehabilitation is when people undergoing scheduled surgery are encouraged to develop a series of salable behaviours to promote therapeutic success. For this, four disciplines (health education, physical exercise, psychological intervention, and nutrition) are integrated within the same action program, making prehabilitation multi- and interdisciplinary [17, 18].

For the support of the patient before, during and after a surgical process, prehabilitation has been developed as a process that pursues the patient's psychological improvement and physical function. In this sense, the development of a pre-rehabilitation program can favor the following:

- favor the acceleration of the patient's recovery process;
- improve clinical results in the short, medium, and long term;
- optimize the resources of the health system;
- improve the patient's clinical experience [19].

Analyzing surgical prehabilitation as a complex and multimodal therapeutic process, it is easy to see how its main objectives are the improvement of mental and physical aspects, focusing, like the more specific ones, on the reduction of risk factors, whether pre-surgical or post-surgical, optimizing, the capacities of the patient, the resources (economic, human, logistic, etc.) of the health system and the improvement, as the ultimate goal of improving the quality of life of the patient and shortening recovery times [20].

On the other hand, prehabilitation pursues progressive empowerment of the patient, making him the center of the therapeutic process and the leading actor in it, beginning his participation long before the surgical intervention and ending long after the said intervention. During the process, the patient will learn much about the pathological process he is suffering from, the best interventions the scientific literature recommends, and how his participation can promote therapeutic success or enhance its positive outcome [17, 19].

In this sense, in order for a pre-surgical rehabilitation program to be designed correctly, it must attend to five specific principles [18–20]:

- use interventions with the most solid scientific evidence;
- make the patient active in the intervention through an educational and participative preparatory (and preoperative) phase;
- establish outcome variables and the methods for their assessment, follow-up, and analysis;
- select prehabilitation programs that are sustainable over time;
- analyze the local community, identify their needs, and seek their satisfaction.

23.2.1 Main Recommendations of the Scientific Literature

According to the literature, a surgical pre-rehabilitation program must be based on four interventions that are differentiated between them and, at the same time, intercorrelated. This multimodal and multidisciplinary intervention should include a health education program, a nutritional intervention, a physical exercise program, and a psychological care program (Fig. 23.1) [17, 18].

23.2.1.1 Health Education Program

Offering the patient helpful information about their pathological process and the different stages they face during a surgical process facilitates, on the one hand, that they become an active part of the therapeutic process, allowing better consensual and informed decision-making. The information must be transferred as soon as possible and, among other aspects, must inform the patient of aspects such as:

- Times:
  - time available before surgery;
  - hospital stay time;
  - expected time from surgical intervention to final discharge.

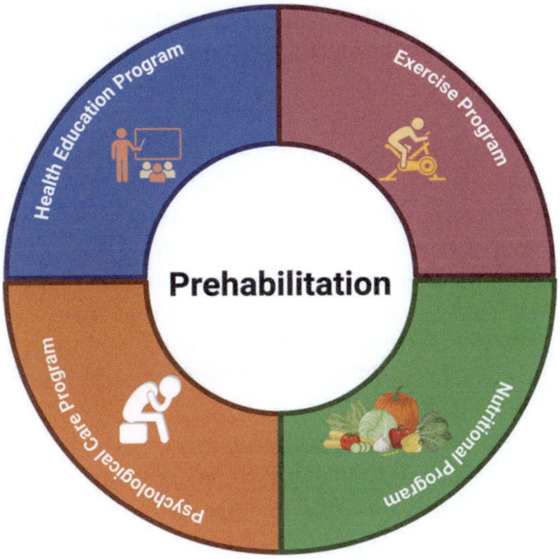

Fig. 23.1 Four pillars on which a prehabilitation program is based

– Potential side effects of surgery and strategies to mitigate or shorten them over time.

When designing the educational material that will be made available to the patient, it will be necessary to consider the different actors that will participate in the process: the clinical team, the patient, the relatives, and in some cases, the caregivers, etc. In this process, the patient must understand that there are three distinct phases [17, 19–22]:

– preparation for the surgical process;
– hospital phase;
– the phase of reincorporation to the activities of daily life.

23.2.1.2 Exercise Program

When carrying out a physical exercise program, it is very important to consider the design of an intervention that can be developed (or adaptable) to the three different environments that the patient will face throughout the therapeutic process: Community environments, hospital, and ambulatory care settings. In this sense, physiotherapy will play a fundamental role as it is a discipline that has the necessary training to know all the relevant aspects of the surgical process, it has transversal training in the four basic pillars of a pre-rehabilitation program, so it could participate as a coordinator of the program [22].

When making a proposal for an exercise program, it is important to consider what type of exercises should be part of the training program. In this sense, a balance must be found between strength, respiratory function, and cardiovascular health, clinical and functional objectives that, as indicated before in terms of their need, can be developed in the previously mentioned settings. In this sense, it is essential to consider the functional possibilities of the patient, the physical possibilities of being able to carry out the proposed exercise program and, at the same time, it is important to have planned the different adaptations that could be necessary during the development of the therapeutic physical exercise program [23].

In order to assess the evolution suffered by the patient during the different stages in which a surgical process breaks down, the clinical professionals who work together in the prehabilitation program have had to decide, prior to the start of the program, what the variables would be, Outcome and how they can be measured. In this sense, it is essential to include at least one functional variable, measurable through the different tests that, due to their psychometric characteristics or the frequency of clinical use, are more frequently found in the literature [24].

23.2.1.3 Nutritional Program

When carrying out a nutritional program as part of the patient's pre-habilitative program, it is essential to consider those aspects that, if not acted correctly, occur regularly in a surgical process. Among the episodes that can be found, sarcopenia and malnutrition stand out above the rest, appearing more frequently in certain population groups, such as older adults or frail people [25, 26].

An assessment and follow-up of the patient's nutritional status are essential before a surgical process to identify eventual states of malnutrition that could condition therapeutic success. Based on this assessment, follow-up can be done to be able to intervene, if necessary, through changes in the patient's diet or even through nutritional supplements.

If a state of malnutrition is identified, intense intervention strategies could be designed with a duration that could last between 7 and 30 days (depending on the case) and could be complemented with the health education program. The main objectives to be pursued are [25, 26]:

- to solve malnutrition prior to the surgical process, or at least minimize it;
- to support the nutritional requirements that the physical training program or a modulation of the corporal composition could need;
- to prepare the patient nutritionally to face the surgical process with guarantees.

It is very important that nutritional programs be developed by a group of clinical professionals who will participate in the surgical process, such as anesthesiologists and surgeons, supported by a nutritionist. The objective will be to recover the correct nutritional status by the patient, but always considering those fundamental aspects that must be taken into account when carrying out the surgical process, such as the regulation of fluid intake or eventual fasting [27].

23.2.1.4 Psychological Care Program

Traditionally, when talking about pre-surgical prehabilitation, great emphasis has been placed on the patient's preparation from a physical point of view. However, the scientific evidence is increasingly solid about the need to incorporate psychological care programs as a necessary strategy to improve clinical results [28].

The psychological care program's main objectives are oriented towards improving anxiety management, preoperative self-efficacy, or depression, which have been associated with a better postoperative quality of life in different patient profiles, such as elderly, frail, or cancer patients [28, 29].

The main aspects that are usually addressed by a psychological care program integrated into a pre-rehabilitation program, before and after surgery, are [28, 29]:

- help the patient to acquire relaxation techniques that allow him to face the surgical episode more serenely;
- evaluate patients to identify potential risks of exacerbation of cognitive impairment or delirium during the preoperative period;
- train the patient in techniques that allow better control of stress, anxiety, or depression and their coping strategies;
- during the postoperative process, interventions should be designed to increase their ability to control emotions and beliefs and improve the patient's attitude and commitment to pain control or certain health behaviors.
- In the same way that has happened with the rest of the programs that make up a process of rehabilitation of the patient in order to face major surgery, in the case of the psychological care program, it is necessary to establish tools for the assessment of the psychological aspects of the patient and thus being able to evaluate their evolution throughout the therapeutic process.

23.2.2 Prehabilitation in Older Patients with Cancer

Fortunately, the number of surviving patients of any cancer has increased significantly in recent years. However, this has also led to a series of symptoms and variables that should be considered when designing an intervention program for cancer patients.

For this, the planning of a clinical intervention process must address all the stages in which a patient is involved. Preparation for the surgical process is a fundamental part of this clinical process. In this sense, pre-awakening is presented as a tool that helps to improve functionality throughout the therapeutic process; correctly considering and evaluating the basal state at the time of making a diagnosis is essential to be able to establish objectives and determine the potential effects that cancer surgery can cause in the patient and thus plan their intervention before it occurs, considering in this perspective both the physical and psychological state of the patient and their functionality or the possible levels of disability that the intervention could cause in it [30, 31].

Although prehabilitation was understood as a single-modal intervention strategy a few years ago, in recent years, different disciplines have been integrated to make a much more holistic intervention for the patient, considering not only the physical aspect but also the nutritional aspect. The emotional aspect, stress management, or even the medical dimension helps control comorbidities [30–32].

The main objective pursued through the intervention with prehabilitation is to favor a faster recovery of the patient in the short term and, at the same time, an improvement in the quality of life of functional independence and community reintegration in the medium and long term, without forgetting that there are studies that have shown the effectiveness of physical exercise and complementary interventions to avoid recurrences of the oncological process [31].

Therefore, the pre-surgical period increases the patient's physiological reserve in anticipation of neoadjuvant therapies and the surgery itself so that the postoperative process is facilitated, contributing to improved clinical results and faster patient recovery [32].

There is solid scientific evidence that shows how the adverse effects that surgery causes in the short and medium term are modifiable through structured and executed interventions before surgery. Among the main adverse effects that surgery causes in cancer patients are fatigue, pain, and weakness. In addition, there are studies in which the different factors that decisively contribute to hospital readmission have been analyzed. Pre-surgical risk factors, such as comorbidities, age of the subject, functional status, or type of diagnosis, must be considered. In addition, other determining factors could negatively determine therapeutic success and, therefore, must be taken into account, such as the patient's family and social situation, perioperative risk factors or even, in the case of transmission, those aspects that have favored this situation, such as dehydration, bleeding, postoperative infection, intestinal obstruction, etc. (Table 23.1) [30–32].

Given these data, it is understood that preactivation could be understood as a strategy aimed at reducing both direct and indirect health and social costs, an increase in post-surgical results as an extension of the different therapeutic options, a decrease in the period of hospitalization, or even a reduction in the number of reactions in the short and medium term [33–35].

However, the heterogeneity of the profiles of patients suffering from different oncological processes means that there is still no established protocol for each cancer type. However, different scientific documents suggest main lines of intervention, in which the activity of physical and psychological intervention and control of food is a fundamental part of this pre-habilitative process. In what there is, however, the consensus is on the main goals that must be achieved through pre-rehabilitation and the benefits that this brings. For this, it is essential to identify the different situations that deserve to be considered and the different objectives that we should consider for each of these situations [31–34].

Below are some objectives that could be considered because of the different situations that must be identified during a pre-habilitative process in cancer patients.

Usually, the intervention that supports the most significant evidence in a preplanning intervention is physical exercise. In this sense, it is essential to differentiate between increasing physical activity and maintaining an active lifestyle. In order to increase physical activity, it is necessary to increase the time that physical activity is carried out to improve one's state of health. However, to maintain an active

Table 23.1 Situations and objectives that must be identified in a pre-habilitative process in cancer patients (Modified from Silver and Baima [33])

Aim	Situation to identify
Increase	Pretreatment physical function
	Pretreatment psychological function
	Treatment options
	Adherence to cancer treatment.
	Results in physical health
	Results in psychological health
	Health-related quality of life
	Occupational function
Identify, assess, and document	Pretreatment deficiencies
	Baseline state prior to treatment
Decrease	Treatment-related deficiencies
	Unnecessary exams
	Time to regain skills
	Hospital stays
	Therapist care at home
	Rehabilitation visits
	Hospital readmissions
	Risk of future comorbidity
	Risk of cancer recurrence
	Risk of second primary cancer
	Disability
	Mortality
	Time to return to work
	Direct health care costs
	Indirect health care costs

lifestyle, reducing the daily sedentary lifestyle permeating modern societies is necessary. In this sense, physically active individuals have a much more positive evolution in many outcome variables compared to those with a sedentary lifestyle. In addition, it has also been shown that patients who perform physical activity have significant improvements compared to those who do not. In this sense, the ideal patient would maintain an active lifestyle and regularly perform physical activity [30, 31, 33, 34].

For all these reasons, and based on the available scientific literature, increasing preoperative physical fitness levels should become a priority when facing scheduled significant surgery. In addition, this increase in the physical activity must be complemented by changes in lifestyles that must be aimed at breaking the sedentary lifestyle during activities of daily life, an improvement in the diet, as well as better management of the psychological aspects of the patient.

It is also essential to consider that patients who present a worse physical condition before starting the pre-aviation process obtain significant improvements concerning those who do have an excellent physical condition. Therefore, acute interventions aimed at specific improvement of the condition. Physical therapy in patients with low physical fitness allows very positive results to be achieved in cancer patients who must undergo major surgery [31, 32, 34].

Table 23.2 shows where different objectives should be achieved during a rehabilitation process in cancer patients and different alternatives to achieve them. Of all those, none require a high level of physical fitness or specific supervision, so any patient who eats under medical supervision could do so independently in their daily environment.

Prehabilitation in elderly cancer patients is, therefore, a multimodal intervention strategy aimed at an acute lifestyle change that aims to promote a better situation for

Table 23.2 Objectives, methodology, and frequency of strategies to be implemented in the activities of daily living in cancer patients in a pre-rehabilitation process (Adapted from Carli et al. [35])

Aim	Methodology	Intensity/Frequency
Improve musculoskeletal strength.	Perform specific exercises for large muscle groups (10–15 reps)	Alternate days for each muscle group
Improved cardiovascular and respiratory capacity	Reach at least the threshold of 150 min/week of moderate-intensity physical exercise	Aerobic exercises (walking, running, cycling)... At an intensity of at least 5/10
Reduction of sedentary lifestyle	Reduce the sitting period throughout the day, both absolutely (total time) and relatively (uninterrupted time sitting), through alarms or strategies that force the patient to get up	Maintain alertness in this regard throughout the day
Increased flexibility	Maximum stretch positions held for a few seconds in daily gestures (touching the back, opening the legs, stretching the legs, etc.)	Perform at least once a day for a total time of 10 min

the patient facing a surgical process and simultaneously improve the process, reduce the risks and recovery times.

23.2.3 Management of Frailty in the Patient with Orthopedic Disease Preoperatively

In the human body, physical exercise plays a vital role in the correct functioning of the organism and maintaining a healthy state of health. Faced with physical stimuli, the human body reacts by acting very efficiently as a consequence of the adaptation to the stimulus that occurs, especially in the musculoskeletal system. In this way, all the elements that make up the neuromusculoskeletal system remain active, renewed, and healthy.

However, in the absence of physical activity, the muscles progressively lose capacity; that is, they weaken, becoming less mobile, less contractile, and weaker, and may even exceed the threshold of musculoskeletal dysfunction. In situations of prolonged bed rest, as usually happens in the postoperative period of surgical processes, the musculoskeletal system undergoes very rapid degradation, resulting in a decrease in muscle mass and a loss of bone mineral mass, which would aggravate the situation in failure to act in a fast, precise, and controlled manner.

It is therefore essential to consider that in musculoskeletal system surgeries, as soon as the structure is sufficiently stable and solid to begin to be functional, seek the early initiation of physical activity to, on the one hand, slow down and stop the process of degradation of the neuromusculoskeletal structures and, on the other hand, gradually recovering functional capacities and integrating them into the development of activities of daily life.

Figure 23.2 shows a diagram of the patient's evolution depending on the stages in which the pre/rehabilitation process begins.

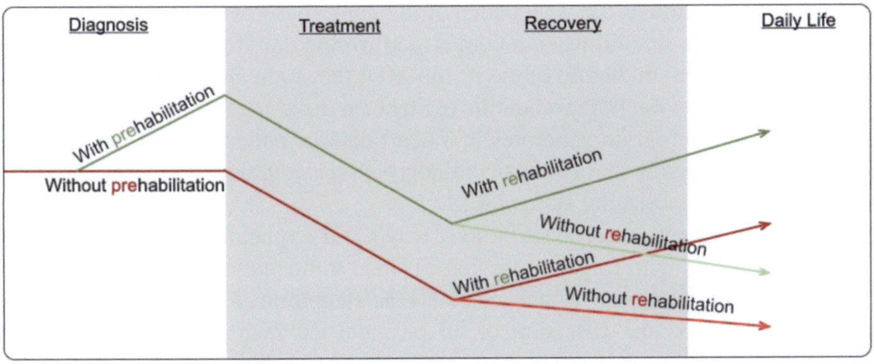

Fig. 23.2 Schematic representation of the evolution of a person who perform the rehabilitation process, considering the moment that rehabilitation begins

23.2.4 Prehabilitation in Geriatric Patients Awaiting Cardiac Surgery

From a demographic point of view, the world population, especially in developed countries, is bringing a change in population distribution. This paradigm shift is due, among other factors, to the progressive population aging, a consequence, among other reasons, of an improvement in the quality of care and more and more specialized surgical procedures, which also favor the postoperative phase. This aging population is leading to older adults increasingly undergoing surgical processes related to their heart health.

This increase in the number of cases is causing cardiac surgeons to have more and more heterogeneity in the cases to be treated due to the particularities of each case. On the other hand, this increase in heart problems is also the progressive result of a physical deconditioning of the population, which is often disproportionate. In this sense, to maintain the therapeutic success that cardiac surgery should promote, physical conditioning protocols must be carried out in the preoperative phase, which, once the patient leaves the hospital, must also be continued with adaptations. However, it must be a protocol that you should follow for life. In this way, the postoperative recovery phase would suffer a decrease in its mortality and morbidity rate. This mortality and morbidity rate has justified the development of these physical conditioning programs, which have been associated with a decrease in this rate in the short and medium term.

Another of the objectives pursued is that, after the surgical intervention, the patient's functional capacity progressively returns to the values before the surgery or even exceeds them. This is posing a challenge since, due to age and cardiac pathology, these patients find it very difficult to carry out activities of daily living, so it is common for these patients to be discharged towards an outpatient clinic that allows them to continue monitoring the patient in the medium and long term [24–26].

In this type of patient, the preoperative evaluation is essential to measure the risk that the patient suffers as a consequence of his cardiac pathology, also due to the potential aggravation as a consequence of the comorbidities he could present. The scientific evidence is solid when it comes to affirming that this type of preoperative evaluation allows a prediction of the results after the surgical intervention.

However, even though the scientific evidence is solid regarding the benefits that a prehabilitation program generates in a heart disease patient before and after the intervention, the index that is most confidently associated with an increase in mortality is poor cardiovascular status [36].

On the other hand, there is still a long way to go in planning rehabilitation programs for patients with cardiac pathologies since some pathologies, such as severe aortic stenosis or coronary lesions, can increase symptoms. Frequently, the medical recommendation is the cessation of all physical exercise until the surgery has occurred. In addition, as in the case of these pathologies, but also others such as left center trunk stenosis, aneurysms, or unstable angina, physical exercise is contraindicated.

23.2.5 Prehabilitation Program in Older Patients Awaiting Abdominal Surgery

Surgical aggression induces a physiological response to stress that activates a series of metabolic, hormonal, and tissue changes directly proportional to the intensity of the stimulus. In response to aggression, the hypothalamic–pituitary system and the sympathetic–adrenal system are activated with the release of corticosteroids and catecholamines. Immunological changes also occur with the production of cytokines, acute phase reactants, leukocytosis or leukopenia, neutrophilia, complement activation, increased prostaglandin and nitric oxide synthesis, endothelial dysfunction, and procoagulant states. All these favor insulin resistance, hyperglycemia, and hypothermia. It has been shown that multimodal rehabilitation programs can attenuate this response to stress and reduce perioperative morbidity and mortality.

These pathophysiological changes generate catabolism, immunosuppression, pain, nausea and vomiting, paralytic ileus, respiratory and cardiac failure, prothrombotic situation, and infection of surgical wounds.

The general costs of major surgery are sometimes significantly threatened due to postoperative complications that force a patient to increase the period of hospital stay. These facts are usually observed in a percentage that oscillates between 20% and 50%, depending on the type of surgery performed. In addition, another added problem is that, after the surgery is performed, patients experience episodes of physical fatigue and inactivity, which generates a degenerative loop, since this problem appears for the period that they have been bedridden but, in case of not breaking the vicious circle, the patient's condition would worsen. In this sense, a fantastic strategy is the development of a prehabilitation protocol so that the patient, before entering surgery, has improved his physical condition, and his margin to cushion the damages of the therapeutic process increases significantly, which will facilitate, in turn, the postoperative phase.

On the other hand, physiotherapy prior to surgical intervention benefits the patient's physical condition and reduces the risk of postoperative complications. In this sense, planning a pre-habilitative protocol following the guidelines previously explained would facilitate the development of this type of intervention, favoring an improvement of the patient in qualitative, quantitative, and temporal terms.

23.3 Physical Therapy after Surgery: The Importance of Early Patient Care

23.3.1 Management of the Geriatric Patient After Cancer Surgery

By 2050, an estimated 6.9 million new cancer cases (21.5% of global cases, all ages combined) are expected to be diagnosed in adults aged 80 years or older worldwide [37].

Surgery is an important treatment modality in the majority of cancers with the exception of hematological malignancies. The role of surgery is vast; it can be utilized for prophylaxis, primary treatment, after neoadjuvant systemic therapy, as well as in the palliation of symptoms and improvement of quality of life in the metastatic setting. Consequently, the average age of the population served by a surgeon is significantly increasing [38].

This has also been made possible by improved surgical techniques and postoperative management techniques. However, elderly cancer patients have a high probability of experiencing a "frail" condition before surgery in combination with comorbidities (such as reduced physical function, respiratory function, presence of chronic obstructive pulmonary disease, heart failure, or diabetes).

And the most important feature of rehabilitation is precisely not to examine patients only at the organ level, but to assess them comprehensively by analyzing the condition at the individual and social level. Therefore, in the surgical treatment of elderly patients with cancer, implementation of preoperative "frailty" assessment and initiation of assessment-based active rehabilitation prior to or shortly after the surgery improves physical and mental functions and AdL of elderly patients with cancer and may contribute to the improvement of the treatment results and prognosis [39].

23.3.1.1 Physical Therapy Treatment After Breast Cancer Surgery

Female breast cancer has now surpassed lung cancer as the leading cause of global cancer incidence in 2020, with an estimated 2.3 million new cases, representing 11.7% of all cancer cases. It is the fifth leading cause of cancer mortality worldwide, with 685,000 deaths. Among women, breast cancer accounts for 1 in 4 cancer cases and for 1 in 6 cancer deaths, ranking first for incidence in the vast majority of countries (159 of 185 countries) and for mortality in 110 countries [40]. Over a third of patients diagnosed with invasive breast cancer, and almost half of breast cancer-related mortalities in Western societies are reported among those over 70 years of age [41].

Surgical resection with proper surgical margins remains the cornerstone of breast cancer therapy and with modern surgery and anesthesia, breast surgeries are considered safe and is usually associated with very low complication rates regardless of extent of surgery [42].

Breast and axillary surgery also appears to be low risk for selected patients in the elderly breast cancer population, although it is not without complications or impact on QoL [43].

In the first year postoperative and at long-term follow-up patients with breast cancer suffer from constraints in arm and shoulder and patients treated with axillary lymph node dissection are most at risk for developing this impairments. Other issues reported following surgical treatment for breast cancer, and particularly after axillary lymph node dissection, include decreased ROM and muscle strength, pain, lymphedema, and decreased activities of daily living. In contrast, radiotherapy and hormone therapy are the main risk factors for pain [44].

Chronic pain after breast surgery (CPBS) is a frequent complication that interferes with patients' daily activities. Evaluation of CPBS according to the International

Association for the Study of Pain (IASP) definition resulted in a 28% incidence at 3 months postoperatively [45].

A timely identification of high-risk patients might allow the implementation of proactive pharmacologic and non-pharmacologic approaches to prevent CPBS.

Therefore, after breast cancer surgery, a multifactorial physiotherapy intervention which is effective in treating nociceptive musculoskeletal pain is essential. It involves tissue, accessory and neurodynamic joint mobilization plus active exercises with increasing intensity. The most effective treatment for drug-induced and radio-induced neuropathic pain appears to be supervised active exercise of moderate intensity. In addition to improving pain sensation, statistically significant improvements were calculated in the WHOQOL, BFI, and ROM scales of the shoulder. Finally, in patients with chronic pain, multidisciplinary rehabilitation is helpful in reducing disability and improving quality of life [46].

Another complication is chronic arm edema after breast cancer whose estimated overall incidence has been found to be 21.4%, indicating that breast cancer-related lymphedema (BCRL) is a widespread problem affecting 1 in 5 patients after breast cancer treatment and due to the lack of diagnostic criteria for BCRL, the reported incidence varies from less than 5% to more than 50% [47]. The conservative treatment of this health issue is based on decongestive physical therapy and physiotherapy.

Physical therapy consists of Comprehensive or Comprehensive Decongestive Therapy (CDT) that is individualized for each patient, but typically includes manual lymphatic drainage (MLD), compression bandaging, exercise, skin care, and patient education [48].

Endermologic therapy, which induces both objective improvement in the form of decreased upper limb swelling and subjective improvements in the form of decreased pain and improved the mobility of the affected limb, may also be useful [49, 50].

23.3.1.2 Pelvic Floor Muscle Training After Radical Prostatectomy

With an estimated almost 1.4 million new cases and 375,000 deaths worldwide, prostate cancer is the second most frequent cancer and the fifth leading cause of cancer death among men in 2020 [40]. For a disease as common as prostate cancer, relatively little is known about its etiology. Established risk factors are limited to advancing age, family history of this malignancy, and certain genetic mutations (e.g., BRCA1 and BRCA2) and conditions (Lynch syndrome) [40]. Advances in prostate cancer diagnosis and treatment have enhanced clinicians' capacities to classify patients by risk and propose therapy based on cancer prognosis and patient preference. Surveillance, prostatectomy, and radiotherapy are recognized as the standard treatments for stage I–III prostate cancer patients [51]. The natural history of radical prostatectomy consists of several side effects. Men tend, in fact, to experience a sharp initial decline in urinary and sexual function immediately after surgery (within the first 2 months), followed by gradual improvement to near or below baseline levels within the first year after surgery. An exception to this pattern is micturition dysfunction (or urinary irritation or obstruction). In some previous studies, improvement in micturition dysfunction symptoms over pre-surgical values has been observed, presumably because of the elimination of urinary obstruction due to prostatectomy in men with both prostate cancer and benign prostatic hyperplasia (BPH) [52]. Multi-disciplinary treatment approach determined by urologists, physiotherapists, and other healthcare professionals is the treatment standard for urinary incontinence after radical prostatectomy. Pelvic floor muscle training is recognized as the physiotherapeutic modality for the treatment of urinary incontinence in men after radical prostatectomy and this method is recommended by the European Association of Urology [53]. Current evidence indicated that advanced pelvic floor muscle training might facilitate the recovery of urinary incontinence after radical prostatectomy according to intermediate-term advantages over conventional pelvic floor muscle training in terms of pad number, ICIQ-SF score, PFME, and pad weight [54].

23.3.1.3 Early Postoperative Treatment of Lung Cancer

With an estimated 2.2 million new cancer cases and 1.8 million deaths, lung cancer is the second most commonly diagnosed cancer and the leading cause of cancer death in 2020; lung cancer is the leading cause of cancer morbidity and mortality in men, whereas, in women, it ranks third for incidence, after breast and colorectal cancer, and second for mortality, after breast cancer [40]. Thoracic surgery is considered the standard of care for people with early-stage lung cancer (stage I, stage II, and some stage IIIA) who are deemed fit enough. Over the past 10 years, surgical resection rates have increased from 9% to nearly 17% and surgeons are now more likely to operate on people who are older than 70 years (the median age of lung cancer diagnosis is 73 years) [55]. Video-assisted thoracoscopic surgery (VATS) as a minimally invasive alternative approach shows remarkable safety, feasibility, and efficacy. Therefore, the decrease in mortality also puts forward higher requirements for patients' quality of life (QoL) after surgery. Still, surgical procedures for lung cancer need to face significant postoperative challenges, such as fatigue, cough, and postoperative pain. Lung cancer survivors may suffer decreased pulmonary function, physical activity level, and psychological distress, which significantly affects the QoL [56].

To date, various treatment strategies and methods such as identification and prevention of risk factors, improvement of the preoperative condition and patient education, intraoperative practices, and postoperative pulmonary care have been developed to reduce the incidence of postoperative pulmonary complications. Fundamental turns out to be an intensive postoperative physical therapy program from the early postoperative period (from the 4th) that includes techniques that improve ventilation such as deep breathing exercises, maximum long-term inspiration with an incentive spirometer and pursed limp breathing; bronchial hygiene techniques such as autogenic drainage methods, effective cough training, huffing, bottle positive expiratory pressure; early ambulation and progressive mobility exercises for shoulder girdle and thoracic cage [57, 58]. Exercise training, including aerobic and resistance exercises, can improve exercise capacity in a clinically important way and improve the physical component score of overall health-related quality of life (HRQoL) and has reduced dyspnea in people who have undergone lung resection for non-small cell lung cancer [59]. Therefore, in all thoracic surgery clinics, more and more importance should be given to simple, cost-effective, and low-risk physiotherapy practices that reduce health costs and increase the success of surgery.

23.3.2 Management of the Geriatric Patient After Orthopedic Surgery

Orthopedic surgery, thanks to scientific advances, technical development of prostheses, equipment, anesthetic technologies, and perioperative controls, is expanding on a large scale to elderly patients. The rate of postoperative complications in the surgical management of the elderly is, however, high, and, therefore, careful considerations are needed for this group of patients after orthopedic surgery. Indeed, possible cognitive impairment, control of postoperative analgesia, pulmonary complications, prevention of falls, urinary tract infections, pressure ulcers, and functional decline should always be considered in postoperative treatment. More attention needs to be paid to early mobilization and patient education, as these factors can contribute significantly to avoiding some of the postoperative complications that commonly affect this population [60].

23.3.2.1 Physical Therapy After Lower Limb Surgery

Osteoarthritis (OA) is a worldwide highly prevalent chronic joint disease that causes pain, disability, and loss of function. Global trends showed a 114.5% increase in years lived with disability due to OA from 1990 to 2019; OA prevalence varies with the joints involved. The knee is the most frequently affected joint, followed by the hand and the hip [61]. OA has a considerable impact on patients' quality of life (QoL), activities of daily living, and general health status. Joint replacement is the only definitive treatment for symptomatic end-stage hip and knee OA, aiming to relieve the pain and restore joint function. Total hip arthroplasty (THA) and total knee arthroplasty (TKA) are usually followed by an intense rehabilitation program focused on muscle strengthening, stretching, range of motion (ROM) recovery, gait rehabilitation, neuromuscular function, and proprioception recovery [62].

After TKA, the patient's movement is limited and restricted due to decreased muscle strength and pain; for instance, muscle function has been found to be reduced by 20–25% at 1 month after surgery, while, after 1 year, it remains lower than in healthy adults, with reports of 18% slower walking speed and 51% slower stair-climbing speed. Furthermore, range of motion (ROM) of the knee joint is reduced due to post-operation pain, hematoma and swelling, and these limits complete functional recovery to only 67% of patients. In addition, the strength of the quadriceps muscle is reduced by 30.7% immediately after TKA, and by 50–60% after 1 month, despite the initiation of rehabilitation within 48 h after surgery [63].

Therefore, postoperative rehabilitation programs are crucial in order to best recover function, mobility, and autonomy for patients after TKA (Fig. 23.3).

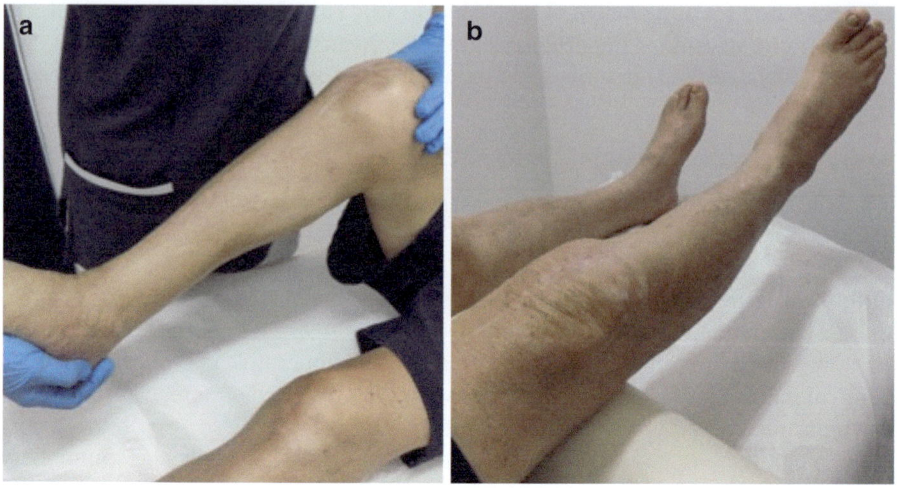

Fig. 23.3 Examples of passive mobilization (**a**) and therapeutic exercise (**b**) after TKA

However, when comparing different rehabilitation programs with standard programs after TKA, there is no clear pattern in the combination of rehabilitation start times and duration that significantly improves clinical outcomes [63].

Among the reasons for needing hip surgery, however, besides OA, are fractures, which are very common in the elderly and whose incidence increases as the population ages. Depending on the characteristics of the fracture, total hip arthroplasty (THA), hemiarthroplasty (HA), or using osteosynthesis means can be performed. However, regardless of the type of surgery performed, active physiotherapy and structural exercises are essential for hip fracture recovery.

Muscle strengthening and balance training turn out to be essential, although weight-bearing exercises have been discussed in terms of timing and progression depending on the type of surgery, although the benefit of treatment appears to be high [64]. In fact, arthroplasty, which allows lifting weights earlier, leads to superior functional outcomes compared with internal fixation in elderly patients with hip fractures [65]. When weight-bearing exercises are proposed, however, close communication between surgeons and physical therapists is necessary to determine the timing and level of exercises [64].

23.3.2.2 Physical Therapy After Upper Limb Surgery

Rotator cuff disease is one of the most common causes of shoulder pain, accounting for up to 70% of shoulder complaints in the adult population and is a leading cause of shoulder-related disability. Etiologies of rotator cuff disease are multifactorial and include a combination of major extrinsic trauma, microtrauma resulting from daily wear and tear, and natural degeneration over time [66]. Despite widespread prevalence in the general population, optimal management remains controversial.

A nonsurgical course with an appropriate physiotherapy program is the first choice in the management of degenerative rotator cuff tears and this is especially the case in patients with significant risk factors for surgery, those who do not wish to go through a surgical treatment, as well as those with small, partial, and irreparable tears. Nevertheless, rotator cuff repair has a good clinical outcome with significant improvements in pain, range of motion, strength, quality of life, and sleep patterns [67]. After rotator cuff surgery, early passive, postoperative exercise can be used without indicating an increased rate of disruption of the healing process or ruptures and cryotherapy is recommended in the first 3 weeks following reconstruction of the rotator cuff in order to support rehabilitation and, in particular, to treat pain. In the later stages, the goals of rehabilitation are recovery of active function, improvement of strength and, eventually, return to sports [68].

Surgical options, in addition to partial repair and/or debridement, repair (open or arthroscopic), reconstruction (transfer of transformed muscle or tissue) also includes arthroplasty (hemi- or reverse shoulder) [69].

Reverse shoulder arthroplasty (RSA) was first developed as an alternative treatment for rotator cuff arthropathy. Since then, it has proven to be an effective implant for many shoulder disorders. For this reason, there has been a gradual increase in the last decade in its use for proximal humerus fractures in elderly patients. Clinical studies of RSA in this kind of fracture have shown improved outcomes when compared with hemiarthroplasty [70].

Postoperative results after RSA may depend on several factors, including: preoperative pathology, surgical technique, implant design, duration of postoperative immobilization, and timeliness of physiotherapy intervention. The prevailing theory of postoperative rehabilitation involves early joint protection with progressive functional mobilization and strengthening, in fact, the restoration of shoulder strength has been shown to be a strong determinant of functional outcomes, shoulder range of motion (ROM), and patient satisfaction. This must be balanced with risks of acromial fracture, scapular spine fracture, instability, deltoid fatigue, and early loosening [71].

Given the rotator cuff deficient nature of postoperative RSA patients, functional outcomes rely largely upon deltoid recruitment. With the newer design advances of the reverse shoulder arthroplasty, there is improved biomechanical efficiency of both the deltoid and the preserved posterior rotator cuff. The combination of these muscle groups allows superior recovery of active motion and patient function [71]. In addition, some authors have purposed possible neuromuscular electrical stimulation (NMES) of the deltoid muscle as a treatment used to improve postoperative outcomes concluding that NMES following RSA could lead to the early restoration of external rotation and recovery of deltoid function [71, 72].

23.3.2.3 Physical Therapy After Spine Surgery

Osteoporosis (OP) is one of the most common metabolic bone disorders in the world and has been defined as a skeletal disorder characterized by reduced bone strength, which predisposes a person to an increased risk of fractures. Among fragility fractures, the most common is vertebral compression fracture (VCF). It represents a major health problem in the elderly population, as the incidence of these fractures increases with age, and it has been shown that patients who have already had one are at substantial risk of suffering others [73]. Most of the osteoporotic fractures of the spine can and should be treated conservatively or in a minimally invasive manner and conservative therapeutic strategies include acute fracture treatment with analgesia, temporary bed rest, or immobilization in a frame corset, as well as mandatory secondary prophylaxis through antiresorptive or osteoanabolic medication [74]. However, for patients who have been diagnosed with spinal fractures, the pain relief is insufficient, the treatment cycle is long, accompanied by possible complications. Therefore, patients with such fractures are often treated by surgery, which can not only relieve pain in a timely and effective manner, but also reduce complications and improve the quality of life. Percutaneous vertebroplasty (PVP) and percutaneous kyphoplasty (PKP) are commonly used clinical surgical modalities in treating elderly osteoporotic spinal compression fractures with high surgical safety and good postoperative pain relief, from which patients can obtain restored vertebral body function and improve mobility [75].

After PKP or PVP for elderly patients with osteoporotic lumbar compression fractures, early regular core strength training has a positive effect on early functional recovery and improvement of life ability, which is in line with the concept of accelerated rehabilitation surgery [76].

As the aging population increases, degenerative spinal diseases such as degenerative spinal stenosis, degenerative spondylolisthesis, and degenerative disc disorder.

Lumbar spinal stenosis (LSS) is one of the most common degenerative spinal diseases in the elderly population. With the aging process, the degeneration of the intervertebral disc, the thickening of the ligamentum flavum and facet joints would eventually lead to the narrowing of the spinal canal. These pathological changes could cause clinical symptoms of low back or leg pain, or neurogenic claudication, which would severely impair the quality of life. If the symptoms do not relieve after conservative therapy, surgical management should be performed and the decompression and fusion surgery is generally considered the golden standard [77]. In case of decompression surgery for lumbar spinal stenosis, active rehabilitation is more effective than usual care in improving both short- and long-term (back-related) functional status, short-term improvement in low back pain and long-term improvement in both low back pain and leg pain, although limited impact was observed in relation to improvements in general health status [78].

Degenerative spondylolisthesis most commonly affects individuals >50 years old and is an especially common indication for spinal surgery in elderly patients. Spondylolisthesis is frequently treated with a single-level lumbar fusion procedure in which adjacent vertebrae are surgically joined to increase spinal stability, eliminating pain caused by the abnormal mobility of the affected segment. The data support that age alone should not exclude a patient for this procedure. However, extra caution is warranted given the slightly increased morbidity [79]. Following spinal fusion surgery, rehabilitation is essential, which combined with psychosocial treatment improves outcomes. Regarding treatment, it is of paramount importance to calibrate treatment choices to the patient and to propose cardiovascular exercises in order to improve aerobic capacity, decrease pain, improve function, and reduce the duration of hospitalization; soft tissue treatment, which is useful in patients who report pain and swelling in the incision area or in patients who seem most anxious or stressed during postoperative recovery; neurodynamic exercises motor control and muscle strengthening exercises, particularly exercises to strengthen the extensors of the spine; joint mobilizations aimed at the thoracic and hip tracts, educational treatment to reduce anxiety, increase patient satisfaction and awareness, especially in a multidisciplinary setting [80].

Percutaneous endoscopic lumbar discectomy (PELD), either transforaminal (PTELD), or interlaminar (PIELD), has proven to be a safe, fast, and practical approach for treating lumbar disc prolapse. Such a technique may be helpful in the treatment of lumbar prolapsed disks in the elderly ($\geq$75 years) because it is minimally invasive, has a shorter recovery time, and is associated with reduced scar tissue formation than open microdiscectomy. Moreover, it may also be performed under spinal anesthesia, allowing for safer operations even in patients with severe comorbidities [81].

Although spine surgery is generally considered a safe and effective treatment, approximately one-in-five of patients experience continued or recurrent chronic post-surgical pain [82].

Even in the case of surgery for lumbar disc herniation, an exercise program started 4–6 weeks after surgery appears to lead to more rapid improvement in pain and disability than no treatment, and that a high-intensity exercise program leads to more rapid improvement in pain and disability than a low-intensity one [83].

23.3.3 Functional Recovery of the Geriatric Patient After Cardiovascular Surgery

Acute-phase cardiac rehabilitation after cardiac surgery is recommended to prevent postoperative complications and declines in physical function, as well as to regain patients' preoperative functional level in activities of daily living (AdL) as early as possible.

Due to the shift in patient population, the profile of patients who are referred to cardiac surgeon changed dramatically. The share of surgically treated elderly patients ($\geq$80 years old) increased from 2.6–7% to 9.3–12% in a period of 10 years due to innovation in cardiac surgery techniques, advance in anesthesiology, and early post-surgery care which have led to a lower risk of cardiac surgery in elderly patients; however, older patients still have higher mortality and morbidity rates, more frequent complications related to surgery, and longer stay in hospital compared to younger patients [84].

Surgery can result in respiratory muscle dysfunction, which can also lead to decreased vital capacity (VC), tidal volume, and total lung capacity. Therefore, postoperative pulmonary complications can be prevented by inspiratory muscle training before surgery; training techniques include preoperative breathing exercises, respiratory muscle training, and spirometric training, while in the postoperative phase, bronchial toileting, early ambulation, lung expansion techniques, and spirometric training may be crucial (Fig. 23.4) [85]. Multiple-intervention pulmonary rehabilitation was, also, associated with significant improvements in Maximal Inspiratory Pressure (MIP), Borg Scale Score, and FEV1/FVC ratio in elderly patients with multimorbidity who underwent coronary artery bypass graft surgery [85, 86].

In addition, physical exercise on a cycle ergometer combined with CPAP as an adjunct to the rehabilitation of hospitalized subjects who underwent myocardial revascularization with coronary artery bypass graft was safe, decreased the length of stay in the intensive care unit, and helped maintain functional capacity [87].

High intensity, long-duration postoperative inspiratory muscle training is highly effective in improving lung function, inspiratory muscle strength, and functional capacity, in the short- and long-term, even in frail valvular heart disease patient [84, 88].

Therefore, exercise significantly improves functional recovery in the post-surgical elderly cardiac population and the combination of aerobic exercise with resistance training is more effective at improving muscle strength and cardiorespiratory fitness compared to isolated aerobic or resistance training [89]; however, uncertainty still exists with regard to which modes of exercise and their specific parameters (frequency, program duration, session duration, mode, and intensity) are most effective in improving cognitive recovery [90].

23.3.4 Physical Therapy Management of the Patients After Abdominal Surgery

The increase of life expectancy at birth increases the proportion of the elderly population and the need for emergency surgery in this age group. Among the conditions

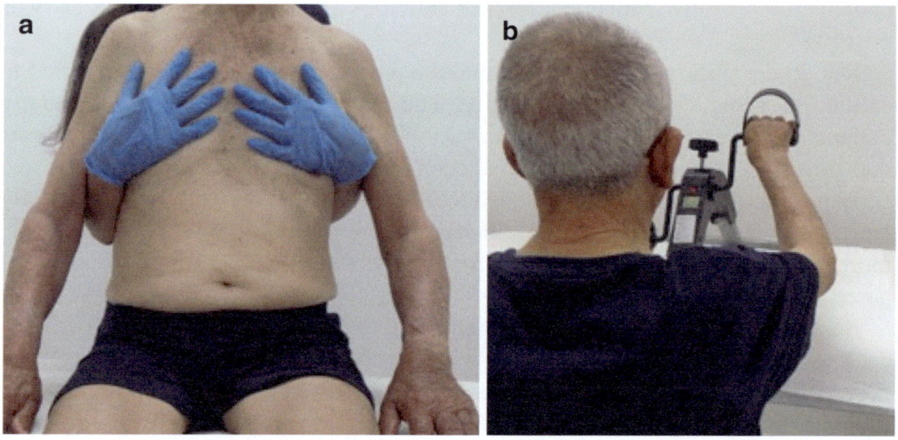

Fig. 23.4 Examples of breathing exercises (**a**) and respiratory muscle training (**b**)

requiring emergency surgery in elderly individuals are gallbladder and biliary tract emergencies, acute bowel obstruction, hernia, and peptic ulcer perforation [91].

This group of patients, therefore, accounts for approximately 50% of all emergency surgeries and 75% of postoperative mortality. It is believed, however, that the presence of comorbidities alone does not have a significant effect on the mortality of elderly patients undergoing emergency abdominal surgery but that in terms of postoperative prognosis, the type of comorbidity (dysthymia, heart failure, renal failure, and chronic obstructive pulmonary disease) is more important [91].

Among complications after abdominal surgery, pulmonary complications—such as atelectasis, pneumonia, and hypoxia—are very prevalent and are associated with several negative factors, including delayed mobilization. Early and intensive mobilization after acute high-risk abdominal surgery is in fact considered essential to reduce postoperative pulmonary complications and prevent loss of function. And the early intensive mobilization protocol is also well tolerated by patients undergoing acute high-risk abdominal surgery, despite patients having significantly decreased physical function after their surgery [92].

Furthermore, mobilization out of bed, with or without breathing exercises, within 2 h after elective abdominal surgery improves SpO_2 and PaO_2 as well as affecting patients' physical and mental well-being. Patients report that they feel more alert, regain their autonomy, recover appetite and thirst, and feel that it is easier to breathe when they sit up in a chair compared with when they lie in bed [93].

23.4 Conclusions

Given the increase in the geriatric population, it is reasonable to assume that in the future the percentage of elderly patients requiring surgery will continue to increase. Having ascertained, within a multidisciplinary perspective, the importance of physiotherapy in this population, it is therefore desirable that within the scientific landscape increasingly accurate preoperative, peri- and postoperative interventions are identified in order to ensure effective care for patients based on the most up-to-date scientific evidence. It is also necessary, given the complexity of the frail patient, that physiotherapists be extremely well trained and continuously updated in order to ensure their optimal management, preventing complications and providing them with the tools to achieve the best level of quality of life.

References

1. Beard BR, Officer A, de Carvalho IA, Sadana R, Pot AM, Michel JP, Lloyd-Sherlock P, Epping-Jordan JE, Peeters G, Mahanani WR, Thiyagarajan JA, Chatterji S. The world report on ageing and health: a policy framework for healthy ageing. Lancet. 2017;387:2145. https://doi.org/10.1016/S0140-6736(15)00516-4.
2. World Health Organization: Geneva, Switzerland. World report on ageing and health. Indian J Med Res. 2017;145(1):150–1. https://doi.org/10.4103/0971-5916.207249.

3. Liu-Ambrose T, Davis JC, Best JR, Dian L, Madden K, Cook W, Hsu CL, Khan KM. Effect of a home-based exercise program on subsequent falls among community-dwelling high-risk older adults after a fall. JAMA. 2019;321(21):2092–100. https://doi.org/10.1001/jama.2019.5795.
4. Kato M, Mori Y, Watanabe A, Onoda H, Fujiyama K, Toda M, Kito K. Relationship between average daily rehabilitation time and decline in instrumental activity of daily living among older patients with heart failure: a preliminary analysis of a multicenter cohort study, suruga-care. PLoS One. 2021;16(7):e0254128. https://doi.org/10.1371/journal.pone.0254128.
5. Shepherd CW, While A. Cardiac rehabilitation and quality of life: a systematic review. Int J Nurs Stud. 2012;49(6):755–71. https://doi.org/10.1016/j.ijnurstu.2011.11.019.
6. Kagioglou O, Mouratoglou SA, Giannakoulas G, Kapoukranidou D, Anifanti M, Deligiannis A, Skarbaliene A, Razbadauskas A, Kouidi E. Long-term effect of an exercise training program on physical functioning and quality of life in pulmonary hypertension: a randomized controlled trial. Biomed Res Int. 2021;2021:8870615. https://doi.org/10.1155/2021/8870615.
7. Ali A, Tabassum D, Baig SS, Moyle B, Redgrave J, Nichols S, McGregor G, Evans K, Totton N, Cooper C, Majid A. Effect of exercise interventions on health-related quality of life after stroke and transient ischemic attack: a systematic review and meta-analysis. Stroke. 2021;52(7):2445–55. https://doi.org/10.1161/STROKEAHA.120.032979.
8. Chang ET, Piegari R. Which patients are persistently high-risk for hospitalization? Am J Manag Care. 2019;25(9):e274–81.
9. Wang MC, Liao WC, Lee KC, Lu SH, Lin YP. Validation of screening tools for predicting the risk of functional decline in hospitalized elderly patients. Int J Environ Res Public Health. 2022;19(11):6685. https://doi.org/10.3390/ijerph19116685.
10. Martínez-Velilla N, Casas-Herrero A, Zambom-Ferraresi F, Sáez de Asteasu ML, Lucia L, Galbete A, García-Baztán A, Alonso-Renedo J, González-Glaría B, Gonzalo-Lázaro M. Effect of exercise intervention on functional decline in very elderly patients during acute hospitalization: a randomized clinical trial. JAMA Intern Med. 2019;179(1):28–36. https://doi.org/10.1001/jamainternmed.2018.4869.
11. Hester AL, Tsai PF, Rettiganti M, Mitchell A. Predicting injurious falls in the hospital setting: implications for practice. Am J Nurs. 2016;116(9):24–31. https://doi.org/10.1097/01.NAJ.0000494688.10004.85.
12. Hallford DJ, Nicholson G, Sanders K, McCabe MP. The association between anxiety and falls: a meta-analysis. J Gerontol. 2017;72(5):729–41. https://doi.org/10.1093/geronb/gbv160.
13. Morris ME, Webster K, Jones C, Hill AM, Haines T, McPhail S, Kiegaldie D, Slade S, Jazayeri D, Heng H, Shorr R, Carey l, Barjer A, Cameron I. Interventions to reduce falls in hospitals: a systematic review and meta-analysis. Age Ageing. 2022;51(5):afac077. https://doi.org/10.1093/ageing/afac077.
14. Gual N, García-Salmones M, Bríez L, Crespo N, Udina C, Pérez LM, Inzitari M. The role of physical exercise and rehabilitation in delirium. Eur Geriatr Med. 2020;11(1):83–93. https://doi.org/10.1007/s41999-020-00290-6.
15. Chen X, Mao G, Leng SX. Frailty syndrome: an overview. Clin Interv Aging. 2014;9:433–41. https://doi.org/10.2147/CIA.S45300.
16. Rezaei-Shahsavarloo Z, Atashzadeh-Shoorideh F, Gobbens RJ, Ebadi A, Ghaedamini HG. The impact of interventions on management of frailty in hospitalized frail older adults: a systematic review and meta-analysis. BMC Geriatr. 2020;20:526. https://doi.org/10.1186/s12877-020-01935-8.
17. Hijazi Y, Gondal U, Aziz O. A systematic review of prehabilitation programs in abdominal cancer surgery. Int J Surg. 2017;39:156–62. https://doi.org/10.1016/j.ijsu.2017.01.111.
18. Macmillan Cancer Support. Principles and guidance for prehabilitation within the management and support of people with cancer [electronic book]. London: Macmillan; 2020.
19. Wynter-Blyth V, Moorthy K. Prehabilitation: preparing patients for surgery. BMJ. 2017;8(358):j3702. https://doi.org/10.1136/bmj.j3702.
20. Kehlet H. Fast-track surgery: an update on physiological care principles to enhance recovery. Langenbeck's Arch Surg. 2011;396(5):585–90. https://doi.org/10.1007/s00423-011-0790-y.

21. Holland AE, Malaguti C, Hoffman M. Home-based or remote exercise testing in chronic respiratory disease, during the COVID-19 pandemic and beyond: a rapid review. Chron Respir Dis. 2020;17:1479973120952418. https://doi.org/10.1177/1479973120952418.
22. Chen S, Li X, Wu Y, Li Y, Cao P, Yin Y, Chen Z. Preoperative respiratory muscle training combined with aerobic exerciseimproves respiratory vital capacity and daily life activity following surgicaltreatment for myasthenia gravis. Cardiothorac Surg. 2023;18(1):160. https://doi.org/10.1186/s13019-023-02283-5.
23. Boyle H, Fullbrook A, Wills A, Veal I, Peat N, Al-Noor Z, Bradshaw R, Raga A, Hegarty A, Hainsworth A, Ilyas M, Banugo P, Bidd H, Guy's and St Thomas' Hospital Prehabilitation team. Multimodal prehabilitation service for patients with colorectal cancer: the challenges of implementation. BMJ Open Qual. 2023;12(2):e002064. https://doi.org/10.1136/bmjoq-2022-002064.
24. Tran D. Cardiopulmonary exercise testing. Methods Mol Biol. 2018;1735:285–95. https://doi.org/10.1007/978-1-4939-7614-0_18.
25. Khan A, Wong J, Riedel B, Laing E, Beaumont A, Kong J, Warrier S, Heriot A. The impact of Peri-operative enteral Immunonutrition on post-operative complications in gastrointestinal cancer surgery: a meta-analysis. Ann Surg Oncol. 2023;30(6):3619–31. https://doi.org/10.1245/s10434-023-13265-1.
26. Pang NQ, Tan YX, Samuel M, Tan KK, Bonney GK, Yi H, Kow WCA. Multimodal prehabilitation in older adults before major abdominal surgery: a systematic review and meta-analysis. Langenbeck's Arch Surg. 2022;407(6):2193–204. https://doi.org/10.1007/s00423-022-02479-8.
27. Griffin SB, Palmer MA, Strodl E, Lai R, Burstow MJ, Ross LJ. Elective surgery in adult patients with excess weight: can preoperative dietary interventions improve surgical outcomes? A systematic review. Nutrients. 2021;13(11):3775. https://doi.org/10.3390/nu13113775.
28. Zhang X, Wang S, Ji W, Wang H, Zhou K, Jin Z, Bo L. The effect of prehabilitation on the postoperative outcomes of patients undergoing colorectal surgery: a systematic review and meta-analysis. Front Oncol. 2022;29(12):958261. https://doi.org/10.3389/fonc.2022.958261.
29. Liu C, Lu Z, Zhu M, Lu X. Trimodal prehabilitation for older surgical patients: a systematic review and meta-analysis. Aging Clin Exp Res. 2022;34(3):485–94. https://doi.org/10.1007/s40520-021-01929-5.
30. Argillander TE, Heil TC, Melis RJF, van Duijvendijk P, Klaase JM, van Munster BC. Preoperative physical performance as predictor of postoperative outcomes in patients aged 65 and older scheduled for major abdominal cancer surgery: a systematic review. Eur J Surg Oncol. 2022;48(3):570–81. https://doi.org/10.1016/j.ejso.2021.09.019.
31. Guo Y, Ding L, Miao X, Jiang X, Xu T, Xu X, Zhu S, Xu Q, Hu J. Effects of prehabilitation on postoperative outcomes in frail cancer patients undergoing elective surgery: a systematic review and meta-analysis. Support Care Cancer. 2022;31(1):57. https://doi.org/10.1007/s00520-022-07541-1.
32. Barnes K, Hladkowicz E, Dorrance K, Bryson GL, Forster AJ, Gagné S, Huang A, Lalu MM, Lavallée LT, Saunders C, Moloo H, Nantel J, Power B, Scheede-Bergdahl C, Taljaard M, van Walraven C, McCartney CJL, McIsaac DI. Barriers and facilitators to participation in exercise prehabilitation before cancer surgery for older adults with frailty: a qualitative study. BMC Geriatr. 2023;23(1):356. https://doi.org/10.1186/s12877-023-03990-3.
33. Silver JK, Baima J. Cancer prehabilitation: an opportunity to decrease treatment related morbidity, increase cancer treatment options, and improve physical and psychological health outcomes. Am J Phys Med Rehabil. 2013;92(8):715–27. https://doi.org/10.1097/PHM.0b013e31829b4afe.
34. Forbes CC, Swan F, Greenley SL, Lind M, Johnson MJ. Physical activity and nutrition interventions for older adults with cancer: a systematic review. J Cancer Surviv. 2020;14(5):689–711. https://doi.org/10.1007/s11764-020-00883-x.
35. Carli F, Gillis C, Scheede-Bergdahl C. Promoting a culture of prehabilitation for the surgical cancer patient. Act Oncol. 2017;56(2):128–33. https://doi.org/10.1080/0284186X.2016.1266081.

36. Hughes MJ, Hackney RJ, Lamb PJ, Wigmore SJ, Christopher Deans DA, Skipworth RJE. Prehabilitation before major abdominal surgery: a systematic review and meta-analysis. World J Surg. 2019;43(7):1661–8. https://doi.org/10.1007/s00268-019-04950-y.
37. Pilleron S, Soto-Perez-de-Celis E, Vignat J, Ferlay J, Soerjomataram I, Bray F, Sarfati D. Estimated global cancer incidence in the oldest adults in 2018 and projections to 2050. Int J Cancer. 2021;148(3):601–8. https://doi.org/10.1002/ijc.33232.
38. Parks R, Cheung KL. Challenges in geriatric oncology—a Surgeon's perspective. Curr Oncol. 2022;29(2):659–74. https://doi.org/10.3390/curroncol29020058.
39. Tsuji T. Rehabilitation for elderly patients with cancer. Jpn J Clin Oncol. 2022;52(10):1097–104. https://doi.org/10.1093/jjco/hyac139.
40. Sung H, Ferlay J, Siegel RL, Laversanne M, Soerjomataram I, Jemal A, Bray F. Global cancer statistics 2020: GLOBOCAN estimates of incidence and mortality worldwide for 36 cancers in 185 countries. CA Cancer J Clin. 2021;71(3):209–49. https://doi.org/10.3322/caac.21660.
41. DeSantis CE, Miller KD, Dale W, Mohile SG, Cohen HJ, Leach CR, Goding SA, Jemal A, Siegel RL. Cancer statistics for adults aged 85 years and older, 2019. CA Cancer J Clin. 2019;69(6):452–67. https://doi.org/10.3322/caac.21577.
42. Abdel-Razeq H, Rous FA, Abuhijla F, Abdel-Razeq N, Edaily S. Breast cancer in geriatric patients: current landscape and future prospects. Clin Interv Aging. 2022;17:1445–60. https://doi.org/10.2147/CIA.S365497.
43. Morgan JL, George J, Holmes G, et al. Breast cancer surgery in older women: outcomes of the bridging age gap in breast cancer study. Br J Surg. 2020;107(11):1468–79. https://doi.org/10.1002/BJS.11617.
44. Hidding JT, Beurskens CHG, Van der Wees PJ, Van Laarhoven HWM, Nijhuis-van der Sanden MWG. Treatment related impairments in arm and shoulder in patients with breast cancer: a systematic review. PLoS One. 2014;9(5):e96748. https://doi.org/10.1371/journal.pone.0096748.
45. Villa G, Mandarano R, Scirè-Calabrisotto C, Rizzelli V, Del Duca M, Pomarè Montin D, Paparella L, De Gaudio AR, Romagnoli S. Chronic pain after breast surgery: incidence, associated factors, and impact on quality of life, an observational prospective study. Perioper Med (Lond). 2021;10(1):6. https://doi.org/10.1186/s13741-021-00176-6.
46. Giacalone A, Alessandria P, Ruberti E. The physiotherapy intervention for shoulder pain in patients treated for breast cancer: systematic review. Cureus. 2019;11(12):e6416. https://doi.org/10.7759/cureus.6416.
47. DiSipio T, Rye S, Newman B, et al. Incidence of unilateral arm lymphoedema after breast cancer: a systematic review and meta-analysis. Lancet Oncol. 2013;14(6):500–15. https://doi.org/10.1016/S1470-2045(13)70076-7.
48. Gillespie TC, Sayegh HE, Brunelle CL, Daniell KM, Taghian AG. Breast cancer-related lymphedema: risk factors, precautionary measures, and treatments. Gland Surg. 2018;7(4):379–403. https://doi.org/10.21037/gs.2017.11.04.
49. Mohamed FA, Hossam E-DM. Effectiveness of endermologie technique in post-mastectomy lymphedema. Med J Cairo Univ. 2011;79(2):1–4.
50. Ahmed ET. Endermologie technique versus decongestive lymphatic therapy on post-mastectomy related lymphedema. J Nov Physiother. 2013;3:3.
51. Sekhoacha M, Riet K, Motloung P, Gumenku L, Adegoke A, Mashele S. Prostate cancer review: genetics, diagnosis, treatment options, and alternative approaches. Molecules. 2022;27(17):5730. https://doi.org/10.3390/molecules27175730.
52. Yang L, Lee JA, Heer E, Pernar C, Colditz GA, Pakpahan R, Imm KR, Kim EH, Grubb RL, Wolin KY, Kibel AS, Sutcliffe S. One-year urinary and sexual outcome trajectories among prostate cancer patients treated by radical prostatectomy: a prospective study. BMC Urol. 2021;21:81. https://doi.org/10.1186/s12894-021-00845-0.
53. Strączyńska A, Weber-Rajek M, Strojek K, Piekorz Z, Styczyńska H, Goch A, Radzimińska A. The impact of pelvic floor muscle training on urinary incontinence in men after radical prostatectomy (RP)—a systematic review. Clin Interv Aging. 2019;14:1997–2005. https://doi.org/10.2147/CIA.S228222.

54. Feng D, Liu S, Li D, Han P, Wei W. Analysis of conventional versus advanced pelvic floor muscle training in the management of urinary incontinence after radical prostatectomy: a systematic review and meta-analysis of randomized controlled trials. Transl Androl Urol. 2020;9(5):2031–45. https://doi.org/10.21037/tau-20-615.
55. Jones GS, Baldwin DR. Recent advances in the management of lung cancer. Clin Med (Lond). 2018;18(Suppl 2):s41–6. https://doi.org/10.7861/clinmedicine.18-2s-s41.
56. Wang J, Li R, Chang J, Wang Y, Lai Y, Dong Y, Che G. Quality of life between home-based and outpatient pulmonary rehabilitation in patients after surgical resection for lung cancer: protocol for a prospective, single-blind, randomised controlled trial. BMJ Open. 2023;13(5):e067845. https://doi.org/10.1136/bmjopen-2022-067845.
57. Ulaş Çınar H, Kefeli Çelik H, Çelik B, Doğan C. Is respiratory physiotherapy effective on pulmonary complications after lobectomy for lung cancer? Turk Gogus Kalp Damar Cerrahisi Derg. 2020;28(4):638–47. https://doi.org/10.5606/tgkdc.dergisi.2020.19693.
58. Wang L, Yu M, Ma Y, Tian R, Wang X. Effect of pulmonary rehabilitation on postoperative clinical status in patients with lung cancer and chronic obstructive pulmonary disease: a systematic review and meta-analysis. Evid Based Complement Alternat Med. 2022;2022:4133237. https://doi.org/10.1155/2022/4133237.
59. Cavalheri V, Burtin C, Formico VR, Nonoyama ML, Jenkins S, Spruit MA, Hill K, Cochrane Lung Cancer Group. Exercise training undertaken by people within 12 months of lung resection for non-small cell lung cancer. Cochrane Database Syst Rev. 2019;6:CD009955. https://doi.org/10.1002/14651858.CD009955.pub3.
60. Gjorgjievski M, Ristevski B. Postoperative management considerations of the elderly patient undergoing orthopaedic surgery. Injury. 2020;51(Suppl 2):S23–7. https://doi.org/10.1016/j.injury.2019.12.027.
61. Long H, Liu Q, Yin H, Wang K, Diao N, Zhang Y, Lin J, Guo A. Prevalence trends of site-specific osteoarthritis from 1990 to 2019: findings from the global burden of disease study 2019. Arthritis Rheumatol. 2022;74(7):1172–83. https://doi.org/10.1002/art.42089.
62. Papalia R, Campi S, Vorini F, Zampogna B, Vasta S, Papalia G, Fossati C, Torre G, Denaro V. The role of physical activity and rehabilitation following hip and knee arthroplasty in the elderly. J Clin Med. 2020;9(5):1401. https://doi.org/10.3390/jcm9051401.
63. Alrawashdeh W, Eschweiler J, Migliorini F, El Mansy Y, Tingart M, Rath B. Effectiveness of total knee arthroplasty rehabilitation programmes: a systematic review and meta-analysis. J Rehabil Med. 2021;53(6):2784. https://doi.org/10.2340/16501977-2827.
64. Min K, Beom J, Lim JY, et al. Clinical practice guideline for postoperative rehabilitation in older patients with hip fractures. Ann Rehabil Med. 2021;45(3):225–59. https://doi.org/10.5535/arm.21110.
65. Yoo JI, Ha YC, Lim JY, Kang H, Yoon BH, Kim H. Early rehabilitation in elderly after arthroplasty versus internal fixation for unstable intertrochanteric fractures of femur: systematic review and meta-analysis. J Korean Med Sci. 2017;32:858–67. https://doi.org/10.3346/jkms.2017.32.5.858.
66. Grusky AZ, Giri A, O'Hanlon D, Jain NB. The relationship of aging and smoking with rotator cuff disease: a systematic review and meta-analysis. Am J Phys Med Rehabil. 2022;101(4):331–40. https://doi.org/10.1097/PHM.0000000000001820.
67. Narvani AA, Imam MA, Godenèche A, Calvo E, Corbett S, Wallace AL, Itoi E. Degenerative rotator cuff tear, repair or not repair? A review of current evidence. Ann R Coll Surg Engl. 2020;102(4):248–55. https://doi.org/10.1308/rcsann.2019.0173.
68. Jung C, Tepohl L, Tholen R, Beitzel K, Buchmann S, Gottfried T, Grim C, Mauch B, Krischak G, Ortmann H, Schoch C, Mauch F. Rehabilitation following rotator cuff repair. Obere Extrem. 2018;13(1):45–61. https://doi.org/10.1007/s11678-018-0448-2.
69. Gutiérrez-Espinoza H, Araya-Quintanilla F, Pinto-Concha S, Zavala-González J, Gana-Hervias G, Cavero-Redondo I, Álvarez-Bueno C. Effectiveness of supervised early exercise program in patients with arthroscopic rotator cuff repair. Medicine (Baltimore). 2020;99(4):e18846. https://doi.org/10.1097/MD.0000000000018846.

70. Izquierdo-Fernández A, Gómez-Rodríguez M, Urbano-Luque M, García-Carmona M, Quevedo-Reinoso R, Minarro JC. Reverse shoulder arthroplasty in complex fractures of the proximal humerus: results after 7 years of follow-up. J Orthop Traumatol. 2021;22:38. https://doi.org/10.1186/s10195-021-00597-5.
71. Howard CM, Trasolini NA, Waterman BR. Optimizing outcomes after reverse Total shoulder arthroplasty: rehabilitation, expected outcomes, and maximizing return to activities. Curr Rev Musculoskelet Med. 2023;16(4):145–53. https://doi.org/10.1007/s12178-023-09823-5.
72. Lee JH, Chun YM, Kim DS, Lee DH, Shin SJ. Effects of neuromuscular electrical muscle stimulation on the deltoid for shoulder function restoration after reverse total shoulder arthroplasty in the early recovery period: a prospective randomized study. Arch Orthop Trauma Surg. 2020;143:3037. https://doi.org/10.1007/s00402-022-04515-0.
73. Kutsal FY, Ergin Ergani GO. Vertebral compression fractures: still an unpredictable aspect of osteoporosis. Turk J Med Sci. 2021;51(2):393–9. https://doi.org/10.3906/sag-2005-315.
74. Koepke LG, Weiser L, Stangenberg M, Dreimann M, Heuer A, Strahl A, Viezens L. Outcome after posterior vertebral column resection in patients with severe osteoporotic fractures—a retrospective analysis from two centers. Medicina (Kaunas). 2022;58(2):277. https://doi.org/10.3390/medicina58020277.
75. Zhang B, Li T, Wang Z. Efficacy and complications of different surgical modalities of treating osteoporotic spinal compression fracture in the elderly. Am J Transl Res. 2022;14(1):364–72.
76. Chen X, Wan D, Xiong XM, Shi HG, Deng XG, Gu T, Song SM, Hou W, Li QL. Application of enhanced recovery after surgery in postoperative rehabilitation of osteoporotic lumbar compression fractures with percutaneous vertebroplasty or percutaneous kyphoplasty. Zhongguo Gu Shang. 2020;33(12):1179–83. https://doi.org/10.12200/j.issn.1003-0034.2020.12.018.
77. Huang R, Pan F, Zhu W, Kong C, Lu S. Predictors for the restoration of the sagittal spinal malalignment in patients with lumbar stenosis after short-segment decompression and fusion surgery. BMC Musculoskelet Disord. 2022;23:711. https://doi.org/10.1186/s12891-022-05666-2.
78. McGregor AH, Probyn K, Cro S, Doré CJ, Burton AK, Balagué F, Pincus T, Fairbank J. Rehabilitation following surgery for lumbar spinal stenosis. Cochrane Database of Syst Rev. 2013;12:CD009644. https://doi.org/10.1002/14651858.CD009644.pub2.
79. Lieber BA, Chiang V, . Prabhu AV, Agarwal N, Henry JK, Lin D, Kazemi N, Tabbosha M. Postoperative complications for elderly patients after single-level lumbar fusions for spondylolisthesis.World Neurosurg 2016;91:149–153. doi: https://doi.org/10.1016/j.wneu.2016.03.052.
80. Madera M, Brady J, Deily S, McGinty T, Moroz L, Singh D, Tipton G, Truumees E. The role of physical therapy and rehabilitation after lumbar fusion surgery for degenerative disease: a systematic review. J Neurosurg Spine. 2017;26(6):694–704. https://doi.org/10.3171/2016.10.SPINE16627.
81. Tacconi L, Giordan E, Baldo S, Serra G, Signorelli F. Percutaneous endoscopic lumbar discectomy in the elderly: an effective treatment for prolapsed disc: consideration on 75 case. Interdisciplinary. Neurosurgery. 2020;20:100655.
82. Weir S, Samnaliev M, Kuo T-C, Ni Choitir C, Tierney TS, Cumming D, Bruce J, Manca A, Taylor RS, Eldabe S. The incidence and healthcare costs of persistent postoperative pain following lumbar spine surgery in the UK: a cohort study using the clinical practice research datalink (CPRD) and hospital episode statistics (HES). BMJ Open. 2017;7:e017585. https://doi.org/10.1136/bmjopen-2017-017585.
83. Oosterhuis T, Costa LO, Maher CG, De Vet HC, van Tulder MW, Ostelo RW. Rehabilitation after lumbar disc surgery. Cochrane Database Syst Rev. 2014;3:CD003007. https://doi.org/10.1002/14651858.CD003007.pub3.
84. Tamuleviciute-Prasciene E, Drulyte K, Jurenaite G, Kubilius R, Bjarnason-Wehrens B. Frailty and exercise training: how to provide best care after cardiac surgery or intervention for elder patients with Valvular heart disease. Biomed Res Int. 2018;2018:9849475. https://doi.org/10.1155/2018/9849475.

85. Chen OJ, Liu JF, Liu YQ, Chen YM, Tu ML, Yu HR, Lin CC LMC, Liu SF. Effectiveness of a perioperative pulmonary rehabilitation program following coronary artery bypass graft surgery in patients with and without COPD. Int J Chron Obstruct Pulmon Dis. 2018;13:1591–7. https://doi.org/10.2147/COPD.S157967.
86. Liu JF, Lee HM, Chen JO, Fang TP, Chen YM, Lo CM, Liu SF, Lin HL. Benefits of multiple-intervention pulmonary rehabilitation to older adults with high-risk multimorbidity after coronary artery bypass grafting. Healthcare (Basel). 2020;8(4):368. https://doi.org/10.3390/healthcare8040368.
87. Windmöller P, Bodnar MT, Casagrande J, Dallazen F, Schneider J, Agnolleto Berwanger S, Borghi-Silva A, Roseli WE. Physical exercise combined with CPAP in subjects who underwent surgical myocardial revascularization: a randomized clinical trial. Respir Care. 2020;65(2):150–7. https://doi.org/10.4187/respcare.06919.
88. Hegazy FA, Mohamed Kamel SM, Abdelhamid AS, Aboelnasr EA, Elshazly M, Hassan AM. Effect of postoperative high load long duration inspiratory muscle training on pulmonary function and functional capacity after mitral valve replacement surgery: a randomized controlled trial with follow-up. PLoS One. 2021;16(8):e0256609. https://doi.org/10.1371/journal.pone.0256609.
89. Khadanga S, Savage PD, Ades PA. Resistance training for older adults in cardiac rehabilitation. Clin Geriatr Med. 2019;35(4):459–68. https://doi.org/10.1016/j.cger.2019.07.005.
90. Pengelly J, Pengelly M, Lin KY, Royse C, Karri R, Royse A, Bryant A, Williams G, El-Ansary D. Affiliations expand exercise parameters and outcome measures used in cardiac rehabilitation programs following median sternotomy in the elderly: a systematic review and meta-analysis. Heart Lung Circ. 2019;28(10):1560–70. https://doi.org/10.1016/j.hlc.2019.05.098.
91. Çinar F, Parlak G, Etí Aslan F. The effect of comorbidity on mortality in elderly patients undergoing emergency abdominal surgery: a systematic review and metaanalysis. Turk J Med Sci. 2021;51(1):61–7. https://doi.org/10.3906/sag-2001-27.
92. Jønsson LR, Foss BN, Orbæk JD, Lauritsen ML, Sejrsen HN, Kristensen MT. Early intensive mobilization after acute high-risk abdominal surgery: a nonrandomized prospective feasibility trial. Can J Surg. 2023;66(3):E236–45. https://doi.org/10.1503/cjs.008722.
93. Svensson-Raskh A, Schandl AR, Ståhle A, Nygren-Bonnier M, Fagevik OM. Mobilization started within 2 hours after abdominal surgery improves peripheral and arterial oxygenation: a single-center randomized controlled trial. Phys Ther. 2021;101(5):pzab094. https://doi.org/10.1093/ptj/pzab094.

Early Identification of Post-Demission Setting

24

Antonietta Castiello

24.1 Introduction

The role of nurses in the care of frail individuals is vital, particularly in the surgical setting. During hospitalization, older people experience significant functional decline, which impairs their future independence and quality of life. The frail surgical patient is defined as a person "at risk" with multiple chronic diseases, an unstable general state of health, and frequently, disability and/or socio-economic and socio-environmental difficulties. Frail and older people have higher rates of hospital admission than the general population and higher rates of readmission due to complications after surgery. In a systematic review, Shepperd and colleagues [1] found evidence that good discharge planning with early identification of the post-discharge setting reduces readmission to the hospital and hospital length of stay for older adults with an acute medical condition such as surgery. A variety of strategies have been used to strengthen discharge planning, such as early screening, specialized geriatric programs, liaison nurses, and case management [2]. Although discharge is not, as one might think, the final phase of the clinical path, it represents a critical phase. The primary objective of the clinical path is, in fact, the achievement of the highest possible level of functional autonomy for that specific patient. Often, in a patient, perhaps frail and complex, such as a geriatric surgical patient, this does not occur within the hospital environment. Even the transition from one hospitalization facility to another is a protected discharge, because the patient while remaining in a structured health environment passes to a different level of care intensity.

A. Castiello (✉)
Division of Gerontology and Geriatrics, Santa Maria della Misericordia Hospital, Perugia, Italy

V. Boccardi, L. Marano (eds.), *The Frail Surgical Patient*, Practical Issues in Geriatrics, https://doi.org/10.1007/978-3-031-77707-3_24

24.2 The Nursing Process

The nurse plays a significant role in several areas, including managing the frail and complex person, providing global and holistic management, maintaining or recovering self-sufficiency, promoting self-care, providing education and support to the family network, and maintaining continuity of care. Everyone is unique and constantly changing, just like their state of health. Similarly, the nurse case manager must follow possible changes in clinical conditions and not be limited to the initial assessment. For the discharge planning process to be successful, early identification of people at high risk of inappropriate access to health services and/or readmission at protected discharge becomes fundamental [3]. The Individualized Care Plan (ICP) is at the heart of the entire protected discharge process; it is born during hospitalization defining the interventions necessary to achieve the objectives of the care and the health needs of the patient, both in the hospital and in the phases after hospitalization; therefore, the ICP is born in the hospital but defines the whole path of care, even at the patient's home. It will then be the district to carry out the plan outside the hospital.

Discharge planning should be early [4] and should begin at admission or, at the latest by the third day of hospitalization as soon as the patient has passed the critical or acute phase, in order to create the conditions for patients and family members to be able to contribute to the best decisions to be made. The patient is always included in the decisions, while the team must:

- Evaluate the patient involving social and health personnel, hospital, and territorial at a multi-professional level. It is a complex phase of extreme importance that must presuppose protocols and paths of intervention and a structured, shared, and integrated approach to the patient of the different professions involved (doctors, nurses, physiotherapists, social workers, etc.).
- Analyze the functional abilities and residual capacities of the subject. In this phase, the nurse analyzes, in simple terms, what the patient cannot do with respect to their state of health, what capacities the disease has reduced, removed, or modified, and which skills of the patient can be used to return to an adequate level of functional autonomy. Care goals are then defined. The right of the patient to participate, in this establishment and during the process, expressing his own opinions, doubts, and beliefs is primary.
- Analyze social support: in this phase, the nurse analyzes the specific family and social context of the subject to understand what resources the patient has and will have available to achieve their goals or, otherwise, to understand the type of support from activate in case of low presence or total absence, for example, of caregivers.
- Choose the right setting: this is done with the comparison between the assessment of the patient and his needs and what is offered by the territorial services, their adequacy, and responsiveness to the needs highlighted. This evaluation is early, and it must be reapplied if there are psychophysical alterations in the

patient. For this reason, the patient will be evaluated periodically during hospitalization and consequently also the discharge plan.

After surgery, the transition from hospital to home is very difficult, especially because subjects require intermediate and continuity of care. Preparing the patient for discharge is therefore a care responsibility, as well as a right of the patient and their family, who must be involved and accompanied throughout the care process. The nurse's discharge plan develops throughout the integrated discharge letter that will accompany the patient to any welcoming structure or service. In the integrated discharge letter, the nurse will summarize the care plan carried out and propose operative solutions relating to the post-operative period and also in collaboration with the team. The aim is, therefore, to highlight the interventions implemented and those possibly planned to meet the residual needs of the patient. In this view, the nurse becomes a linking figure between different care structures, home, or long-term care, according to the principles of guaranteeing "continuity of care," "equality, globality, and territoriality," established by Law 833/78 (law establishing by the National Health Service).

Post-operative complications are more common in frail patients due to an increased occurrence of comorbid illnesses and age-related physiologic impairments in pulmonary, cardiovascular, and kidney function. Therefore, competent assessment is necessary to recognize early signals of deterioration. To identify and solve or prevent patient problems, the nurse must carry out a logical sequence of five phases according to the nursing process:

1. Nursing assessment
2. Formulation of nursing diagnoses
3. Intervention planning
4. Implementation of interventions
5. Evaluation of the results

24.2.1 Nursing Assessment

To promote patient well-being, a holistic assessment through multidimensional and multidisciplinary assessment (MDA) is fundamental. For older persons, the geriatric multidimensional approach finds the geriatric evaluation unit (GEU) to be the most important tool to promote care for the frail person, which recognizes and combines health and social needs to create personalized care plans. The nurse in the geriatric evaluation unit has a global vision of the person being assisted, starting from the reception and respecting the frail person's times, ways, values, fears, expectations, limits, and problems.

Every patient has their own peculiarities, and the nurse has a duty to personalize the care process. The main tool for implementing the individualized care plan is the nursing record. It certifies and organizes, with logic and effectiveness, all the information and care activities of the person collected and/or performed by the nurse.

The nursing record is an integral part of the medical record, as it completes the health documentation of the user/client and will be reunited with the archiving. Formally recognized by art. 69 of Presidential Decree 384/90, it is legally considered a public act. In the nursing record, you can document the nursing process through assessment, definition of objectives, nursing interventions, formulation of the care plan, implementation, and evaluation. Nursing diagnoses are formulated to allow greater objectification of nursing problems and the adoption of care protocols. Being a standardized tool, it also helps in communication with other operators in the care process.

As the very first step toward an efficient discharge process, during the patient's admission and evaluation phase, a nurse (either a primary nurse or a case manager nurse) has the responsibility of assessing the risk of discharge. Assessing the risk of difficult discharge from the moment of hospitalization is not a simple task. A systemic approach is required that considers the individual and their peculiarities in such a way that the best treatment outcomes are identified, even for patients with similar pathologies. At the time of discharge, the nurse must re-evaluate all the information kept during the pre-operative management and collected in the nursing record. A valuable aid for healthcare providers is the Blaylock Risk Assessment Screening Scale (BRASS), a standardized assessment scale that identifies the risk of discharge and helps the nurse define the best treatment path by detailing the patient and their needs (Table 24.1). The BRASS index investigates ten dimensions: age, life situation, social support, functional status, cognitive status, behavioral model, sensory deficits, previous hospitalizations, access to the emergency room, active clinical problems, and the number of drugs taken. The evaluation is made through the information provided by a family member or person who knows the patient well. Three risk classes are identified: low (0–10), medium (11–19), and high (≥20). This scale has proven to be a quick and effective tool in framing patients at higher risk after discharge [5, 6]. As can be seen, the BRASS index evaluates the patient considering various dimensions. For a good discharge risk assessment, the subject must be assessed from a multidimensional point of view periodically, both at the time of admission, during the hospital stay, and at the time of discharge.

24.2.2 Formulation of Nursing Diagnoses

Thanks to the assessment phase, the nurse will elaborate on a series of nursing diagnoses aimed at identifying the best interventions for the surgical patient. "Nursing diagnosis is a judgment on the answers given by the individual, family, or community, to health problems and life processes, real or potential. The nursing diagnosis provides the basis for making a choice of nursing care interventions, which will lead to the achievement of the objectives for which the nurse is responsible." This definition of diagnosis was given by the North American Nursing Diagnosis Association (NANDA, of which the first president was Marjory Gordon), in March 1990, during its ninth conference (even if the first nurse talking about nursing diagnosis was Virginia Fry, in 1953). Nursing diagnosis is based on the concepts of Nursing

Table 24.1 Blaylock Risk Assessment Screening (BRASS) scale

Blaylock Risk Assessment Screening (choose only one option)			
Age	**Score**	**Living situation**	**Score**
55 years or less	0	Lives with family	0
From 56 to 64 years	1	Lives only with spouse	1
From 65 to 79 years	2	Lives alone with family support	2
80 years or more	3	Lives alone with friends' support	3
		Nursing home/residential care	4
Mobility	**Score**	**Sensory deficit**	**Score**
Ambulatory	0		
Ambulatory with mechanical assistance	1	None	0
Ambulatory with human assistance	2	Visual or hearing deficits	1
Nonambulatory	3	Visual and hearing deficits	2
Behavior pattern	**Score**	**Number of drugs**	**Score**
Appropriate	0		
Wandering	1	Fewer than three drugs	0
Agitated	1	3–5 drugs	1
Confused	1	More than five drugs	2
Other	1		
Cognition	**Score**	**Number of active medical problems**	**Score**
Oriented	0		
Disoriented to some spheres + some of the time	1	Three medical problems	0
Disoriented to some spheres all the time	2	3–5 medical problems	1
Disoriented to all spheres some of the time	3	More than five medical problems	2
Disoriented to all spheres some all of the time	4		
Functional status	**Score**	**Number of previous admission/emergency room visits**	**Score**
Independent basic ADLs/IADLs	0		
		None in the last 3 months	0
		One in the last 3 months	1
		Two in the last 3 months	2
		More than two in the last 3 months	3
Dependent in			
Eating/fooding	1		
Bathing/grooming	1		
Toileting	1		
Transferring	1		

(continued)

Table 24.1 (continued)

Blaylock Risk Assessment Screening (choose only one option)		
Incontinent of bowel function	1	**Risk factor index**:
Incontinent of bladder function	1	**Score of 10** = at risk for home care resources **Score of 11–19** = at risk for extended discharge planning **Score greater than 20** = at risk for placement other than home if the patient's score is 10 or greater, refer the patient to the discharger planning coordinator or discharger planning team
Meal preparation	1	
Responsible for own medication administration	1	
Handing own finances	1	
Grocery shopping	1	
Transportation	1	

Interventions Classification (NIC) and Nursing Outcomes Classification (NOC). In relation to the objectives set (NOC), the appropriate nursing interventions (NIC) are implemented.

Examples of nursing diagnoses (NOC) in a surgical geriatric patient could be: "risk for fall," "constipation," "risk for deficient fluid volume," "risk for injury," "risk for infection," "risk for impaired skin integrity," "disturbed sleep pattern," "ineffective health maintenance," "deficient knowledge," and "acute pain". The use of these standardized nursing diagnoses helps the nurse to precociously identify the needs of the surgical patients [7].

Also, it is essential to consider the possible presence (previous or occurred) of external devices such as stomas (urinary/intestinal), tracheostomy, bladder catheter, suprapubic catheter, and percutaneous endoscopic gastrostomy that can affect the patient's quality of life if not adequately managed both in hospitalization and in other settings, which would require further actions.

24.2.3 Intervention Planning

After thoroughly understanding the complex needs of older patients, nurses are expected to prescribe appropriate nursing interventions (NIC) to enhance their health outcomes. It is fundamental to identify an individual in the patient's family/social context who will take care of them. With this person, the healthcare personnel will interface to make the care path as simple, effective, and efficient as possible.

The caregiver, therefore, becomes a pivotal point, even at the time of discharge. The inclusion of this figure within the discharge plan will facilitate its success. In this context, the nurse case manager assumes the management of the case and becomes the reference figure for the patient, family members and/or caregivers, and other health and social workers, with the responsibility to:

- Present and explain the process and the phases that compose it.
- Ensure and coordinate the application of the process.
- Identify and help overcome any critical issues.

After analyzing the results of the evaluation by the BRASS index, in the first few days of hospitalization, the nurse, in collaboration with the GEU, after a structured interview with the patient (if possible) and the caregiver, identified the patient's destination for discharge:

- Return home without specific measures.
- Return home with the help of a caregiver.
- Return home with a prescription of principles.
- Return home with activation of forms of integrated home care (IHC).
- Return home with the activation of social services.
- Return home and activation of the palliative care unit and/or entry into hospice for cancer patients.
- Entry into territorial structures (community hospital, nursing home, or retirement home).
- Return to a retirement home with or without aggravation.
- Transfer to long-term care (post-acute or rehabilitative).

24.2.4 Implementation of Interventions

The nurse case manager collaborates with the geriatric assessment team and social and territorial services and accompanies the patient and family during hospitalization. They support them from a welfare and educational perspective and identify the best extra-hospital path suited to the individual patient [8]. The nurse case manager and the multidisciplinary team work together toward the common goal of choosing the right dismissive setting based on objective and subjective parameters (Table 24.2). The patient and family members' right to choose is never excluded. Everyone has the right to take part in the discharge process and choose among the various opportunities most suited to them, provided they are able to understand and want to [9]. If the patient is unable to understand and want, the family members or support guardians have the same right. Therapeutic education toward patients and their families/caregivers is essential to guarantee a better discharge process and minimize readmission. Through therapeutic education, the patient (considering adherence regarding self-management) or the caregiver must know how and where to seek support and manage care at home. The caregiver will have a good preparation to provide care after surgery. Communication is also essential although it is often underestimated or ignored. Throughout the process, operators must communicate with each other, the patient, family members, and/or caregivers, and local services. If communication is not effective, there will be a flaw in the whole process. With advanced age and a high degree of frailty, communication efficacy may be compromised.

Studies have shown the importance of having suitable tools to facilitate communication with relatives and patients during the treatment process, especially at the time of discharge. A bedside "leaving hospital information sheet" can potentially improve communication between patients, families, and their treating team [10]. Research has also been done on the use of printed material and

Table 24.2 Intermediate and continuity of care setting in the surgical frail patient

Intermediate and continuity of care setting in the surgical frail patient	
Type	Features and users
Integrated home care (IHM)	Service for: • Older and disabled adults in fragile conditions with chronic degenerative diseases that severely limit their autonomy • Patients discharged from hospital wards who require social and health support • Patients in advanced stages of oncological or degenerative diseases
Residential facilities, as a protected residence or assisted health residence	These residential accommodations are organized to prioritize individual needs for confidentiality and privacy while also promoting socialization among the residents. This enables the patients to feel at home and maintain a lifestyle as similar as possible to their previous living arrangements. The facility provides all the necessary medical, nursing, and rehabilitative interventions to prevent and treat chronic diseases and potential exacerbations The number of beds in these facilities is limited to a maximum of 120, divided into smaller units of approximately 20–30 older individuals each. They cater to older individuals who require assistance with daily activities and are not fully independent. Hospitalizations in these facilities can be either temporary or indefinite
Nursing home	In a nursing home, various forms of support and care are provided, including protective assistance, meal administration, recreational and social activities, and assistance with daily tasks and functions, as well as nursing care and medication administration, if required
Hospice	A residential social health facility serves as a place of welcome and temporary shelter for terminally ill patients, providing them with the opportunity to experience this natural phase of their existence with appropriate medical, welfare, psychological, and spiritual support. The facility emphasizes the values of value, dignity, and participation as key focal points
Rehabilitation facilities	Specialized in post-traumatic interventions, they focus on the rehabilitation of various types of pathological events commonly experienced by disabled and older individuals, such as stroke, hip fracture, femur fracture, and more
Community (or territorial) hospitals	Intermediate care inpatient facilities are intended for short-term admissions for patients who require low-intensity clinical interventions. They help provide more appropriate care by, for example, reducing improper access to the emergency room or other health services. Additionally, they facilitate the transfer of patients from acute care facilities to their homes, allowing families time to adapt to the home environment and make it more suitable for patients' care needs
Home palliative care	Care is provided by home palliative care units that guarantee, depending on the complexity of the needs and the different care intensities, both basic interventions coordinated by the general practitioner and interventions by multidisciplinary specialist teams. They are provided at the expense of the health system and therefore do not involve any cost for the sick person and their family. However, it is not possible to provide this home care to all types of patients and at every stage of the disease: There are, in fact, requirements that must be met according to a previous multidimensional evaluation. Even, the patient's home must meet specific requirements

person-based discharge communication methods, including verbal instructions (either in person or via telephone calls). Several studies have examined the use of information technology (IT), such as computer-generated and video-based discharge communication practices. Utilizing technology to deliver discharge information is preferred by healthcare providers and patients and improves patients' understanding of their medical conditions and discharge instructions. Effective discharge summaries reduce adverse drug events, unplanned hospital readmission, post-discharge complications, and mortality and increase patient and carer satisfaction [11]. However, for discharge summaries to be effective, they must be well-structured, precise, and easy to understand, even if summarized, which is not always the case. Delivery of discharge instructions is often rushed, and patients frequently do not understand aspects of their discharge, particularly medication management. This can cause readmission and failure of the clinical process. To avoid this, it is necessary to train all operators to provide complete discharge cards by providing all necessary information for the patient's management once discharged from a given care setting [12].

Obviously, the content and structure of integrated discharge letters depend on the specialty, type of hospital care, and the individual preferences and style of the physician who authored the content. When well-structured and personalized, the integrated discharge letter can become an effective tool for patient satisfaction, as well as achieving the purpose of the care process [13]. In this context, the development of a "centralized nurse" figure who acts as a bridge between the hospital nurse and the community nurse plays a vital role in ensuring seamless continuity of care. This connecting point serves as a crucial link in the healthcare chain, facilitating effective communication and information flow between different care settings.

24.2.5 Evaluation of the Results

Before discharge, the nurse must verify that the educational process has been successful. They will summarize the highlights of the home care plan, explain how to manage therapy and devices, and fill any gaps in understanding. The nurse will remain available for any necessary information, even after the patient is discharged from the hospital environment, and provide all the contact details that may be needed. Following discharge, the nurse will establish rapport with patients and family members, monitor their progress, and arrange for any further intervention that may be necessary. The nurse will also remain in contact with intermediate care facilities, providing support during the post-discharge period. Periodic phone calls after discharge can also be of great help to assess the effectiveness of the planning carried out and to correct any errors in advance. Telemedicine, tablets, and other apps have revolutionized healthcare in the post-discharge phase, providing invaluable support to both patients and caregivers. These technological advancements may play a crucial role in ensuring a seamless transition from the hospital to home care, enhancing convenience, accessibility, and overall patient outcomes. Through video calls or online chats, patients can discuss their recovery progress, address concerns, and receive personalized recommendations without the need for physical visits to the hospital or clinic. By staying "up to date with the times," healthcare systems can harness these technologies to improve patient outcomes.

24.3 Conclusions and Final Remarks

The discharge of a patient from the hospital to home is not an easy process. It can be characterized by several problems, such as reduced independence in activities of daily living, a deficit of care, problems in the management of medications, social problems, the need for information, and emotional problems. The literature review shows that the essential elements for discharge planning are communication, coordination, education, patient participation, and collaboration between medical personnel. Multidimensional assessment is the prerequisite for any care process for the older people with frailty. It allows for the improvement of diagnostic accuracy, the selection of interventions necessary to preserve health and recovery, the recommendation of the most appropriate care context, the prediction of outcomes, the monitoring of clinical changes over time, and the making of consequent decisions. In addition, older patients are more likely to be alive and in their homes at follow-up if they receive a complete geriatric assessment (CGA) at the time of hospitalization [14, 15]. Once the patient has been framed as an "individual," it is necessary to analyze the social context around them. Usually, the closest family members take care of their care needs directly or by entrusting their care to a third person during this delicate phase of life. The reduction of stress and anxiety for the patient, family, nurse, doctor, hospital, and community services helps achieve the success of the process. Considering the variety and organizational complexity of the various structures and lacking validated parameters to be used for "good communication," it would be interesting and useful to encourage related studies, as has already been done in a few realities [16]. Interviewing patients and their families (where possible), caregivers, and even collaborators in various settings can help to try to find the right communicative approach for each specific reality. This could be done through questionnaires administered during hospitalization in various settings but also once back home, even through periodic phone calls [17]. The use of the BRASS scale combined with the nursing record can concretely help in the discharge planning process. The medical literature typically identifies the first day of admission as the time to begin discharge planning to minimize the patient's length of stay in the acute care hospital. This strategy has its limitations as older patients are often confused by unfamiliar surroundings, surgical anesthesia, post-operative pain, and the rapid pace of hospital recovery typically expected today. Consequently, options for discharge may be limited to the most expedient plan that will ensure safety and continued recovery [18].

References

1. Gonçalves-Bradley DC, Lannin NA, Clemson LM, Cameron ID, Shepperd S. Discharge planning from hospital. Cochrane Database Syst Rev. 2016;2016(1):CD000313. https://doi.org/10.1002/14651858.CD000313.pub5. PMID: 26816297; PMCID: PMC7073416.
2. Courtney MD, Edwards HE, Chang AM, Parker AW, Finlayson K, Hamilton K. A randomised controlled trial to prevent hospital readmissions and loss of functional ability in high risk older adults: a study protocol. BMC Health Serv Res. 2011;11:202. https://doi.org/10.1186/1472-6963-11-202. PMID: 21861920; PMCID: PMC3224378.
3. Suter-Gut D, Metcalf AM, Donnelly MA, Smith IM. Post-discharge care planning and rehabilitation of the elderly surgical patient. Clin Geriatr Med. 1990;6(3):669–83.
4. Styrborn K. Early discharge planning for elderly patients in acute hospitals—an intervention study. Scand J Soc Med. 1995;23(4):273–85. https://doi.org/10.1177/140349489502300409.
5. Cammilletti V, Forino F, Palombi M, Donati D, Tartaglini D, Di Muzio M. BRASS score and complex discharge: a pilot study. Acta Biomed. 2018;88(4):414–25. https://doi.org/10.23750/abm.v88i4.6191. PMID: 29350655; PMCID: PMC6166170.
6. Dal Molin A, Gatta C, Derossi V, Guazzini A, Cocchieri A, Vellone E, Alvaro R, Rasero L. Hospital discharge: results from an Italian multicenter prospective study using Blaylock risk assessment screening score. Int J Nurs Knowl. 2014;25(1):14–21. https://doi.org/10.1111/2047-3095.12016. Epub 2013 Dec 3.
7. Cesare M, D'agostino F, Maurici M, Zega M, Zeffiro V, Cocchieri A. Standardized nursing diagnoses in a surgical hospital setting: a retrospective study based on electronic health data. SAGE Open Nurs. 2023;9:23779608231158157. https://doi.org/10.1177/23779608231158157. PMID: 36824318; PMCID: PMC9941607.
8. Armold S. Case management: an overview for nurses. Nursing. 2019;49(9):43–5. https://doi.org/10.1097/01.NURSE.0000577708.49429.83.
9. Birmingham J. Patient choice in the discharge planning process. Prof Case Manag. 2009;14(6):296–309. https://doi.org/10.1097/NCM.0b013e3181c3d3c5.
10. New PW, McDougall KE, Scroggie CP. Improving discharge planning communication between hospitals and patients. Intern Med J. 2016;46(1):57–62. https://doi.org/10.1111/imj.12919.
11. Newnham H, Barker A, Ritchie E, Hitchcock K, Gibbs H, Holton S. Discharge communication practices and healthcare provider and patient preferences, satisfaction and comprehension: a systematic review. Int J Qual Health Care. 2017;29(6):752–68. https://doi.org/10.1093/intqhc/mzx121.
12. Yemm R, Bhattacharya D, Wright D, Poland F. What constitutes a high quality discharge summary? A comparison between the views of secondary and primary care doctors. Int J Med Educ. 2014;5:125–31. https://doi.org/10.5116/ijme.538b.3c2e. PMID: 25341221; PMCID: PMC4207187.
13. Lindhardt CL, Maerkedahl M, Brandt CE, Madsen SR. The personalised discharge letter: the experience of patients and parents from the Filadelfia epilepsy hospital. Scand J Caring Sci. 2021;35(1):67–74. https://doi.org/10.1111/scs.12846. Epub 2020 Apr 2.
14. Ellis G, Gardner M, Tsiachristas A, Langhorne P, Burke O, Harwood RH, Conroy SP, Kircher T, Somme D, Saltvedt I, Wald H, O'Neill D, Robinson D, Shepperd S. Comprehensive geriatric assessment for older adults admitted to hospital. Cochrane Database Syst Rev. 2017;9(9):CD006211. https://doi.org/10.1002/14651858.CD006211.pub3. PMID: 28898390; PMCID: PMC6484374.
15. Zurlo A, Zuliani G. Management of care transition and hospital discharge. Aging Clin Exp Res. 2018;30(3):263–70. https://doi.org/10.1007/s40520-017-0885-6. Epub 2018 Jan 8.
16. Weetman K, Dale J, Scott E, Schnurr S. The discharge communication study: research protocol for a mixed methods study to investigate and triangulate discharge communication experiences of patients, GPs, and hospital professionals, alongside a corresponding discharge letter sample. BMC Health Serv Res. 2019;19(1):825. https://doi.org/10.1186/s12913-019-4612-1. PMID: 31711500; PMCID: PMC6849198.

17. Tan M, Lang D. Effectiveness of nurse leader rounding and post-discharge telephone calls in patient satisfaction: a systematic review. JBI Database System Rev Implement Rep. 2015;13(7):154–76. https://doi.org/10.11124/jbisrir-2015-2013.
18. Merriman ML. Pre-hospital discharge planning: empowering elderly patients through choice. Crit Care Nurs Q. 2008;31(1):52–8. https://doi.org/10.1097/01.CNQ.0000306397.25024.d6.

25 Continuity of Care: A Multidimensional Vision for the Frail Patient

Alberto Castagna, Giuseppe Sena, Giuseppe Gallelli, Carmen Ruberto, Anna Maria Condito, and Giovanni Ruotolo

25.1 Background

Time after discharge is critical, especially for individuals with complex care needs such as frail surgical patients. A possible answer is employing care transition programs aimed to guarantee the coordination among healthcare practitioners and continuity of medical care on moving among different settings and different levels of care. It is a question of creating and implementing a collaborative model that "breaks down" the hospital/territory boundaries and acts with a strong integration of the professionals involved not only in the territorial context closest to the person and the family but also for the management of the crises that lead often to inappropriate hospitalizations.

The implementation of this work is in line with the interventions indicated in Italian Mission 6 of the PNRR (National Recovery and Resilience Plan) [1] oriented toward "physically" structuring a new model of territorial assistance based on needs identified as "priority." In summary, the objective of the PNRR Health Mission is to strengthen prevention and health services in the area, modernize and digitize the health system, and guarantee equity and uniformity of access to treatment. In Italy, another opportunity is the PNNA (Piano Nazionale Non-Autosufficienza e

A. Castagna (✉)
Cure Primarie, Distretto di Soverato, Azienda Sanitatia Provinciale di Catanzaro, Catanzaro, Italy

G. Sena · G. Gallelli
SOC Chirurgia Vascolare, AOU" R. Dulbecco" di Catanzaro, Catanzaro, Italy

C. Ruberto
SOC di Geriatria, AOU "R. Dulbecco" di Catanzaro, Catanzaro, Italy

A. M. Condito
Direzione Medica di Presidio, AOU "R. Dulbecco" di Catanzaro, Catanzaro, Italy

G. Ruotolo
Giovanni Ruotolo, SOC di Geriatria, AOU "R. Dulbecco" di Catanzaro, Catanzaro, Italy

V. Boccardi, L. Marano (eds.), *The Frail Surgical Patient*, Practical Issues in Geriatrics, https://doi.org/10.1007/978-3-031-77707-3_25

Riabilitazione) [2]. The PNNA is a national plan in Italy that focuses on caring for and rehabilitating non-self-sufficient individuals, including older adults and those with disabilities. The program aims to improve the quality and availability of intermediate care services, including skilled nursing facilities, rehabilitation centers, and other residential care settings. In addition, the PNNA recognizes the importance of providing comprehensive, person-centered care that is tailored to the needs of everyone [3]. The usefulness of protected discharge programs to guarantee continuity of care between the hospital and the territory is increasingly evident. Continuity of care implies a "taking charge" shared by several actors and several services from different environments in the context of care management and case management, through the transmission of all the information useful in the setting transition phase. The transmission of clinical and social health data is essential for the agreed planning of discharge according to the principle of the therapeutic alliance [4]. The literature data, in fact, support that therapeutic education and communication between health professionals and family are particularly important in discharge planning [5]. The structure of a country's healthcare system is of the utmost importance. Global standards require a healthcare system to have three tiers such as primary, secondary, and tertiary healthcare. Basic primary health care is the first level of health services that first comes into contact with a patient. Patients identified as having any abnormalities by primary health services are then referred to secondary health services for specialist curative management. When patient management requires more advanced facilities and skills, they are referred to tertiary centers. The search for continuity of care has led to the creation of a new treatment setting, the "intermediate" structure between the hospital and the territory. The international community has not yet reached a single definition of "intermediate care" [6].

Within the intermediate care path, several elements play a central and priority role [3]:

1. Comprehensive geriatric assessment (CGA) and an individualized as well as personalized path.
2. Bidirectional communication between a hospital and territorial services.
3. Uniform operational modalities between a hospital and a territory.
4. The sharing of patient information.
5. The establishment of an integrated team composed of different professional figures (nurses, physiotherapists, nutritionists, etc.)
6. Ensuring the continuity of care [3]·

There are very different interpretations of the pitch. In our opinion, it would be more correct to consider intermediate care as a modality of intervention, a care process to be carried out through the concurrence of multiple services in a dynamic and modular way and not as a structure. The work we have developed aims to ensure a path of continuity that guarantees the fragile surgical patient discharged from each node of the complex care network a timely response toward the appropriate setting. In fact, an innovative model is described for the management of fragile surgical patients with complex discharge, i.e., those who can only be discharged by activating high-intensity assistance measures (e.g., admission to long-term care facilities or hospital rehabilitation) or medium-low intensity (e.g., intermediate care, out-of-hospital residential rehabilitation, and activation of home assistance).

25.2 The Decision-Making Process

In the literature, the concept of frailty does not seem to be well-defined; however, an international group has designated it as a multifactorial clinical syndrome characterized by decreased strength, endurance, and reduced physiological function that increases an individual's vulnerability to developing increased dependency and/or death [7]. Frailty is, therefore, a condition predictive of adverse outcomes in surgical patients [8]. Defining and quantifying frailty in surgical patients therefore makes it possible to modify their management, especially at discharge. In fact, there are several critical points that worsen the outcome in this subgroup of patients.

25.2.1 Cognitive Status and Decision-Making Capacity

Conditions characterized by cognitive impairment and dementia are associated with increased morbidity and mortality. Under these conditions, identifying the patient's social support system, including family members or other caregivers, is also crucial for the postoperative course.

For example, a meta-analysis conducted on over 9.000 frail patients undergoing elective surgery demonstrated that caregiver support is essential in reducing the risk of complications and re-admissions [9]. Mild to moderate cronic kidney disease (CKD) is highly pervasive among frail elderly individuals, and the severity of renal dysfunction is independently correlated with that of cognitive impairment [10].

25.2.2 Cardiac Complications

Myocardial infarction after noncardiac surgery remains the leading cause of mortality up to 6 months after surgery with a rate ranging from 15% to 25% [11]. Therefore, tools for risk stratification such as the geriatric sensitive perioperative cardiac risk index or the Gupta MICA (GSPCRI) must be used at discharge for better management [12].

25.2.3 Pulmonary Complications

In frail patients undergoing noncardiac surgery, the risk of developing pulmonary complications is 33% [13]. Several risk prediction tools exist to predict the development of pulmonary complications [14]. After discharge, continued mobilization, pulmonary respiration exercises, and pain control can reduce the risk of these complications [15]. Noninvasive positive-pressure ventilation could treat and reduce the risk of respiratory failure [16]. We want to emphasize that, even more difficult to carry out in the emergency state of the COVID-19 pandemic, especially in several national health systems, the use of multidimensional assessment tools may be useful in planning the management of hospitalized COVID-19 older patients with dementia [17]. Moreover, higher multidimensional prognostic index (MPI) can be an excellent core set to identify older adults with dementia at a greater risk of in-hospital mortality and non invasive ventilation failure [18].

25.2.4 Fluid and Electrolyte Management

An optimal fluid and electrolyte balance is essential for maintaining good perfusion and oxygen transport. However, the frail patient could easily experience fluid overload due to various comorbidities such as cardiac and renal failure. A positive fluid and electrolyte balance is usually marked by adverse outcomes [19]. Conversely, a restrictive fluid intake is characterized by fewer complications [20]. Alterations in sodium and potassium concentrations are also common in surgically frail patients and are characterized by increased mortality [21]. Regular evaluations are, therefore, essential in this subset of patients.

25.2.5 Nutrition Management

An excellent nutritional status generally contrasts the catabolic state of the surgical patient and favors healing and recovery. However, despite the association between macro- and micronutrient deficiencies and frailty, there is no evidence that nutritional supplementation improves outcomes in frail surgical patients. However, careful and close monitoring of the nutritional status of elderly, frail patients undergoing surgery is rational [22].

25.2.6 Wound Complication

The risk of wound infection or wound infections with dehiscence is significantly increased in frail patients and constitutes one of the main causes of outpatient and hospital access [23]. Effective wound management in the community is therefore mandatory to reduce hospital overload and prevent complications.

25.3 Model of Continuity of Care

The frail surgical patient requires a multi-professional and multidisciplinary team, with territorial and hospital specialists, who can jointly evaluate the patient's needs, suggesting the ideal care setting. It is important to underline how the care settings

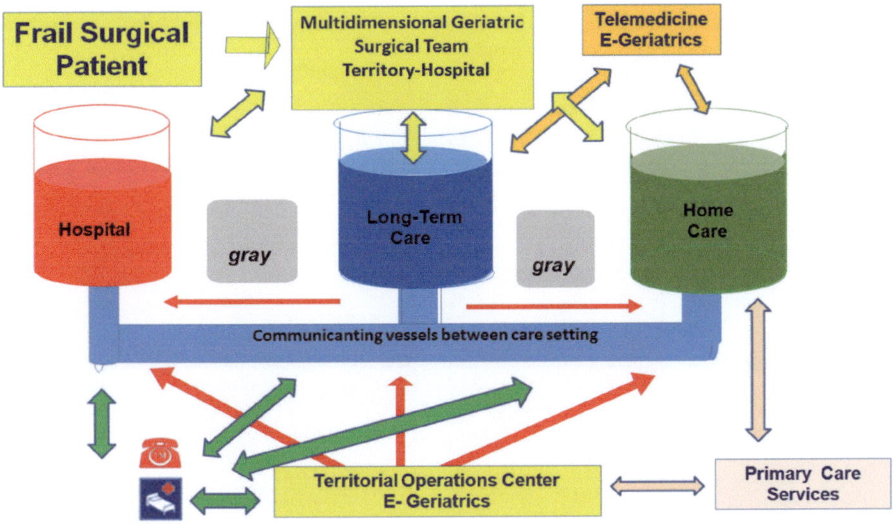

Fig. 25.1 Continuity of care: a model for the frail surgical patient

must be considered as communicating vessels, with the possibility of continuous dialogue (Fig. 25.1). However, some aspects must be clarified, including the role of the Territorial Operations Center. In our opinion, these structures should be understood as an active element of territorial hospital management, with the close collaboration of all primary care services (Fig. 25.1). A few years ago, we used the term "E-Geriatrics" with reference to geriatrics as a science of complexity accustomed to interdisciplinary and intergenerational dialogue, which opens up to the use of telemedicine and artificial intelligence in order to facilitate the management of older persons, evidently also useful for the possibilities in diagnosing and following up frail surgical patient [24].

25.4 SWOT Analysis of a Multidimensional Vision for the Frail Surgical Patient

The complete set of positive (benefits) and negative (risks) effects expected from the implementation of the project for the reorganization of assistance to frail surgical patients can be examined concisely with the support of a SWOT matrix which provides a quick and intuitive reading key. SWOT analysis is a strategic planning tool used to evaluate the strengths, weaknesses, opportunities, and threats of a project or in any other situation where an organization or an individual has to make a decision to achieve a goal. The analysis can concern the internal (analyzing strengths and weaknesses) or external environment of an organization (analyzing threats and opportunities). The representation of this type of analysis is shown in Fig. 25.2.

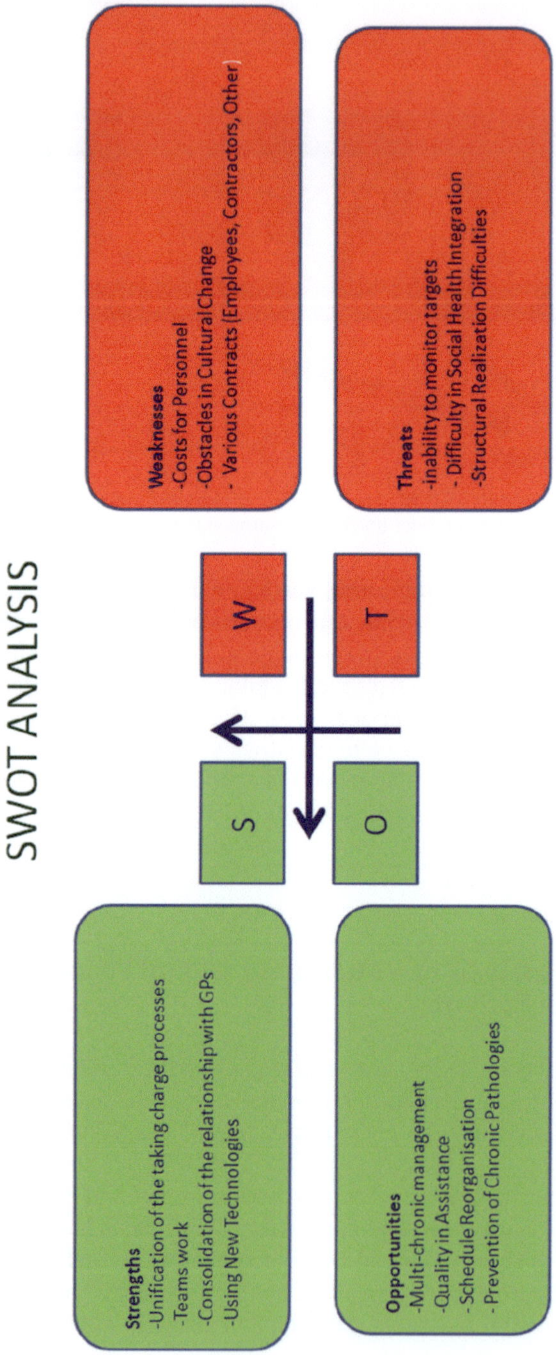

Fig. 25.2 SWOT analysis chart of a multidimensional vision for the frail surgical patient

25.5 Conclusions and Future Perspectives

The expected results of the reorganization process are greater suitability and social health integration, thanks to the possibility of responding in a personalized way to the needs of the person and the family (strengthening home care and the network of community hospitals). The stronger the territorial assistance, the better the systems for taking charge of the most complex situations (even in a timely and continuous manner), and the lower the total costs of the health system. The home (compatible with the family and social context which must be supported on a par with health care) can become the first place of care by exploiting technological innovation, and integrated, multidisciplinary, and multi-professional assistance. The supply of services must be diversified to be able to respond to the changing health needs of the population. Other expected results are the increase in personalized assistance, from prevention to treatment, also thanks to the use of big data and artificial intelligence support systems and the promotion of health services close to the citizens and easily accessible. Strengthening citizen's self-determination (empowerment) is more difficult in a frail and elderly population but it is a challenge to be taken up above all thanks to systems for intercepting frailty and the promotion of active aging interventions. Performance indicators must produce information capable of supporting decision-making processes, measuring, detecting, and communicating company results, as well as monitoring the objectives present in the reorganization project.

References

1. Ministero della Salute. Piano Nazionale della Cronicità (PNC). 2016. www.salute.gov.it/imgs/C_17_pubblicazioni_2584_allegato.pdf. Accessed 29 June 2023.
2. Italian Recovery and Resilience Plan #RestartingItaly. https://www.lavoro.gov.it. Accessed 29 June 2023.
3. Boccardi V, Mecocci P. Intermediate Care in Italy: addressing the challenges and opportunities for person-tailored care. Geriatrics. 2023;8(3):59. https://doi.org/10.3390/geriatrics8030059.
4. Shepperd S, McClaranJ PCO, et al. Discharge planning from hospital to home. Cochrane Database Syst Rev. 2010;1:CD000313.
5. Bauer M, Fitzgerald L, Haesler E, et al. Hospital discharge planning for frail older people and their family. Are we delivering best practice? A review of evidence. J Cln Nurs. 2009;18:2539–46.
6. Melis RJ, Olde Rikkert MG, Parker SG, Van Eijken ML. What is intermediate care? Br Med J. 2004;329:360–1.
7. Morley JE, Vellas B, Abellan van Kan G, et al. Frailty consensus: a call to action. J Am Med Dir Assoc. 2013;14:392–7.
8. Fried LP, Tangen CM, Walston J, et al. Frailty in older adults: evidence for a phenotype. J Gerontol A Biol Sci Med Sci. 2001;56:M146.
9. Watt J, Tricco AC, Talbot-Hamon C, et al. Identifying older adults at risk of delirium following elective surgery: a systematic review and meta-analysis. J Gen Intern Med. 2018;33(4):500–9.
10. Coppolino G, Bolignano D, Gareri P, Ruberto C, Andreucci M, Ruotolo G, Rocca M, Castagna A. Kidney function and cognitive decline in frail elderly: two faces of the same coin? Int Urol Nephrol. 2018;50:1505–10.
11. Chow WB, Rosenthal RA, Merkow RP, et al. Optimal preoperative assessment of the geriatric surgical patient: a best practices guideline from the American college of surgeons national

surgical quality improvement program and the American geriatrics society. J Am Coll Surg. 2012;215(4):453–66.
12. Alrezk R, Jackson N, Al Rezk M, et al. Derivation and validation of a geriatric-sensitive perioperative cardiac risk index. J Am Heart Assoc. 2017;6(11):Nov.
13. Fernandez-Bustamante A, Frendl G, Sprung J, et al. Postoperative pulmonary complications, early mortality, and hospital stay following non cardiothoracic surgery: a multicenter study by the perioperative research network investigators. JAMA Surg. 2017;152(2):157–66.
14. Canet J, Gallart L, Gomar C, et al. Prediction of postoperative pulmonary complications in a population-based surgical cohort. Anesthesiology. 2010;113(6):1338–50.
15. Ramly E, Kaafarani HM, Velmahos GC. The effect of aging on pulmonary function: implications for monitoring and support of the surgical and trauma patient. Surg Clin North Am. 2015;95(1):53–69.
16. Stephan F, Barrucand B, Petit P, et al. High-flow nasal oxygen vs noninvasive positive airway pressure in hypoxemic patients after cardiothoracic surgery: a randomized clinical trial. JAMA. 2015;313(23):2331–9.
17. Castagna A, Manzo C, Ruotolo G. Comprehensive Geriatric Assessment in hospitalized older patients with COVID-19. Geriatr Gerontol Int. 2021;21:118–9. https://doi.org/10.1111/ggi.14103.
18. Castagna A, Manzo C, Fabbo A, Cerra RP, Greco L, Ruberto C, Ruotolo G. Multidimensional prognostic index in hospitalized COVID-19 patients with dementia and its relationship with non-invasive ventilation failure. Arch Gerontol Geriatr. 2022;98:104578. https://doi.org/10.1016/j.archger.2021.104578. Epub 2021 Nov 14.
19. Bagshaw SM, Brophy PD, Cruz D, et al. Fluid balance as a biomarker: impact of fluid overload on outcome in critically ill patients with acute kidney injury. Crit Care. 2008;12(4):169.
20. El-Sharkawy AM, Sahota O, Maughan RJ, et al. The pathophysiology of fluid and electrolyte balance in the older adult surgical patient. Clin Nutr. 2014;33(1):6–13.
21. McCluskey SA, Karkouti K, Wijeysundera D, et al. Hyperchloremia after noncardiac surgery is independently associated with increased morbidity and mortality: a propensity-matched cohort study. Anesth Analg. 2013;117(2):412–21.
22. Lorenzo-Lopez L, Maseda A, de Labra C, et al. Nutritional determinants of frailty in older adults: a systematic review. BMC Geriatr. 2017;17:108.
23. Panayi AC, Orkaby AR, Sakthivel D, Endo Y, Varon D, Roh D, Orgill DP, Neppl RL, Javedan H, Bhasin S, Sinha I. Impact of frailty on outcomes in surgical patients: a systematic review and meta-analysis. Am J Surg. 2019;218(2):393–400. https://doi.org/10.1016/j.amjsurg.2018.11.020. Epub 2018 Nov 27.
24. Castagna A, Manzo RG. Comment on: Coronavirus 2019 in Geriatrics and Long-Term Care: The ABCDs of COVID-19. J Am Geriatr Soc. 2020;68:1166. https://doi.org/10.1111/jgs.16795.

Continuity of Care: Territory and General Practitioner

26

Alessandro Brunini, Luigi Maria Bracchitta, Ferdinando Petrazzuoli, and Jacopo Demurtas

The continuity of care is a concept whose definition is not universally agreed upon, despite publications on this topic since the 1970s [1–4]. Its definition and conceptualization may vary depending on whether they have been approached by different medical disciplines or from the perspectives of patients, physicians, or institutions.

We need to consider two essential and overarching elements of the definition: continuity of care is a patient-centered concept and is built over time [5]. Continuity of care considers the established relationship between a patient and a healthcare provider over a period of care that extends beyond a single encounter or visit.

The concept of continuity of care can be broken down into multiple dimensions. We can consider three main dimensions: informational continuity, relational continuity, and managerial continuity [5]. The following are the suggested definitions for these dimensions:

– Informational continuity: the use of information about past experiences and personal considerations to provide appropriate and personalized care to everyone.

A. Brunini
The Dementia Diagnosis and Treatment Center USL Sud-Est, Tuscany, Italy

L. M. Bracchitta
ATS, Milan, Italy

Department of Biomedical Sciences, Humanitas University, Milan, Italy

F. Petrazzuoli
School of Specialization in Community Medicine and Primary Care, University of Naples "Federico II", Naples, Italy

Center for Primary Health Care Research, Department of Clinical Sciences, Lund University, Malmö, Sweden

J. Demurtas (✉)
Family Medicine Department, USL Sud-Est Toscana, Tuscany, Italy
e-mail: jacopo@medi-ca.it

V. Boccardi, L. Marano (eds.), *The Frail Surgical Patient*, Practical Issues in Geriatrics, https://doi.org/10.1007/978-3-031-77707-3_26

- Relational or longitudinal continuity: a lasting therapeutic relationship between a patient and one or more healthcare professionals.
- Managerial continuity: a consistent and logical management of a health problem that meets the changing needs of the patient.

There is an implicit hierarchy among these three dimensions: informational continuity is necessary for relational continuity to exist, and relational continuity is a prerequisite for establishing a patient-physician relationship (interpersonal continuity).

Continuity of care lies at the core of general medicine characteristics, as defined by the European Society of General Practice/Family Medicine (WONCA—World Organization of Family Doctors, Europe) in 2022: the family physician "promotes continuity of doctor-patient relationships as a central organizing principle" [6].

In the detailed description of this definition, we find the various dimensions of continuity of care. The definition specifically mentions that "the doctor-patient relationship is based on personal involvement and confidentiality; continuity of care helps build mutual trust and enable high-quality, person-centered care" and "GPs seek to maintain this continuity of care when organizing their practices, regardless the size, composition and nature of the primary care team." In the previous WONCA definition of 2002, longitudinal continuity was described as an "approach (that) must be constant (allowing for) care provision during a substantial period of patients' lives, across different episodes of illness." Relational continuity is the "story of the doctor-patient relationship." Lastly, informational continuity focuses on the "medical record, (...) memory of consultations."

Continuity of care in general medicine is valued by patients and general practitioners. According to Stange and Ferrer's seminal editorial, primary care has "the added value of integrating, prioritizing, contextualizing, and personalizing health care across acute and chronic illness, psychosocial issues and mental health, disease prevention, and optimization of health and meaning" [7].

In England, approximately two-thirds of a sample of doctors and patients surveyed through a questionnaire considered the principle of having a personal primary care physician as "very important" or "extremely important" [8].

Hospital discharge is a critical moment in the care pathway, particularly at risk of disrupting the usual continuity of care in general medicine, especially for older patients [9]. The risk of readmission in the weeks or months following discharge increases. In France, in 2008, the rate of early readmission within 30 days of hospital discharge was estimated at 14.2% for patients aged 75 and older [10].

Various strategies have demonstrated a reduction in the risk of readmission through complex interventions in the hospital-to-home transition: patient and family education, medication reconciliation, sending a standardized transfer document on the day of discharge, discharge coordination, and home visits by a nurse or social worker [11–14].

Their effect can be measured up to 1 year after discharge [13–15].

A U.S. study showed a reduction in the risk of early readmission from 12% to 24% in Medicare beneficiaries who had seen a primary care physician within 7 days of their hospital discharge [16].

In France, the High Authority of Health/Haute Autorité de Santé (HAS) issued recommendations in 2013 regarding optimal conditions for the hospital-to-home transition. It advised multiple interventions in the three phases of the transition: early identification of patients at high risk of readmission, discharge preparation with the primary care team, and close follow-up by the general practitioner (GP) starting from the first week after discharge, with transmission of documents on the day of discharge [10].

In more complex cases, various nations have different but essentially homogeneous organizational systems.

It should be noted that the continuity of care varies according to the country under consideration. Healthcare systems can be broadly classified into three types:

1. Insurance-based (the United States).
2. Public and universally funded through general taxation—Beveridge models (Italy and Great Britain).
3. Mixed public-private—Bismarck (most other European countries).

The organization of continuity of care between hospitals and community settings also varies according to healthcare systems. Leaving aside the United States, where continuity is also influenced by the coverage provided by various insurance systems, although recent reforms (such as Medicare) have improved the care pathway, it can be stated that the care pathway, while placing the patient at the center, must also consider the sustainability of the system.

In the United States, continuity of care and assistance is also influenced by the individual's economic capabilities, resulting in a loss of appropriateness of care pathways. In other countries, different models of diagnostic, therapeutic, and care pathways have been proposed for the management of complex patients after discharge from the hospital.

Such pathways are also based on the appropriateness of responses to individual needs [17].

In Italy, there is a system of regional health autonomy, and the Tuscany Region has implemented its own system for the care of patients with high complexity referred by various medical or surgical hospital departments.

In this regard, the Tuscany Region has established the Hospital-Territory Continuity Agency.

The care pathway involves the referral of a patient with high socio-assistance complexity (in one or both domains) through an IT platform.

The referred patient is then assessed by a referring physician assigned to one of the 24 district areas of the region.

The territory-based physician coordinates a multidisciplinary team composed mainly of:

- Social worker.
- Home nurse.
- Physiotherapist.

Each member of this team carries out their professional assessment, and at the end, the physician coordinates the responses, primarily informing the primary care physician and selecting the most appropriate response to the individual's needs.

The responses, in turn, can be of various types and depend on the level of care intensity, whether it is healthcare or social.

In the case of end-of-life situations, a hospice pathway will be provided.

In case of chronicization of a situation with high clinical complexity that still requires nursing care (e.g., management of drainage, intravenous therapies, etc.), admission to a community hospital will be proposed.

In case of difficulties in returning home primarily due to social reasons, a stay (temporary or permanent) in assisted health residence is proposed.

For rehabilitation needs (e.g., after a femoral fracture), a residential rehabilitation pathway will be offered.

The responses to the needs of older individuals with high socio-assistance complexity can have different solutions established through precise pathways based on social and healthcare appropriateness [18].

In Europe, the situation is generally homogeneous.

In France, in more complex situations involving medical and social issues or when there has been a significant decline in patient autonomy during hospitalization, continuity of care by the same healthcare professional during and after hospitalization is recommended by the HAS [10]. In these cases, systematic discharge planning with the entire primary care team, as well as potential home support, should be the norm. In the French healthcare context, continuity of management can be ensured by independent practice nurses trained in advanced practices, mobile geriatric teams for elderly patients, case managers (such as an MAIA—method of action for the integration of healthcare and support services in the field of autonomy), network coordinators (such as a primary care intervention coordinator who can be in contact with a hospital intervention coordinator), or social workers [10]. Additionally, the primary care physician should remain systematically involved in these hospital-to-home transitions.

Therefore, factors to be considered are determined by the general aging of the population, the increase in age-related and lifestyle-related chronic diseases, and the fact that older individuals can also experience both acute and elective surgical conditions.

Given the "silver tsunami" [19], it is not feasible to have a strategy aimed at avoiding the problem by choosing not to operate. Instead, it is necessary to prioritize the patient who, in this case, has specific needs in terms of both healthcare and assistance and sometimes social needs as well.

The approaches taken, such as those in the case of the Tuscany region in Italy [18] or France [10], clearly show an initial attempt to take charge of the complex healthcare needs of older patients through an integrated and multidisciplinary approach at the time of discharge.

However, what is lacking is the consideration of the purely surgical aspects. The integrated approaches currently in place focus more on medical rather than surgical aspects, which tend to become chronic and unresolved, such as stroke or congestive heart failure.

What needs to be developed is an approach aimed at improving the outcome of the surgical intervention, not only as a technical procedure but also in terms of the patient's overall recovery, including their functional independence, to the possible extent.

Surgery induces significant physiological stress, even in healthy individuals. Therefore, it is not surprising that the presence of frailty before a procedure is regularly associated in the literature with a doubling of the risk of major morbidity, mortality, and rehospitalization in different types of surgery [20–22]. Postoperative complications (cardiac, pulmonary, renal, hematologic, infectious, and surgical) are common in older frail subjects [20, 23, 24], with a higher incidence of 25% [21]. In a literature review, frailty is one of the most important independent risk factors for the occurrence of postoperative morbidity in elderly patients [25].

Delirium is one of the most frequent postoperative complications; the incidence of which is between 10 and 50% depending on the type and urgency of the surgery. Its occurrence is accompanied remotely by the intervention of an increased risk of cognitive decline and functional dependence.

Postoperative mortality is increased in frail patients [20, 26–28]. In a cohort that included more than 2.7 million patients from two North American databases data, frailty is associated with postoperative mortality at 1 month and 6 months in all types of surgery regardless of the operative stress they generate, assessed by the operative stress score (OSS) [23].

In the immediate postoperative and longer term, fragility also doubles the risk appearance of a new functional limitation [24], degrades the quality of life [21, 22], and increases the risk of institutionalization on discharge from the hospital by a factor of 5 [20].

In months and years following heart surgery, patients' time spent at home is reduced proportionally to the impairment of their frailty [29].

26.1 Strategies for Managing Frail Patients

Given that frail patients have a higher risk of complications and death in the short and medium term after a surgical event, it is important to provide multidisciplinary care for them in the perioperative setting.

The reversal or reduction of frailty in the preoperative period, with the objective of impacting the prognosis and outcome of these patients, is the subject of prehabilitation approaches [30–32].

In a North American, monocentric, prospective cohort of over 9000 patients [33], it was found that the knowledge by medical and surgical teams of the existence of frailty and associated surgical risk before noncardiac surgery is independently associated with a decrease in mortality at 30, 180, and 365 days after surgery, regardless of any protocolization of perioperative care [33]. The magnitude of the effect increases over the later time points of the study [33]. This effect is not due to the exclusion of a greater number of patients, as the frailty score is higher in patients where the existence of frailty is communicated to the healthcare team. The authors attribute this effect to an overall optimization of pre-, peri-, and postoperative care [33].

26.2 Prehabilitation

Prehabilitation refers to any intervention delivered before surgery that optimizes function by increasing physiological reserves and/or potentially reducing postoperative risk, allowing for faster or more complete recovery. Despite a clear association between frailty, decreased functional reserves, and increased postoperative morbidity, evidence for the benefit of prehabilitation for frail patients is limited, while the literature is more abundant and these benefits are documented in non-frail older adults [34–36]. Several recently published systematic reviews of the literature confirm this [36].

The main determinants of reduced reserves and functional capacity in frail individuals are physical, nutritional, and psychological factors [37]. These three elements are the hallmarks of prehabilitation: physical exercise, nutritional advice and supplementation, and psychological support. Prehabilitation should therefore be multimodal and multidisciplinary. These interventions should be structured and personalized, considering the specific characteristics and comorbidities of the patient, in order not to compromise adherence and tolerance to these interventions.

The recommended basic physical activity for older adults is 150 minutes per week if the intensity is moderate or 75 min if it is intense. Aerobic exercises and relaxation maneuvers should be added to this activity. Inspiratory muscle training can also be included among these interventions.

Nutritional optimization includes screening for malnutrition (defined as a weight loss of more than 10% in 6 months or 5% in the last 3 months, or a BMI below 20), advice on nutritional balance, oral supplementation to ensure a protein intake of 1.5 g per kilogram of body weight to ensure anabolism, correction of iron deficits if present, and promotion of immunonutrition with products containing arginine, omega-3 fatty acids, and antioxidants [38].

The goal of neuropsychological support is to reduce anxiety, stress, as well as depression secondary to the disease (e.g., cancer) and surgery. This may also include cognitive stimulation [24]. Neuropsychological support relies on a non-pharmacological approach.

Finally, it allows for clear and personalized information and facilitates shared decision-making, an essential element of the care of older adults [39].

26.3 Standardized Geriatric Assessment and Individualized Multimodal Intervention

This diagnostic approach determines the management of comorbidities and pharmacological therapies, dependencies, anemia, and social living conditions, as well as the optimization of physical, nutritional, and neuropsychological activity [37] and has been shown to have a positive impact on mortality, length of hospitalization, and institutionalization of patients hospitalized for a femoral fracture, without prejudicing the existence of associated fragility [40].

The benefit is less documented for other types of surgery [40]; although in some studies of vascular surgery and planned cardiac surgery, the multimodal approach has reduced cardiovascular complications, delirium, infections, and length of hospitalization [41, 42].

The multimodal approach is therefore the ideal context for a shared decision on the care strategy [43].

Some optimization measures of anesthesia have been proposed for the elderly, considering the increase in postoperative morbidity and mortality related to age, regardless of any comorbidities. Often, these measures validated in patients or for "high-risk" surgeries have not been specifically evaluated in the elderly or fragile patients. Their cumulative benefit has not been evaluated [44].

While the impact of neurophysiological monitoring of the depth of anesthesia on morbidity and particularly on the incidence of postoperative delirium is debated [45, 46], such monitoring is still recommended in elderly patients as it allows limiting overdosing and overly deep anesthesia, facilitating the titration of anesthetic agents. In surgical patients considered "high-risk," titration of intraoperative vascular filling based on systolic ejection volume measurement is also recommended to reduce postoperative morbidity [47].

However, this strategy does not reduce the incidence of complications in elderly patients suffering from an upper femoral fracture in a general literature review although it is based on a limited number of studies with poor power [48].

The prevention or treatment of hypotension is legitimate in the elderly to reduce the incidence of cardiac, renal, and neurological complications [49].

However, the harmful thresholds, the effect of comorbidities (including hypertension), and treatments on such thresholds are poorly defined in this population. Prevention or treatment of hypotension with an individualized approach aimed at a systolic blood pressure of ±10% of the patient's reference pressure has demonstrated its interest in the onset of postoperative organic dysfunction compared to treatment of hypotension below 80 mmHg or in case of a decrease greater than 40% compared to the reference pressure in middle-aged elderly subjects [50].

In major surgery, the benefit of protective ventilation combining low lung volume, positive end expiratory pressure (PEEP), and recruitment maneuvers is also established in patients at high risk of postoperative respiratory complications, including the elderly. Prevention of hypothermia, management of anemia, and a restrictive transfusion strategy are also recommended in this population [51, 52].

26.4 Postoperative

Older patients benefit from enhanced recovery after surgery (ERAS) protocols in surgery [53]. This approach encompasses the pre and perioperative period and overlaps with the measures previously mentioned (nutritional support, preoperative optimization of comorbidities and treatments, prevention of hypothermia, etc.) but also allows for their integration (morphine-sparing strategy, use of locoregional analgesia, etc.).

This protocol can be applied in the postoperative period in frail patients. A benefit of these protocols has been found in colorectal surgery with a decrease in complications and length of hospital stay, but this benefit is even greater as the degree of frailty increases [54, 55].

There is a clear interest in postoperative geriatric care for upper femur fractures, which reduces postoperative morbidity and mortality [56].

More recently, it has been demonstrated that shared management of elderly patients undergoing cancer surgery allows for a reduction in mortality at 3 months [57] in an analysis adjusted for major risk factors including frailty. These results confirm the importance of integrating the postoperative course of these frail patients in a multidisciplinary approach [58] with objectives of optimizing comorbidities, early oral hydration and nutrition, multimodal analgesia, limiting the risk of confusion and cognitive decline, reducing iatrogenic harm, mobilization to reduce physical frailty, and prevent loss of autonomy.

26.5 Conclusions

It is clear, therefore, that both "Beveridge"-type and "Bismarck"-type healthcare systems need to implement hospital-to-community continuity of care pathways, considering the surgical aspect as an emerging issue alongside the "traditional" conditions of older patients, as an increase in absolute value can be expected.

Addressing this problem can lead to improvements in the individual's quality of life and result in a reduced burden on healthcare system budgets.

References

1. Hansen MF. Continuity of care in family practice. J Fam Pract. 1975;2(6):439–44.
2. Wall EM. Continuity of care and family medicine: definition, determinants, and relationship to outcome. J Fam Pract. 1981;13(5):655–64.
3. Freeman G. Continuity of Care in General Practice: a review and critique. Fam Pract. 1984;1(4):245–52.
4. Rogers J, Curtis P. The concept and measurement of continuity in primary care. Am J Public Health. 1980;70(2):122–7.
5. Haggerty JL, Reid RJ, Freeman GK, Starfield BH, Adair CE, McKendry R. Continuity of care: a multidisciplinary review. BMJ. 2003;327(7425):1219–21.

6. Europe W. The European definition of general practice/family medicine. Barcelona: WONCA Europe; 2002.
7. Stange KC, Ferrer RL. The paradox of primary care. Ann Fam Med. 2009;7:293.
8. Kearley KE, Freeman GK, Heath A. An exploration of the value of the personal doctor-patient relationship in general practice. Br J Gen Pract. 2001;51(470):712–8.
9. Kripalani S, Jackson AT, Schnipper JL, Coleman EA. Promoting effective transitions of care at hospital discharge: a review of key issues for hospitalists. J Hosp Med. 2007;2(5):314–23.
10. de Santé HA. Note méthodologique et de synthèse documentaire: Prendre en charge une personne âgée polypathologique en soins primaires. Marsyas. 2015;2015:2015–04.
11. Rennke S, Nguyen OK, Shoeb MH, Magan Y, Wachter RM, Ranji SR. Hospital-initiated transitional care interventions as a patient safety strategy: a systematic review. Ann Intern Med. 2013;158(5_Part_2):433–40.
12. Allen J, Ottmann G, Roberts G. Multi-professional communication for older people in transitional care: a review of the literature. Int J Older People Nursing. 2013;8(4):253–69.
13. Parker S, Peet S, McPherson A, Cannaby A. A systematic review of discharge arrangements for older people. Clinical Governance. 2003;8(1):79.
14. Shepperd S, Lannin NA, Clemson LM, McCluskey A, Cameron ID, Barras SL. Discharge planning from hospital to home. Cochrane Database Syst Rev. 2013;1:1.
15. Halfon P, Eggli Y, van Melle G, Chevalier J, Wasserfallen J-B, Burnand B. Measuring potentially avoidable hospital readmissions. J Clin Epidemiol. 2002;55(6):573–87.
16. Shen E, Koyama SY, Huynh DN, Watson HL, Mittman B, Kanter MH, Nguyen HQ. Association of a dedicated post–hospital discharge follow-up visit and 30-day readmission risk in a medicare advantage population. JAMA Intern Med. 2017;177(1):132–5.
17. Wallace LS. A view of health care around the world. Ann Fam Med. 2013;11:84.
18. Maccari M, Salutini L, Mariotti M, Quercioli C. L'invecchiamento attivo: l'esperienza nella Regione Toscana. Revisione e considerazioni sulla normativa di riferimento, vol. 1. Mondo Sanitario; 2020.
19. Demurtas J, Mereu A, Veronese N, Maeseneer JD. Family doctors and the silver tsunami: team up to survive the storm. In: The role of family physicians in older people care. Cham: Springer; 2022. p. 1–13.
20. McIsaac DI, Taljaard M, Bryson GL, Beaulé PE, Gagné S, Hamilton G, Hladkowicz E, Huang A, Joanisse JA, Lavallée LT. Frailty as a predictor of death or new disability after surgery: a prospective cohort study. Ann Surg. 2020;271(2):283–9.
21. Lin H-S, Watts J, Peel N, Hubbard R. Frailty and post-operative outcomes in older surgical patients: a systematic review. BMC Geriatr. 2016;16(1):1–12.
22. Kim DH, Kim CA, Placide S, Lipsitz LA, Marcantonio ER. Preoperative frailty assessment and outcomes at 6 months or later in older adults undergoing cardiac surgical procedures: a systematic review. Ann Intern Med. 2016;165(9):650–60.
23. McIsaac DI, Bryson GL, van Walraven C. Association of frailty and 1-year postoperative mortality following major elective noncardiac surgery: a population-based cohort study. JAMA Surg. 2016;151(6):538–45.
24. McIsaac DI, MacDonald DB, Aucoin SD. Frailty for perioperative clinicians: a narrative review. Anesth Analg. 2019;130(6):1450–60.
25. Watt J, Tricco AC, Talbot-Hamon C, Pham B, Rios P, Grudniewicz A, Wong C, Sinclair D, Straus SE. Identifying older adults at risk of harm following elective surgery: a systematic review and meta-analysis. BMC Med. 2018;16(1):1–14.
26. Fu D, Tan X, Zhang M, Chen L, Yang J. Association between frailty and postoperative delirium: a meta-analysis of cohort study. Aging Clin Exp Res. 2021;34:1–13.
27. Gracie TJ, Caufield-Noll C, Wang N-Y, Sieber F. The association of preoperative frailty and postoperative delirium: a meta-analysis. Anesth Analg. 2021;133(2):314.
28. Castillo-Angeles M, Cooper Z, Jarman MP, Sturgeon D, Salim A, Havens JM. Association of frailty with morbidity and mortality in emergency general surgery by procedural risk level. JAMA Surg. 2021;156(1):68–74.

29. McIsaac DI, Fottinger A, Sucha E, McDonald B. Association of frailty with days alive at home after cardiac surgery: a population-based cohort study. Br J Anaesth. 2021;126(6):1103–10.
30. Durrand J, Hackett R, Yates D, Danjoux G. Prehabilitation. In: Perioperative medicine–current controversies. Cham: Springer; 2016. p. 15–47.
31. Hanna K, Ditillo M, Joseph B. The role of frailty and prehabilitation in surgery. Curr Opin Crit Care. 2019;25(6):717–22.
32. Milder DA, Pillinger NL, Kam PC. The role of prehabilitation in frail surgical patients: a systematic review. Acta Anaesthesiol Scand. 2018;62(10):1356–66.
33. Hall DE, Arya S, Schmid KK, Carlson MA, Lavedan P, Bailey TL, Purviance G, Bockman T, Lynch TG, Johanning JM. Association of a frailty screening initiative with postoperative survival at 30, 180, and 365 days. JAMA Surg. 2017;152(3):233–40.
34. George EL, Hall DE, Youk A, Chen R, Kashikar A, Trickey AW, Varley PR, Shireman PK, Shinall MC, Massarweh NN. Association between patient frailty and postoperative mortality across multiple noncardiac surgical specialties. JAMA Surg. 2021;156(1):e205152.
35. Alvarez-Nebreda ML, Bentov N, Urman RD, Setia S, Huang JC-S, Pfeifer K, Bennett K, Ong TD, Richman D, Gollapudi D. Recommendations for preoperative management of frailty from the Society for Perioperative Assessment and Quality Improvement (SPAQI). J Clin Anesth. 2018;47:33–42.
36. Buta BJ, Walston JD, Godino JG, Park M, Kalyani RR, Xue Q-L, Bandeen-Roche K, Varadhan R. Frailty assessment instruments: systematic characterization of the uses and contexts of highly-cited instruments. Ageing Res Rev. 2016;26:53–61.
37. Carli F, Baldini G. From preoperative assessment to preoperative optimization of frail older patients. Eur J Surg Oncol. 2021;47(3):519–23.
38. Chan S, Ip K, Irwin M. Peri-operative optimisation of elderly and frail patients: a narrative review. Anaesthesia. 2019;74:80–9.
39. Bruijnen CP, Heijmer A, van Harten-Krouwel DG, van den Bos F, de Bree R, Witteveen PO, Emmelot-Vonk MH. Validation of the G8 screening tool in older patients with cancer considered for surgical treatment. J Geriatr Oncol. 2021;12(5):793–8.
40. Eamer G, Taheri A, Chen SS, Daviduck Q, Chambers T, Shi X, Khadaroo RG. Comprehensive geriatric assessment for older people admitted to a surgical service. Cochrane Database Syst Rev. 2018;1(1):CD012485.
41. Partridge J, Harari D, Martin F, Peacock J, Bell R, Mohammed A, Dhesi J. Randomized clinical trial of comprehensive geriatric assessment and optimization in vascular surgery. J Br Surg. 2017;104(6):679–87.
42. McIsaac DI, Huang A, Wong CA, Wijeysundera DN, Bryson GL, van Walraven C. Effect of preoperative geriatric evaluation on outcomes after elective surgery: a population-based study. J Am Geriatr Soc. 2017;65(12):2665–72.
43. Norris CM, Close JC. Prehabilitation for the frailty syndrome: improving outcomes for our most vulnerable patients. Anesth Analg. 2019;130(6):1524–33.
44. Molliex S, Passot S, Futier E, Bonnefoi M, Rancon F, Lemanach Y, Pereira B. Stepped wedge cluster randomised controlled trial to assess the effectiveness of an optimisation strategy for general anaesthesia on postoperative morbidity and mortality in elderly patients (the OPTI-AGED study): a study protocol. BMJ Open. 2018;8(6):e021053.
45. Shan W, Chen B, Huang L, Zhou Y. The effects of bispectral index–guided anesthesia on postoperative delirium in elderly patients: a systematic review and meta-Analysis. World Neurosurg. 2021;147:e57–62.
46. Wildes TS, Mickle AM, Abdallah AB, Maybrier HR, Oberhaus J, Budelier TP, Kronzer A, McKinnon SL, Park D, Torres BA. Effect of electroencephalography-guided anesthetic administration on postoperative delirium among older adults undergoing major surgery: the ENGAGES randomized clinical trial. JAMA. 2019;321(5):473–83.
47. Vallet B, Blanloeil Y, Cholley B, Orliaguet G, Pierre S, Tavernier B. Guidelines for perioperative haemodynamic optimization Stratégie du remplissage vasculaire périopératoire. Ann Fr Anesth Reanim. 2013;32:e151–8.

48. Lewis SR, Butler AR, Brammar A, Nicholson A, Smith AF. Perioperative fluid volume optimization following proximal femoral fracture. Cochrane Database Syst Rev. 2016;3(3):CD003004.
49. Wesselink E, Kappen T, Torn H, Slooter A, Van Klei W. Intraoperative hypotension and the risk of postoperative adverse outcomes: a systematic review. Br J Anaesth. 2018;121(4):706–21.
50. Futier E, Lefrant J-Y, Guinot P-G, Godet T, Lorne E, Cuvillon P, Bertran S, Leone M, Pastene B, Piriou V. Effect of individualized vs standard blood pressure management strategies on postoperative organ dysfunction among high-risk patients undergoing major surgery: a randomized clinical trial. JAMA. 2017;318(14):1346–57.
51. Aceto P, Antonelli Incalzi R, Bettelli G, Carron M, Chiumiento F, Corcione A, Crucitti A, Maggi S, Montorsi M, Pace MC. Perioperative Management of Elderly patients (PriME): recommendations from an Italian intersociety consensus. Aging Clin Exp Res. 2020;32:1647–73.
52. Mahmoudi R, Novella J, Jaidi Y. Transfusion in elderly: take account frailty. Trans Cliniq Biol. 2017;24(3):200–8.
53. Ljungqvist O, Hubner M. Enhanced recovery after surgery—ERAS—principles, practice and feasibility in the elderly. Aging Clin Exp Res. 2018;30:249–52.
54. Millan M, Espina-Perez B, Caro-Tarrago A, Jorba-Martin R. ERAS programs in elderly patients: is there a limit? Int J Color Dis. 2018;33:1313.
55. Studniarek A, Borsuk DJ, Marecik SJ, Park JJ, Kochar K. Enhanced recovery after surgery protocols. Does frailty play a role? Am Surg. 2021;87(7):1054–61.
56. Grigoryan KV, Javedan H, Rudolph JL. Ortho-geriatric care models and outcomes in hip fracture patients: a systematic review and meta-analysis. J Orthop Trauma. 2014;28(3):e49.
57. Shahrokni A, Tin AL, Sarraf S, Alexander K, Sun S, Kim SJ, McMillan S, Yulico H, Amirnia F, Downey RJ. Association of geriatric comanagement and 90-day postoperative mortality among patients aged 75 years and older with cancer. JAMA Netw Open. 2020;3(8):e209265.
58. Van Grootven B, Flamaing J, Dierckx de Casterlé B, Dubois C, Fagard K, Herregods M-C, Hornikx M, Laenen A, Meuris B, Rex S. Effectiveness of in-hospital geriatric co-management: a systematic review and meta-analysis. Age Ageing. 2017;46(6):903–10.

Shared Decision-Making at the End of Life

27

Simone Cernesi, Victoria Hewitt, Mathieu Jackson, Maria Stella Padula, Francesca Rossi, and Ilaria Rossiello

27.1 Introduction

According to the International Association for Hospice and Palliative Care (IAHPC), palliative care is the active holistic care of individuals across all ages with serious health-related suffering due to severe illness, especially those near the end of life [1]. It aims to improve the quality of life of patients, their families, and their caregivers. This definition was agreed by a consensus of experts and is augmented by the following objectives, taken from the Palliative Care Advisory Council of the United States of America in 2018 [2], stating that palliative care:

- Provides support to help patients live as fully as possible until death by facilitating effective communication, helping them and their families determine goals of care.

S. Cernesi (✉)
Primary Care AUSL Modena, Palliative Care and Geriatric Medicine, Modena and Reggio Emilia University (UNIMORE), Laboratorio EduCare, Unimore, Modena, Italy
e-mail: s.cernesi@unimore.it

V. Hewitt
School of Pharmacy, Newcastle University, Newcastle upon Tyne, UK
e-mail: victoria.hewitt@newcastle.ac.uk

M. Jackson
Centre of Excellence on Partnerships with Patients and the Public, University of Montreal Hospital Research Centre, Montreal, QC, Canada
e-mail: mathieu.jackson@ceppp.ca

M. S. Padula · F. Rossi
Laboratirio EduCare, Unimore, Modena, Italy
e-mail: mspadula@unimore.it

I. Rossiello
AST303, Marche, Italy

V. Boccardi, L. Marano (eds.), *The Frail Surgical Patient*, Practical Issues in Geriatrics, https://doi.org/10.1007/978-3-031-77707-3_27

- Is applicable throughout the course of an illness, according to the patient's needs.
- Is provided in conjunction with disease-modifying therapies whenever needed.
- May positively influence the course of illness.
- Intends neither to hasten nor postpone death, affirms life, and recognizes dying as a natural process.
- Provides support to the family and the caregivers during the patient's illness and in their bereavement.
- Is delivered recognizing and respecting the cultural values and beliefs of the patient and the family.
- Is applicable throughout all healthcare settings (place of residence and institutions) and at all levels (primary to tertiary).
- Can be provided by professionals with basic palliative care training.
- Requires specialist palliative care with a multi-professional team for referral of complex cases.

Surgical palliative care is the treatment of suffering and promotion of quality of life for seriously ill patients undergoing surgical care [3]. Within the context of geriatrics, it is a specialized approach aimed at enhancing the quality of life for older individuals facing serious illnesses or life-limiting conditions. Unlike traditional surgical interventions focused on curative measures, surgical palliative care prioritizes the relief of symptoms, the improvement of functional status, and the promotion of overall well-being in older patients. Surgical palliative care assumes a holistic approach, addressing suffering across physical, emotional, social, and spiritual domains. Importantly, it acknowledges that surgical interventions may play a role in achieving relief and comfort during this critical phase of a patient's journey and integrates therapies aimed at both extending life and improving its quality. The unit of care extends to not only the patient but also encompasses their family, recognizing the interconnectedness of their experiences and needs. This approach underscores the commitment to providing compassionate and comprehensive care that acknowledges the multidimensional nature of a patient's well-being.

Prognostication in this context considers a comprehensive range of factors, including morbidity, mortality, and patient-centered outcomes such as quality of life, functional ability, and independence. Surgical interventions are carefully evaluated based on their potential to align with the patient's goals and aspirations, unrestricted by the sole capacity to alter the trajectory of the disease. The decision to avoid performing surgery on older individuals requires a comprehensive approach that prioritizes their overall well-being [4]. A shift toward a palliative or supportive approach becomes crucial to ensure the individual's comfort, dignity, and personal preferences that are achieved with a focus on symptom management, pain control, and enhancing the overall quality of life.

Supportive care (in cancer) has traditionally focused on the treatment of antineoplastic therapy-related adverse effects and has now expanded its scope to include palliative care, as well as survivorship care [5]. Supportive care includes palliative care although it is sometimes used interchangeably [6] to describe palliative care programs or services. However, palliative care is more than supportive care, based on a holistic approach, including emotional support, addressing psychosocial aspects [7] of the different trajectories of illness [8, 9], and ensuring effective communication to facilitate shared decision-making with the patient and/or their caregivers. The latter aspect of palliative care is the focus of this chapter.

Although several tools to identify patients who could potentially benefit from a palliative approach exist, they lack specificity for frailty in geriatric surgical palliative care. One of the main barriers is the existence of structural inequities in service provision that hamper the voices of older people being expressed and heard [10]. Yet older people must be able to find their voice to understand their own palliative care needs and priorities. Identifying the palliative care needs that matter most to older people with multimorbidity requires the recognition of their concerns, as well as their symptoms, across a continuum of living and dying. Supporting end-of-life provision for this growing and underserved population necessitates a shift to tailored multidimensional tools and community-focused integrated care services [11].

Frailty is a progressive physiological decline in multiple organ systems marked by loss of function, reduction in physiological reserve, and increased vulnerability to disease and death [12, 13]. Frail older persons are more susceptible to adverse health outcomes, including delirium, falls, functional decline, reduced mobility, social withdrawal, institutionalization, and death [12–14]. Frailty is a dynamic process, but transition to a level of worse frailty is more common than improvement [12, 14]. It is most common in older persons and in those with multiple comorbidities but can occur independently of these factors and, therefore, differs from normal aging [15]. There is no single widely accepted definition of frailty. It is commonly described as a clinical syndrome in which three or more of the following are present: unintentional weight loss, self-reported fatigue, slow walking, muscular weakness, and low levels of energy. If one or two are present, the patient is defined as pre-frail [15]. Alternatively, the concept of frailty has been described as a consequence of an accumulation of deficits over time. Deficits include disabilities, diseases, cognitive impairment, psychosocial risk factors, and geriatric syndromes (i.e., falls, delirium, and urinary incontinence) [12].

Pre-clinical and clinical frailties are different entities, and therefore, should be evaluated by different methods, such as Fried's (pre-clinical) frailty phenotype [16] and Rockwood's method for assessing clinical frailty. Clinical frailty is characterized by four factors (physical, mental, nutritional, and social frailty). Each frailty factor should be evaluated by definite instruments. Rockwood's method is reliable and feasible, especially if preceded by a geriatric comprehensive assessment. A tool that may help in the identification process is the clinical frailty scale (CFS) [17] which suggests the best approach is based on functional status.

It is also important to understand which illness trajectory (frailty/dementia, cancer, and/or organ failure) [18] the patient is following and whether the clinical condition or conditions are stable. Clinical deterioration is important to consider in the palliative care approach. Tools such as SPICT™ [19] and NECPAL (Necesidades Paliativas) [20] are useful for identifying palliative care needs. SPICT™ was developed and validated in 2010 by a Scottish primary care research group. This tool supports healthcare professionals in identifying people with deteriorating health conditions who may benefit from a palliative approach. Furthermore, it allows the evaluation of palliative care already in place to detect any unmet needs of the patient or if the patient shows clinical signs of deterioration, leading to a review of current care planning.

NECPAL is a screening tool that aims to identify patients with an advanced and serious chronic condition to activate an early palliative approach aimed at improving patients' quality of life. It is indicated when there is a negative answer to the surprise question [21] "Would you be surprised if this patient died within the next 12 months?" and if at least one of the clinical or laboratory criteria is simultaneously present. There is no minimum number of indicators to establish the need for basic or specialist palliative care, but it can be assumed that the presence of two general indicators of clinical deterioration and a specific indicator of pathology significantly correlate to the need to establish a palliative approach to the patient.

To assess prognosis, the palliative performance scale (PPS) correlates well with survival time for patients with cancer. The PPS evaluates walking, life activities, the ability to take care of oneself, oral intake, and level of consciousness [22]. The phase of illness tool relates distinct characteristics of the illness trajectory with the needs and resources used by the individual and family as the unit of care [23].

Frailty is a clinical syndrome associated with an increased risk of functional disability, dependency, institutionalization, and death [12].
Frailty is a dynamic process, but transition to a level of worse frailty is more common than improvement [12].
The palliative care needs of older people are often under-assessed and undertreated [12].
Comprehensive specialist assessment during acute admissions reduces the risk of cognitive or functional decline and death [12].
Palliative care in the form of anticipatory care planning, consideration of addition to the general practitioner's palliative care register, and symptom control should be initiated early and can include curative treatments, which might improve functioning and quality of life [12].

27.2 Shared Decision-Making

Shared decision-making (SDM) is defined as "a formal process or tool that helps physicians and patients work together to choose the treatment option that best reflects both medical evidence and the individual patient's priorities and goals for his or her care" (American Medical Association, 2012). Coulter and Collins (2012) [24] augment this definition to include evidence-based discussions of outcomes and uncertainties and the documentation of the patient's informed preferences. SDM is a collaboration between a patient and their healthcare professionals to reach the best decision for the individual by sharing information, knowledge, and values, discussing preferences and goals of care, and negotiating treatment options [25, 26].

Because decision-making at the end of life is affected by individual patient values, cultures, and preferences, SDM is a crucial part of palliative care. The desire for people with palliative care needs and their caregivers to participate in decisions applies to issues beyond medical interventions. Choosing between life-prolonging treatments with side effects and improving the quality of life with less aggressive treatments involves complex medical care options and high emotional distress. This should be addressed in future research and practice [27]. Although SDM may also involve the patient's family and friends, it is the person concerned who ultimately makes the decision, if they can do so. A patient is presumed to have decision-making capacity unless proven otherwise. A frail older person can have intact intellectual faculties that are not always evident.

Decision-making capacity can be temporarily compromised by delirium, dementia, metabolic imbalances, severe pain, life-threatening infections, and shifting levels of consciousness. In palliative care, it is not uncommon for the level of consciousness to fluctuate due to advancing disease and the effects of medication. Furthermore, psychological factors can impede concentration and engagement, including existential distress and denial of a serious, progressive illness [28].

In medical settings, it is usually the physician's responsibility to determine the patient's capacity to make a specific decision. Capacity may change depending on the patient's condition and the complexity of the decision. He/she needs to be able to:

- Understand relevant information and the implications of treatment choices.
- Reflect in accordance with personal values and draw conclusions.
- Make and communicate a choice to healthcare professionals.

In cases where the patient is unable to participate in the decision-making process, it is important to be familiar with national legislation; in many countries, there is the possibility of defining who can decide for the patient in case of impediment, considering their previous wishes.

Patient engagement in healthcare is essential for patient-centered care planning and medical decision-making; yet in modern society, the fear of opening a conversation on the subject of illness and end of life is still often taboo. Very few patients (and even healthcare professionals) document their wishes in writing regarding treatment choices. This remains a major limitation to the development of palliative care globally [29].

27.3 Ethical Considerations in Shared Decision-Making

As with surgical interventions, a treatment plan oriented toward the palliative approach must rest upon clear ethical foundations. Bioethical fundamentals may assist the evaluation, communication, and definition of goals and plans of care regarding surgical treatment options in palliative care.

The palliative care approach involves the following:

1. The goal is not healing but (holistic) patient care.
2. It is essential to avoid global suffering (total pain).
3. Attention and relief of major symptoms.

4. Nutrition and hydration are health treatments (they can be maintained or suspended).
5. Patient consent and/or discussion with legal representatives or proxies of the risks and benefits of each medical procedure.

It is important in the discussion to emphasize that increasing the intensity of care does not always lead to a benefit in terms of control of suffering and quality of life. It is also possible to die from futile treatments. The belief that only intensive care can be a solution to complexity while the palliative approach is perceived as a kind of defeat or abandonment is false. It should be explained that the choice not to endanger is a choice of care that does not take away rights. On the contrary, the person can contribute to a dignified end of life. The limit on the intensity of a care intervention is related to the individual's values of quality of life and dignity.

It is also crucial to emphasize that the palliative care approach is based on open and transparent communication, anchored in the four ethical principles of Childress and Beauchamp [30]. These principles, widely recognized in the field of bioethics, are essential for guiding medical practice and ensuring the respectful and conscientious treatment of patients. The principle of autonomy underscores the patient's right to be actively involved in decisions regarding their health. In the palliative context, this translates into empowering the patient to express their preferences, desires, and values concerning the care they receive. Non-maleficence requires healthcare professionals to avoid causing unnecessary harm to the patient. This principle is applied in palliative care through careful symptom management and scrupulous attention to the patient's well-being, minimizing any negative impact resulting from the care provided. Beneficence emphasizes the obligation to provide care that maximizes benefit for the patient. In the palliative context, this means promoting optimal quality of life, alleviating pain, and enhancing comfort, as well as fulfilling the patient's individual care goals. The principle of justice necessitates the fair distribution of resources and care, avoiding unjust discrimination. Ensuring equitable and dignified access to palliative care for all patients, regardless of socioeconomic background or other disparities is an enactment of the principle of justice.

In summary, the palliative approach is not merely a medical practice but an ethical commitment based on respectful communication and the promotion of fundamental values of autonomy, non-maleficence, beneficence, and justice. The understanding and conscious application of these principles ensures that each patient receives attentive and respectful palliative care tailored to their unique needs and desires [31].

27.3.1 The Importance of Communication

Effective communication is a cornerstone of the palliative approach, as highlighted by Smith and Field (2011) [32]. This element is not only perceived as crucial by family members and patients but also emerges as a top educational priority among healthcare professionals. Communication in the palliative context is inherently complex, involving words, thoughts, and emotions. Its centrality lies in the decision-making process related to care choices, aiming to define a comprehensive care plan by clearly outlining care objectives and the actions required for their achievement.

In palliative care, effective communication is essential to adequately meet the needs and preferences of patients and their relatives, requiring adequate time and preparation. After a thorough case review by the medical team, it is essential to delve further into care choices and prepare for the conversation, considering some key communication suggestions. Evidence-based tools to assist communication include the SPIKES [33] and REDMAP [34, 35] protocols. Effective communication includes exchanging information, facilitating shared decision-making, and promoting an empathic care relationship [36].

The SPIKES protocol is a standardized approach to presenting distressing information to patients and families. REDMAP is a six-step guide to future care planning conversations with people who are living with serious illness, health conditions, progressive disability, or frailty in old age. Future care planning involves the person and people who are close to them.

The main responsibility for successful patient participation in shared decision-making lies with the healthcare professionals and the organizations providing palliative care [37]. In clinical settings, physicians should first assess the patient's mental and cognitive status and then, if necessary, look for treatable physical conditions that may be interfering with his/her ability to process information and draw conclusions.

During the conversation, it is crucial to present information about care options clearly and understandably, actively involving the patient and their family in the decision-making process. This fosters a collaborative and informed approach. Open-ended questions should be promoted and understanding checked. Sensitivity and empathy are crucial to managing expectations in the delicate context of palliative care, carefully balancing realism and compassion. The educational aspect of communication should address the handling of difficult conversations and the ability to communicate sensitive information empathetically. In conclusion, the role of communication in the palliative approach goes beyond the simple transmission of information; it is a fundamental catalyst for building trusting relationships, actively involving patients in care decisions, and creating an empathetic and respectful context in such a delicate moment of life [38].

27.3.2 Advance Care Plan (ACP)

An advance care directive involves documenting a patient's preferences for future care. It aims to ensure that the patient's values, goals, and treatment preferences are clearly communicated and respected, even when the patient may no longer be able to express their wishes.

It is important to know the legislative context in each country and the specific national laws. In Italy, advance healthcare directives, commonly referred to as "testamento biologico" or "biotestamento" (biological testament), are regulated by

Article 4 of Law 219 dated December 22, 2017. This legislation provides the opportunity for every individual to express their wishes regarding healthcare treatments, as well as consent to or refusal of diagnostic assessments, therapeutic choices, and individual healthcare treatments, in the event of future inability to self-determine and after acquiring adequate medical information about the consequences of one's choices.

In the UK, advance statements are general and cover any aspect of future health or social care, whereas an advance decision (also known as an advanced decision to refuse treatment or living will) is a documented legally binding decision to refuse specific treatments in the future. Advance decisions in the UK are legally binding but advance statements are not although the contents of the latter must be taken into account when a "best decision" is made on behalf of a person lacking decision-making capacity. It is illegal to refuse basic care (such as nursing care and pain relief) and the offer of food or drink by mouth.

In Italy, patients can also formally appoint a substitute decision-maker in an advance care directive. An advance care plan is created by someone else on behalf of a person with diminished or no capacity to make decisions for themselves. In the UK, only the person concerned can make the decision, but they can appoint a health and welfare attorney to make decisions about their care should they lose the capacity to do so.

Anyone can consider advance care planning, regardless of age or health. It has been argued that people should start planning when they are in a state of good health and well-being before the need for a plan is urgent. This is particularly important in chronic illness, multiple diseases, cognitive impairment, and approaching the end of life. Affording people affected by serious or life-threatening illnesses the opportunity "to express in advance their values and preferences about life-sustaining treatment and the care they will receive" is recognized by the World Health Organization as an indicator of the strength of a country's palliative care provision [39].

Advance care planning is a team effort, involving conversations with family, care workers, and other health professionals. These conversations guide the patient and their loved ones to consider what is important to them. The process of advance care planning does not need to be complicated but it does require sensitive consideration of a person's values and preferences for care and acceptable outcomes, appropriate discussion with others, possible proxy decision-makers, and clear, comprehensive, and accurate documentation. Advance care planning benefits everyone (family, carers, and health professionals). ACP helps to ensure you receive the care you choose; families of people who have undertaken advance care planning have less anxiety, depression, and stress and are more satisfied with care; and for healthcare professionals and organizations, it reduces unnecessary transfers to acute care and unwanted treatment [40].

27.4 Realistic Medicine

Shared decision-making is at the heart of realistic medicine, an emerging healthcare approach to personalized care that was developed in Scotland [41, 42]. Current models of health and social care services are stretched and do not always suit patients, their carers, or the aspirations of the workforce. Realistic medicine aims to improve patient care by ensuring that people receive appropriate, beneficial, and evidence-based care aligned with their personal preferences.

Realistic medicine rests upon six core principles:

1. Building a personalized approach to patient care.
2. Shared decision-making.
3. Reducing harm and waste.
4. Tackling unwarranted variation in practice and outcomes.
5. Managing risk better.
6. Becoming improvers and innovators in healthcare.

To deliver realistic medicine, all health and social care professionals must be empowered to work together in teams and networks, in partnership with people.

27.5 Patient Partnership

Partnership with patients has been an emerging model of care for over 10 years and is increasingly recognized as a solution to multiple problems modern healthcare systems are faced with. The Montreal Model of patient partnership, as it is referred to in the literature considers patients and caregivers as full-fledged members of the healthcare team rather than passive receivers of a service [43]. This is the main distinction with so-called *patient-centered* approaches [44], which do not go as far as to consider the patient as a full member of the team and caregivers to themselves. The patient partnership model promotes the co-creation or co-production of healthcare and services at all levels of society, including research, education, quality improvement, governance, and clinical treatment plans [45]. It recognizes and develops patients' competencies to co-produce treatment plans and mobilizes their expertise to improve quality and for peer-to-peer education and support [45]. Patient partnership's framework can be a powerful vector for favoring shared-decision making. For example, a new innovative methodology developed in Quebec called the *patient learning pathway* (PLP) involves both patients as experts, community groups, such as patient societies, and medical associations in identifying key learning objectives for patients throughout a given healthcare pathway. These learning objectives are then integrated into the patient's journey with illness, using available technology [46].

The PLP methodology has been used in multiple specialties, including pediatrics, oncology, mental health, and dermatology [47]. It could represent a useful tool to support patient empowerment throughout a geriatric surgical palliative care trajectory.

The principles and tools of both realistic medicine and patient partnership, combined, could represent a powerful lever for improving SDM in advance care planning.

27.6 Conclusions

In conclusion, shared decision-making at the end of life within the fields of geriatrics, family medicine (general practitioners are often consulted by patients and/or caregiver) and surgical settings represents an important approach that prioritizes the collaborative involvement of patients, their families, and healthcare professionals. The unique challenges presented by aging and surgical interventions require an individualized approach that promotes patient autonomy, respects their values, and acknowledges the complex medical condition. In both geriatric care and palliative care, shared decision-making acknowledges the multifaceted nature of ageing, encompassing not only medical considerations but also the psychosocial and emotional dimensions of the patient and their family unit.

Engaging older persons in open and clear discussions about their healthcare goals, preferences, and expectations fosters a sense of empowerment and ensures that the care provided aligns with their unique needs. Within the surgical context, shared decision-making takes on added significance as patients navigate complex treatment options, potential risks, and the impact on their quality of life.

Collaborative discussions involving surgeons, patients, and, when applicable, family members, allow for a comprehensive exploration of choices. This process ensures that decisions regarding surgical interventions are informed, reflective of the patient's values, and aligned with their overall goals of care. This collaborative approach not only enhances the overall quality of care but also serves as a testament to the respect and compassion owed to individuals as they navigate these challenging and sensitive phases of their lives [41, 48–50]. As mentioned previously, complementary approaches, such as patient partnership and the PLP methodology, could be explored and integrated into advanced care to better support patient and family empowerment and foster a context conducive to SDM in advanced care planning

References

1. Radbruch L, De Lima L, Knaul F, Wenk R, Ali Z, Bhatnaghar S, Blanchard C, Bruera E, Buitrago R, Burla C, Callaway M, Munyoro EC, Centeno C, Cleary J, Connor S, Davaasuren O, Downing J, Foley K, Goh C, Gomez-Garcia W, Harding R, Khan QT, Larkin P, Leng M, Luyirika E, Marston J, Moine S, Osman H, Pettus K, Puchalski C, Rajagopal MR, Spence D, Spruijt O, Venkateswaran C, Wee B, Woodruff R, Yong J, Pastrana T. Redefining palliative care-a new consensus-based definition. J Pain Symptom Manag. 2020;60(4):754–64. https://

doi.org/10.1016/j.jpainsymman.2020.04.027. Epub 2020 May 6. PMID: 32387576; PMCID: PMC8096724.
2. Ferrell BR, Twaddle ML, Melnick A, Meier DE. National consensus project clinical practice guidelines for quality palliative care guidelines 4th Edition. J Palliat Med. 2018;21:1684–9. https://doi.org/10.1089/jpm.2018.0431.
3. Mosenthal AC. Principles of surgical palliative care. In: Surgical palliative care. Oxford: Oxford University Press; 2019. p. 13.
4. Boccardi V. Enriching lives: Geriatricians' Mission of supportive Care for Older Persons. Geriatrics (Basel). 2023;8(6):106. https://doi.org/10.3390/geriatrics8060106. PMID: 37987466; PMCID: PMC10660685.
5. Bruera E, Higginson IJ, von Gunten CF, Morita T. Textbook of palliative medicine and supportive care. 3rd ed. Boca Raton: CRC Press; 2021. eBook ISBN 9780429275524.
6. Hui D, et al. Concepts and definitions for "supportive care," "best supportive care," "palliative care," and "hospice care" in the published literature, dictionaries, and textbooks. Support Care Cancer. 2013;21:659–85.
7. Murray SA, Moine S, Boyd K. Palliative care as a primary care issue. In: Textbook of palliative medicine and supportive care. 6000 broken Sound Parkway NW, suite 300. Boca Raton, FL: CRC Press; 2021. p. 17–24.
8. Murray SA, Kendall M, Boyd K, Sheikh A. Illness trajectories and palliative care. BMJ. 2005;330(7498):1007–11.
9. Cernesi S, Demurtas J, Centeno C, Pettus K, Murray SA, Bruera E. Supportive and palliative approach to the older persons. In: The role of family physicians in older people care. Cham: Springer; 2022. p. 343–56.
10. Nicholson CJ, Combes S, Mold F, King H, Green R. Addressing inequity in palliative care provision for older people living with multimorbidity. Perspectives of community-dwelling older people on their palliative care needs: a scoping review. Palliat Med. 2023;37(4):475–97. https://doi.org/10.1177/02692163221118230. Epub 2022 Aug 24. PMID: 36002975; PMCID: PMC10074761.
11. Murray SA, Firth A, Schneider N, Van den Eynden B, Gomez-Batiste X, Brogaard T, Moine S. Promoting palliative care in the community: production of the primary palliative care toolkit by the European Association of Palliative Care Taskforce in primary palliative care. Palliat Med. 2015;29(2):101–11.
12. Pal LM, Manning L. Palliative care for frail older people. Clin Med. 2014;14(3):292.
13. Moorhouse P, Rockwood K. Frailty and its quantitative clinical evaluation. J R Coll Physicians Edinb. 2012;42:333–40. https://doi.org/10.4997/JRCPE.2012.412.
14. Fried LP, Tangen CM, Walston J, et al. Frailty in older adults: evidence for a phenotype. J Gerontol A Biol Sci Med Sci. 2001;56:M146–56. https://doi.org/10.1093/gerona/56.3.M146.
15. Fulop T, Larbi A, Witkowski, et al. Aging, frailty and age-related diseases. Biogerontology. 2010;11:547–63. https://doi.org/10.1007/s10522-010-9287-2.
16. Bieniek J, Wilczyński K, Szewieczek J. Fried frailty phenotype assessment components as applied to geriatric inpatients. Clin Interv Aging. 2016;11:453–9.
17. Church S, Rogers E, Rockwood K, Theou O. A scoping review of the clinical frailty scale. BMC Geriatr. 2020;20(1):1–18.
18. Murray SA, Kendall M, Boyd K, Sheikh A. Illness trajectories and palliative care. Int Perspect Public Health Palliat Care. 2013;330:s.
19. Maas EAT, Murray SA, Engels Y, Campbell C. What tools are available to identify patients with palliative care needs in primary care: a systematic literature review and survey of European practice. BMJ Support Palliat Care. 2013;3(4):444–51.
20. Turrillas P, Peñafiel J, Tebé C, Amblàs-Novellas J, Gómez-Batiste X. NECPAL prognostic tool: a palliative medicine retrospective cohort study. BMJ Support Palliat Care. 2021;2021:bmjspcare-2020-002567.
21. Moroni M, Zocchi D, Bolognesi D, Abernethy A, Rondelli R, Savorani G, SUQ-P group. The 'surprise'question in advanced cancer patients: a prospective study among general practitioners. Palliat Med. 2014;28(7):959–64.

22. Baik D, Russell D, Jordan L, Dooley F, Bowles KH, Masterson Creber RM. Using the palliative performance scale to estimate survival for patients at the end of life: a systematic review of the literature. J Palliat Med. 2018;21(11):1651–61.
23. Mather H, Guo P, Firth A, Davies JM, Sykes N, Landon A, Murtagh FE. Phase of illness in palliative care: cross-sectional analysis of clinical data from community, hospital and hospice patients. Palliat Med. 2018;32(2):404–12.
24. Coulter A, Collins A. Making shared decision-making a reality: no decision about me without me. London: King's Fund; 2011.
25. Rosca A, Karzig-Roduner I, Kasper J, et al. Shared decision making and advance care planning: a systematic literature review and novel decision-making model. BMC Med Ethics. 2023;24:64. https://doi.org/10.1186/s12910-023-00944-7.
26. Van de Pol MH, Fluit CR, Lagro J, Slaats YH, Rikkert MGO, Lagro-Janssen AL. Expert and patient consensus on a dynamic model for shared decision-making in frail older patients. Patient Educ Couns. 2016;99(6):1069–77.
27. Akdeniz M, Yardımcı B, Kavukcu E. Ethical considerations at the end-of-life care. SAGE open medicine. 2021;9:20503121211000918.
28. Jaffe E, Knight CF. Unipac six: ethical and legal dimensions of treating life-limiting illness. Hospice and palliative care training for physicians: a self-study program. 3rd ed. Chicago: American Academy of Hospice and Palliative Medicine; 2008. p. 15.
29. Eng V, Hewitt V, Kekalih A. Preference for initiation of end-of-life care discussion in Indonesia: a quantitative study. BMC Palliat Care. 2022;21:6. https://doi.org/10.1186/s12904-021-00894-0.
30. Beauchamp TL. Standing on principles: collected essays. Oxford: Oxford University Press; 2010.
31. Varkey B. Principles of clinical ethics and their application to practice. Med Princ Pract. 2021;30(1):17–28. https://doi.org/10.1159/000509119. Epub 2020 Jun 4. PMID: 32498071; PMCID: PMC7923912.
32. Smith TJ, Dow LA, Virago EA, Khatcheressian J, Matsuyama R, Lyckholm LJ. A pilot trial of decision aids to give truthful prognostic and treatment information to chemotherapy patients with advanced cancer. J Support Oncol. 2011;9(2):79–86.
33. Buckman RA. Breaking bad news: the SPIKES strategy. Commun Oncol. 2005;2(2):138–42.
34. Mason B, Canny A, Carduff E, Spiller J, Patterson R, Boyd K. 50 making ACP work for people in practice: implementation of a structured advance/anticipatory care planning intervention in Scottish primary care (4ACP). BMJ. 2023;13:1.
35. Cernesi S, Bonesi MG, Cancian M, Guerroni A, Lora Aprile P, Salvetti A. General practice opens the door to primary palliative care in Italy: an Italian version of red map. Palliat Med. 2021;1:184.
36. Payne S, Ahmad N, Albone R, Van den Block L, Burlá C, Cernesi S, Pettus K (2020). Palliative care for older persons infected with COVID-19.
37. Kuosmanen L, Hupli M, Ahtiluoto S, Haavisto E. Patient participation in shared decision-making in palliative care—an integrative review. J Clin Nurs. 2021;30(23–24):3415–28. https://doi.org/10.1111/jocn.15866. Epub 2021 May 24. Epub 2021 May 24.
38. Doyle D. Guidelines and suggestions for those starting a hospice/palliative care service. 3rd ed. IAHPC Press; 2009.
39. Age UK. Advance decisions, advance statements and living wills. 2023. https://www.ageuk.org.uk/globalassets/age-uk/documents/factsheets/fs72_advance_decisions_advance_statements_and_living_wills_fcs.pdf [online]. Accessed 19 Feb 2024.
40. World Health Organization. Assessing the development of palliative care worldwide: a set of actionable indicators [online]. 2021. https://www.who.int/publications/i/item/9789240033351. Accessed 19 Feb 2024.
41. Fenning SJ, Smith G, Calderwood C. Realistic medicine: changing culture and practice in the delivery of health and social care. Patient Educ Couns. 2019;102(10):1751–5.
42. https://learn.nes.nhs.scot/18350/realistic-medicine [online]. Accessed 9 Mar 2024.

43. Brinkman-Stoppelenburg A, Rietjens JA, Van der Heide A. The effects of advance care planning on end-of-life care: a systematic review. Palliat Med. 2014;28(8):1000–25.
44. Pomey M, Flora L, Karazivan P, Dumez V, Lebel P, Vanier M, Jouet E. Le « Montreal model » : enjeux du partenariat relationnel entre patients et professionnels de la santé. Sante Publique. 2015;1:41–50. https://doi.org/10.3917/spub.150.0041.
45. Philippe K, Dumez V, Luigi F, Marie-Pascale P, Del Grande C, Philip GD, Nicolas F, Emmanuelle J, Olivier LV, Paule L. The patient-as-partner approach in health care: a conceptual framework for a necessary transition. Acad Med. 2015;90(4):437–41. https://doi.org/10.1097/ACM.0000000000000603.
46. Boivin A, Dumez V, Castonguay G, Berkesse A. The ecology of engagement: fostering cooperative efforts in health with patients and communities. Health Expect. 2022;25:2314–27. https://doi.org/10.1111/hex.13571.
47. Pomey MP, Paquette J, Nelea MI, et al. Integrating accompanying patients into clinical oncology teams: limiting and facilitating factors. BMC Health Serv Res. 2024;24:150.
48. Jackson M, Clovin T, Montiel C, Bogdanova E, Côté C, Descoteaux A, Wong C, Dumez V, Pomey MP. Adopting a learning pathway approach to patient partnership in telehealth: a proof of concept. PEC Innov. 2023;3:100223. https://doi.org/10.1016/j.pecinn.2023.100223. PMID: 37842174; PMCID: PMC10570687.
49. Rietjens JA, Sudore RL, Connolly M, van Delden JJ, Drickamer MA, Droger M, Korfage IJ. Definition and recommendations for advance care planning: an international consensus supported by the European Association for Palliative Care. Lancet Oncol. 2017;18(9):e543–51.
50. Colley A, Lin JA, Pierce L, Finlayson E, Sudore RL, Wick E. Missed opportunities and health disparities for advance care planning before elective surgery in older adults. JAMA Surg. 2022;157(10):e223687.

Living with Frailty: Psychological Stress and Support for Emotional Tension 28

Patrick Bini

28.1 Stress in Frail Patients

Why associate the concept of stress with frail and geriatric patients? Often, these individuals have been grappling with various issues related to their physical condition for an extended period. However, facing the possibility of a medical procedure or the course of an illness can impose significant pressure on them, eliciting emotions such as anxiety, distress, anger, and frustration. If not managed effectively, these emotions can lead to stress and, in some cases, even trigger serious health conditions. Therefore, it is crucial to comprehend the nature of stress and the underlying sensations that commonly accompany the pre-surgery period and extended hospitalization. This understanding enables us to develop strategies to mitigate its effects when working with patients.

28.1.1 What Is Stress?

The term "stress" originally originated in physics and engineering, where it referred to a force or load acting on a specific point of an object, such as a beam or column. This pressure generates a response that can be elastic, plastic, or even lead to the object's breakage. Later, this concept was adopted in psychology by Selye in the mid-1950s [1]. He simply substituted the object with a person and the stress-inducing load with a significant problem weighing on them. Similar to physics, this constant load can result in various potential outcomes, particularly:

- Elastic bending, which burdens the individual but eventually leads to the resolution of the initial issue.

P. Bini (✉)
Center of Psychology and Psychotherapy, Perugia, Italy

V. Boccardi, L. Marano (eds.), *The Frail Surgical Patient*, Practical Issues in Geriatrics, https://doi.org/10.1007/978-3-031-77707-3_28

- Plastic bending, where the individual remains inert, gradually growing accustomed to enduring the load.
- Breaking, representing the incapacity or impossibility of problem resolution, potentially leading to psychopathological conditions such as depression.

Under the same stress-inducing load, often represented by a challenging problem with no easy solution, different individuals may react profoundly differently over time. Some individuals, adaptable and accustomed to handling challenging situations, will adjust to the effort. While they may experience anxiety, sleeplessness, fear, and tension, they will employ functional attempted solutions that, despite adversity, ultimately lead to problem resolution. This is what Selye defines as "eustress" or positive stress, which activates one to be more efficient. On the other hand, there are those who experience the same physiological activation reactions but direct them toward dysfunctional problem-solving attempts, which are not suitable for resolving the issue or who may not have the means to resolve it quickly. Often, physiological issues initially faced with a positive outlook and emotions, when encountered over an extended period or in conjunction with other problems that may arise or in cases of relapse or recurrence, which are more likely to occur in geriatric settings, can influence one's mood with all possible consequences and repercussions. After having fought and resisted for a long time, reaching the end and realizing that all our efforts have been counterproductive can trigger feelings of inadequacy and resignation. But why is stress, which ignites when we are subjected to prolonged periods of pressure, so important from a psychological perspective? First, because there are significant physiological consequences. Tsigos C et al [2] stated that the entire endocrine system is involved, starting with the adrenal glands that release neuro-mediators to the pituitary gland, which responds excessively and disrupts the entire metabolic principle, such as that of the thyroid. Furthermore, if these intense sensations stem from poorly managed emotions, especially fear, pain, and anger, they can, in the long run, trigger actual psychopathologies, often compounding already challenging clinical conditions.

28.2 Emotions Associated with Hospitalization and Pre-Intervention

28.2.1 Basic Sensations

When we are born, nature endows us with basic abilities that are later refined through experiences. This holds true for communication, movement, logic, and more. For instance, at birth, we possess the potential to develop spoken language. However, without learning and structuring it through direct experience, we will never acquire the ability to speak. The same principle applies to the realm of emotions; we are equipped with fundamental sensations, upon which various subclasses of emotions are constructed through experience, branching out from these basic ones. To illustrate, imagine that as a child, during your initial encounter with a cat, it scratched you, evoking a profound fear. From this incident, a spontaneous association forms: cat = pain = fear = avoidance. By following these fear-based emotions without assessing the actual threat posed by cats, you gradually develop a perception of their dangerousness. The more you avoid them, the more menacing they appear, potentially leading to the development of phobic disorders. In essence, it is us who construct our subsequent experiences. However, it is crucial to recognize that in the construction of our reactive perceptual system [3], emotions consistently serve their fundamental function. It is our interpretation of the signals received that can go awry. Therefore, it is not the emotions themselves that malfunction; rather, it is the way we perceive and construct them. Returning to the fear of the cat, its core function is well-oriented as it alerts us to potential harm. However, it is our choice between flight or confrontation that shapes our emotions and perceptions. By consistently opting for flight, the cat transforms into an increasingly terrifying entity to be avoided, as our perception is continually shaped by our feelings and imagination. Since fear is our fundamental sensation, we continue to construct fear upon fear, eventually creating a monstrous image. Conversely, with caution and courage, we can confront the cat, verifying its actual danger and beginning to construct our perceptions based on factual reality. Through this process, we may discover that the cat is not merely a scratching monster but can also be playful, affectionate, and charming. Hence, basic sensations represent the potential for each individual to construct their unique range of emotions through experiences, aligning with both internal and external life events. This contributes to building an individual's perceptual reactive model, mediating perceptions while simultaneously constructing them. Various theories support this thesis. According to Ekman P [4], there are six basic emotions: joy, anger, sadness, disgust, fear, and shame. Meanwhile, Plutchik R [5] identifies eight emotions divided into four pairs: anger and fear, sadness and joy, disgust and acceptance, and surprise and anticipation. It is suggested that the range of emotions experienced, with their nuances and combinations of basic sensations, exceeds 180. However, what is meant by the combination of emotions? Conventionally, in theories such as those of Ekman P [4] or Plutchik R [5], the wide range of experienced emotions results from the combination of different basic emotions. Nonetheless, these theories do not explain how these emotions actually come to be and become integral parts of each individual's perceptual reactive system. From clinical practice, particularly through research interventions that elucidate the workings of a problem, it becomes evident that individuals themselves, through their subjective perceptions and reactions, shape the reality they simultaneously construct and experience. The same applies to the entire spectrum of emotions, which become real for the individual when experienced, either through lived or imagined experiences. Analyzing each emotion as a single variable in the perceptual field would be extremely limiting and methodologically incorrect. In reality, at every moment, myriad sensors and perceptual filters are active within us, analyzing and shaping our subjective reality. Concurrently, as we react to perceived reality, we introduce variations that reciprocally influence us in an ongoing exchange. In this interplay, the entirety of the person is engaged, with all their facets, rather than just a single emotion. Understanding how emotions function empowers us to develop tools that can help manage or effectively utilize them, rather than merely being subject to them with all ensuing consequences. From my perspective, the fundamental basic sensations, in line with the studies of Nardone G [3], are four from which all other emotions stem:

- *Pleasure*
- *Fear*
- *Pain*
- *Anger*

Therefore, we will analyze these basic sensations along with their related emotions, constructed from life experiences, whether lived or avoided. These emotions tend to establish circular mechanisms for maintaining problems when perceptual-reactive structures become rigid and dysfunctional. The emotions most frequently associated with hospitalization and pre-surgery conditions are fear, often coupled with anxiety and panic; pain, leading to distress; and anger, accompanied by feelings of frustration and injustice. Initially, we will examine the functioning of basic sensations in a general sense and then delve into specific emotions to understand how to utilize them, teaching patients tools for their management.

28.3 Fear

Fear is perhaps the most common emotion we encounter. It manifests in various forms: fear of confronting something we dread, making decisions, death, or losing loved ones due to medical outcomes, among others. Each of us has experienced fear in our lives, and indeed, this emotion has proven fundamental for our ancestors' survival. A proto-simian without fear would likely have met a swift demise, perhaps at the jaws of a lion. Fear is vital as it enables us to interact with the world effectively. Imagine not fearing your boss's reaction to a poorly executed job or recklessly dashing across a busy road without concern for traffic. In both scenarios, disaster looms, underscoring the essential nature of fear. As mentioned earlier, fear, like other basic sensations, serves as the foundation upon which emotions are built through subjective experiences.

Emotions stemming from fear include:

- Future-oriented: Anxiety, an anticipatory form of fear that arises in preparation for a potentially frightening event, fueled by the fear of impending danger
- Present-oriented: Panic or horror, the typical reaction displayed in the face of immediate danger
- Past-oriented or constructed: Phobia, developed based on past experiences but sustained by imagination rather than direct encounters, leading to avoidance behaviors

For our discussion, we will focus on anxiety, an emotion known to profoundly impact individuals if mismanaged or prolonged. The systems triggering and perpetuating the problem are complex and multifaceted. Nonetheless, I will attempt to elucidate their basic functions and provide simple tools for their management.

Pre-surgery and geriatric patients often experience:

- Performance or anticipatory anxiety related to potential outcomes (fear of the procedure's course, death, or intervention)
- Anxiety and panic disorders (generalized fear and apprehension)
- Anxiety and pathological doubt (persistent rumination about health concerns)

What is anxiety? Many experience it constantly, yet few truly understand its nature. On a sensory level, anxiety is the somatic manifestation of fear—a tightness in the stomach and a persistent sense of impending doom. Patients often describe it as a dark shadow enveloping their perceptions. Anxiety stems not from actual events but from imagined possibilities, from the fear of losing control or facing adverse outcomes. While anxiety is often viewed negatively due to its discomfort and hindrance to performance, it serves a critical function. It directs our attention to potential future dangers, alerting us to impending threats. Thus, anxiety represents fear in its anticipatory form, preparing us for potential dangers. Consider the pressure before a significant procedure, where obsessive thoughts about potential complications trigger sensations of dread, disrupting sleep and affecting mood. While anxiety prompts physiological reactions to prepare us for danger, it becomes problematic when it arises inappropriately, without imminent threats. Persistent anxiety leads to internal tension, hindering focus and prompting futile attempts to alleviate it. Anxious individuals often believe that avoiding triggers preserves their well-being, but avoidance exacerbates fears. Avoidance behaviors reinforce anxiety, making feared objects or situations appear even more menacing. In fragile patients facing challenging clinical conditions, anxiety often becomes chronic, leading to persistent rumination or obsessive-compulsive behaviors. If left unchecked, chronic anxiety can lead to significant avoidance of life events and various somatic symptoms. In summary, anxiety, though uncomfortable, plays a crucial role in our survival by alerting us to potential dangers. However, when mismanaged or prolonged, it can severely impact one's well-being. Understanding its nature and implementing effective coping strategies are essential for managing anxiety in clinical settings.

28.3.1 Anxiety and Panic Disorder

Panic attacks represent an extreme form of anxiety and are defined in the DSM IV as "a distinct period of intense fear that occurs suddenly." The symptoms are primarily physical and resemble the sensations experienced in the early stages of a heart attack, with symptoms such as tachycardia, rapid breathing, sweating, chest constriction, blurred vision, fear of fainting or losing control, and a sense of impending doom. Panic attacks usually begin with an initial episode of intense anxious somatization, leading to the symptoms described above. The physical reaction is so overwhelming that the individual starts to view the exception as the rule, constantly monitoring their physical condition for fear of a recurrence of the attack. Panic is a natural response to fear materializing in the present. However, it is quite different when facing a furious bear in the woods, diverting attention from fear to the need for confrontation or escape. In such a scenario, worrying about being scared is entirely natural. Conversely, if the same sudden fear reaction occurs while sitting on the couch, perhaps watching a favorite movie, reason and emotion become chaotic. The rational mind searches for causes it cannot find, leading the person to fear itself.

28.3.2 Therapeutic Guidelines for Anxiety and Panic

28.3.2.1 Management of Complaints

Among the most common dysfunctional solutions adopted by fragile patients is incessantly discussing their health problems and dragging others into their web of fear. While some may try to console them, it often perpetuates a cycle of depression. Hence, discussions about politics, gossip, or sports are preferable, avoiding topics related to their condition or surgery. If they seek reassurance or anticipate outcomes, redirect the conversation. For example:

> Patient: "Do you think it will go well?"
> Therapist: "Why do you think it will go well?"

28.3.3 Worst Fantasy Technique

In cases where individuals attempt to avoid anxious thoughts, escalating them to panic, a paradoxical approach can be effective. By voluntarily exaggerating fears in an imaginary ritual, fears are confronted and eventually dissipate. This technique is implemented in two ways:

1. *Prescribed Worst Fantasy*: The patient confronts worst-case scenarios for 5 minutes every 3 h, imagining catastrophic outcomes associated with their fears. Intentional exposure to these fears reduces their intensity and diminishes anxiety.
2. *User-Guided Worst Fantasy*: The patient verbalizes their fears with guidance, allowing them to articulate their worst fantasies without adding new elements to the narrative.

Before applying these techniques, ensure the patient genuinely seeks relief from anxious thoughts. If they engage in rumination or pathological doubt, different approaches are necessary.

28.3.4 Anxiety and Pathological Doubt

Pathological doubt arises from attempts to dispel anxiety by seeking definitive answers to unanswerable questions. The mind fixates on unsolvable queries, leading to incessant rumination. Patients often question past events, future outcomes, or present sensations, attempting to maintain control over uncontrollable events.

28.3.5 Breaking the Obsessive Questioning Cycle

Since questioning becomes obsessive, actively responding may perpetuate the cycle. Instead, blocking responses inhibits further questioning. Replace the obsession with a mantra such as, "There are no intelligent answers to stupid questions," shifting attention away from the obsession and allowing it to fade.

28.4 Pain

Pain is a fundamental sensation innate to human nature, experienced from the earliest moments of life, but it evolves into an emotion based on life experiences. It is a sharp sensation that emerges whenever we are deprived, whether temporarily or irreversibly, of something tangible or abstract. From the loss of a loved one to the anxiety over a surgery's outcome, from the departure of a child to feeling trapped in resolving pressing issues, pain shrouds the lives of those who endure it. Prolonged suffering can plunge individuals into a genuine state of depression, where they perceive no escape from the abyss and resign themselves to the pain of loss. The primary emotions associated with pain across different temporal orientations include:

- Anticipatory pain: Anxiety about future pain
- Present pain: Despair and affliction
- Postponed pain: A sense of powerlessness regarding past losses

Anxiety represents the anticipatory form of pain, where individuals anticipate experiencing pain due to an impending loss. Unlike anxiety, which revolves around potential future events, anxiety anticipates inevitable pain, such as death, leading individuals to anticipate the associated suffering.

Anxiety is often prevalent in fragile patients for various reasons:

- Advanced age brings physical and pathological concerns, fostering anxiety about deteriorating health and mortality.
- Aging prompts individuals to confront mortality, leading to anxiety about their own demise and that of loved ones.

28.4.1 Therapeutic Guidelines for Managing Anxiety

Unfortunately, there is no magic solution to eradicate anxiety, as life comprises both joyous and sorrowful events. Prolonged anxiety can lead to stress-related and pathological consequences, compelling individuals to implement counterproductive solutions. For instance, comforting someone by urging them to go out and enjoy life may exacerbate their depression if their low mood prevents them from following such advice. Robert Frost's assertion, "if you want to get out of the pain, you have to go through it," underscores the necessity of confronting pain rather than avoiding it. Encouraging patients to confront their anxieties through writing without ruminating on them helps them gradually detach from their fears, making them more manageable.

28.5 Anger

Anger serves a crucial evolutionary function by activating internal resources to overcome obstacles and achieve goals. Despite being perceived as unpleasant, anger is necessary for maintaining balance with the world. However, culturally, those who succumb to anger are often viewed as weak due to its significant relational impact. Irritability and explosive anger can lead to social conflicts, complicating relationships with bosses, friends, spouses, or family members. Additionally, anger distorts perceptions, narrowing focus and impairing rational judgment. It encompasses various related emotions constructed through experiences:

- Anticipatory anger: Frustration and exasperation
- Present anger: Expressed or suppressed rage
- Past anger: Resentment, revenge, or guilt

Frustration emerges when we feel physically or mentally restricted, unable to fulfill our needs due to external or internal factors. According to Dollard J [6], aggressive behavior, the response to frustration, is always triggered by a frustrating event, the stimulus. We may feel frustrated with ourselves due to our limitations, with others when they impede us, or with the world when circumstances prevent us from achieving our desires. Frustration does not always manifest as anger; instead, it often leads to irritability, melancholy, and persistent rumination about the situation. In geriatric patients and individuals awaiting surgery, frustration often manifests as anger due to prolonged hospitalization, previous unsuccessful surgeries, or extended stays in hospitals. Frustration does not necessarily culminate in anger; rather, it entails a persistent sense of discomfort. Additionally, individuals affected by illness or accidents may find themselves frustrated with their unfortunate circumstances. Thus, frustration serves as the anticipatory precursor to anger, similar to how anxiety anticipates fear, warning us to proceed cautiously. This activation may either lead to problem resolution or, if unresolved, result in the expression or suppression of anger, accompanied by stress-related or psychopathological consequences. Accumulated frustration can severely impact one's self-relationship. Those who suppress their anger keenly feel it but struggle to express it, leading to a cycle of escalating frustration. In such cases, ongoing frustration may lead to anxiety and stress or result in explosive outbursts akin to a balloon reaching its breaking point. Constant rumination on unresolved events loads the metaphorical spring, and when tension accumulates without release, it eventually reaches a breaking point, overwhelming inhibitory mechanisms.

28.5.1 Managing Repressed Anger

To address repressed anger without causing harm, a tool is needed to release tension safely. The "anger letter" technique, part of the brief strategic model, offers an effective strategy. To begin, write a letter addressed to the source of your anger, expressing all the negative feelings and thoughts without inhibition. Repeat this exercise daily until a sense of relief is felt, without revisiting what has been written. This approach allows anger to dissipate without causing harm, preserving relationships and preventing the public expression of resentment.

28.6 Conclusion

In conclusion, the exploration of stress, anxiety, and anger in frail and geriatric patients underscores the complexity of emotional experiences during hospitalization and pre-surgery periods. By delving into the psychological mechanisms underlying these emotions, the text offers valuable insights into their management and therapeutic approaches. From understanding stress as a response to challenging situations to exploring the anticipatory nature of anxiety and the dynamics of anger in response to frustration, the text provides a comprehensive framework for supporting patients facing medical challenges. Moreover, the emphasis on tailored therapeutic interventions, such as redirecting discussions, employing worst fantasy techniques, and addressing pathological doubt, highlights the importance of personalized care in mitigating the adverse effects of these emotions. Ultimately, by fostering a deeper understanding of emotional experiences and offering practical strategies for intervention, the text serves as a valuable resource for healthcare professionals striving to enhance the well-being of frail and older patients navigating medical care.

References

1. Selye H. The stress of my life. Toronto: McClelland and Stewart; 1977. p. 85.
2. Tsigos C, Kyrou I, Kassi E, Chrousos GP. In: Feingold KR, Anawalt B, Boyce A, et al., editors. Stress: endocrine physiology and pathophysiology. Endotext, MDText.com, Inc.; 2020.

3. Capogna G, Capogna E, Nardone G. The strategic debriefing. Incorporating strategic dialogue in the standard debriefing after the scenario. Med Ed Publish. 2020;9:210. https://doi.org/10.15694/mep.2020.000210.1.
4. Ekman P. An argument for basic emotions. Cognit Emot. 1992;6:169–200.
5. Plutchik R. The Nature of Emotions: Human emotions have deep evolutionary roots, a fact that may explain their complexity and provide tools for clinical practice. American Scientist. 2001;89(4):344–50.
6. Dollard J, Doob L, Miller N, Mowrer O, Sears R. Frustration and aggression. New Haven, CT: Yale University Press; 1939.

Informed Consent Challenges in Frail Surgical Patients

29

Alessandro Feola, Antonietta Porzio, Mariavictoria De Simone, Omero Pinto, Graziamaria Corbi, and Carlo Pietro Campobasso

29.1 Introduction

The principle of informed consent is one of the most controversial aspects of clinical bioethics and the core of contemporary patient-centered healthcare, embodying the values of autonomy or self-determination, freedom, and respect for human life, dignity, and the rights of the patient.

The acquisition of consent or dissent is an act of specific and exclusive competence of every physician, not delegable to anybody. The physician does not undertake or continue in diagnostic procedures and/or therapeutic interventions without the preliminary acquisition of informed consent or in the presence of an informed dissent. The physician is recommended to acquire the consent or dissent of the patient in written form and signed or with other methods of equal effectiveness in documents.

In memory of Prof. Luigi D'Ancora, University of Campania "Luigi Vanvitelli", via Luciano Armanni 5, 80138 Naples, Italy.

A. Feola (✉) · M. De Simone · C. P. Campobasso
Department of Experimental Medicine, University of Campania "Luigi Vanvitelli", Naples, Italy
e-mail: alessandro.feola@unicampania.it; mariavictoria.desimone@unicampania.it; carlopietro.campobasso@unicampania.it

A. Porzio
Department of Mental and Physical Health and Preventive Medicine, University of Campania "Luigi Vanvitelli", Naples, Italy
e-mail: antonietta.porzio@unicampania.it

O. Pinto
Forensic Medicine Unit, "Sant'Anna e San Sebastiano" Hospital, Caserta, Italy

G. Corbi
Department of Translational Medical Sciences, University of Naples Federico II, Naples, Italy
e-mail: graziamaria.corbi@unina.it

V. Boccardi, L. Marano (eds.), *The Frail Surgical Patient*, Practical Issues in Geriatrics, https://doi.org/10.1007/978-3-031-77707-3_29

For frail surgical patients, ethical and legal issues are mainly related to the increased vulnerability to adverse outcomes when exposed to endogenous and/or exogenous stressors. Surgical interventions can represent a real challenge for all frail patients who may experience risks of falls, hospitalization, physical disability, and early mortality. The poor outcomes in frail surgical patients are often the object of medical malpractice claims, mainly due to poor information or an inappropriate pre-operative frailty assessment. To ensure that these individuals possess a comprehensive understanding of the potential benefits, risks, and alternatives, complete information should be addressed comprehensively and efficiently, with patients encouraged to actively participate in their care whenever possible. This chapter regards the importance of informed consent within the context of frail surgical patients, emphasizing the need for healthcare professionals to navigate the intricate complexities and considerations associated with respecting autonomy, protecting vulnerability, and promoting wellness.

29.1.1 Historical Background of Consent

For thousands of years, the Hippocratic Oath has represented the only expression of medical ethics in the world, instructing physicians and other medical professionals to the first principle of "do not harm." The medical profession regulated its conduct through this statement, for which, however, the patient participation in decision-making for medical treatment was not encouraged. The principle of informed consent has undergone significant development throughout the past century. The traditional approach to medical decision-making was paternalistic, which assumed that physicians, like caring fathers, would act in the patient's best interests. This approach was prevalent until the early 1900s. The modern regulations for informed consent in the US have their origins soon after World War II, when Nazi physicians conducted inhumane experiments on Jewish deported people and prisoners without their consent. At the Nuremberg trial dealing with war crimes and crimes against humanity, ten ethical principles were assessed. They represent the so-called Nuremberg Code, among which the principle of voluntary informed consent was declared to protect individuals' right to control their own bodies. In the Code of Medical Ethics approved in 1949 by the World Medical Association, physicians were requested to respect a competent patient's right to accept or refuse treatment. Individuals have the right to request and be provided with information about their data. The Helsinki Declaration (1964) also highlighted the importance of respecting the principle of individual autonomy and the right to informed decision-making, specifically acknowledging that the free choice of medical treatments is a fundamental principle. Articles 25 and 26 of the Declaration of Helsinki address the principle of voluntary informed consent, highlighting the need for adequate information prior to participation in clinical trials. Participation by individuals capable of giving valid consent for medical research must be voluntary. It is essential that each individual who may take part in the trial be fully informed about the "aims, methods, sources of funding, any possible conflicts of interest, institutional affiliations of the researcher, the anticipated benefits and potential risks of the study, and the discomfort it may entail, and any other relevant aspects of the study. The potential subject must be informed of the right to refuse to participate in the study or to withdraw consent to participate at any time without reprisal." The principle of informed consent has also been clearly assessed by the Oviedo Convention (1997) for the protection of human rights and dignity of the human being regarding the application of biology and medicine, which is the only international legally binding instrument for the protection of human rights in the biomedical field. Article 5 reports as a general rule that "an intervention in the health field may only be carried out after the person concerned has given free and informed consent to it. This person shall beforehand be given appropriate information as to the purpose and nature of the intervention, as well as on its consequences and risks. The person concerned may freely withdraw consent at any time." Therefore, medical treatments may only be given if the individual has provided their consent after full information about his/her health. According to Article 9, everyone has the right to respect for their private life in relation to information about his/her health, and he/she is entitled to know any information collected about his/her health. To protect persons unable to consent, the Oviedo Convention (Article 6) requires that if a patient is a minor or someone who does not have the capacity to consent due to mental disability or other diseases, the authorization of his/her representative by law is necessary. Moreover, the previously expressed wishes relating to medical intervention by a patient who is not, at the time of the intervention, in a state to express his or her wishes shall be taken into account (Article 9). The most important personal freedom and rights enjoyed by European citizens are also reported in the European Union's Charter of Fundamental Rights (CFR), declared in 2000. According to the EU charter, the "free and informed consent" of a person is the expression of the individual right to integrity. It is crucial to obtain informed consent or dissent from patients before applying medical and biological treatments. This policy acknowledges the patient's integrity and rights.

29.1.2 Ethical Principles and Legal Framework of Informed Consent

Informed consent is the core of a well-functioning healthcare system. From an ethical point of view, it represents the expression of the human right to decide about medical care. Consent is a crucial part of care since the doctor-patient relationship is based on it. The impact of the pandemic on the healthcare system and the spread of medical misinformation through social media contributed to creating an atmosphere of general mistrust toward science, with a relevant increase in malpractice claims. Based on the previously reported ethical principles, consent should be informed, clearly expressed, personal, voluntary, participatory, specific, current, and revocable at any time. The expression of consent by a patient is a process that can be divided into several stages, including the information phase, comprehension, voluntary decision-making, and authorization. The primary endpoint of proper consent is to provide basic and complete information about the diagnosis, treatment options, potential risks, and benefits of the proposed pharmacological therapy or surgery, as well as alternatives to the procedure that patients can choose. Significant focus needs to be placed on the occurrence of poor outcomes, including adverse drug reactions, postoperative mortality or other complications, and extended hospital stay. Communication should be tailored to the patient's individual comprehension level. It is recommended to minimize written materials and use simple language, considering the participants' abilities and limitations. Transparency and empathy during communication are essential when the physician explains, establishing trust in medical care and clinical assistance. To define the patient as "correctly informed," an assessment of decision-making capacity is also needed. Any decline in cognitive ability has the potential to hinder the informed consent process. An individual must possess both the ability to understand and the ability to choose. The ability of an individual to make an informed decision is also called the decision-making capacity, which the physician should be able to assess. The patient's decision-making autonomy is made manifest by the process underlying informed consent, but sometimes this is not enough as for older or frail patients. Obtaining valid informed consent in frail surgical patients represents a challenging aspect of medical practice. Many studies reported that frailty is highly common among elderly patients undergoing surgical interventions due to an increased risk of adverse postoperative outcomes. Therefore, an evaluation of physical frailty status is always required to identify disabilities/vulnerabilities that make patients less susceptible to restoring their previous state of health.

29.1.3 Definition of Frailty

For many years, the definition of "frailty" has not been uniform, and a large number of attempts to define frailty have been reported. In the early 1980s, the term frailty was used to express the concept of institutionalization. According to this position, fragile individuals can be minors, the elderly, or disabled people but also every subject with mental or physical disease. The main ethical duty of a physician is to protect their health and rights without discrimination.

Brown et al. [1] compared the frailty status to cognitive and functional decline conditions occurring near the end of life. In 1999, the term frailty was used to define the combinations of aging, disease, and other factors contributing to making people more vulnerable [2]. Fried et al. [3], in 2001, proposed a more specific definition of frailty as a standardized clinical phenotype based on the presence of three or more than five items (Table 29.1).

According to Fried's criteria, frailty is an older adult's physiologic syndrome distinguished from disability and comorbidity entities, previously used as frailty synonyms. Comorbidities and disabilities are commonly the result of frailty. They could be considered as frailty etiologic risk factors, contributing to accelerating the progression of frailty. Furthermore, supporting geriatricians' hypothesis, disability could be both a precursor and a consequence of frailty. The impact of weakness, reduced endurance, and slowed performance on mobility, with decreased energy

Table 29.1 Fried's criteria of frailty phenotype

Shrinking	Weight loss, unintentional (i.e., not due to dieting or exercise), evaluated in the prior year or at follow-up (calculated as weight in the previous year—current measured weight/weight in the previous year) *A subject is frail when have lost more than 10 pounds unintentionally or at follow-up, an unintentional weight loss of at least 5% of the previous year's body weight*
Weakness	Grip strength adjusted for gender and body mass index (BMI) *A man is frail when the cutoff for grip strength is*: ≤29 (if BMI is ≤24) ≤30 (if BMI is 24.1–26) ≤30 (if BMI is 26.1–28) ≤32 (if BMI is >28) *A woman is frail when the cutoff for grip strength is*: ≤17 (if BMI is ≤23) ≤17.3 (if BMI is 23.1–26) ≤18(if BMI is 26.1–29) ≤21 (if BMI is >29)
Poor endurance and energy	As indicated by self-report of exhaustion identified by two questions from the CES–D scale [a]: (1) I felt that everything I did was an effort and (2) I could not get going. [0 = rarely or none of the time (<1 day), 1 = some or a little of the time (1–2 days), 2 = a moderate amount of the time (3–4 days), or 3 = most of the time] *A subject is frail when the answer is "2" or "3" to either of these questions*
Slowness	Based on time to walk 15 feet, adjusting for gender and standing height *A man is frail when the cutoff for time to walk 15 feet is:* ≥7 s (if height ≤ 173 cm) ≥6 s (if height ≤ 173 cm) *A woman is frail when the cutoff for time to walk 15 feet is*: ≥7 s (if height ≤ 159 cm) ≥6 s (if height > 159 cm)
Low physical activity level	Based on the short version of the Minnesota leisure time activity questionnaire, a weighted score of kilocalories expended per week is calculated at baseline; the lowest quintile of physical activity was identified for each gender. *A man is frail when kcals of physical activity per week < 383* *A woman is frail when kcals of physical activity per week < 270*

[a] Center for Epidemiologic Studies Depression Scale (CES–D scale), originally published by Radloff in 1977, is a 20-item measure that asks caregivers to rate how often over the past week they experienced symptoms associated with depression, such as restless sleep, poor appetite, and feeling lonely. Response options range from 0 to 3 for each item. Scores range from 0 to 60, with high scores indicating greater depressive symptoms

[b] The Minnesota Leisure Time Physical Activity Questionnaire (LTPAQ) is an instrument that was created by Taylor et al. (1978) to assess the level of physical activity, sports, and leisure according to energy expenditure (i.e., asking about walking, chores (moderately strenuous), mowing the lawn, raking, gardening, hiking, jogging, biking, exercise cycling, dancing, aerobics, bowling, golf, singles tennis, doubles tennis, racquetball, calisthenics, and swimming)

and speed of execution, could lead to difficulties in activities of daily living (ADL) with consequent disability. However, end-stage functions (i.e., self-feeding and personal hygiene) could not be impaired, and the disability could be the result of other pathological pathways. From another point of view, frailty is a "dynamic process" determined by the progressive accumulation of age-related deficits in medical, functional, and psychosocial areas. The cumulative impact of these deficits can be expressed as the Frailty Index (FI), developed by Rockwood et al. (1999), which is a set of 70 clinical deficits from the Canadian Study of Health and Aging. Each deficit is assigned a value between 0 and 1 to indicate the severity of the issue [4] (Table 29.2).

Table 29.2 List of variables used by the Canadian Study of Health and Aging to construct the 70-item CSHA Frailty Index

1. Changes in everyday activities	15. Problems going out alone	29. Depression (clinical impression)	43. Postural tremor	57. Myocardial infarction
2. Head and neck problems	16. Impaired mobility	30. Sleep changes	44. Intention tremor	58. Arrhythmia
3. Poor muscle tone in the neck	17. Musculoskeletal problems	31. Restlessness	45. History of Parkinson's disease	59. Congestive heart failure
4. Bradykinesia, facial	18. Bradykinesia of the limbs	32. Memory changes	46. Family history of degenerative disease	60. Lung problems
5. Problems getting dressed	19. Poor muscle tone in limbs	33. Short-term memory impairment	47. Seizures, partial complex	61. Respiratory problems
6. Problems with bathing	20. Poor limb coordination	34.. Long-term memory impairment	48. Seizure, generalized	62. History of thyroid disease
7. Problems carrying out personal grooming	21 poor coordination, trunk	35. Changes in general mental functioning	49. Syncope or blackouts	63. Thyroid problems
8. Urinary incontinence	22. Poor standing posture	36. Onset of cognitive symptoms	50. Headache	64. Skin problems
9. Toileting problems	23. Irregular gait pattern	37. Clouding or delirium	51. Cerebrovascular problems	65. Malignant disease
10. Bulk difficulties	24. Falls	38. Paranoid features	52. History of strokes	66. Breast problems
11. Rectal problems	25. Mood problems	39. History relevant to cognitive impairment or loss	53. History of diabetes mellitus	67. Abdominal problems
12. Gastrointestinal problems	26. Feeling sad, blue, depressed	40. Family history of degenerative disease	54. Arterial hypertension	68. Presence of snout reflex
13. Problems cooking	27. History of depressed mood	41. Impaired vibration	55. Peripheral pulses	69 presence of the palm omental reflex
14. Sucking problems	28. Tiredness all the time	42. Tremor at rest	56. Cardiac problems	70. Other medical history

Many versions of the FI scale have been proposed: Searle et al. (2008) [5], developed a 40-item FI, later simplified to 38 items by Munster et al. (2016) [6]. The Groningen Frailty Indicator (15 items) [7], G-8 (eight items), and a modified FI consisting of only five comorbidities have also been proposed as short procedure for FI assessment [8, 9]. In 2005, the Canadian Study of Health and Aging (CSHA) developed also the Clinical Frailty Scale (CFS) with the aim to summarize the evaluation of older adults' overall health status (level of fitness or frailty condition) after being examined by an experienced clinician [4]. Although initially intended for epidemiological use, the CFS has become a widely used tool for clinical assessment. The original CFS included both severe frailty and terminal illness in its highest grade (level 7). In 2007, CFS was expanded from a 7-point scale to the current 9-point scale, distinguishing three different groups with different related care plans: severely frail, very severely frail, and terminally ill individuals. Table 29.3 reported the CSF updated by Rockwood et al. (2020) [10].

Less concentrated on physical condition, the measure of frailty based on CFS is more "subjective" than IF. In 2008, a different concept of frailty was also proposed [11] as a "pre-disability phase" in older individuals with an inadequate response to stress and a high risk of adverse outcomes, such as the onset of disabilities, illnesses, institutionalization, or mortality. This conceptualization does not exclude that frailty could coexist with a previous disability status. A wide consensus has

Table 29.3 Clinical Frailty Scale 2005–2020 Rockwood Version 2.0

1. Very fit	People who are robust, active, energetic, and motivated. They tend to exercise regularly and are among the fittest for their age
2. Fit	People who have no active disease symptoms but are less fit than category 1. Often, they exercise or are very active occasionally
3. Managing well	People whose medical problems are well controlled, even if occasionally symptomatic, but often are not regularly active beyond routine walking
4. Living with very mild frailty	Previously "vulnerable," this category marks an early transition from complete independence. While not dependent on others for daily help, often, symptoms limit activities. A common complaint is being "slowed up" and/or being tired during the day
5. Living with mild frailty	People who often have more evident slowing and need help with high-order instrumental activities of daily living (finances, transportation, and heavy housework). Typically, mild frailty progressively impairs shopping and walking outside alone, meal preparation, and medication and begins to restrict light housework
6. Living with moderate frailty	People who need help with all outside activities and with keeping house. Inside, they often have problems with stairs, need help with bathing, and might need minimal assistance (cuing and standby) with dressing
7. Living with severe frailty	Completely dependent on personal care, from whatever cause (physical or cognitive). Even so, they seem stable and not at high risk of dying (within about 6 months)
8. Living with very severe frailty	Completely dependent on personal care and approaching end of life. Typically, they could not recover even from a minor illness
9. Terminally ill	Approaching the end of life. This category applies to people with a life expectancy <6 months, who are not otherwise living with severe frailty (many terminally ill people can still exercise until very close to death.)

gradually converged into the multidisciplinary diagnostic process of the comprehensive geriatric assessment (CGA) for frailty assessment [12]. This is actually reported as the gold standard for evaluating the health status and care needs of older adults [13]. The core domains of CGA (Table 29.4) are physical and cognitive function, nutritional status, polypharmacy, and socioeconomic factors.

The comprehensive nature of CGA makes it an optimal instrument for patient management in clinical practice but, at the same time, a difficult tool to use in clinical practice for the time required for the assessment and the need for specific operator experience. In geriatric assessment, it is also essential to consider gender differences in long-term survival rates among frail elderly individuals. A recent Italian observational study reported that, although the female gender is associated with a longer survival rate than the male gender in the elderly, frailty has a negative impact on the survival rate in women minimizing the female advantage over males in terms of survival [14].

The pandemic has brought renewed attention and further understanding of frailty and its impact on health. In particular, frailty consistently correlated with COVID-19 mortality both before and after the introduction of SARS-CoV-2 vaccination [15]. COVID-19 has highlighted how the elderly and frail individuals are particularly vulnerable to the severe consequences of the virus. There is general agreement that frailty is a state of decrease in physiological reserves resulting in increased vulnerability to adverse outcomes when exposed to endogenous and/or exogenous stressors [16].

Table 29.4 Domains of the comprehensive geriatric assessment and corresponding instrument for clinical assessment

Domain	Topic investigated	Clinical assessment instruments
Health status	Chronic diseases, multimorbidity, and polypharmacy	Charlson index Cumulative illness rating scale Number of medications
Nutritional status and sarcopenia	Malnutrition	Mini nutritional assessment Geriatric nutritional risk index Serum albumin levels anthropometric measures handgrip strength Bioelectrical impedance analysis
Cognition and mood	Cognitive status and affective disorders	Mini-mental state examination Montreal cognitive assessment Geriatric depression scale
Functional status	Basal and instrumental activities of daily living	Activities of daily living Instrumental activities of daily living
Mobility	Gait and balance	Gait speed Chair stand test Short physical performance battery
Socioeconomic status and quality of life	Home care, long-term care services, nursing homes, income	Cohabitation status Short form health survey 36

29.1.4 The Frail Surgical Patient

As a direct consequence of the growing aging population, the demand for anesthetic and surgical procedures is increasing. Surgery can easily reveal the hidden frailty of the patient, or it can exacerbate a previous fragility state [17], especially in elderly people, in which the ability to face stressor events such as surgery treatment can be reduced. According to a systematic review of 70 studies, the prevalence of frailty in older people undergoing general surgery ranged from 8% to 77.8% [18]. Frailty can represent a significant risk for adverse outcomes of any surgery. It seems that from 25% to 50% of postoperative adverse outcomes in older people have been accounted for and related to frailty [19]. The decreased physiological reserve and the impaired response to stressors in frail elderly are particularly relevant in the context of hospitalization for anesthesia and surgical interventions. Several studies [20–22] report that a higher modified frailty index score is associated with increased postoperative complications, extended length of stay, disability, and mortality. Velanovich et al. [23] reported an increase in the risk of both morbidity and mortality for each unit increase in the modified frailty index across different surgical specialties and levels of operational complexity. Frailty is an effective predictor of poor outcomes and may also suggest the likelihood of an extended hospital stay as well as the need for subsequent readmissions. To ensure the best possible outcome for these patients, healthcare providers are recommended to follow these steps [17]:

1. Preoperative frailty assessment: A prompt assessment of the patient's medical history, current health status, and potential risks should be conducted before the surgery to develop a personalized treatment plan and optimize the care. Assessing general health status, physical and cognitive functions, nutritional state, skeletal muscle mass, strength and mobility, mood, social support, and relationships is crucial in defining a frailty condition.
2. Perioperative management: A multidisciplinary coordinated approach involving surgeons, anesthesiologists, nurses, and physical therapists is crucial for these patients. The working team can optimize the patient's perioperative management which includes preoperative education, proper nutrition, and pain management.
3. Postoperative care: After surgery, frail patients may require extra care and attention to ensure the best possible outcome, reducing the risk of future complications, and improving the patient's recovery.

There are several potential benefits of identifying frail patients before surgery. This approach can improve patient outcomes and patient management strategies tailored to various stages of the clinical history, ranging from risk assessment to pre-habilitation programs and surgical decisions.

The use of preoperative assessments for frailty has proven to be highly beneficial across numerous surgical specialties, particularly in orthopedics [24], cardiovascular [25], and oncological surgery. Frailty has been associated with high postoperative mortality in patients undergoing surgery for pelvic and lower extremity fractures, adult spinal deformity, femoral neck fracture, primary hip arthroplasty, and primary knee arthroplasty [26]. The Six-Item Modified Frailty Index (MF-6) has been proposed for orthopedic surgery as it is a significant predictor of postoperative complications [24]. A higher MF-6 score seems strongly related to readmission, non-home discharge, and mortality following open reduction and internal fixation procedures for lower extremity, pelvis, and acetabular fractures [19]. Preoperative assessment of frailty in geriatric hip surgery is essential to prevent postoperative delirium in elderly patients with hip fractures [27]. Feng et al. [27] recommend the importance of identifying potential risks and implementing targeted interventions to address frailty factors, which can ultimately reduce the incidence of postoperative delirium.

The field of geriatric cardiology has expanded to include the use of a CGA within cardiology practices. The role of geriatricians in the improvement of the cardiovascular specialists' approach to older patients' management has been emphasized [28]. The assessment of frailty is also fundamental in valve surgery. In patients undergoing aortic valve replacement, several studies [29, 30] showed that frailty trajectories can predict functional outcomes. Ongoing clinical trials are exploring perioperative care and interventions to optimize functional outcomes in the field of cardiology.

Unfortunately, the incidence of frailty among older cancer patients is particularly high. Cancer and its therapies can play a significant role in stressing a patient's physiological reserve. It is estimated that more than half of the older patients with cancer have frailty or pre-frailty. Frail patients seem to have a higher risk of all-cause mortality, postoperative complications, and chemotherapy-related adverse events [31]. Chemotherapy intolerance and disease recurrence or progression are cancer-specific risks of frailty status. The US National Comprehensive Cancer Network, the International Society of Geriatric Oncology, and the European Organization for Research and Treatment of Cancer all recommend conducting frailty assessments and CGAs for older cancer patients [32].

29.2 Informed Consent in Frail Surgical Patient

Obtaining valid informed consent in frail surgical patients represents a challenging aspect of medical practice. Frail patients may face complex decisions regarding surgical procedures. They cannot fully understand the risks, benefits, and alternatives associated with surgical interventions due to cognitive impairment, disability, and comorbidities. Healthcare professionals must be sure that patients and their families are adequately informed and supported during the entire process of decision-making. A cautious approach that considers the patient's capacity to provide informed consent with respect to the patient's rights and dignity is recommended. Addressing informed consent in frail surgical patients requires a patient-centered approach based on adequate information and respect for patient autonomy. Several key considerations must be taken into account when addressing informed consent in frail surgical patients:

1. Preoperative assessment of frail patients: Evaluation of frailty status is crucial for healthcare professionals to assess the patient's physical, cognitive, and functional capabilities to fully understand the surgical procedure and its consequences. This assessment may involve cognitive tests, functional assessments, and discussions with family members or caregivers with the aim of personalizing the consenting process by suiting the unique requirements of these patients.
2. Communication techniques: According to the Italian Code of Medical Ethics and Law 24/17, communication time is time spent for cure. Simplified and clear communication is essential for healthcare professionals when discussing surgical procedures, potential risks, and expected outcomes in frail patients. Difficulties in obtaining valid informed consent can arise due to various factors, including communication barriers and emotional and psychological conditions. The communication should be conducted in a quiet, private room, and sufficient time for questions and comments must be ensured. Linguistic and cultural barriers should be overcome by speaking clearly and simplifying explanations to facilitate understanding. Physicians should use plain language, avoid medical jargon, and consider using visual aids, such as diagrams or videos, to enhance understanding. Empathy and patience are also needed. Communication must also respect patient privacy and be confined to necessary information. Strategies to enhance the understanding of information are suggested by using different formats and media, including simplified storybooks, videos, and vignettes. Physicians should streamline the consent process by eliminating relevant information that participants are unlikely to read or understand. Information documents should be simple and brief focusing on the risks and benefits of surgery. Contact information for questions or reporting injuries needs to be provided.
3. Decision-making process: The interaction between healthcare professionals, frail patients, and their families is fundamental to getting a care pathway as close as possible to the patient's needs. Patients should be encouraged to express their preferences, desires, and goals of care. When decision-making capacity is lacking, surrogate decision-makers, such as legally appointed guardians or family members, may be involved in the informed consent process. However, it is crucial to ensure that proxies make decisions based on patients' best interests.
4. Documentation: All discussions related to informed consent should be thoroughly documented in the patient's medical record, including the information provided, the patient's understanding, any questions or concerns raised, and the patient's or proxy's decision, if applicable. After ensuring that the patient has understood the information, the physician or another appropriately qualified individual must then seek the potential subject's freely given informed consent, preferably in writing. If the consent cannot be expressed in writing, the non-written consent must be formally documented and witnessed.
5. Ongoing reassessment: Informed consent is not a one-time event but rather an ongoing process that may require periodic reassessment, especially in the context of evolving patient preferences, clinical status changes, or the emergence of new information about treatment options. As already mentioned, according to Article 5 of the Oviedo Convention (1997), the person concerned may freely withdraw consent at any time.

29.2.1 Comprehension and Decision-Making Capacity Assessment

Informed consent assumes that an individual fully understands the information presented. He should be able to make an appropriate decision, accepting the risks and benefits. In the case of frail patients incapable of giving informed consent, the physician must seek informed consent from a legally authorized representative. Unfortunately, obtaining informed consent in cases where patients have limited capacity to understand medical information can be a complex process. The assessment of the patient's capability to understand the information and to give consent is the necessary premise for any kind of surgery. According to Ruske et al. [33], frailty emerged as the only characteristic independently linked to a lack of knowledge despite other factors, such as decisional conflict, educational background, and provider level. The prevalence of cognitive impairment in frail patients has raised concerns about the capability of these patients to give consent. Impaired hearing or vision is also common in frail individuals. Individuals with aphasia, dysarthria, or bradykinesia may lack the ability to ask questions. Some medications may also impair attention and concentration. It is essential to discuss the potential risks in older individuals with physical disabilities or sensory deficits to avoid misunderstandings or any form of coercion.

The nature of frailty makes it difficult to assess the patient's ability to make autonomous decisions. Dementia, delirium, psychosis, intellectual disability, or other neuropsychiatric illnesses can impair patients' decision-making capacity. Frailty and cognitive impairment or dementia have been found to be closely related. This relationship has been demonstrated by some cross-sectional and longitudinal studies [34]. The International Academy of Nutrition and Aging (IANA) and the International Association of Gerontology and Geriatrics (IAGG) proposed in 2013 a definition of "cognitive frailty" as the simultaneous presence of physical frailty (frailty phenotype) and cognitive impairment (clinical dementia rating [CDR] = 0.5) in older individuals without a definite diagnosis of dementia independent of other frailty dimensions (e.g., social, psychological, and oral frailty). Assessing a cognitive impairment in elder patients is a crucial step of clinical practice. Due to the lack of standardized evaluation tools, a variety of instruments have been developed to assess the patient's capacity. One of the first tests developed to evaluate the validity of the decision-making process was the Hopkins Competency Assessment Test (HCAT) [35]. The HCAT is an assessment tool used to analyze the patient's capability to provide consent and is a brief questionnaire to evaluate the patient's comprehension of the main issues of the questionnaire. The MacArthur Competence Assessment Tool for Treatment (MacCAT-T) is a semi-structured interview developed to assess all aspects of a patient's capability to understand. It has been used in psychiatric patients with conditions such as schizophrenia, major depressive disorder, and anorexia nervosa, as well as in patients with dementia and hospitalized patients. However, the interview lasts approximately 15–20 min, and it is based on the patient's clinical information to individualize the assessment for each patient. Although the Mini-Mental State Examination (MMSE) is commonly used in capacity assessments, some studies have shown that the MMSE may not be an accurate measure, as some patients may score normally on the test but still have significant cognitive deficits. For example, Fitten and Waite [36] found that elderly hospitalized patients who had normal MMSE scores still had greater deficits in their understanding of treatment options compared to healthy controls. The MMSE may not be a sensitive instrument for detecting specific cognitive dysfunction related to impaired capacity but it can be useful in identifying patients whose capacity status may be questionable.

29.2.2 Loss of Autonomy and the Involvement of Family Members

Individuals with frailty may necessitate additional support and attention to ensure that they are adequately informed and comforted regarding their treatment. The involvement of family members and caregivers is necessary to help the patient understand treatment options and to support decision-making. Joint decision-making or shared decision-making approaches, which involve the patient, his/her family, and caregivers, have been recommended. However, some ethical issues can be raised, mainly dealing with the importance of protecting the privacy and confidentiality of the patients, the patient's best interest, and the respect of his/her autonomy. The tendency to treat elderly patients in a paternalistic manner already exists, and frailty may exacerbate this approach. Caregivers and family members showing paternalistic behavior toward frail patients may undermine the individual's autonomy and the right to self-determination. This can result in caregivers and family members making decisions on behalf of individuals, even if they have the capacity to express informed consent themselves. The frail patients' dependence on a caregiver can also lead to "coerced consent." The loss of patients' decisional autonomy can also be favored by physicians providing more information to caregivers or family members than to the individuals themselves. A study [37] based on 200 patients over 65 years of age interviewed about the quality of information provided by physicians reported that this information was mainly directed toward the accompanying family members, and the main issues given to elderly patients were insufficient. Furthermore, due to the limited understanding of the risks and benefits, frail patients often base their decisions more on trust in their doctor or deference to authority than on information. In these cases, the given consent is the result of passive acceptance of treatment risks and blind adherence to experts' recommendations. Therefore, many older and frail patients tend to delegate responsibility to their doctors for assessing medical information and making medical decisions. It is important for healthcare professionals to avoid imposing their choices on them; this is a crucial ethical principle in medicine, which ultimately promotes patient-centered healthcare.

29.3 Conclusion and Future Strategies

Incorporating informed consent into daily surgical practice is a difficult task, and there is a recognized gap between the theoretical goals of informed consent and actual practice. It is important to recognize that obtaining informed consent from elderly patients with frailty poses additional complex challenges that require careful consideration of the material risks associated with their frailty and potential cognitive impairments. Evaluating frailty requires time, training, and human resources, and ideal tools may not yet be available in busy preoperative surgery assessment clinics. These include an understanding of the patient's capacity and autonomy and the need for shared decision-making or delegation to a legally authorized representative when necessary. Rushing through the informed consent process as a quick add-on to a medical evaluation is not an appropriate approach. If surgeons cannot fulfill these requirements, the informed consent process may not be valid, and incorrect decisions can result in the denial of the patient's legal and ethical rights. To avoid this risk, modifying the informed consent process to make it more practical for frail older patients could be necessary.

References

1. Brown I, Renwick R, Raphael D. Frailty: constructing a common meaning, definition, and conceptual framework. Int J Rehabil Res. 1995;18(2):93–102.
2. Rockwood K, Stadnyk K, MacKnight C, McDowell I, Hébert R, Hogan DB. A brief clinical instrument to classify frailty in elderly people. Lancet. 1999;353(9148):205–6. https://doi.org/10.1016/S0140-6736(98)04402-X.
3. Fried LP, Tangen CM, Walston J, Newman AB, Hirsch C, Gottdiener J, Seeman T, Tracy R, Kop WJ, Burke G, McBurnie MA. Cardiovascular health study collaborative research group. Frailty in older adults: evidence for a phenotype. J Gerontol A Biol Sci Med Sci. 2001;56(3):M146–56. https://doi.org/10.1093/gerona/56.3.m146.
4. Rockwood K, Song X, MacKnight C, Bergman H, Hogan DB, McDowell I, Mitnitski A. A global clinical measure of fitness and frailty in elderly people. CMAJ. 2005;173(5):489–95. https://doi.org/10.1503/cmaj.050051. PMID: 16129869; PMCID: PMC1188185.
5. Searle SD, Mitnitski A, Gahbauer EA, et al. A standard procedure for creating a frailty index. BMC Geriatr. 2008;8:24. https://doi.org/10.1186/1471-2318-8-24.
6. Munster BCV, Drost D, Kalf A, Vogtlander NP. Discriminative value of frailty screening instruments in end-stage renal disease. Clin Kidney J. 2016;9(4):606–10. https://doi.org/10.1093/ckj/sfw061.
7. Steverink N, Slaets J, Schuurmans H, Lis M. Measuring frailty: developing and testing the GFI (Groningen frailty indicator). Gerontologist. 2001;41:236–7.
8. Baitar A, Van Fraeyenhove F, Vandebroek A, De Droogh E, Galdermans D, Mebis J, Schrijvers D. Evaluation of the Groningen frailty indicator and the G8 questionnaire as screening tools for frailty in older patients with cancer. J Geriatr Oncol. 2013;4(1):32–8. https://doi.org/10.1016/j.jgo.2012.08.001. Epub 2012 Aug 24.
9. Weaver DJ, Malik AT, Jain N, Yu E, Kim J, Khan SN. The modified 5-item frailty index: a concise and useful tool for assessing the impact of frailty on postoperative morbidity following elective posterior lumbar fusions. World Neurosurg. 2019;124:e626–32. https://doi.org/10.1016/j.wneu.2018.12.168. Epub 2019 Jan 11.

10. Rockwood K, Theou O. Using the clinical frailty scale in allocating scarce health care resources. Can Geriatr J. 2020;23(3):210–5.
11. Abellan van Kan G, Rolland Y, Bergman H, Morley JE, Kritchevsky SB, Vellas B. The I.A.N.A task force on frailty assessment of older people in clinical practice. J Nutr Health Aging. 2008;12(1):29–37. https://doi.org/10.1007/BF02982161.
12. Lee H, Lee E, Jang IY. Frailty and comprehensive geriatric assessment. J Korean Med Sci. 2020;35(3):e16. https://doi.org/10.3346/jkms.2020.35.e16. PMID: 31950775; PMCID: PMC6970074.
13. Mazya AL, Garvin P, Ekdahl AW. Outpatient comprehensive geriatric assessment: effects on frailty and mortality in old people with multimorbidity and high health care utilization. Aging Clin Exp Res. 2019;31:519–25. https://doi.org/10.1007/s40520-018-1004-z.
14. Corbi G, Cacciatore F, Komici K, Rengo G, Vitale DF, Furgi G, Pagano G, Bencivenga L, Davinelli S, Ferrara N. Inter-relationships between gender, frailty and 10-year survival in older Italian adults: an observational longitudinal study. Sci Rep. 2019;9(1):18416. https://doi.org/10.1038/s41598-019-54897-2. PMID: 31804552; PMCID: PMC6895198.
15. Dash D, Mowbray FI, Poss JW, et al. The association between frailty, long-term care home characteristics and COVID-19 mortality before and after SARS-CoV-2 vaccination: a retrospective cohort study. Age Ageing. 2023;52(12):afad229. https://doi.org/10.1093/ageing/afad229.
16. Fried LP, Cohen AA, Xue QL, Walston J, Bandeen-Roche K, Varadhan R. The physical frailty syndrome as a transition from homeostatic symphony to cacophony. Nat Aging. 2021;1(1):36–46. https://doi.org/10.1038/s43587-020-00017-z. Epub 2021 Jan 14. PMID: 34476409; PMCID: PMC8409463.
17. Pozzi M, Mariani S, Scanziani M, Passolunghi D, Bruni A, Finazzi A, Lettino M, Foti G, Bellelli G, Marchetto G. The frail patient undergoing cardiac surgery: lessons learned and future perspectives. Front Cardiovasc Med. 2023;10:1295108. https://doi.org/10.3389/fcvm.2023.1295108. PMID: 38124896; PMCID: PMC10731467.
18. Aucoin SD, Hao M, Sohi R, Shaw J, Bentov I, Walker D, et al. Accuracy and feasibility of clinically applied frailty instruments before surgery: a systematic review and meta-analysis. Anesthesiology. 2020;133(1):78–95.
19. McIsaac DI, Jen T, Mookerji N, Patel A, Lalu MM. Interventions to improve the outcomes of frail people having surgery: a systematic review. PLoS One. 2017;12(12):e0190071.
20. Rabelo LG, Bjornsdottir A, Jonsdottir AB, Einarsson SG, Karason S, Sigurdsson MI. Frailty assessment tools and associated postoperative outcomes in older patients undergoing elective surgery: a prospective pilot study. Acta Anaesthesiol Scand. 2023;67(2):150–8. https://doi.org/10.1111/aas.14162. Epub 2022 Nov 9.
21. Gong S, Qian D, Riazi S, Chung F, Englesakis M, Li Q, Huszti E, Wong J. Association between the FRAIL scale and postoperative complications in older surgical patients: a systematic review and meta-analysis. Anesth Analg. 2023;136(2):251–61. https://doi.org/10.1213/ANE.0000000000006272. Epub 2022 Nov 29. PMID: 36638509; PMCID: PMC9812423.
22. Lin HS, Watts JN, Peel NM, et al. Frailty and post-operative outcomes in older surgical patients: a systematic review. BMC Geriatr. 2016;16:157. https://doi.org/10.1186/s12877-016-0329-8.
23. Velanovich V, Antoine H, Swartz A, Peters D, Rubinfeld I. Accumulating deficits model of frailty and postoperative mortality and morbidity: its application to a national database. J Surg Res. 2013;183(1):104–10. https://doi.org/10.1016/j.jss.2013.01.021. Epub 2013 Feb 1.
24. Pean CA, Thomas HM, Singh UM, DeBaun MR, Weaver MJ, von Keudell AG. Use of a six-item modified frailty index to predict 30-day adverse events, readmission, and mortality in older patients undergoing surgical fixation of lower extremity, pelvic, and acetabular fractures. J Am Acad Orthop Surg Glob Res Rev. 2023;7:e22.00286. https://doi.org/10.5435/JAAOSGlobal-D-22-00286.
25. Li R, Sidawy A, Nguyen BN. The 5-factor modified frailty index is a concise and effective predictor of 30-day adverse outcomes in carotid endarterectomy. J Surg Res. 2024;7:507. https://doi.org/10.1016/j.jss.2024.01.024.

26. Mamtora PH, Fortier MA, Barnett SR, Schmid LN, Kain ZN. Peri-operative management of frailty in the orthopedic patient. J Orthop. 2020;22:304–7. https://doi.org/10.1016/j.jor.2020.05.024. Erratum in: J Orthop 2020 Dec 14;23:274. PMID: 32616993; PMCID: PMC7322091.
27. Feng C, Wu H, Qi Z, et al. Association of preoperative frailty with the risk of postoperative delirium in older patients undergoing hip fracture surgery: a prospective cohort study. Aging Clin Exp Res. 2024;36(1):16. Published 2024 Jan 31. https://doi.org/10.1007/s40520-023-02692-5.
28. Forman D, Rich M, Alexander K, et al. Cardiac care for older adults: time for a new paradigm. J Am Coll Cardiol. 2011;57(18):1801–10. https://doi.org/10.1016/j.jacc.2011.02.014.
29. Afilalo J, Lauck S, Kim DH, Lefèvre T, Piazza N, Lachapelle K, et al. Frailty in older adults undergoing aortic valve replacement: the FRAILTY-AVR study. J Am Coll Cardiol. 2017;70(6):689–700. https://doi.org/10.1016/j.jacc.2017.06.024.
30. Strange JE, Christensen DM, Sindet-Pedersen C, Schou M, Falkentoft AC, Østergaard L, Butt JH, Graversen PL, Køber L, Gislason G, Olesen JB, Fosbøl EL. Frailty and recurrent hospitalization after transcatheter aortic valve replacement. J Am Heart Assoc. 2023;12(8):e029264. https://doi.org/10.1161/JAHA.122.029264. Epub 2023 Apr 12. PMID: 37042264; PMCID: PMC10227237.
31. Handforth C, Clegg A, Young C, Simpkins S, Seymour MT, Selby PJ, Young J. The prevalence and outcomes of frailty in older cancer patients: a systematic review. Ann Oncol. 2015;26(6):1091–101. https://doi.org/10.1093/annonc/mdu540. Epub 2014 Nov 17.
32. Goede V. Frailty and cancer: current perspectives on assessment and monitoring. Clin Interv Aging. 2023;18:505–21. https://doi.org/10.2147/CIA.S365494. PMID: 37013130; PMCID: PMC10066705.
33. Ruske J, et al. Patient comprehension necessary for informed consent for vascular procedures is poor and related to frailty. J Vasc Surg. 2021;73(4):1422–8. https://doi.org/10.1016/j.jvs.2020.06.131.
34. Sugimoto T, et al. An update on cognitive frailty: its definition, impact, associated factors and underlying mechanisms, and interventions. Geriatr Gerontol Int. 2022;22(2):99–109. https://doi.org/10.1111/ggi.14322.
35. Janofsky JS, McCarthy RJ, Folstein MF. The Hopkins competency assessment test: a brief method for evaluating patients' capacity to give informed consent. Hosp Community Psychiatry. 1992;43(2):132–6. https://doi.org/10.1176/ps.43.2.132. PMID: 1572608.
36. Fitten LJ, Waite MS. Impact of medical hospitalization on treatment decision-making capacity in the elderly. Arch Intern Med. 1990;150:1717–21.
37. Osuna E, Lorenzo MD, Pérez-Cárceles MD, Luna A. Informed consent: evaluation of the information provided to elderly patients. Med Law. 2001;20(3):379–84.

Bioethical Issues in Gerosurgery

30

Giampaolo Ghilardi, Francesco De Micco, and Laura Leondina Campanozzi

During the spring of 2020, when COVID was raging at its full strength in Italy, the Italian Society of Anesthesia, Analgesia, and Intensive Care (SIAARTI) published a controversial document named: *Clinical ethics recommendations for admission to and withdrawal from intensive treatment under exceptional conditions of mismatch between the needs and the available resources*. In these recommendations, it was suggested that:

> It may become necessary to place an age limit on intensive care unit (ICU) entry. This is not a matter of making purely value-based choices, but of reserving resources that may be in short supply to those who are primarily most likely to survive and secondarily to those who may have the most years of life saved, with a view to maximizing benefits for the greatest number of people [1].

This statement has given rise to long and harsh debates about the legitimacy of establishing such criteria. Moreover, it has been argued that setting up an extra clinical criterion as a filter to access ICU is not only discriminatory, for those who fall under this exclusion criterion, but it is also unacceptable from a more internal and clinical point of view. In fact, age has always been considered among the clinical elements, but one thing is to evaluate it within the clinical framework, together with many other indicators such as comorbidity, respiratory distress, ongoing treatments,

G. Ghilardi
Research Unit of Bioethics and Humanities, Department of Medicine and Surgery, Università Campus Bio-Medico di Roma, Rome, Italy
e-mail: g.ghilardi@unicampus.it

F. De Micco (✉) · L. L. Campanozzi
Research Unit of Bioethics and Humanities, Department of Medicine and Surgery, Università Campus Bio-Medico di Roma, Rome, Italy

Department of Clinical Affair, Fondazione Policlinico Universitario Campus Bio-Medico, Rome, Italy
e-mail: L.Campanozzi@unicampus.it; f.demicco@unicampus.it

V. Boccardi, L. Marano (eds.), *The Frail Surgical Patient*, Practical Issues in Geriatrics, https://doi.org/10.1007/978-3-031-77707-3_30

etc., and a completely different thing is to isolate age from the clinical context to think of it as something bad: the older you are, the less deserving to receive the cure you should be [2].

We have started this chapter remembering this issue to showcase how age can be a tricky topic when it comes to clinical reasoning. It can be both an important element of clinical assessment and an a priori criterion to judge the appropriateness of specific treatments. The argumentative line we will follow will be the first one, considering age as an important and specific tool to build an appropriate assessment of the clinical condition, within the clinical framework, but we will strongly reject the second line of reasoning, according to which the age *per sé* should be considered as a meaningful parameter to rule in or out different patients. Clinical history and the health context of the patient cannot be neglected because of his/her age; we think that this argument is not rational and suffers from huge myopia, reducing the complexity of health to the simple linear and external parameters of age.

This chapter is mainly divided into two parts: the first one addresses the topic of appropriateness from an epistemological and ethical point of view and the second one will look into this same concept from a forensic angle since it is our strong belief that both these perspectives integrate one another and need, therefore, to be developed together.

30.1 Appropriateness as a Multi-Layered Approach

Over the past decades, the number of older patients undergoing elective and emergency surgery has increased, due to the growth in the aging population, along with ongoing advances in surgical and anesthetic techniques, holding more positive expectations in both patients and professionals about healthcare delivery in adulthood [3, 4]. While geriatric surgery is receiving more attention, new challenges arise for the decision-making process not only in terms of adequately assessing the risks and benefits but also and primarily of moving beyond uncritical and preconceived approaches when it comes to defining the criteria by which evaluating the appropriateness or not of treatments in this domain.

Adopting reductive stances in the clinical reasoning process about gerosurgery leads to overlooking the complexity of the health condition and the specific needs of each older and often frail patients, thereby neglecting the fact that this is a broad and diversified category of individuals, in spite of common misconceptions. Among these, ageism seems still widespread in our society, as the SIAARTI document previously mentioned shows, and its classic or primary expression is precisely the denial of appropriate and effective treatments due to advanced age, which amounts to what can be considered a form of tacit rationing in healthcare [5]. Likewise, more recent ways of labeling older adults under the generic terms of "frail or vulnerable," that is, as patients at risk especially when it comes to surgery, seem to reintroduce ageism in more modern terms: a simplifying approach that neglects other important variables, both clinical and nonclinical, thereby complying more for the concerns of healthcare professionals and economics than for those of patients [6].

In this vein, a recent article entitled "The less is more crusade—Are we over-medicalizing or oversimplifying?" has revived the controversial issue of healthcare appropriateness at the international level, a very topical subject in times when the challenge of curbing healthcare costs is highly charged [7]. At times, something less can yield something more. This was the view of Ludwig Mies van der Rohe, one of the most influential architects of the twentieth century and representative of the minimalist design style, who made known the dictum "Less is more." He meant it to convey the need to overturn the thought that it is pomp and complexity that made works great. By learning to subtract the superfluous, perfection can be achieved, which ultimately occurs when a building—but this applies to any kind of product—is functional in providing a simple solution to a complex need [8]. In the decades since van der Rohe's work, the adage "Less is more" has become a benchmark far beyond the boundaries of architecture, reaching across many different contexts, from technology to clothing, and the medical realm has not been exempt. For the latter, many research studies and movements have sprung up since the early 2000s to revisit the issue of the appropriate use of medical resources, while hinting that higher quality of care is not closely related to higher healthcare costs or the provision of more treatments. In other words, doing more is not always the same as doing better, hence the notion "Less is more," which resulted in books, educational proposals aimed at streamlining medical resources, talks on overdiagnosis or overtreatment, or design efforts devoted to raising awareness about the risks associated with inappropriate medical decisions, like the Choosing Wisely or Slow Medicine initiatives [9, 10]. These efforts inspired by the slogan "Less is more" have raised both optimism and apprehension within healthcare as it can be understood in different and potentially troubling ways. On the one hand, this view is generally welcomed when it is not merely proposing to do less to reduce waste in healthcare but means to improve the quality and safety of care by identifying interventions that might not provide value or even harm patients and by promoting shared decision-making between patients and healthcare providers [11]. On the other hand, when this motto is implemented literally and rigorously in daily clinical practice, it leads to oversimplification, consistent with the logic of extreme reductionism, exposing patients to the risk of being undertreated or, even worse, not receiving the care they would need. Additionally, blindly following the philosophy of "Less is more" disregards individual differences, sociocultural variables, and patient preferences, compromising the quality of care provided [12]. These perils are clearly acknowledged in medicine, even in the field of geriatric surgery, where it was firmly reiterated that denying elderly patients surgery purely on the basis of age is scientifically unacceptable as well as morally. Several studies have reported how age-based stereotypes or biases can affect clinical decisions and treatment of older patients, resulting in different kinds of discrimination, namely: being excluded or not considered as suitable candidates for some surgical procedures, including more invasive ones; underestimating their potential benefits in older adults, to focus instead on the risks and complications associated with the procedure, thus biasing the decision to undertake or recommend surgery; being less involved in decisions regarding their surgical treatment, with less participation in planning and understanding of available options;

and doubting their ability to understand medical information or make informed decisions [13–15]. Broadly speaking, concerns raised about the adage that "Less is more" in geriatric surgery stem mainly from extreme or context-free renditions, which could lead to standardized care and lack of personalization. It is critical to strike a balance between avoiding excess and ensuring high-quality, tailored care for each individual patient, working to promote equitable, evidence-based care and multidimensional assessment for all patients.

Besides, clinical decisions that aspire to be taken under a wise approach, for that is the issue at stake hereto, should bear in mind that sometimes doing less is the best thing to do, but in other cases doing more is the most appropriate choice. This means that decisions about treatments must be reached based on a careful evaluation of each geriatric case, within a spectrum of other considerations, rather than through a dogmatic and therefore reductive approach. Reductionism in gerosurgery occurs when there is a narrow focus on the treatment of individual age-related conditions or diseases, without considering the broader context of aging as a complex biological process, sorting it into isolated components and addressing them separately, instead of taking a comprehensive approach. This rationale can lead to fragmented care regardless of the overall well-being of the person, thereby neglecting the interconnections and cumulative effects of multiple health conditions and failing to address the complex needs of elderly patients thoroughly [16].

Thus, it is imperative for the surgeon and his team to adopt a sound philosophy regarding the geriatric patient. Such a philosophy should include, first, raising awareness among health professionals on issues related to discrimination, whether age-based or not explicitly. There is no doubt that the central point in any decision to operate or not is medical in nature. However, in actual day-to-day clinical practice, other issues may be involved, at conscious and unconscious levels, such as economic considerations, underestimation of outcomes, and unwillingness to take risks, among others [17]. This has prompted the claim that movements appealing uncritically to "Less is more" are neglecting the myriad factors that can inform final decisions and are failing to best express the complexity in which medicine operates. And that is why the author of the above article concludes the work by stating that:

> Until we learn how to better manage the uncomfortable uncertainties inherent in clinical case, "less is more" may be an aphorism better suited to telling coherent stories than to complex decisions faced by doctors and patients [18].

Nevertheless, within the framework of such a philosophy, surgeons should rely on a proper understanding of reduction, lest it slide toward an uncritical and simplistic reductionism. Ultimately, what is at stake is the life and death of the elderly, hence their dignity as human beings.

The action of reduction is at home in scientific practice and thus in any discipline based on science, such as medicine. It belongs to the logic of scientific explanation, which seeks to know the unknown by breaking it down into more known elements, according to a principle we might call simplicity, whereby the complex is explainable and reducible from the simplest. The reduction has as its necessary corollary synthesis or composition, an action by which elements previously obtained by decomposition are recomposed into a unity that gives them significance. In selecting a particular point of view on a given object, an operation that is crucial for any scientific practice that aims to carry out a careful and rigorous analysis of it, the reductionist approach has come, over time, to reduce to this particular point of view all the possible aspects in which this object can be studied. In this way, a legitimate and fruitful practice, that of reduction, transmutes into an ideological and therefore fruitless practice, that of reductionism, to overcome which a continuous dialogue between analysis and synthesis, between the part and the whole, is deemed necessary [19]. In his criticism of over-specialization, which is a form of reductionism, the French philosopher Bergson pointed out that:

> You do not grasp a particular truth until you have seen how it relates to others. Do you know a building until you have been shown the stones? But there are only stones in the building. All the art is in the arrangement, and what is important is not to know the stone, but the place it will take. [...]. if you do not start by looking at the whole, if you go straight to the parts to look them over, you may see very well, but you will not even know what you have looked at [20].

The Bergsonian lesson is well suited to capture the focus of reductionism still ingrained in the practice of geriatric surgery, suggesting a path to follow in order to overcome it. According to a multidimensional approach respectful toward the complexity of each individual clinical situation, which is never ordinary but always multifaceted, the assessment of the appropriateness of treatment must necessarily take into account several parameters, rather than being reduced to a single one, such as age. To summarize this line of thought on reductionism in geriatric surgery, we can say that reduction is a useful and necessary operation, but there are reductions and reductions. It is up to the wise surgeon, i.e., the one who is aware of the epistemological dimension of his work, to understand that reductions are necessary, on the one hand, but that these are partial and require methodological precautions on the other hand. It follows that reduction must be aware and cooperative, that is, open to both shared decision-making among multidisciplinary teams, patients, and their families, and to other perspectives that temper its one-dimensional view, restoring, if not reality in its entirety, which is not possible, at least an understanding that is more faithful to its structural complexity. Failing this, healthcare providers would not be practicing good medicine but a counterfeit of it, ideology; they would not be respecting their intelligence since it is proper for humans to know reality by attempting to make it transpire for what it is, not by imposing preconceived beliefs upon that; and yet they would not even honor reality in its own nature but would enforce their own narrow category on it [21].

This is consistent with the true meaning of the saying "Less is more," which, according to the German architect Ludwig Mies van der Rohe, was intended to rid architecture of all those superstructures that do not allow its form, its authentic meaning, to be grasped [22].

Dealing with a reduction in an accurate way also allows us to gain a broader view of appropriateness in medicine, in its different and intertwined levels, without flattening it to cost-benefit assessment alone. There is also an epistemological appropriateness that should assess the correspondence between reality and its conceptual apprehension, in line with the realism criterion of "*adequation rei et intellectus*" [23].

Over the centuries, aging has been perceived as a time of human life marked by immutability and profoundly troubled by many difficulties, whether related to psycho-physical decline or to situations of economic, social, and psychological distress. In this regard, the ancient adage of the Latin poet Terence, *senectus ipsa morbus* [24], is well-known, whereby advanced age was equated with a pathological event, without distinguishing between physiological or natural aging and pathological aging. Today, it is no longer possible to uncritically embrace such a stereotypical hermeneutic perspective regarding the understanding of old age although it is still widely pervasive.

People around the world are living longer, with general improvements in life conditions and technological advances in medicine, giving people access to health services that promise to improve the quality and length of their lives [25]. Legitimized also by the World Health Organization (WHO), which is particularly sensitive to the medical and ethical implications of old age, taking a firm stance against widespread misconceptions that negatively impact choices even in the health domain, a different sensibility toward the elderly has thus spread for several years [26]. Starting from the recognition, grounded in scientific evidence, that the elderly are not individuals in the grip of a progressive and inexorable psycho-physical decline that destroys their lives, we must increasingly broaden the range of references, also in terms of health and disease, beyond mere quantitative aspects. In other words, old age appears today as a stage of life accompanied by particular frailties (like any other stage of life), and as such it requires specific and necessary hygienic, biomedical, and social attention but certainly not as an age in which the right to health, as a fundamental human right to therapy and care in general, must be diminished or disappear [27]. In this respect, bioethical reflection needs to gain room to engage in the field of geriatric surgery, championing a more realistic conceptualization of aging in its biological aspects and the rights associated with it but even before that of his ontology. In his seminal view of the human life cycle, the German philosopher Romano Guardini pointed out that:

> The distinction between the beginning of life, birth and childhood [...] does not mean that life starts from a starting point then left behind, but that this starting point accompanies life as it unfolds. [...]. Inversely, the end acts backward to the first beginning. Likewise the attack of the melody determines its form throughout its subsequent development, just as the end also gives form to the melody by traversing its unfolding backward. Life is not a jumble of parts, but a totality that [...] is present at every point of development [28].

Doing the good and right thing implies considerations of a technical and scientific as well as an ethical-normative nature [29]. Keeping this sense of complexity in view, framing appropriateness in its different levels, will help to understand that evaluating a medical treatment, such as surgery for frail, means above all deciding on many interacting worlds, as well as on what is best for the individual patient.

30.2 A Comprehensive and Multidimensional Assessment: Risk-Benefit Assessment, Decision-Making Autonomy, and Access to Care

The population aging is causing a radical transformation of the demographic structure in many parts of the world [30]. The increase in life expectancy is directly correlated with advances in medicine and improvements in socioeconomic conditions [31, 32]. However, this generated new challenges with significant implications for society, the economy, and health systems [33]. Within this complex scenario, geriatric surgery is confronted with a number of peculiar ethical challenges, considering the specific characteristics of elderly patients and the complexities associated with their surgical treatments, among which we consider: risk-benefit assessment, decision-making autonomy of the elderly patient, and equity of access to care.

Risk-benefit assessment in geriatric surgery is a crucial step that requires a thoughtful evaluation of the potential consequences of surgery for vulnerable patients [34]. The elderly are more susceptible to physical frailty and impaired functional reserve, i.e., they have a reduced ability to adapt to stressors, including those associated with surgery. This results in an increased risk of postoperative complications, such as infections, cognitive dysfunction, delirium, falls, and functional decline [35–37]. Therefore, the risk assessment should carefully consider the patient's frailty and its impact on surgical outcome.

Addressing the frailty of the elderly patient requires a multidisciplinary and multidimensional approach to assess and optimize the physical, cognitive, and psychosocial state of the elderly patient prior to surgery and to provide comprehensive support during the perioperative and postoperative periods [38–40]. This approach is based on the realization that the effective management of persons requires a comprehensive assessment and planning that considers not only the physical and psychological health but also the social and functional aspects of the patient. It is, therefore, necessary to involve not only the patients but also their families and caregivers in the decision-making process as a key element of effective care that respects individual wishes [41–44].

In the surgical setting, the comprehensive assessment of patients enables the recognition of frailty in order to implement appropriate management strategies during the surgical planning phase and minimize the risk of postoperative complications. This assessment should also extend during the hospitalization and recovery period. The elderly patient's complexity requires a narrow medical assessment of physical and cognitive function, nutritional status, and specific medical conditions, given a clinical scenario frequently characterized by the presence of several chronic diseases and the simultaneous intake of multiple drugs [45–48]. This complexity requires a systemic assessment of the patient in which the global evaluation cannot be limited to a list of pathologies and drugs but must consider the impact of comorbidities and drug treatments on the surgical outcome in the specific case.

Useful support tools for a comprehensive assessment are the Frailty Screening Test (FRAIL), the Phenotypic Frailty Test, or the Comprehensive Geriatric Assessment (CGA). These tools can help to identify frail elderly patients and to pursue individualized surgical treatment in order to minimize surgical trauma and minimize the risk of postoperative complications [49–51].

Although comprehensive, an assessment of older patients can only be said to be global if it also considers social support and available resources. The social support of the family and caregivers is a key point to the well-being of the elderly patient in the perioperative and recovery phases [52, 53]. Involving family members can help ensure better adherence to treatment, provide emotional and practical support, and ease the transition from the hospital to the home setting after surgery [54, 55]. In some cases, the elderly patient may require home care or palliative care after surgery. These services provide medical support and personal assistance at home to help the elderly patient recover and manage daily activities during the rehabilitation period. The comprehensive assessment examines the older patient's access to community support services, such as support groups for the elderly, daycare centers, transport services, and home meal programs. These services can help promote the elderly patient's independence and social involvement during the recovery period [56–59]. Social support should promote the empowerment of the person, enabling him/her to maintain an active role in decision-making and to manage his/her own recovery.

As shown, the "age factor" is only one of the elements to be considered when dealing with an assessment of the expectations of therapeutic outcomes for older patients. The older adults, like any other patient, must be assessed as a whole, i.e., considering the patient not only as a set of physical or biological characteristics but as a complex and unique individual, characterized by physical, psychological, social, cultural, spiritual, and ethical dimensions. Otherwise, using age as the single criterion in the cost-benefit ratio can lead to distortions and erroneous decisions such as intervening only in favor of those who are, at the end of medical treatment, productive and useful for society. This is a utilitarian approach to the allocation of resources in healthcare, one of the possible consequences of which is the risk of discriminating in the treatment of the elderly if they are seen as a "burden" on society and violating their individual rights, especially if it leads to decisions that sacrifice their well-being in favor of the collective well-being.

Even in cases of exceptional imbalance between the real clinical needs of the population and the actual availability of intensive resources, criteria for access to treatment inspired by principles of distributive justice based on age do not appear ethically licit, since priority should rather be given to persons whose lives are in immediate danger. On the contrary, such an admission to medical treatment would clearly contradict both the right to health protection and the deontological principle according to which the protection of human life is part of the physician's duties without any discrimination whatsoever, whatever the institutional or social conditions in which he or she operates.

In the case of having to choose to whom to offer the only available means first, having first screened all possible solutions in order to increase the availability of deliverable therapeutic resources, a proportional approach based on a multidisciplinary and multidimensional, case-specific assessment can be envisaged, without any reference to abstract and a priori deliberate criteria. The decision-making process should be shared, justified, communicated, and documented.

A comprehensive, multidimensional assessment of the elderly patient, conducted by a multidisciplinary team, makes it possible to evaluate the proportionality of interventions according to the patient's state. This assessment includes an in-depth analysis of the patient's state of health, an evaluation of the potential benefits expected from the proposed intervention, an assessment of the associated risks and complications, and a consideration of psychological and social aspects. Furthermore, the patient's individual opinions, wishes, and values are crucial elements in balancing the potential benefits and harms of an intervention, taking into account the patient's overall well-being. A multidimensional approach to the elderly patient allows an accurate assessment to determine whether a treatment should be considered ordinary or extraordinary. In the first case, we include treatment that is considered standard for the patient's medical condition, offering a reasonable expectation of benefit without causing undue burden or suffering. In the second case, we include treatments that entail an excessive burden or risk disproportionate to the expected benefits, or that offer no real hope of improving the patient's health. It is in the latter area that we should remember the risks of futile treatment when a treatment of proven ineffectiveness plus a high risk of suffering or additional burden to the patient is undertaken that is clearly disproportionate to the risk-benefit ratio [60].

30.3 Bioethical Evaluation

Our new healthcare scenario presents a different demographical outfit, where aged people are covering larger areas than we were used to observing.

This new epidemiological evidence needs to be considered, that is, we need to understand how to face the challenges this change entails. On the other side, we are also observing a steady growth in the global population, meaning that for one aging society there are different ones with greater birth rates rising. We need to also keep this piece of evidence in mind to correctly assess the issue at hand, which otherwise would be out of context.

It is worth noting that for human beings it is possible to flourish at every age, of course, this human flourishing has specific connotations in different stages of life; nonetheless, this task is always achievable for our species. In fact, there is a specific flourishing also for elder people that can be fostered and enhanced by the appropriate care. The bioethical focus therefore should be pointed to recognize and promote those practices aimed at such a goal and, on the other hand, to criticize those that result in impairing this flourishing.

References

1. Cf. Siaarti. Raccomandazioni di etica clinica per l'ammissione a trattamenti intensivi e per la loro sospensione, in condizioni eccezionali di squilibrio tra necessità e risorse disponibili, March 6 2020. p. 5.
2. Windish D. Searching for the right evidence: how to answer your clinical questions using the 6S hierarchy. Evid Based Med. 2013;18:93–7.
3. Etzioni DA, Liu JH, Maggard MA, Ko CY. The aging population and its impact on the surgery workforce. Ann Surg. 2003;238:170–7.
4. Partridge J, Sbai M, Dhesi J. Proactive care of older people undergoing surgery. Aging Clin Exp Res. 2018;30(3):253–7.
5. Banerjee AK. Ethical dilemmas facing the practicing geriatrician. J Royal Coll Phys Edinburgh. 1998;28(1):4–14.
6. Barbagallo M, Dominguez LJ, Cucinotta D. The place of frailty and vulnerability in the surgical risk assessment: should we move from complexity to simplicity? Aging Clin Exp Res. 2018;30:237–9.
7. Rosenbaum L. The less is more crusade. Are we overmedicalizing or oversimplifying? N Engl J Med. 2017;24:2392–7.
8. Blaser W, Van Der Rohe M. Less is more. Waser: University of Michigan; 1986.
9. Rosenbaum L. The less is more crusade. Are we overmedicalizing or oversimplifying? N Engl J Med. 2017;377:2392.
10. Bobbio M, Vernero S, Colimberti D, Giardini A. Slow medicine and choosing wisely: a synergistic alliance. J Evid Based Healthcare. 2022;4:e4222.
11. Korenstein D, Falk R, Howell EA, Bishop T, Keyhani S. Overuse of health care services in the United States: an understudied problem. Arch Int Med. 2012;172(2):171–8.
12. Ñamendys-Silva SA. Less is more, but are we doing enough? Intensive Care Med. 2020;46(1):113–5.
13. Bettelli G, Maggi S. Decision-making about surgery in the elderly. Aging Clin Exp Res. 2018;30(3):225–7.
14. Baggett ND, Schulz K, Buffington A, et al. Surgeon use of shared decision-making for older adults considering major surgery: a secondary analysis of a randomized clinical trial. JAMA Surg. 2022;157(5):406–13.
15. Latifi R, Gogna S, George G. Decision-making in geriatric surgery: more surgery or less surgery? In: Latifi R, editor. Surgical decision making in geriatrics. Cham: Springer; 2020. p. 3–13.
16. Preston SD, Southall AR, Nel M, Das SK. Geriatric surgery is about disease, not age. J R Soc Med. 2008;101(8):409–15.
17. Reiss R. Moral and ethical issues in geriatric surgery. J Med Ethics. 1980;6:71–7.
18. Rosenbaum L. The less is more crusade. Are we overmedicalizing or oversimplifying? N Engl J Med. 2017;377:2329.
19. Tambone V, Ghilardi G. Philosophy and deontology of medical practice. Ethics of the job well done in bio-medical sciences. Roma: Società Editrice Universo; 2020. p. 99–117.
20. Bergson H. La specializzazione. In: Russo MT, editor. Educazione, cultura, scuola. Roma, Armando: Saggi pedagogici; 2020. p. 55. (our translation).
21. Tambone V, Ghilardi G. Philosophy and deontology of medical practice. In: Ethics of the job well done in bio-medical sciences. p. 99–117.
22. Hershberger RG. Architecture and meaning. J Aesthet Educ. 1970;4(4):37–55.
23. Tambone V, Ghilardi G. For a concise understanding of this epistemological view see, philosophy and deontology of medical practice. In: Ethics of the job well done in bio-medical sciences. p. 55–63.
24. Publius terentius afer, Phormio, V 575.
25. United Nations, Department of Economic and Social Affairs, Population Division. 2015. World Population Ageing. 2015 (ST/ESA/SER.A/390).

26. Gutman GM. Healthy population ageing. World Health. 1997;4:20–1.
27. Italian Committee for Bioethics. Bioethics and the rights of the elderly. https://bioetica.governo.it/en/opinions/opinions-responses/bioethics-and-the-rights-of-the-elderly/. Accessed 28 Mar 2024.
28. Guardini R. Le età della vita. Milano: Vita e Pensiero. p. 73–4. (our translation).
29. Boudreau JD, Cassell EJ. Medical wisdom. Perspect Biol Med. 2021;64(2):251–70.
30. Bloom DE, Zucker LM. Aging is the real population bomb. 2023. https://www.imf.org/en/Publications/fandd/issues/Series/Analytical-Series/aging-is-the-real-population-bomb-bloom-zucker.
31. Kaplan RM, Milstein A. Contributions of health care to longevity: a review of 4 estimation methods. Ann Fam Med. 2019;17(3):267–72. https://doi.org/10.1370/afm.2362. PMID: 31085531; PMCID: PMC6827626.
32. Miladinov G. Socioeconomic development and life expectancy relationship: evidence from the EU accession candidate countries. Genus. 2020;76:2. https://doi.org/10.1186/s41118-019-0071-0.
33. Ince Yenilmez M. Economic and social consequences of population aging the dilemmas and opportunities in the twenty-first century. Appl Res Qual Life. 2015;10:735–52. https://doi.org/10.1007/s11482-014-9334-2.
34. Oresanya LB, Lyons WL, Finlayson E. Preoperative assessment of the older patient: a narrative review. JAMA. 2014;311(20):2110–20. https://doi.org/10.1001/jama.2014.4573. PMID: 24867014.
35. McIsaac DI, Moloo H, Bryson GL, van Walraven C. The Association of frailty with outcomes and resource use after emergency general surgery: a population-based cohort study. Anesth Analg. 2017;124(5):1653–61. https://doi.org/10.1213/ANE.0000000000001960. PMID: 28431425.
36. McIsaac DI, Bryson GL, van Walraven C. Association of Frailty and 1-year postoperative mortality following major elective noncardiac surgery: a population-based cohort study. JAMA Surg. 2016;151(6):538–45. https://doi.org/10.1001/jamasurg.2015.5085. PMID: 26791334.
37. Lin HS, Watts JN, Peel NM, Hubbard RE. Frailty and post-operative outcomes in older surgical patients: a systematic review. BMC Geriatr. 2016;16(1):157. https://doi.org/10.1186/s12877-016-0329-8. PMID: 27580947; PMCID: PMC5007853.
38. Pilotto A, Custodero C, Maggi S, Polidori MC, Veronese N, Ferrucci L. A multidimensional approach to frailty in older people. Ageing Res Rev. 2020;60:101047. https://doi.org/10.1016/j.arr.2020.101047. Epub 2020 Mar 21. PMID: 32171786; PMCID: PMC7461697.
39. Cruz-Jentoft AJ, Daragjati J, Fratiglioni L, Maggi S, Mangoni AA, Mattace-Raso F, Paccalin M, Polidori MC, Topinkova E, Ferrucci L, Pilotto A, MPI_AGE Investigators. Using the multidimensional prognostic index (MPI) to improve cost-effectiveness of interventions in multimorbid frail older persons: results and final recommendations from the MPI_AGE European project. Aging Clin Exp Res. 2020;32(5):861–8. https://doi.org/10.1007/s40520-020-01516-0. Epub 2020 Mar 16. PMID: 32180170.
40. Veronese N, Custodero C, Cella A, Demurtas J, Zora S, Maggi S, Barbagallo M, Sabbà C, Ferrucci L, Pilotto A. Prevalence of multidimensional frailty and pre-frailty in older people in different settings: a systematic review and meta-analysis. Ageing Res Rev. 2021;72:101498. https://doi.org/10.1016/j.arr.2021.101498. Epub 2021 Oct 23. PMID: 34700009.
41. Saadeh M, Welmer AK, Dekhtyar S, Fratiglioni L, Calderón-Larrañaga A. The role of psychological and social Well-being on physical function trajectories in older adults. J Gerontol A Biol Sci Med Sci. 2020;75(8):1579–85. https://doi.org/10.1093/gerona/glaa114. PMID: 32384140; PMCID: PMC7357580.
42. Yoshizawa T, Makram AM, Elsheikh R, Nakamura S, Makram EM, Kubota K, Huy NT, Moji K. Spirituality, quality of life, and health: a Japanese cross-sectional study. Eur J Investig Health Psychol Educ. 2024;14(3):767–81. https://doi.org/10.3390/ejihpe14030050. PMID: 38534911; PMCID: PMC10969095.

43. Bernabei R, Venturiero V, Tarsitani P, Gambassi G. The comprehensive geriatric assessment: when, where, how. Crit Rev Oncol Hematol. 2000;33(1):45–56. https://doi.org/10.1016/s1040-8428(99)00048-7. PMID: 10714961.
44. Ellis G, Langhorne P. Comprehensive geriatric assessment for older hospital patients. Br Med Bull. 2005;71:45–59. https://doi.org/10.1093/bmb/ldh033. PMID: 15684245.
45. Rizzuto D, Melis RJF, Angleman S, Qiu C, Marengoni A. Effect of chronic diseases and multimorbidity on survival and functioning in elderly adults. J Am Geriatr Soc. 2017;65(5):1056–60. https://doi.org/10.1111/jgs.14868. Epub 2017 Mar 17. PMID: 28306158.
46. Quiñones AR, Markwardt S, Botoseneanu A. Multimorbidity Combinations and Disability in Older Adults. J Gerontol A Biol Sci Med Sci. 2016;71(6):823–30. https://doi.org/10.1093/gerona/glw035. Epub 2016 Mar 11. PMID: 26968451; PMCID: PMC4888400.
47. Juurlink DN, Mamdani M, Kopp A, Laupacis A, Redelmeier DA. Drug-drug interactions among elderly patients hospitalized for drug toxicity. JAMA. 2003;289(13):1652–8. https://doi.org/10.1001/jama.289.13.1652. PMID: 12672733.
48. Hines LE, Murphy JE. Potentially harmful drug-drug interactions in the elderly: a review. Am J Geriatr Pharmacother. 2011;9(6):364–77. https://doi.org/10.1016/j.amjopharm.2011.10.004. Epub 2011 Nov 11. PMID: 22078863.
49. Gleason LJ, Benton EA, Alvarez-Nebreda ML, Weaver MJ, Harris MB, Javedan H. FRAIL questionnaire screening tool and short-term outcomes in geriatric fracture patients. J Am Med Dir Assoc. 2017;18(12):1082–6. https://doi.org/10.1016/j.jamda.2017.07.005. Epub 2017 Aug 31. PMID: 28866353; PMCID: PMC6611671.
50. Cesari M, Gambassi G, van Kan GA, Vellas B. The frailty phenotype and the frailty index: different instruments for different purposes. Age Ageing. 2014;43(1):10–2. https://doi.org/10.1093/ageing/aft160. Epub 2013 Oct 16. PMID: 24132852.
51. Parker SG, McCue P, Phelps K, McCleod A, Arora S, Nockels K, Kennedy S, Roberts H, Conroy S. What is comprehensive geriatric assessment (CGA)? An umbrella review. Age Ageing. 2018;47(1):149–55. https://doi.org/10.1093/ageing/afx166. PMID: 29206906.
52. Chappell NL, Funk LM. Social support, caregiving, and aging. Can J Aging. 2011;30(3):355–70. https://doi.org/10.1017/S0714980811000316. Epub 2011 Jul 18. PMID: 21767465.
53. Brown SL, Nesse RM, Vinokur AD, Smith DM. Providing social support may be more beneficial than receiving it: results from a prospective study of mortality. Psychol Sci. 2003;14(4):320–7. https://doi.org/10.1111/1467-9280.14461. PMID: 12807404.
54. Reinhard SC, Given B, Petlick NH, Bemis A. Supporting family caregivers in providing care. In: Hughes RG, editor. Patient safety and quality: an evidence-based handbook for nurses. Rockville: Agency for Healthcare Research and Quality (US); 2008.
55. Bevan JL, Pecchioni LL. Understanding the impact of family caregiver cancer literacy on patient health outcomes. Patient Educ Couns. 2008;71(3):356–64. https://doi.org/10.1016/j.pec.2008.02.022. Epub 2008 Mar 26. PMID: 18372142.
56. Sağlam Aksüt R, Kiliç D. Effect of home care after cardiac surgery. Am J Manag Care. 2023;29(4):e96–e103. https://doi.org/10.37765/ajmc.2023.89349. PMID: 37104835.
57. Naylor MD, Brooten D, Campbell R, Jacobsen BS, Mezey MD, Pauly MV, Schwartz JS. Comprehensive discharge planning and home follow-up of hospitalized elders: a randomized clinical trial. JAMA. 1999;281(7):613–20. https://doi.org/10.1001/jama.281.7.613. PMID: 10029122
58. Naylor MD, Brooten DA, Campbell RL, Maislin G, McCauley KM, Schwartz JS. Transitional care of older adults hospitalized with heart failure: a randomized, controlled trial. J Am Geriatr Soc. 2004;52(5):675–84. https://doi.org/10.1111/j.1532-5415.2004.52202.x. Erratum in: J Am Geriatr Soc 2004 Jul;52(7):1228. PMID: 15086645.
59. Bell M, Eriksson LI, Svensson T, Hallqvist L, Granath F, Reilly J, Myles PS. Days at home after surgery: an integrated and efficient outcome measure for clinical trials and quality assurance. EClinicalMedicine. 2019;11:18–26. https://doi.org/10.1016/j.eclinm.2019.04.011. PMID: 31317130; PMCID: PMC6610780.
60. Sgreccia E. Manuale di Bioetica, vol. 2. Milano: Vita e Pensiero; 2002.

MIX
Papier aus verantwortungsvollen Quellen
Paper from responsible sources
FSC® C105338

If you have any concerns about our products,
you can contact us on
ProductSafety@springernature.com

In case Publisher is established outside the EU,
the EU authorized representative is:
Springer Nature Customer Service Center GmbH
Europaplatz 3, 69115 Heidelberg, Germany

Printed by Libri Plureos GmbH
in Hamburg, Germany